This volume is the second in a series of annotated bibliographies covering research into psychological and behavioral interventions for medical disorders. Each volume is a self-contained guide to the scientific literature on a specific set of disorders; the series as a whole will review behavioral and psychological interventions across all medical disorders. Once the series is completed, there will be regular updates of new research.

The aim of the series is to provide information about relevant research to practitioners of behavioral medicine, and to physicians and nursing personnel interested in the application of mind-body techniques. We hope that the series will also prove useful to the growing group of researchers, medical consumers, and interested lay people who see the area of mind-body health as one with important potential.

We ask that readers and authors call to our attention articles that we may have overlooked or that are forth-coming. Address your letters to: Steven E. Locke, M.D., c/o Institute for the Advancement of Health, 16 East 53rd Street, New York, NY 10022.

For
Richard C. Mason,
George A. Perera,
Harvey L. Shein, and
Shervert H. Frazier

Psychological and
Behavioral Treatments for
Medical Disorders

Volume 2

Psychological and Behavioral Treatments for Disorders Associated with the Immune System

An Annotated Bibliography

Steven E. Locke, M.D.

Dept. of Psychiatry, Beth Israel Hospital
Harvard Medical School

Elizabeth D. Power
Associate Editor

Linda N. Cabot
Assistant Editor

A Publication of the
Institute for the Advancement of Health

16 East 53rd Street, New York, New York 10022

Library of Congress Catalog Number 86-00000
ISBN 0-914533-02-9

Published by:
Institute for the Advancement of Health
16 East 53rd Street
New York, N.Y. 10022

Designed by:
Modi & Beckler Design

Printed in the United States of America

Contents

Foreword

Halsted R. Holman
Stanford University School of Medicine

Practitioners of medicine have long recognized that patients with the same diagnosis vary enormously in many manifestations of their disease, including its severity, its fluctuation of intensity, and the frequency of spontaneous healing and disability. Among people with streptococcal infection, for example, only a few develop such long-term consequences as rheumatic fever or glomerulonephritis. Among patients with deforming rheumatoid arthritis, for another example, many function very well and independently while others are significantly impaired. In the first example, where infection is an integral part of the disease, differences in outcome are ascribed to "host resistance," often considered a purely biological phenomenon. In the second example, the differences in function are usually attributed to differences in emotional strength, often considered a purely psychological phenomenon. The difficulty with these explanantions is that we do not now understand adequately the mechanisms whereby either host resistance or psychological responses influence disease or health.

This issue—the same diagnosis but widely varying disease manifestations—can be framed more broadly by characterizing disease as a biological aberration and illness as the sum of that aberration and the human response to it. The disease process would include (1) the primary insult to the body (infection, allergen, malignant transformation), (2) the body's resistance to the insult, and (3) the body's healing capacity. Illness would include the foregoing plus the ways the individual responds or is able to respond to the disease (depression or will to overcome, access to health care, availability of appropriate nutrition and/or rest, presence or absence of financial difficulty).

This admittedly simplified picture serves to highlight the many variables that determine the nature of a disease or illness and raises the serious possibility that interaction among the variables is a major determinant of disease outcome. But do the variables really interact, especially between the realms that appear to be purely biological or purely psychological? In some instances they clearly do. Classical examples include evidence for emotional influences on gastric acid secretion and peptic ulcer formation, and for the effect of emotional state on blood pressure levels. Similarly relevant are the studies of Reilly demonstrating that in susceptible mice the appearance time of a genetically determined and environmentally provoked breast cancer is profoundly affected by the animals' living conditions.[1]

Recent research on the nature of the immune response and on the endocrine system reinforces the importance of multivariate interactions. The immune system has at least three major components: antibody formation, cellular immunity, and the process of inflammation. Each component has proved to be highly complex in its own right, and immune resistance involves interactions among all of them. Further, cells involved in each component are now known to be responsive both to soluble factors elaborated by other components in the system and to hormones, such as corticosteroids, elaborated by the endocrine system. Hormone release in turn appears to be affected by emotional responses. These interactions evoke notions of complex networks in which the various ingredients influence the activities of other ingredients, bringing into some common realm both the psychological and the biological. A tantilizing aspect of such networks is the role of memory. At least the brain and the immune system possess memory, and it is reasonable to suppose that memory of past experience influences responses to the present.

These bare comments underscore the complexity of events that lead to the appearance of disease and illness, and their resolution. Unfortunately, while we currently glimpse the complexity of the process, we understand little of its actual operation. Worse yet, our clinical ability to affect the interactions is small.

High on our list of needs is a fuller understanding of these matters. This is where the editors of the present volume make a significant contribution. They have complied a compendium of research information about psychological and behavioral approaches to disorders associated with the immune system, a field that has been fraught with controversy: hard information has been submerged by inadequate evidence, hopes have been been transmuted into conclusions, and speculation has been rampant. This well-organized compendium allows one to appraise the objective state of the field and to extract from it relevant references, which is the necessary prelude to studies that will generate deeper understanding and richer practical applications. Given the importance of the subjects, and the emerging recognition of the inordinate complexity of disease and illness processes, one can expect the present volume to shed more light and less heat on a matter central to health care.

Reference

1. Reilly V. Mouse mammary tumors: alternation of incidence as apparent function of stress. Science 1975;189:465.

Preface

This is the second volume of a series that compiles research studies on psychosomatic and behavioral medicine. The first volume addressed treatment of heart and blood vessel disorders (*Psychological and Behavioral Treatments for Disorders of the Heart and Blood Vessels*, Institute for the Advancement of Health, 1985). The present volume covers psychological and behavioral treatments for disorders associated with the immune system. In the case of blood diseases and skin disorders, we have also included—to group in one place all the papers on these subjects—a few studies on problems that are not immune associated.

Although scientific interest in modifying the neural control of the immune system through psychological and behavioral techniques has grown considerably during the last decade, the use of psychic factors in healing is an ancient tradition. Today, this tradition not only survives in modern folk medicine but also in the research facilities of our finest academic medical centers. As Mark Twain said: "The ancients have stolen all our best ideas."

In the historical effort of physicians to disavow their unscientific origins as shamans and priests, the role of psychic factors in physical illness was largely rejected while medicine focused on increasingly effective "physical" interventions. The scientific investigation of the placebo response allowed for psychic factors in healing but for the most part the use of psychological and behavioral approaches has been dismissed as unproven and unscientific. Despite the resurgence of scientific interest in such approaches, the attitude of disapproval remains strong. If some segments of the medical research community today take their lead from the great physician and teacher, Sir William Osler, who in 1909 admonished that "the care of tuberculosis depends more on what the patient has in his head than what he has in his chest," other segments subscribe to the views expressed in a recent editorial in the *New England Journal of Medicine* (June 13, 1985): "The evidence for mental state as a cause and cure of today's scourges is not much better than it was for the afflictions of earlier centuries . . . it is time to acknowledge that our belief in disease as a direct reflection of mental state is largely folklore."

In this volume we are attempting to bring together for the first time descriptions of all relevant research and medical writings on the use of psychological treatments for the various disorders related to immune function. The work is widely scattered and but surprisingly plentiful. Covering the period from 1848 to July 1985, the current volume contains 1479 entries, drawn from 530 journals and 225 books and book chapters. The entries include 219 foreign language citations (many with English abstracts), representing 18 different languages. We believe this collection will be useful to the practicing clinician, the active investigator, and the casual observer eager to learn more about mind-body links and health.

Our primary concern has been to compile research examining the medical effects of (1) noninvasive psychological and behavioral interventions on (2) human beings. Given this perspective, we excluded articles that examined nonallopathic interventions with a direct physical aspect (for example, acupuncture, massage, and herbal remedies), even though these techniques may contain a psychological and/or behavioral component. We also excluded studies on exercise and nutritional interventions. Put broadly, the interventions examined here emphasize psychological processes. For each abstract we have included a legend that identifies the types of psychological interventions covered in the article.

We focus on papers investigating the effects of psychological and behavioral techniques on an individual's medical symptoms, as opposed to papers examining the psychological rehabilitation of patients with medical disorders. In most cases, the research deals with disease states in patients rather than with normal physiological processes in healthy humans.

Within our central perspective, a variety of considerations guided our search and our choices. For example, what is considered essential for good research design today was not always evident in early studies, and our criteria for selecting early papers were somewhat relaxed. In choosing early papers, we looked for studies that treated the emotions or the personality to improve recovery.

Major on-line bibliographic databases are the primary source of our recent material. Since the databases do not contain entries from before 1965, we located earlier material by hand searching the literature, an extensive and laborious process. Existing computerized systems also proved inadequate for locating relevant medical books and book chapters, and we culled most of the material again by hunting through library stacks (in the Countway Medical Library of Harvard Medical School, the Lamar Soutter Library of the University of Massachusetts Medical Center, and the Brown University Sciences Library).

Because of the limited availability of published proceedings from national or international scientific meetings, we elected not to include abstracts from these sources unless the papers had been published in a major journal. Foreign language citations were included either on the basis of their translated titles or the contents of English abstracts.

This book reflects the combined efforts of three groups: the editorial staff, the Joint Center for Clinical Computing (JCCC) at Beth Israel and Brigham and Women's Hospitals, and the Institute for the Advancement of Health. Our involvement with the JCCC, led by Drs. Howard Bleich and Warner Slack, began with the production of the annotated bibliography, *Mind and Immunity; Behavioral Immunology* (New York: Institute for the Advancement of Health, 1983). For that book, the JCCC generously donated its efforts by developing software that enabled us to sort citations and by facilitating our ability to transmit the complete text of the book via telecommunication to the typesetter. For the current series, the JCCC's involvement has been greatly expanded, and the JCCC created computer software that can produce annotated bibliographies in any scientific field.

The software is now capable of utilizing magnetic tape outputs of searches from on-line bibliographic databases (Medline and PsycINFO were used here), transferring abstracts to word-processor files via a user-friendly system (PaperChase,™ Beth Israel Hospital, Boston, Massachusetts), and allowing the entry of items culled from hand searching of the literature. The JCCC has developed an extensive automated system for obtaining the rights and permissions to original abstracts, reducing dramatically the time this task would otherwise take.

Readers are advised that the appearance of an abstract in this book in no way alters the copyright ownership of the abstracts and that the articles can be duplicated only under the provisions of the Copyright Code. The appearance of the abstracts here does not constitute permission from the original publisher to photo-duplicate the original articles. Although we have made every effort to reproduce citations and abstracts accurately, we also advise readers to check the original publication before quoting the material. Readers should also note that an author's name may appear in slightly different forms, depending on the citation.

Finally, while we provide no evaluation of the abstracts, we have developed a journal assessment index that appears at the end of the book.

Steven E. Locke

Acknowledgments to Staff

Many people deserve credit for their valuable assistance during the editing of this book, which was the product of a team effort. This acknowledgement is but a token of our deep appreciation for the cooperation and assistance of the people involved.

The skills and dedication of the editorial staff were essential to the successful completion of the book and to the continuation of this series on psychological and behavioral treatments of medical disorders. The management of the editorial work was the responsibility of Elizabeth D. Power, whose leadership, editorial talent, and penchant for excellence were of the highest order. Linda N. Cabot's responsibilities were extensive. Demonstrating a rich capacity for organization and research, she executed a comprehensive search for relevant books and book chapters, administered the copyright permissions process, and prepared the Journal Assessment Index. Susan J. Avery's editorial assistance and diligent reference searching were instrumental in completing the project on time. The word-processing skills of Karen Rapuano, Jane A. Power, and Patti Andrews were invaluable. Ruth Lloyd helped to develop the table of contents for the volume as well as for the remainder of the series, and the impact of her contribution is evident. The review of earlier versions of the manuscript by Drs. Bernard Fox and Hans Baltrusch provided useful feedback and enabled us to make improvements in the final book. Nancy Newman again did an excellent job in preparing the comprehensive and impressive subject index.

To make our survey as exhaustive as possible, we used electronic bibliographic databases, searched by hand the holdings of three university library systems, and requested interlibrary loans when our other efforts were insufficient. Once again, the skills of Cherie Haitz, our search consultant, and her intimate knowledge of the databases enabled us to tap efficiently several world-wide electronic resources. Her fine tuning of the computer search algorithm was an impressive accomplishment. Our ability to conduct searches and obtain computer tapes of the output was facilitated through the cooperation of Bibliographic Retrieval Services (BRS) and PsycINFO. We are grateful to Kathy Doyle (PsycINFO) and Hillary Buckland (BRS) for their support and assistance.

In the demanding task of hand searching the literature, library researcher Judith C. Watkins waded through volumes of scientific writings at the Countway Medical Library, analyzing the material for possible inclusion. Emil I. Shieh searched for hard-to-locate citations in the libraries of Brown University. We also gratefully acknowledge Dennis Rourke whose proficiency in European languages enabled him to translate our foreign titles. The staff at the Countway Medical Library, our principal resource, has been enormously helpful and cooperative. The Copy Service Center efficiently photocopied the large volume of abstracts not available on-line. Lance Higgins and Peggy Hall processed numerous interlibrary loan requests. The assistance of Maria Velaudia and Stephanie Moye and the support of Susan Whitehead, director of the Reference Department, provided important help. The Agoos Medical

Library of the Beth Israel Hospital was another key resource, and there the assistance of James Daly, Henrietta Green, and the recently retired librarian, Martha Cole, were critical. The Lamar Soutter Library of the University of Massachusetts Medical Center was an additional source for retrieving hard-to-find journals and abstracts, and the catalog of their holdings, prepared by Gael A. Evans, made our work easier and should serve as a model for other libraries.

The support of the Joint Center for Clinical Computing (formerly the Division of Computer Medicine) at Beth Israel and Brigham and Women's Hospitals has been vital to the production of these books. Drs. Howard L. Bleich and Warner V. Slack continue to provide the necessary support to permit this project to thrive. The creativity of our computer programmer, Valerie Portway, is hidden from the view of the reader, yet all of us who have worked on the project have benefited from the growing efficiency and automation with which her programming skill enabled us to work. We are indebted to her. Jerome D. Jackson helped maintain and improve the software upon which we depend, especially the PaperChase resource. The fine computer operations staff, including Michael Card, Richard Mocera, Thomas McDonough, Sandra Mitchell, Ellen Eichorn, Jean Maguire, and Marilyn Meuninck, helped to set up and maintain our equipment. Karen Rapuano and John Kirk jointly oversaw the financial administration of our effort at Beth Israel Hospital.

We wish to express our appreciation of the support provided by the Department of Psychiatry at Beth Israel Hospital, the Department of Medicine at Beth Israel and Brigham and Women's Hospitals, and the Institute for the Advancement of Health. The Department of Medicine lent our project a temporary home while we awaited our own space generously provided by the Department of Psychiatry. We thank Drs. Eugene Braunwald and William Grossman for the space they loaned to the project, while Dr. Fred Frankel, Acting Chairman of the Department of Psychiatry, and Howard Hoople, Administrator for Psychiatry, arranged for the space that permitted us to complete this work. Frank Harris, Assistant Manager of Environmental Services, and his staff did yeoman's work in moving our equipment and files to our present quarters atop two flights of stairs. We are indepted to the Beth Israel Hospital Senior Volunteers headed by Trudy Agress, for their ongoing assistance.

And lastly we wish to thank our primary supporter, the Institute for the Advancement of Health, and in particular, Harris Dienstfrey and M. Barry Flint for their continued support of this effort.

About the Institute

The Institute for the Advancement of Health, a non-profit organization, was established in 1983 to further the scientific understanding of how mind-body interactions affect health and disease. The Institute seeks to promote sound research; to encourage fuller interdisciplinary exchange among researchers, clinicians, and the larger health-care community; and to inform the interested public about developments in this swiftly emerging field.

For full information on the Institute's publications, workshops, and other programs, contact: Programs, Institute for the Adancement of Health, 16 East 53rd Street, New York, N.Y. 10022. Phone: (212) 832 8282.

About the Author

Steven E. Locke, M.D., is on the faculty of the Harvard Medical School and the staff of Beth Israel Hospital. He is the co-editor of *Mind and Immunity* (Institute for the Advancement of Health, 1983), an editor of *Foundations of Psychoneuroimmunology* (Aldine, 1985), and, most recently, co-author of *The Healer Within* (Dutton, 1986). He maintains a private psychiatric practice in Newton, Massachusetts.

Immunologic
Disorders

Allergic Disorders

Asthma

Behavior Therapy

1
Cooper AJ. **A case of bronchial asthma treated by behaviour therapy.** Behav Res Ther 1:351-356, 1964.

▶ desensitization, reciprocal inhibition

Desensitization employing the reciprocal inhibition principle was applied to a case of intractable bronchial asthma. Therapy has resulted in dramatic and maintained improvement. An explanation, in terms of learning theory, is given on the development of the psychosomatic symptom, and the rationale of the treatment explained. It is suggested that should relapse occur, booster treatments administered on an out-patient basis would be a feasible proposition.

2
Courteheuse C. **Educating the asthmatic patient.** Schweiz Med Wochenschr 114:1336-1339, 1984. (in German)

▶ behavior therapy

Education of the asthmatic patient by an appropriate program is an important tool in achieving optimal management. The program should include not only lectures on the physiopathology and treatment of asthma, but also self-management skills through a behavioural approach to the disease. The education program aims to assist the patient in preventing symptoms and coping with asthma attacks.

3
Creer TL. **The use of a time-out from positive reinforcement procedure with asthmatic children.** J Psychosom Res 14:117-120, 1970.

▶ reinforcement

This study demonstrated the use of the time-out from positive reinforcement in effectively curtailing the fre-quency and duration of hospitalizations in two asthmatic children.

4
Creer TL, Burns KL. **Self-management training for children with chronic bronchial asthma.** Psychother Psychosom 32:270-278, 1979.

▶ review: behavior therapy, milieu therapy

We have described examples of behaviors that occur antecedent to, concurrent with, or as a consequence of childhood asthma. Ways these patterns can be altered have also been described. Three points should be emphasized: first, social learning techniques can contribute to a child acquiring self-monitoring and self-management skills over his or her affliction. Thus, youngsters with asthma can learn self-responsibility over their affliction. Second, while we do have follow-up data indicating that youngsters continue to perform similar behaviors once they leave the Center and return to their families, such generalization does not automatically occur. For this reason, we have initiated several programs for working with a child's family. Finally, what about the youngster who is never admitted to an asthma facility such as the national Asthma Center? It is here where we are beginning to focus most of our efforts. By teaching a child and his or her family ways that the youngster can learn to manage asthma means that the disease will become less of a disruptive influence within the home, that costs of the affliction can be contained, and that the youngster can remain within the mainstream of both his or her family and community. Future reports from the Center will describe efforts we are making in this direction.

5
Creer TL, Renne CM, Christian WP. **Behavior contributions to rehabilitation and childhood asthma.** Rehab Lit 37:226-232, 1976.

▶ milieu therapy, behavior therapy, psychotherapy, relaxation, family therapy

In light of the above knowledge, the aims of the treatment and rehabilitation program at the Children's Asthma Research Institute and Hospital (CARIH), a Division of the National Asthma Center in Denver, Colorado, are twofold: First, every effort is directed toward establishing control over the symptoms of the affliction. This is accomplished through manipulations of medications, diets, and environment variables. The second aim is to rehabilitate the child with asthma behaviorally.

6
Danker PS, Miklich DR, Pratt C, Creer TL. **An unsuccessful attempt to instrumentally condition peak expiratory flow rates in asthmatic children.** J Psychosom Res 19:209-213, 1975.

▶ biofeedback, conditioning, relaxation

Two unsuccessful attempts to operantly condition bronchial relaxation with spirometry in asthmatics are reported. Only one of eleven subjects showed definite signs of conditioning; none showed any resulting changes in their asthmatic condition. The implications of this research for previously reported successful conditioning of this response are discussed.

7
Dekker E, Pelser HE, Groen J. **Conditioning as a cause of asthmatic attacks: a laboratory study.** J Psychosom Res 2:97-108, 1957.

▶ deconditioning, supportive psychotherapy

Two patients suffering from severe bronchial asthma who had a skin sensitivity to grass-pollen and house-dust extract, respectively, reacted to the inhalation of an aerosol of these allergens in the laboratory, with an attack of asthma. After these exposures they also showed attacks of asthma after the inhalation of the neutral solvent, or of oxygen, or even after the introduction of the glass mouthpiece, when this was not connected to the inhalation apparatus. These phenomena were interpreted as a result of conditioning by the simultaneous exposure of the patient to the inhalation of the allergen and to the situation in which this took place. Deconditioning by psychotherapeutic supportive interviews proved difficult and its success was temporary. The relative importance of conditioning in the genesis of attacks of asthma in general and of psychogenic attacks in particular is discussed.

8
Franks CM, Leigh D. **The theoretical and experimental application of a conditioning model to a consideration of bronchial asthma in man.** J Psychosom Res 4:88-98, 1959.

▶ behavior therapy, conditioning

Some research workers believe that asthmatics tend basically to be introverts; others believe that asthmatics tend to be extraverts. These beliefs were investigated in terms of an experimentally supported theory which relates ease of conditionability to the personality dimension of introversion-extraversion. When asthmatics, neurotics and normal subjects were compared on questionnaire measures of introversion-extraversion and on laboratory tests of eyelid conditioning, none of the groups were found to differ on either of these measures. The only trend apparent was for the asthmatics to occupy an intermediate position between the normal subjects and the neurotic patients on the neuroticism scale of the personality questionnaires. These findings provide further support for the belief that there is no specific asthmatic personality apart from a common core of neuroticism which may be reactive to the dysfunction itself. Although asthma can apparently occur in patients with any kind of personality, it seems probable, from the literature, that some attacks of this disorder may be understood and treated in terms of learning theory and conditioning model.

9
Gardner JE. **A blending of behavior therapy techniques in an approach to an asthmatic child.** Psychother Theory Res Pract 5:46-49, 1968.

▶ desensitization, operant conditioning, reinforcement, placebo

Broadly speaking, behavior therapy is a logical extension of the principles of learning. In practice, however, behavior therapists have often successfully relied on the desensitization paradigm or on operant conditioning. In some cases, it may be useful to blend elements of both as well as vicarious reinforcement and modeling. This paper describes such a blending of procedures in working with a severely emotionally disturbed, asthmatic child.

10
Hochstadt NJ, Shepard J, Lulla SH. **Reducing hospitalizations of children with asthma.** J Pediatr 97:1012-1015, 1980.

▶ positive reinforcement, behavior therapy

This study sought to determine if the amount of in-hospital time could be reduced for a selected population of asthmatic children by using a behavioral intervention ("time-out" from positive reinforcement) in a general pediatric hospital. The measurements of hospital use selected were duration and frequency of hospitalization, and the time needed after admission to reverse airflow obstruction, as reflected by peak expiratory flow rates. Seven patients were selected because their use of the hospital appeared to be appreciably in excess of the severity of their asthma. All seven had been followed for at least one year prior to intervention, and were then followed for at least one year after the initial intervention. Intervention was a time-out procedure consisting of a program that removed many of the social rewards for being hospitalized. The results indicated that each of the measures of hospital use tested was reduced during and following the intervention.

11
Khan AU, Olson DL. **Deconditioning of excercise-induced asthma.** Psychosom Med 39:382-392, 1977.

▶ deconditioning, extinction

The majority of asthmatic children develop a significant degree of bronchospasm after a moderate amount of exercise. Etiology of this phenomenon has remained unknown. Pulmonary function tests, measurements of blood gases, and immunological assessments have been essentially normal. This study was designed to investigate the role of conditioning process in the development of exercise-induced bronchospasm (EIB). Fifty asthmatic children, between the ages of 8 and 15, were subjected to a standardized test of exercise. Thirty-six of the children who developed EIB were divided into an experimetnal and a control group. The experimental procedure was designed as a classical extinction procedure in which the conditioned stimulus (exercise) was presented without the occurrence of conditioned response of EIB. Only the experimental group received Isoproterenol inhalation before the exercise to prevent the occurrence of EIB, while the control groups received plain air in a similar manner. The experimental group showed a significant improvement after the extinction procedure. A 6 month follow-up indicated that the majority of the children in the experimental group maintained the gains that were acquired during the experimental procedure.

12
Khan AU, Staerk M, Bonk C. **Role of counterconditioning in the treatment of asthma.** J Psychosoc Res 18:89-92, 1974. (also J Ast Res 11:57-61, 1973)

▶ conditioning, biofeedback

Twenty asthmatic children between the ages of 8 and 16 were given a counterconditioning treatment. The treatment involved the instigation of bronchial constriction followed by training in bronchial dilation through biofeedback reinforcement. The results of a follow-up for one year indicated that the improvement in the experimental group was significantly greater than in the control group with regard to the frequency of asthmatic attack, emergency room visits and the amount of medication during that period.

13
Knapp TJ, Wells LA. **Behavior therapy for asthma: a review.** Behav Res Ther 16:103-115, 1978.

▶ review: relaxation, desensitization, conditioning

The paper reviews 24 case studies and experiments which assess behavior therapy for asthma or some collateral behavior management problem. The reports are examined in terms of treatment population, design, dependent variable, technique, outcome, and follow-up. Methodological and instrumentation suggestions are made for future research.

14
LeBaron S, Zeltzer L. **The treatment of asthma with behavioral intervention: does it work?** Tex Med 79:40-42, 1983.

▶ review: relaxation, biofeedback, hypnosis

Behavioral techniques such as relaxation, biofeedback, and hypnosis have been studied in individuals with asthma. While many of these studies have demonstrated statistically significant reductions in asthma attack frequency and/or enhancement of pulmonary function, actual sustained clinical improvement resulting from such techniques has not yet been demonstrated. Since studies of behavioral strategies for enhancing compliance and reducing stress have demonstrated positive clinical improvements, behavioral intervention can help asthmatic patients cope with illness by reducing problems related to medication compliance and by reducing stress.

15
Lukeman D. **Conditioning methods of treating childhood asthma.** J Child Psychol Psychiatry 16:165-168, 1975.

▶ conditioning, biofeedback

A review of the literature shows that studies of treatment of childhood asthma by conditioning are few, numbers of patients are small and follow-up inadequate. It is clear, however, that conditioning methods have had some success in the treatment of asthma both by intervention at the precipitant stage and by treatment of the disturbance produced by the presence of the asthma. Further systematic investigation is required, particularly of the variables involved in the selection of cases and in the choice of treatment method, so that the efficacy of conditioning methods in the treatment of asthma can be more fully evaluated.

16

Miklich DR. **Operant conditioning procedures with systematic desensitization in a hyperkinetic asthmatic boy.** J Behav Ther Exp Psychol 4:177-182, 1973.

▶ operant conditioning, systematic desensitization, relaxation, milieu therapy

Panic during asthma attacks interfered with medical treatment of an asthmatic boy. His hyperkinesis and youth (6 yr) prevented the use of ordinary systematic desensitization procedures in treating his panic, therefore an operant conditioning procedure was used. First, it was used to shape relaxed sitting. Then the boy was able to earn tokens by remaining relaxed while the therapist described to him his having progressively worsening asthma. After working through descriptions ranging from mild asthma to death from status asthmaticus, the nurses and physicians attending the boy reported no further difficulties in treating his asthma. Moreover, the hyperkinesis also showed considerable improvement in the first few months following therapy.

17

Miklich DR, Renne CM, Creer TL, Alexander AB, Chai H, Davis MH, Hoffman A, Danker-Brown P. **The clinical utility of behavior therapy as an adjunctive treatment for asthma.** J Allergy Clin Immunol 5:285-294, 1977.

▶ systematic desensitization, reciprocal inhibition

A behavior therapy, Systematic Desensitization by Reciprocal Inhibition (SDRI), was used to reduce the anxiety 19 children reported experiencing before and during asthmatic symptoms. Seven control subjects received no behavioral treatment. Complete records were kept of all medications, treatments, and hospitalizations for asthma, twice daily one-second forced expiratory flow rates (FEV_1) and symptom reports. These data were collected before, during, and after SDRI treatment and at 5-mo follow-up. Posttreatment results showed differences between controls and SDRI-treated children only on the FEV_1 measures. In the face of comparably reduced steroids, treated patients maintained their pretreatment FEV_1 levels while controls' FEV_1s declined slightly. At follow-up, the treated subjects were more like the controls but still maintained some stability in FEV_1 in the face of reduced maintenance medications. On the average the effect was small and of little clinical significance. However, a few patients appeared to show a clinically useful response to SDRI.

18

Mook J, Van der Ploeg HM. **Behavior therapy in bronchial asthma: systematic desensitization applied to 3 patients.** Ned Tijdschr Geneeskd 120:1065-1069, 1976. (in Dutch)

▶ systematic desensitization

Detailed description is given of the application of the behaviour-therapeutic method of systematic desensitization (SD) in three patients with asthma. Following a brief description of the characteristics of these three patients and of the therapeutic schedule, the evolution and the effects of treatment are discussed at length for each patient in succession. At the termination of the treatment, two of the three patients showed substantial improvement (which persisted), whereas no effect could be observed in the third patient. In conclusion, the possible causes of this discrepancy are discussed in some detail.

19

Moore N. **Behaviour therapy in bronchial asthma: a controlled study.** J Psychosom Res 9:257-276, 1965.

▶ reciprocal inhibition, relaxation, suggestion

Bronchial asthma is a conditioned response with complex higher order conditioning and generalization, in which bronchospasm is the final common path. A method of specific deconditioning by behaviour therapy with reciprocal inhibition is described. A report is given of a controlled study to isolate the crucial factor in this treatment, by giving twelve asthmatic patients either relaxation with reciprocal inhibition, relaxation with suggestion, or relaxation alone, in a balanced incomplete block design, using patients as their own controls. Reciprocal inhibition is found to be the crucial factor, having a very significantly greater effect on respiratory function tests than the other treatments, which do not differ from each other. All three treatments produce subjective improvement, but do not differ statistically in this respect. Subjective report and respiratory function tests improved together during reciprocal inhibition, but during the other treatments the subjective improvement outweighed the objective.

20

Neisworth JT, Moore F. **Operant treatment of asthmatic responding with the parent as therapist.** Behav Ther 3:95-99, 1972.

▶ conditioning

Pronounced reduction of chronic asthmatic responding in a 7-year-old boy was achieved through parental management of "therapeutic" contingencies. Treatment was begun with professional guidance by the mother after she had attended several instructional sessions in operant conditioning. Reinstatement of original consequences and return to treatment contingencies produced corresponding changes in the duration of asthmatic behavior. An 11-month follow-up confirmed the stability of the therapeutic changes, general improvement in the child's health, and the absence of any demonstrable deleterious side-effects. The results suggest closer and extended scrutiny of operant techniques in the treatment of asthma and other allergic responses.

21

Nolte D. **Psychogenic asthma—does it exist? Med Klin 77:14-20, 1982.** (in German: no English abstract)

▶ behavior therapy, conditioning

22

Rakos RF, Grodek MV, Mack KK. **The impact of a self-administered behavioral intervention program on pediatric asthma.** J Psychosom Res 29:101-108, 1985.

▶ bibliotherapy, behavior therapy, family therapy, relaxation

This study evaluated the benefits produced by "Superstuff," a self-help program for asthmatic children aged 7-12. Forty-three children with a confirmed diagnosis of moderate to severe asthma were randomly assigned to either the totally self-administered Superstuff condition or to a no-contact Control condition. Self-report, parental, physician, and school data were collected at pre-intervention, and two, six, and twelve months post-intervention. Children receiving Superstuff reported increased asthma self-control skills, but no gains in general self-control abilities or self-esteem. Superstuff subjects also evidenced fewer interruptions of parents, greater improvement in the progression of asthma as reported by physicians (but not in the severity of the disease or intensity of average attack), and tended toward decreased school absenteeism. Superstuff did not reduce scheduled or emergency medical contacts. The demonstration of important, but modest, benefits from a low-cost, easily disseminated, self-administered intervention is discussed in the context of self-help treatment in general.

23

Rathus SA. **Motoric, autonomic, and cognitive reciprocal inhibition of a case of hysterical bronchial asthma.** Adolescence 8:29-32, 1973.

▶ reciprocal inhibition, group psychotherapy, relaxation

In the case of Miss S an attempt was thus made to purposefully utilize the patient's cognitive processes as a factor in the treatment of an apparent case of hysterical bronchial asthma. Treatment was successful. Whether the cognitive concomitant was an essential element in the treatment is unknown since there was no control treatment that relied on motoric and autonomic processes alone, but the employment of structured counterconditioning on a cognitive level would appear to point to a profitable direction for clinical research.

24

Sergeant HGS. **Verbal desensitisation in the treatment of bronchial asthma.** Lancet 2:1321-1323, 1969.

▶ desensitization

A woman with severe late-onset asthma, which had not responded to corticosteroid treatment in hospital, recovered and has remained completely free of asthma for the five years since she was desensitised to descriptions of her asthma attacks and of the circumstances in which they occurred. The term verbal desensitisation distinguishes this from other methods such as desensitisation to allergens, or graduated practice. The patient was relaxed, and then the disturbing items were described to her in precisely controlled steps until she no longer reacted to them. Later, she gradually returned to the situations which had once disturbed her.

25

Spevack M. **Behavior therapy treatment in bronchial asthma: a critical review.** Can Psychol Rev 19:321, 1978.

▶ review: psychotherapy

Behaviour therapy techniques have been applied to asthmatic individuals with some apparent success. The definitive studies isolating a) the critical ingredients of treatments, b) the efficacy of treatment over the long term, have yet to be done. There can be an autonomic conditioning component in asthma, and pulmonary function is improved when subjects are in a relaxed state. Studies reporting results of behavior therapy treatments are examined from an outcome and experimental design viewpoint. With the methodological deficiencies of these studies in mind, proposals for future research are generated.

26

Sribner VA. **Pathological conditioned reflexes in clinical internal diseases.** Vrach Delo 1:140-142, 1965. (in Russian: no English abstract)

▶ conditioning

27

Van der Hal I. **Treatment of asthma by imitation of asthmatic breathing.** Ned Tijdschr Geneeskd 100:767-769, 1966. (in Dutch)

▶ suggestion, conditioning

When children are taught to imitate asthmatic breathing, their fear of the true asthmatic breathing during an attack is reduced. In many cases this treatment also has a favourable effect on the incidence, severity and duration of the attacks. Initially this therapy may be only suggestive and reassuring, but in course of time it may well be that a conditioning or reconditioning takes place.

28
Van der Ploeg HM, Mook J. **Behavior therapy in bronchial asthma.** Ned Tijdschr Geneeskd 120:1083-1087, 1976. (in Dutch)

▶ review: behavior therapy, relaxation, biofeedback, desensitization, assertiveness training

In this article, a survey is presented of the literature on behaviour therapy (case histories and research) for patients with bronchial asthma. Asthma, conceived as a learned response, may be modified by manipulating the environment. Relaxation exercises, if necessary combined with biofeedback training have been found effective for short- as well as long-term therapy. A particular sub-group of patients may be treated by systematic desensitization with very good results. Assertive training, also, has been successfully used in asthma patients.

29
Weinstein AG. **Crying-induced bronchospasm in childhood asthma: combined pharmacologic and behavioral management.** Del Med J 56:473-476, 1984.

▶ behavior therapy

Crying-induced bronchospasm (CIB) in childhood asthma has been reported to be a relatively common clinical syndrome, affecting approximately 40% of asthmatic children seen in an allergist's practice. These patients appear to be more severely affected than those with noncrying-induced bronchospasm in that they require more medication and have onset of asthma at less than one year of age. Crying for any reason, either due to physical or emotional injury, may precipitate bronchospasm. Behavioral issues that can provoke crying-related asthma include parental separation and discipline, as well as sibling, school, and peer interactions. Bronchodilators will significantly reduce these symptoms for many children; however, a smaller percentage will continue with crying-related asthma. To address this problem of crying-induced asthma refractory to pharmacologic management, behavioral strategies were developed to prevent and to stop the crying behavior. Two case reports review specific behavioral factors that produce crying-induced bronchospasm and interventions that may be employed.

30
Wohl TH. **Behavior modification: its application to the study and treatment of childhood asthma.** J Asthma Res 9:41-45, 1971. (address)

▶ behavior modification, reciprocal inhibition, milieu therapy, biofeedback

31
Yorkston NJ, Eckert E, McHugh RB, Philander DA, Blumenthal MN. **Bronchial asthma: improved lung function after behavior modification.** Psychosomatics 20:325-327, 330-331, 1979.

▶ desensitization, relaxation

A systematic, controlled study of psychological desensitization treatment for asthma is described. Relaxation training alone was compared with a combination of relaxation training and either of two types of desensitization in terms of their effect on lung function. In patients receiving steroids, desensitization was significantly more effective than relaxation alone, leading to objective pulmonary function improvement in more than half the patients in the study group. In patients not receiving steroids, treatment was less effective, and there was no significant differences among the treatments.

32
Yorkston NJ, McHugh RB, Brady R, Serber M, Sergeant HGS. **Verbal desensitisation in bronchial asthma.** J Psychosom Res 18:371-376, 1974.

▶ desensitization, relaxation

Of fourteen patients who were having medical treatment for bronchial asthma but who had no obvious psychological difficulties, a group of six improved significantly when they were treated by verbal desensitisation, whereas a group of eight treated by relaxation did not. During verbal desensitisation, the therapist made carefully graded statements, making sure that the patient adapted completely to one statement before progressing to the next. The statements began with a standard description of the symptoms of asthma and tension, followed by the individual's own description. The patient was also desensitised to his disturbing thoughts, to descriptions of the circumstances of the attacks, and then to all these details together, so that eventually he remained quite calm while listening to a vivid description of the asthmatic attacks. Finally, he faced the disturbing situations in practice. While both groups said that they felt better immediately after, only the desensitised group showed significant improvement in the lung function. Two years later, the desensitisation group had reduced the dosage of all drugs, including steroids, significantly more than the group who received relaxation alone.

Biofeedback

33
Abdullah S. **Biofeedback for asthmatic patients.** N Engl J Med 291:1037, 1974. (letter)

▶ biofeedback, meditation, relaxation

34

Creer TL. **Biofeedback and asthma.** Adv Asthma Allergy 1:6-11, 1974.

▶ biofeedback, relaxation

It is wise to remember the advice noted by Risley (1969): "Therapy is a human endeavor with a long history, but one characterized by cycles and fads. New therapeutic approaches gain acceptance, become widely used, and quickly lose adherents as yet another new approach gains popularity. These recurring new approaches were not necessarily ineffective. Some were probably quite effective when they were initiated, but their initial effectiveness was not maintained, or effectiveness alone was not sufficient to maintain their use." The use of biofeedback is now at the apex of its popularity. Whether or not it remains in this position depends on its ultimate ability to benefit those who require alleviation of their suffering. While initial data are encouraging, it must still be confirmed that biofeedback can be used to benefit those afflicted with asthma. This constitutes the goal of current work in the Behavior Science Division of CARIH [Children's Asthma Research Institute and Hospital, Denver].

35

Davis MH, Saunders DR, Creer TL, Chai H. **Relaxation training facilitated by biofeedback apparatus as a supplemental treatment in bronchial asthma.** J Psychosom Res 17:121-128, 1973.

▶ biofeedback, relaxation

This study demonstrated that relaxation training, particularly if aided by biofeedback, resulted in a reduction of asthma symptoms with children considered as experiencing non-severe asthma. This effect was not obtained from children who were regarded as experiencing severe asthma. Data regarding the generalization of symptom reduction, age level of S's, changes in self-reported affect, and the correlation between relaxation and peak flow measurements were also presented and discussed.

36

Feldman GM. **The effect of biofeedback training on respiratory resistance of asthmatic children.** Psychosom Med 38:27-33, 1976.

▶ biofeedback

In a pilot study four children with severe asthma were trained to lower their respiratory resistance by means of biofeedback training techniques. Total respiratory resistance measured continuously by the forced oscillation method was used as the feedback signal. Each child demonstrated lowered respiratory resistance after most sessions. Results were comparable with the improvement seen after bronchodilator inhalation therapy. A nonasthmatic child demonstrated no significant changes of respiratory resistance after using the same techniques. Arguments are presented in support of the hypothesis that changes in total respiratory resistance were primarily due to changes in lower airway resistance. Lowering of airway resistance in asthmatic children by use of biofeedback appears possible; its promise calls for further clinical evaluation.

37

Harding AV, Maher KR. **Biofeedback training of cardiac acceleration; effects on airway resistance in bronchial asthma.** J Psychosom Res 26:447-454, 1982.

▶ biofeedback

Twenty-four volunteer adolescent and adult asthmatics were pre-tested for suggestibility and retained for an investigation of the airway effects of biofeedback induced voluntary cardiac acceleration. Eight subjects were successful in achieving large magnitude voluntary cardiac acceleration after 2-5 training sessions. Eight matched control group subjects received one session of biofeedback assisted training in cardiac constancy. Results revealed that large magnitude heart rate increase was accompanied by a statistically significant increase in Peak Expiratory Flow Rate for experimental group subjects. Control group subjects showed a drop in heart rate and a statistically insignificant drop in PEFR. Clinical records for experimental and control group subjects during the pre- and post-training periods revealed that a significant reduction in the incidence of attacks, the use of p.r.n. medication, and the index of medication use per attack occurred in trained subjects. No change on any of these criteria occurred for control group subjects. The acquisition of the cardiac acceleration response of asthmatic experimental group subjects was compared with the acquisition rate of a matched group of normal subjects receiving one session of biofeedback training. No differences were revealed between the groups in the rate of acquisition. However, symptom-free asthmatics were shown to have PEFR readings significantly below those of the normal group, thus supporting previous findings. The possible implications of these findings for the clinical management of bronchial asthma are discussed.

38

Janson-Bjerklie S, Clarke E. **The effects of biofeedback training on bronchial diameter in asthma.** Heart Lung 11:200-207, 1982.

▶ biofeedback

Extracted summary: [N]o definite conclusions about the effectiveness of biofeedback in changing the bronchial diameter of asthmatics can be made. The magnitude of the observed change in TRR was small and variable within subjects and, therefore, should not be overestimated. The variabiity of results among experimental subjects may be due, in part, to the differences in severity of asthma and hence motivation to cooperate and participate. Under the double-blind conditions of the study, neither subjects nor researchers were aware of which subjects were receiving contingent feedback. Under these circumstances, the findings appear to support the contention that autonomic learning depends on information feedback to the individual rather than on expectations held by the subjects.

39
Kotses H, Glaus KD. **Applications of biofeedback to the treatment of asthma: a critical review.** Biofeedback Self Regul 6:573-593, 1981.

▶ review: biofeedback, relaxation

Both muscular and respiratory biofeedback procedures have been employed in attempts to reduce symptoms of bronchial asthma. Research relating to these approaches is reviewed in the present article. Biofeedback training both for facial muscle relaxation and for respiratory resistance decrease improves short-term pulmonary function in asthmatic individuals. These forms of training represent promising avenues for the management of asthma. However, unqualified endorsement of these procedures is premature, at the present time, since their influence on asthma-related variables other than pulmonary function has not been determined and since their long-term effects have not been investigated.

40
Lerro FA, Hurnyak MM, Patterson C. **Successful use of thermal biofeedback in severe adult asthma.** Am J Psychiatry 137:735-736, 1980.

▶ biofeedback, relaxation

Most research on the use of behavioral techniques to treat bronchial asthma has focused on children. Davis and associates concluded that behavioral procedures are more applicable to adults whose asthma is not severe than to those who asthma is severe. Our paper describes the dramatic and persistent improvement of an adult who had severe asthma and who responded fairly rapidly to thermal biofeedback and relaxation training after experiencing a protracted period of recurrent hospitalizations for acute asthma attacks.

41
Levendel L, Lakatos M. **Application of the biofeedback method in asthmatic patients.** Allerg Immunol (Leipz) 27:35-39, 1981. (in German)

▶ biofeedback

Principle and research with the biofeedback method, their relations to the techniques of relaxation and possibilities of the therapeutical use in the clinic were described. The practical importance of this method is based on the possibility to measure the ability to relax and their degree and to mediate the relaxation more rapidly. For this purpose a biofeedback apparatus (electromyograph) was the best. Studies were carried out with a mini-suitcase apparatus. The first experiences with this method were described.

42
Levendel L, Lakatos M. **Biofeedback studies in asthmatic patients.** Orv Hetil 121:2193-2195, 1980. (in Hungarian: no English abstract)

▶ biofeedback

43
Pratt C, Danker P, Miklich DR, Chai H, Creer TL. **An investigation of the use of peak expiratory flow rate for feedback treatment of asthmatic children.** CARIH Res Bull 4, 1974.

▶ biofeedback

Vachon's impressive research suggests that operant techniques of biofeedback have promise for the treatment of asthma. Consequently, the research reported in this paper was undertaken to assess its therapeutic value in the treatment of asthmatic children. This research attempted to show single session improvements similar to those found by Dr. Vachon, to determine if these improvements persist across time; and to assess what effect these improvements might have on the severity of the Ss' asthmatic condition.

44
Scherr MS, Crawford PL, Sergent CB, Scherr CA. **Effect of biofeedback techniques on chronic asthma in a summer camp environment.** Ann Allergy 35:289-295, 1975.

▶ biofeedback, relaxation, milieu therapy

Bio-feedback mediated deep muscle relaxation procedures produced significant results as compared with a control group. Behavior ratings and medical staff evaluations were made without knowledge of group subject assignments. Asthma attacks and infirmary visits information was independently obtained from the medical records. Pulmonary function readings in terms of peak-flow rate were obtained three times daily for all campers. Positive improvement occurred in the asthmatic status of bronchial asthma in most of the campers during the summer camp session. The experimental group which received the biofeedback relaxation procedures demonstrated significantly greater improvement than the control group. Statistically significant improvement was demonstrated in terms of (1) behavior rating, (2) improvement in peak-flow rates, (3) reduction in infirmary visits, (4) reduction in number of asthma attacks and (5) reduction in steroid usage. Medical staff rating of severity of asthma tended to be more severe for the control group ($R^2 = .545$). Caution in interpreting these findings is indicated pending a replication of the research with the introduction of more rigorous controls.

45
Steptoe A, Phillips J, Harling J. **Biofeedback and instructions in the modification of total respiratory resistance: an experimental study of asthmatic and non-asthmatic volunteers.** J Psychosom Res 25:541-551, 1981.

▶ biofeedback

The ability of asthmatic and non-asthmatic subjects to exert voluntary control over pulmonary function was assessed in a short-term experimental context. Total respiration resistance (R1) was monitored using the forced oscillation technique with a Siemens Siregnost FD5, while peak flow (PF) and forced expiratory volume (FEV1) were also recorded periodically. Sixteen non-asthmatic and eight asthmatic volunteers attended one introductory and four experimental sessions. Each experimental session consisted of four 3-min trials, during which the participants tried to lower airways resistance, separated by rest periods. The asthmatic subjects, and eight of the non-asthmatics, were provided with visual and auditory analogue feedback of R1 throughout each trial in all sessions. The second non-asthmatic group attempted voluntary control without feedback (instruction only) in sessions 1 and 2, and feedback was subsequently introduced for the final two sessions. Analysis of sessions 1 and 2 indicated that R1 was lower in the non-asthmatics given feedback compared with those in the instruction condition. During the final two sessions, differences between the two non-asthmatic groups disappeared. Trends also emerged within sessions, since R1, was higher in trials than rests early in sessions, while later this pattern was reversed. The average change between trials 1 and 4 in the last session was 7.1%. These effects were reflected to a limited extent in PF data. The asthmatic response was more variable. Two members of this group produced consistent decreases in R1 of 15-20% during trials compared with rests, while modifications in the reverse direction were recorded in two others. Patients may therefore have to be carefully selected for this approach to asthma management. The mechanisms responsible for these responses are uncertain.

46
Zanus L, Cracco A, Mesirca P, Ronconi GF. **Biofeedback in asthmatic children.** Pediatr Med Chir 6:247-251, 1984. (in Italian)

▶ biofeedback, counterconditioning

This paper reports the results of the treatment of continuous bronchial asthma in children, 7-14 years old, by means of biofeedback and counter-conditioning. We observed the remission of the symptomatology in all the cases, with a statistical significance.

Group and Family Therapy

47
Abramson HA. **Reversed parentectomy.** J Asthma Res 7:109, 1970. (editorial)

▶ family therapy

48
Abramson HA, Peshkin MM. **Psychosomatic group therapy with parents of children with intractable asthma: sibling rivalry and sibling support.** Psychosomatics 6:161-165, 1965.

▶ group therapy, family therapy

Extracted summary: This report covers eleven families (the total number of families in the three groups that evening was comprised of sixteen families). When eleven families can unleash in one evening the material that lay hidden all this while, then one can safely say that such spontaneous pouring forth of vital information was truly spectacular. Moreover, the integrated value of the material indicates that these parents definitely benefited from the learning process that they went through during group therapy. It is therefore recommended that adequate treatment of the intractably asthmatic child must include some type of psychotherapy for the parents. Without provision for this, treatment must be considered inadequate.

49
Abramson HA, Peshkin MM. **Psychosomatic group therapy with parents of children with intractable asthma: adaptation mechanisms.** Ann Allergy 18:87-91, 1960.

▶ group therapy, family therapy, milieu therapy

Two hundred psychotherapeutic group sessions with parents of intractably asthmatic children hospitalized in Denver are briefly summarized. The parents resided in the area of New York City, with their children, therefore, two thousand miles away. There were always two discussion leaders who co-ordinated both the immunologic and psychologic aspects of the adaptation process required by the parents, connected with the removal of their children to Denver. The following briefly outlined items are the subject matter of this paper: (1) the "illness-centered" nature of the discussion groups; (2) the effect of communications from the children, visitors, and office reports from the institute; (3) the effect on sibling relationships, as well as relationships with grandparents and other relatives; (4) the relationship of the parents with one another, incidental to the removal of the asthmatic child; (5) the transference problems with the therapist; (6) the structured neurotic needs of the members of the group, partly with respect to the concept that parental influence must carry punitive authority; (7) the narcissistic needs of the parents; (8) cultural and religious factors; (9) anxiety produced in the parents by attending the group sesions; (10) attitudes toward physical changes in the children while they were in the Denver Institute; and (11) the need for development of insight.

50
Abramson HA, Peshkin MM. **Group psychotherapy of the parents of intractably asthmatic children.** J Child Asthma Res Inst Hosp 1:77-91, 1961. (interviews continued J Asthma Res 11(3), 1974; 12(1), 1974; 12(2), 1974; 13 (3), 1976; 16(1), 1978; 16(2), 1979; 16(3), 1979; 16(4), 1974; 17(1), 1979; 17(2), 1980; 17(3), 1980)

▶ group psychotherapy, family therapy, milieu therapy

Extracted summary: In conclusion: We have described for you the scope of the problem with which we had to cope in the creation of the group therapy sessions with parents of intractably asthmatic children. We have described some general psychological phenomena encountered in these group sessions and the methods we have improvised in the management and orientation of the parents. We know that as a result of the parent group discussions, there will be developed a valuable adjunct, not only to therapy but also to our future knowledge of the basic mechanisms. Our data will also provide a rich body of source material. Our findings may lead to improved treatment for anxious parents of intractably asthmatic children, not only at the institutional level but also in the child's home.

51
Barendregt JT. **The effect of group therapy with asthma patients.** Ned Tijdschr Psychol 12:57-67, 1957. (in Dutch)

▶ group psychotherapy

52
Barendregt JT. **A psychological investigation of the effect of group psychotherapy in patients with bronchial asthma.** J Psychosom Res 2:115-119, 1957.

▶ group psychotherapy

The hypothesis of the existence of an effect of psychotherapy was tested. Thirty-six asthmatics, eighteen of them receiving group psychotherapy, were examined twice with an interval of 19 months by means of the Rorschach test.

53
Bertrand R. **Group psycho-kinetic rehabilitation of asthmatics.** Bronches 16:240-243, 1966. (in French: no English abstract)

▶ group therapy, relaxation, psychotherapy

54
Bien RF. **Remission of intractable asthma in a child during psychotherapy of the mother.** J Asthma Res 7:47-51, 1969. (case report)

▶ family therapy, psychotherapy

55
Cain J, Charpin J, Planson C. **Psychosomatic consideration on 50 cases of allergic asthma: attempted group psychotherapy.** Acta Allerg (Kbh) 14:134, 1959. (in French: no English abstract)

▶ group psychotherapy

56
Clapham HI, Sclare AB. **Group psychotherapy with asthmatic patients.** Int J Group Psychother 8:44-54, 1958.

▶ group psychotherapy

1. An account is given of a year's group therapy with six asthmatic patients; the group met once weekly. 2. The development of the group, from initial guardedness and non-understanding through to the production of affect-laden material from the members' past and present lives, is described. 3. Difficulties in interpersonal relationships and emotional conflicts. 4. Group therapy through transference and identifications provided a framework which led to better reality adaptation and to amelioration of asthma. 5. Though not statistically significant, the results suggest that group therapy is of value in the treatment regime of psychogenic asthma.

57
Combrinck-Graham L. **Structural family therapy in psychosomatic illness: treatment of anorexia nervosa and asthma.** Clin Pediatr (Phila) 13:827-833, 1974.

▶ family therapy

This account of the treatment of anorexia nervosa in a child with asthma stresses the importance of restructuring the family system. Even though the treatment was focused on the management of one psychosomatic problem (anorexia), the other problem (asthma) improved remarkably as well. This supports the hypothesis that psychosomatic symptoms in children serve a function in maintaining dysfunctional patterns in the family system, and that when the system is restructured to alter these dysfunctional patterns, the psychosomatic symptoms improve regardless of the physiology of the illness or its expression.

58
Coolidge JC. **Asthma in mother and child as a special type of intercommunication.** Am J Orthopsychiatry 26:165-178, 1956.

▶ psychotherapy

Of 52 asthmatic children studied in the Massachusetts General Hospital, 3 were chosen for this presentation because their mothers were likewise asthmatic. They demonstrated in strong relief certain dynamic features pertaining to the basic conflicts of the mother-child relationship of the other asthmatic children in the series. Fragments of 3 cases are presented.

59
Deter HC, Allert G. **Group therapy for asthma patients: a concept for the psychosomatic treatment of patients in a medical clinic—a controlled study.** Psychother Psychosom 40:95-105, 1983.

▶ group therapy, autogenic training, relaxation, family therapy

Asthma patients pose special problems as far as the medical supervision, danger of symptoms and the course of the disease are concerned. Some 90 asthma patients were registered for the treatment in the Heidelberg Medical Clinic. 31 patients who were interested in taking part were randomized into 3 groups: two treatment groups consisted of the exchange of information, discussion sessions on the illness as well as "autogenic training" or "functional relaxation". The third group was the control group. Before and after treatment the patients were submitted to a thorough examination both of lungs and other internal organs as well as from the psychodiagnostical point of view. The average age of the patients was 43.5 years and the average duration of illness 16.8 years. Nevertheless, the treatment group's sympathomimetics use was significantly reduced by 1 year of treatment (p less than 0.05); the use of steroids decreased as well. The number of visits of the general practitioner also decreased. These results support the conclusion that psychosomatic group therapy can make an important contribution to the treatment of asthma patients. Body therapy practised in "autogenic training" and "functional relaxation" seems to be another important healing factor for the treatment in addition to the discussion sessions and the exchange of information.

60
Forth MW, Jackson M. **Group psychotherapy in the management of bronchial asthma.** Br J Med Psychol 49:257-260, 1976.

▶ group psychotherapy, psychoanalysis

In this paper the authors present their theoretical view of the place of psychogenic factors in asthma. They review the experience they had in conducting weekly analytically orientated group therapy with a group of asthmatic women for 18 months and review the difficulties they met in this work. From this experience they attempt to reconcile some of the contradictions in previously published work in this area.

61
Gauthier Y, Fortin C, Drapeau P, Breton JJ, Gosselin J, Quintal L, Weisnagel J, Tetreault L, Pinard G. **The mother-child relationship and the development of autonomy and self-assertion in young (14-30 months) asthmatic children: correlating allergic and psychological factors.** J Am Acad Child Psychiatry 16:109-131, 1977.

▶ family therapy, psychotherapy

This study has a threefold purpose: (1) to focus on the very young asthmatic (14-30 months) and to evaluate his autonomous and self-assertive strivings; (2) to study the mother-child relationship as a transactional, reciprocal process of mutual adaptation; and (3) to look for a possible relationship between allergic factors and the psychological variables. We evaluated 40 asthmatic children and their mothers, following an observational methodology, both at home and in the hospital. The results led us to question the theory of a "psychosomatic type" of mother-child relationship in childhood asthma as well as the inverse reciprocity between allergy and psychopathology which has been described in the literature. The implications of this study for pediatric and child psychiatric practice and for future research are also described.

62
Gauthier Y, Fortin C, Drapeau P, Breton JJ, Gosselin J, Quintal L, Weisnagel J, Lamarre A. **Follow-up study of 35 asthmatic preschool children.** J Am Acad Child Psychiatry 17:679-694, 1978.

▶ family therapy, psychotherapy

We reevaluated 35 asthmatic children at age 4 to 6 years, focusing on the child's strivings for autonomy and opposition and the mother-child relationship. Measures were made of an allergy potential score, and pulmonary function tests were performed. A majority of children and mothers were found to be coping very adequately, though a greater number of conflictual mother-child relationships are becoming apparent in the opposition sector. Significant correlations were established between some indicators of psychopathology and a high allergy potential. Although most of the children are now symptom-free, they remain potential asthmatics as evidenced by their reaction to a bronchodilating drug. Prevailing psychosomatic concepts of the psychogenic role of the mother and a disturbed mother-child relationship in childhood asthma should be revised.

63

Geiger AK. **Analysis of family milieu of asthmatic children (family explorations).** Acta Paediatr Acad Sci Hung 15:165-173, 1974.

▶ family therapy, psychotherapy

Exploration within the families of 40 asthmatic children revealed that the child's disease has an important role in maintaining family homeostasis. Since recovery of the child would endanger the family's security, intrafamiliar forces are inhibiting his recovery and play a role in the precipitation of asthmatic attacks. The findings indicated that the characteristic attitudes termed in recent literature as maternal rejection, maternal overprotection and Chronos complex are motivated by a discrepancy of the mother's genuine ego and her ego-ideal.

64

Ghory JE. **Physical rehabilitation of the asthmatic child.** Allergol Immunopathol (Madr) Suppl 9:95-98, 1981.

▶ group psychotherapy, family therapy, couples therapy

Extracted summary: It is a mistake to ascribe too great importance to the role of emotions in the development of bronchial asthma in children. However, it is almost inevitable that an allergic child who endures recurring episodes of severe bronchial asthma will develop some emotional feeling about his chronic illness. This psychologic component, minimal at first, may become of increasing importance as the child gets older and his disease progresses. Rather than viewing asthma as a psychosomatic disease, it is more proper to view asthma in children as a somatopsychic disease, with the emotional overlay developing as a complication of his chronic illness. Over a span of 20 years observation in the Asthma Rehabilitation Program in the Cincinnati Convalescent Hospital for Children, we have yet to observe a single case of asthma caused by psychologic disorder. There can be no doubt, however, that the emotional factors can act as an aggravating or triggering mechanism, similar to many other nonimmunologic factors which influence the existing allergic reaction ... We have placed much less emphasis on psychotherapy for the child and much more emphasis on psychotherapy for the parents. To this end we have

instituted group psychotherapy sessions for the mothers of the asthmatic children, and frequently we have brought in the fathers as well. In addition to the prime value of educating the parents to the disease itself, these group sessions have allowed the parents to ventilate their feelings of anxiety, apprehension, and concern over their children, and where it exists, their own frustrated feelings of anger and hostility. Our general goals with these group psychotherapy sessions were: (1) to help mothers acquire an understanding of the problems of the severely asthmatic child; (2) to promote self-inspection and insight into emotional problems; (3) to examine closely the clinical family pattern of childhood asthma and the personalities of the parents of severely asthmatic children; (4) to help eliminate serious interference by the mothers in the treatment of their children, and (5) to provide a main source of help for parents after their children have been discharged from the hospital. The application of a group-psychotherapeutic technique as an integrated part of a general rehabilitation program must be viewed as having at least functional utility, and supports the opinion that the family must be treated concurrently with the intractable asthmatic child.

65

Groen JJ, Pelser HE. **Experiences with, and results of group psychotherapy in patients with bronchial asthma.** J Psychosom Res 4:191-205, 1960.

▶ group psychotherapy

The writers report the results of a therapeutic trial with eighteen male and fifteen female asthma patients who were treated with group psychotherapy combined, if necessary, with ACTH and symptomatic therapy over a period of 4 and 2 years, respectively. The results were compared with two control groups, who were treated, respectively, with symptomatic therapy only, and a combination of symptomatic therapy and ACTH. Although a significant difference was found in favour of the patients treated by group psychotherapy (supporting the hypothesis that psychic factors play a role in the causation and course of the disease) the results are not yet entirely satisfactory. Further intensive research will be necessary to find more effective methods of treatment in this disease.

66

Gustafsson P. **Psychological and family dynamic aspects of bronchial asthma in children.** Lakartidningen 78:1878-1880, 1981. (in Swedish)

▶ family therapy

The article constitutes a literary review of theories and empirical results relating to the effect of psychological factors on asthma. Theories concerning an "asthmatic personality" are abandoned in favour of a model which regards the asthmatic child as part of a family system, based on the principle that the disease affects all members of the family.

67
Krejci E. **Development of mother-child relations in the picture series of a 5-year-old asthmatic boy.** Prax Kinderpsychol Kinderpsychiatr 18:161-172, 1969. (in German: no English abstract)

▶ family therapy

68
Lange-Nielsen AF, Retterstol N. **Group therapy in asthmatic patients in a medical department: preliminary experience.** Nord Medicin 61:270-273, 1959. (in Norwegian)

▶ group therapy

Asthma patients are considered to maintain a negative attitude towards psychiatric treatment. By applying group therapy in a general medical department, about 10 asthma patients were observed for about a year after discharge from hospital. The group advanced slowly, because of an unusually strong inclination to cling to the somatic aspects of the disease. The group members have, however, taken a gradually increasing interest in the psychogenesis of asthma. Certain general traits in the personality of asthma patients are discussed. The advantages of having two professional group members, one being an internist and the other a psychiatrist, are pointed out.

69
Lask B, Matthew D. **Childhood asthma: a controlled trial of family psychotherapy.** Arch Dis Child 54:116-119, 1979.

▶ family psychotherapy

In an attempt to evaluate the effectiveness of family psychotherapy as an adjunct conventional treatment in childhood asthma, children with moderate to severe asthma were randomly allocated to a control group or to an experimental group; the latter group received 6 hours of family treatment during a 4-month period, and both groups had standard medical treatment. While there was no significant difference between the two groups on three parameters, the experimental group were significantly better in day-wheeze score and thoracic gas volume. These results suggest that family treatment in selected cases may have a place in the overall management of childhood asthma, and that more research with larger numbers of children is necessary.

70
Liebman R, Minuchin S, Baker L. **The use of structural family therapy in the treatment of intractable asthma.** Am J Psychiatry 131:535-540, 1974.

▶ family therapy, behavior therapy

The authors identify characteristics of family organization and functioning associated with psychosomatic illness in children—specifically chronic, severe, relapsing asthma—and report on a successful therapeutic approach designed to change these family characteristics. Weekly outpatient family therapy sessions focused on alleviating asthmatic symptoms, identifying and changing family patterns that exacerbate symptoms, and intervening to change the family system to prevent a recurrence of the symptoms.

71
Mascia AV, Reitner SR. **Group therapy in the rehabilitation of the severe chronic asthmatic child.** J Asthma Res 9:81-85, 1971.

▶ group therapy

We have attempted to utilize group therapy in a multidisciplinary approach in the rehabilitation of the intractable asthmatic adolescent patient. The focus of the program is to bring about a reversal of the patient's pattern of total dependence on his family and medical personnel by helping him achieve a greater sense of independence, adequacy, and control over himself. In terms of the patient's physical management, this is accomplished by helping him understand and correctly use his medications. It involves educating the patient about the specific potential triggering factors of his asthmatic symptoms. Good orientation and proper medical guidance assist the patient in making, by himself, the appropriate decisions which will control his wheezing. Through group therapy we attempt to provide the asthmatic patient with sufficient emotional insight and self-awareness to reduce his anxiety level. Special emphasis is given to the patient's understanding of his attitudes and feelings vis-a-vis authority-dependency relationships. Through relief of feelings of frustration and guilt, the patient's self-concept is enhanced, thus promoting a more self-assertive attitude and decreasing the need to utilize dependency channels for gratification. With the reduction of the patient's anxiety level, a reduction in asthmatic symptoms has been observed.

72
Mayer L, Isbister C. **Report on group therapy for mothers of children with intractable asthma.** Med J Aust 1:887-889, 1970.

▶ group therapy, family therapy, milieu therapy, psychotherapy

A report is presented on group therapy for mothers of children with intractable asthma. The content of the group sessions is briefly presented and evaluated. The sharing of problems and the support offered by members in the group situation seem to be of value. Group therapy is seen in this context as an alternative to individual therapy, as increasing numbers of patients will preclude the offering of individual therapy in every instance.

73

McLean JA, Ching AYT. **Follow-up study of relationships between family situation and bronchial asthma in children.** J Am Acad Child Psychiatry 12:142-161, 1973.

▶ psychotherapy, family therapy

Extracted summary: Child psychiatry is seen to have a selective role in the treatment of the asthmatic child. Routine referral is unnecessary. On the other hand, the disturbed asthmatic child requires psychiatric help, and medical-psychiatric treatment is clearly indicated for a good many of the parents. The deciding factor is not the child's asthma but the emotional status of both child and family, with the recognition that the asthma may add new problems requiring therapeutic intervention through the coordinated efforts of allergists, child psychiatrists, and case workers.

74

Minuchin S, Fishman HC. **The psychosomatic family in child psychiatry.** J Am Acad Child Psychiatry 18:76-90, 1979.

▶ family therapy, psychotherapy

This paper contrasts the individual and contextual approaches to the psychiatric treatment of psychosomatic diseases of children. In contrasting the conceptualizations of the "self", the authors discuss an expanded self inherent in the family-oriented approach. An investigation involving psychosomatic and normal diabetic children and their families demonstrates this concept. The authors present a case of an asthmatic child and discuss and contrast approaches to the areas of diagnosis, etiology, maintainance of symptoms, ideas of change, and treatment.

75

Neraal A. **Bronchial asthma in a female child of 3 1/2: the role of family dynamics.** Monatsschr Kinderheilkd 128:476-479, 1980. (in German)

▶ family psychotherapy

An attempt is made to show the connection between bronchial asthma and interaction within the family in the case of a 3 1/2 years old girl. Relationships within the family structure giving rise to illness should be taken into account during treatment, and dissolved at the same time by therapeutic means within the family.

76

Overbeck A, Overbeck G. **Bronchial asthma in relation to family dynamic processes: case report and comparison with the literature.** Psyche (Stuttg) 32:929-955, 1978. (in German)

▶ family therapy

A five-year-old girl reacted to her familial and psychic situation with bronchial asthma. By reference to the family therapy it is shown that the symptoms can be explained equally as well on the role-theoretical, familial-dynamic level as on the psychoanalytic-psychosomatic level. Various bridging concepts serve to further the understanding of the interpenetration of the inter- and intra-personal fields.

77

Peshkin MM, Abramson HA. **Psychosomatic group therapy with parents of children having intractable asthma.** Ann Allergy 17:344-349, 1959.

▶ group therapy, family therapy, milieu therapy

In conclusion, we have described for you the scope of the problem with which we had to cope in the creation of the group therapy sessions with the parents of intractable asthmatic children. We have described some general psychological phenomena encountered in these group sessions and the methods we have improvised in the management and orientation of the parents. We know that as a result of the parent group discussions a valuable adjunct not only to therapy but also to our future knowledge of the basic mechanisms will develop. Our findings may lead to improved treatment for anxious parents of intractably asthmatic children not only at the institutional level but also in the child's home.

78

Reckless J. **The deconditioning of conversion reactions in a modified group therapy situation.** Act Nerv Super (Praha) 12:167, 1970.

▶ group psychotherapy

Somatic illnesses of psychogenic origin may be deconditioned by verbal interaction in a modified group therapy setting. One example is asthma where the acute onset of bronchial lumen changes were found to be precipitated by discussion of a specific conflict relating to aggression and dependency. By viewing the bronchial change not only as the conditioned response but rather as the conditioning stimulus, it was possible to reverse the psychological conditioned response and trace back in the patient's thinking the original conditioned stimulus. This recall method also externalized the patient's repressed affects. The specific technique requires that the group psychotherapy process be arrested at the point of the wheezing and direct attention be directly focused on the patients. This direct confrontation catalyzes the patient to avoid the unpleasant nature of the attention by meeting the group leader's expectation. In this way, recovery of the affect and conflicts meets the therapist's expectations and provides an example of conditioned avoidance to an aversive stimulus, namely the group attention. While this technique is applicable to certain psychosomatic conditions, its applicability will depend on the personality pattern and reactions of the patient.

79
Reckless J. **A behavioral treatment of bronchial asthma in modified group therapy.** Psychosomatics 12:168-173, 1971.

▶ group psychotherapy, reciprocal inhibition, desensitization

Asthmatic attacks which develop within a group-therapy setting have been treated by a method which trains the patient to inhibit and extinguish the respiratory symptoms without recourse to pharmacological treatment. This method combines psychological insight in the cognitive sense with a deconditioning procedure utilizing the theory of reciprocal inhibition. The desensitization is unsystematic and is engendered spontaneously and erratically by the nature of conflicts produced in the course of group therapy. While the method described is specifically correlated to asthma-like behavior, it can be useful in other psychosomatic conditions involving the autonomic nervous system, as well as in conversion reactions affecting the neuromuscular system. Three years of follow-up suggest that the inhibition and extinction of the asthma-like behavior in the group setting also serves to reduce the incidence of asthmatic attacks outside the group.

80
Reed JW. **Group therapy with asthma patients.** Geriatrics 17:823-830, 1962.

▶ group therapy, psychotherapy

The results of eight years' experience in the comprehensive treatment of 125 patients with severe chronic asthma in the outpatient clinics of the Johns Hopkins Hospital are presented. Psychologic treatment consisted of individual and group psychotherapy. It is suggested that a decrease in morbidity will ensue if this approach is more widely utilized.

81
Sclare AB, Crocket JA. **Group psychotherapy in bronchial asthma.** J Psychosom Res 2:157-171, 1957.

▶ group psychotherapy

(1) 16 female asthmatic patients, considered to have preponderant emotional factors in their illness, were treated by means of group psychotherapy on an outpatient basis. The treatment was given by a psychiatrist, while physical treatments were concurrently given by a physician. (2) Six control groups of varying composition were set up, all having routine medical treatment. One of the control groups also had group psychotherapy and is described in detail elsewhere. (3) The experimental group was treated by a modified analytic technique which closely followed that of Foulkes (1948). (4) The development and content of the group sessions are described in detail. (5) The results of treatment were assessed on a clinical basis. The experimental group did not fare significantly better than the control groups in respect of asthmatic symptomatology: marked diminution of anxiety, tension and inhibition were, however, noted in this group. (6) The group dynamics are discussed and the problems of therapy are reviewed in the light of recent work by others in this field. (7) Group psychotherapy may prove to be a valuable addition to the treatment regime in those asthmatic patients who manifest a significant emotional factor in their illness.

82
Stokvis B. **Group psychotherapy and sociotherapy as adjuvant treatments for asthma.** Evol Psychiatr 4:695-710, 1955. (in French)

▶ group psychotherapy

83
Stokvis B. **Group psychotherapy for asthmatics.** Acta Psychother 7:220-232, 1959. (in German)

▶ group psychotherapy, psychotherapy, suggestion

Extracted summary: As a statistical catamnestic report concerning mainly asthmatic-allergic patients shows, about 40-50 per cent reacted very favourably to individual psychosomatic therapy. There was no significant difference between the results obtained with uncovering and covering individually applied therapy. The result of combined individual and groupwise treatment was better: improvement in 50-60 percentage of cases. The catamnestic investigation revealed, of those that responded, that the improvement, in most of the cases, remained constant. The control time varied between 1/2 and 3 years.

84
Tinkelman DG, Brice J, Yoshida GN, Sadler JE. **The impact of chronic asthma on the developing child: observations made in a group setting.** Ann Allergy 37:174-179, 1976.

▶ group therapy, milieu therapy

Fourteen asthmatic children between ll and 14 years of age participated in weekly group discussion sessions for nine months. The purposes were to allow open discussion about asthma, to mutually educate the children and staff about the medical and social implications of their disease and to give the patients a chance to deal with adults without fear of reprimand or betrayal of trust. Anger, envy, fear, sadness and guilt were the emotions predominant in the sessions. Group sessions may offer a further modality in the total care of the asthmatic child.

85
Ulrich I, Taneli S. **Psychotherapy of children with bronchial asthma, including the family.** Prax Kinderpsychol Kinderpsychiatr 25:4-8, 1976. (in German)

▶ psychotherapy, family therapy

50 children between 4 and 14 years of age suffering from bronchial asthma were treated together with their families with combined psychotherapeutic methods. The degree of severity and the course of the illness within this group of patients ranged from mild to serious bronchial asthma. In follow-ups varying between six months and four years the described therapeutic approach resulted in freedom of symptom for two-thirds of the patients and lower frequency of attacks or at least stabilisation of the psychic development in the last third. The developed approach takes into account the importance of an intensive psychotherapy with quick-resulting effectiveness especially in the treatment of children with bronchial asthma. Emphasis is put upon the necessity of including the social environment in the psychotherapy.

86
Wendt H. **Psychotherapy of the mother as the treatment of bronchial asthma in her child.** Allerg Asthma (Leipzig) 10:366-371, 1964. (in German: no English abstract)

▶ family psychotherapy

87
Wohl TH. **The group approach to the asthmatic child and family.** J Asthma Res 4:237-239, 1967. (address)

▶ group therapy, family therapy

88
Wohl TH. **The role of group psychotherapy for mothers in a rehabilitative approach to juvenile intractable asthma.** Ment Hygiene 47:150-155, 1963.

▶ family therapy, group psychotherapy, milieu therapy

Extracted summary: The focus of this paper is on the contributions that can be made by group psychotherapy with mothers of asthmatic children toward: (1) the understanding of family processes, (2) helping the mother to face and accept relevant emotional factors, and (3) in-

suring that the patient gets the optimum benefit from his hospital and post-hospital experience.

Hypnosis and Suggestion

89
Anonymous. **Asthma and hypnotherapy.** Lond Clin Med J 11:7-9, 1970.

▶ hypnosis, autohypnosis

Extracted summary: Hypnosis helps not only in treating asthma, but many of the ailments that accompany it: insomnia whether primary or related to nocturnal bronchospasm responds well; so do migraine, atopic eczema, vasomotor rhinitis and hay fever, as well as peptic ulceration, premenstrual tension and vomiting of pregnancy. All these conditions share a common autonomic imbalance, and hypnosis, which is effective in restoring balance in asthma can reasonably be expected to achieve the same objective in other respects. Autohypnosis perpetuates the effect and makes the patient feel that he is contributing towards his own recovery, thus helping to restore confidence that the condition itself so often undermines.

90
Anonymous. **Hypnosis for asthma: a controlled trial: a report to the research committee of the British Tuberculosis Association.** Br Med J 4:71-76, 1968.

▶ hypnosis, autohypnosis, progressive relaxation

Investigated the use of hypnosis in the treatment of asthma in patients 10-60 yr. old with paroxysmal attacks of wheezing or tight chest capable of relief by bronchodilators. 1 group was given hypnosis monthly and used autohypnosis daily for 1 yr. Comparisons were made with a control group prescribed a specially devised set of breathing exercises aimed at progressive relaxation. Treatment was randomly allocated and Ss were treated by physicians in 9 centers. Results were assessed by daily diary recordings of wheezing and the use of bronchodilators, and by monthly recordings of forced expiratory volume (FEV) and vital capacity (VC). Independent clinical assessments were made by physicians unaware of Ss' treatment. 176 out of 252 patients completed the program. Both treatment groups showed some improvement. Among men the assessments of wheezing score and use of bronchodilators showed similar improvement in the 2 groups; among women, however, those treated by hypnosis showed improvement similar to that observed in the men, but those given breathing exercises made much less progress, the difference between the 2 groups reaching statistical significance. Changes in FEV and VC between the control and hypnosis groups were closely similar. Independent clinical assessors considered the asthma to be better in 59% of the hypnosis group and in 43% of the controls, the difference being significant. There was little difference between the sexes. Physicians with previous experience of hypnosis obtained significantly better results than did those without such experience.

91
Aronoff GM, Aronoff S, Peck LW. **Hypnotherapy in the treatment of bronchial asthma.** Ann Allergy 34:356-362, 1975.

▶ hypnosis, autohypnosis, milieu therapy

The efficacy of hypnotherapy in aborting acute asthmatic attacks was studied in 17 children ranging in age from six to 17. All had as their primary diagnosis bronchial asthma. Prior to hypnotic induction pulmonary function was assessed, then monitored in the immediate posthypnotic period and at two intervals thereafter. The average improvement for all subjects was greater than 50% above the baseline measurement as documented by spirometry, monitored dyspnea, wheezing and subjective ratings by the subjects. It is suggested that hypnotherapy may be an important tool in ameliorating asthma, improving ventilatory capacity and promoting relaxation without recourse to pharmacologic agents. One explanation offered is that hypnosis affects an autonomic response, thereby diminishing bronchospasm.

92
Ben-Zvi Z, Spohn WA, Young SH, Kattan M. **Hypnosis for exercise-induced asthma.** Am Rev Respir Dis 125:392-395, 1982.

▶ hypnosis

Hypnosis has been used for many years in the treatment of asthma, but studies of its usefulness have been controversial. We assessed the efficacy of hypnosis in attenuating exercise-induced asthma (EIA) in 10 stable asthmatics. The subjects ran on a treadmill while mouth breathing for 6 min on 5 different days. Pulmonary mechanics were measured before and after each challenge. Two control exercise challenges resulted in a reproducible decrease in forced expiratory volume in one second (FEV1). On 2 other days, saline or cromolyn by nebulization was given in a double-blind manner with the suggestion that these agents would prevent EIA. Hypnosis prior to exercise resulted in a 15.9% decrease in FEV1 compared with a 31.8% decrease on the control days (p less than 0.001). Pretreatment with cromolyn resulted in a 7.6% decrease in FEV1. We conclude that hypnosis can alter the magnitude of a pathophysiologic process, namely, the bronchospasm after exercise in patients with asthma.

93
Brown EA. **The treatment of bronchial asthma by means of hypnosis: as viewed by the allergist.** J Asthma Res 3:101-119, 1965.

▶ hypnosis, suggestion, doctor-patient relationship

Extracted summary: Hypnosis is a multiple-purpose therapeutic tool. The physician can help the patient to learn to control the symptoms and therefore to lessen if not obviate the use of drugs. The physician can also use hypnosis to explore the background in which the causes of the symptoms are to be discovered. When instrumental in diagnosis, hypnosis serves to separate some functional from some organic disorders. Obversely, hypnosis may be employed to motivate the patient to become well.

94
Clarke PS. **Effects of emotion and cough on airways obstruction in asthma.** Med J Aust 1:535-537, 1970.

▶ hypnosis, suggestion

Under hypnosis the effects of suggesting fear, anger, cough and an asthmatic attack, alone or in combination, have been studied in three asthmatic patients, using a spirometric method of assessment of airways obstruction. A significant decrease in forced expiratory volume at one second was observed with the suggestion of asthma alone, and more particularly on the combined suggestions of asthma, fear, anger and cough. No statistically significant decrease in ventilatory capacity occurred on coughing by itself, or the suggestion of fear and anger. On the average, these effects were reversed by suggestions of relaxation, but the scatter of post-experimental measurements was wide. The experiments were not designed to study the relationship between chronic emotional tension and the initial onset of asthma, neither were they an assessment of the value of hypnosis in the treatment of asthma.

95
Collison DR. **Hypnotherapy in the management of asthma.** Am J Clin Hypn 11:6-11, 1968.

▶ hypnosis, psychotherapy

Following a brief history of the use of hypnosis in the management of asthma, hypnotherapy with 20 ambulant non-hospitalized patients is described. Of the 7 females and 13 males, 11 had an excellent response, 5 a good response, and 4 a poor response.

96
Collison DR. **Which asthmatic patients should be treated by hypnotherapy?** Med J Aust 1:776-781, 1975.

▶ hypnosis, psychotherapy, autohypnosis, relaxation

Certain patients with bronchial asthma can benefit, often greatly, from hypnotherapy. This report is based on a retrospective analysis of 121 asthmatic patients who were treated by hypnotherapy. Hypnotic techniques and treatment procedure are described. Of the total number, 21% had an excellent response to treatment, becoming completely free from asthma and requiring no drug therapy. A further 33% had a good response, with worthwhile decrease in frequency and severity of the attacks of asthma, or a decrease in drug requirements. About half of the 46% who had a poor response had a marked subjective improvement in general well-being. Statistical evaluation of the six variables (age, sex, result, trance depth, psychological factors and severity of the asthma) confirmed the clinical impression that the ability to go into a deep trance (closely associated with the youthfulness of the subject) gives the best possibility of improvement, especially if there are significant aetiological psychological factors present and the asthma is not severe. Subjective improvement in well-being and outlook is a potential outcome at all age levels, independent of severity of the illness or entranceability of the patient.

97
Collison DR. **Hypnosis for asthma.** Br Med J 1:584, 1968. (letter)

▶ hypnosis, autohypnosis, suggestion

98
De la Parra R. **Treatment of bronchial asthma by hypnosis.** Acta Hipnol Lat Amer 1:60-71, 1960.

▶ hypnosis

Hypnosis is found to be of significant value in the treatment of acute and chronic asthma, small children and elderly patients making the least response. Consideration should be given concomitantly to both psychological and medical aspects.

99
Diamond HH. **Hypnosis in children: the complete cure of forty cases of asthma.** Am J Clin Hypn 1:124-129, 1958.

▶ hypnosis

Extracted summary: [Hypnosis] is but another form of therapy in our medical armamentarium and . . . it is not a short-cut cure for asthma, supplementing vaccine therapy. Moreover, never is it to be used simply to suppress the asthmatic attacks without thoroughly explaining the causation of the asthma. The asthmatic syndrome might very well be the visible manifestation of some well hidden deep-rooted psychosis, which if not handled properly could very well cause some much more serious symptom than asthma. Thorough understanding of this fact is vital, and sympathetic and competent handling is necessary.

100
Edwards G. **Hypnotic treatment of asthma: real and illusory results.** Br Med J 2:492-497, 1960.

▶ hypnosis, suggestion

Six patients admitted to hospital with severe asthma were treated by hypnotic suggestion. Five were subsequently followed up for not less than one year. Patients were assessed both by their subjective testament and objectively by spirometry: it was found that an adequate assessment could be based only on a combination of these methods. With this double assessment it was apparent that hypnosis benefited a patient in one of two entirely different ways—either by effecting physiological improvement (decrease of airways resistance) or by producing psychological improvement (decreased awareness of airways resistance). The distinction between these two responses has not often been adequately stressed. The implications of these findings for psychosomatic theory are discussed. While in hospital one patient failed completely to respond to hypnosis, and one responded poorly. Four had subjectively complete remissions, but in only two of these was remission objectively complete. Immediate response to hypnosis (before and after sessions) was usually poor, but this could be explained by the content of the suggestion. Speed of remission could be as fast with hypnosis as with physical methods. Three patients relapsed within days of going home, but two of these again went quickly into remission. Of the four patients originally responding well, two thought that their condition during the year after was much better than in previous years. Two out of these four patients were readmitted because of asthma. These results cannot be interpreted as valid evidence for or against the value of hypnosis: an uncontrolled series of six patients can be regarded only as pilot study. The results do, however, strongly suggest that a controlled clinical trial of hypnosis would repay the effort. The particular value of hypnosis may be as an alternative to steroid treatment.

101
Godfrey S, Silverman S. **Demonstration of placebo response in asthma by means of exercise testing.** J Psychosom Res 16:293-297, 1973.

▶ placebo

Exercise provokes a brief attack of bronchoconstriction in patients with asthma which can be inhibited by premedication with bronchodilator drugs or disodium cromoglycate. The exercise induced asthma was also significantly reduced by premedication with placebo in 20 out of 44 children with asthma. The reduction in exercise induced asthma varied from 28-46 per cent depending upon the type of placebo used. It is suggested that the placebo blocking of the exercise response might serve to identify a group of asthmatic children with significant emotional factors in their disease.

102

Hossri CM. **The treatment of asthma in children through acupuncture massage.** J Am Soc Psychosom Dent Med 23:3-16, 1976.

▶ hypnosis, suggestion, relaxation

Asthmatic crises in children have been successfully treated by manual stimulation of the acupuncture points in combination with hypnosis. With this treatment, it is possible to alleviate respiratory distress; nasal breathing returns and the bodily defenses against disease are restored.

103

Houghton HE. **Hypnotherapy in asthma.** Nurs Times 61:482-483, 1965.

▶ hypnosis, autohypnosis, suggestion, desensitization

Hypnosis as such is not a treatment for asthma. A situation is induced, however, in which patient and physician, working in accord, sometimes over a long period, can effect a cure. For the physician each patient is a challenge, and success or failure depends upon his insight into the patient's difficulties and his ability to suggest means of overcoming them. Most of all, however, success depends upon the willingness of the patient to co-operate in his own treatment. For both doctor and patient hypnotherapy in asthma is very time-consuming, but very rewarding.

104

Jacobi E. **The treatment of asthma by hypnosis.** Dtsch Med Wochenschr 52:452, 1926. (in German: no English abstract)

▶ hypnosis

105

Kinnell HG. **Hypnosis.** Br Med J 1:1563, 1979. (letter)

▶ hypnosis

106

Laudenheimer R. **Hypnotic exercise therapy of bronchial asthma.** Ther Ggw 67:339, 1926. (in German)

▶ hypnosis

The significance of the psyche in the treatment of asthma has become more and more recognized in the last decade, without capturing the interest, for the most part, of internal specialists. They find the interrelationship between "real bronchial asthma" and psychic disturbances to be negligible. Also, it is interesting that notable modern psy-chotherapists speak very little of asthma treatment through hypnosis. The author studied cases of bronchial asthma for four years and worked out his combination of hypnosis and breathing exercise techniques after coming across the idea quite by accident.

107

Lewis RA, Lewis MN, Tattersfield AE. **Asthma induced by suggestion: is it due to airway cooling?** Am Rev Respir Dis 129:691-695, 1984.

▶ placebo

The effect of suggestion on the airway response to 10 inhalations of normal saline followed by doubling concentrations of isoproterenol was assessed in 12 normal and 30 asthmatic subjects. It was suggested that the first 5 saline solutions contained a bronchoconstrictor and that the second 5 contained a bronchodilator, or vice versa, and that the first 4 isoproterenol solutions were inert, whereas the last was a bronchodilator. Nine asthmatic, but no normal subjects, bronchoconstricted after saline inhalation, with a mean fall in specific airway conductance (SGaw) of 40%. This was dose-dependent and was abolished when inhalations were carried out at 37 degrees C 100% relative humidity. Suggestion did not affect the airway response to saline or isoproterenol in either group, but it did influence the subjective impression of airway caliber recorded on a visual analogue scale. In this study, the bronchoconstriction after saline inhalation, previously attributed to the effect of suggestion, was caused by airway cooling.

108

Luparello TJ, Lyons HA, Bleeker ER, McFadden ER Jr. **Influences of suggestion on airway reactivity in asthmatic subjects.** Psychosom Med 30:819-825, 1968.

▶ suggestion, placebo

The effect of suggestion on bronchomotor tone was evaluated in a setting in which accurate, rapid, and reproducible measurements of airway resistance (Ra) could be made. Subjects with asthma, emphysema, and restrictive lung disease, as well as normal subjects, were studied. All subjects were led to believe that they were inhaling irritants or allergens which cause bronchoconstriction. The actual substance used in all instances was nebulized physiologic saline solution. Nineteen of 40 asthmatics reacted to the experimental situation with a significant increase in Ra. Twelve of the asthmatic subjects developed full-blown attacks of bronchospasm which was reversed with a saline solution placebo. The 40 control nonasthmatic subjects did not react.

109

Magonet AP. **Hypnosis in asthma.** Int J Clin Exp Hypn 8:121-128, 1960.

▶ hypnosis, suggestion

Asthma is a symptom in which personality disturbances are due to psychogenic factors, therefore there must be a return to the treatment of the sick patient instead of the symptoms from which he suffers. If we are to carry out treatment efficiently, we cannot afford to neglect any aspect of the patient's personality. The patient has a mind and the patient has a body, but we must also think of him as a social being in relation to his personal and material environment.

110

Maher-Loughnan G. **Hypnosis.** Br Med J 2:208, 1979. (letter)

▶ hypnosis, autohypnosis

111

Maher-Loughnan GP. **Problems with asthma.** Br Med J 3:173, 1972. (letter)

▶ hypnosis, autohypnosis

112

Maher-Loughnan GP. **Hypnosis and autohypnosis for the treatment of asthma.** Int J Clin Exp Hypn 18:1-14, 1970.

▶ hypnosis, autohypnosis

Two controlled studies were conducted in the use of hypnosis in asthma patients. Several different control procedures were used. The methods and results of both studies were summarized, and the same conclusion was reached: that hypnosis supplemented by autohypnosis was significantly more effective than control procedures. An outline is given of details of treatment methods. A current analysis of patients treated at one center, involving up to six years of follow up, is presented to provide a working guide to the regime in regular practice. To be fully effective, hypnosis should be employed before steroids are started. Steroid-dependent asthma is rarely totally relieved by hypnotherapy.

113

Maher-Loughnan GP, MacDonald N, Mason AA, Fry L. **Controlled trial of hypnosis in the symptomatic treatment of asthma.** Br Med J 2:371-374, 1962.

▶ hypnosis

The results show great symptomatic improvement in the hypnotherapy group in that the wheezing was reduced on an average by about half within three months, but there was very little alteration in the condition of the controls. Controlled trials of asthma are hard to plan because of the problem of therapy for the "controls." Here it was decided for the controls to use treatment by an antispasmodic which was new to the patient . . . Male and female patients progressed equally well. Those under 30 years of age and those whose asthma has lasted 20 years or less fared the best. The severity of asthma and the type of trigger also provided differences in response to hypnosis; mild cases and those with emotional triggers did best, but good responses were observed in the other categories. Patients who were easily hypnotized, those who achieved deep trances, and, perhaps most important, those who could practice the daily use of autohypnosis did best. Despite the many questions yet to be answered, hypnosis is of value in the symptomatic treatment of asthma as assessed by the reduction in wheezing and in the use of drugs.

114

Marchesi C. **The hypnotic treatment of bronchial asthma.** Br J Med Hypn 1:14-17, 1950.

▶ hypnosis

This paper, a short summary of the treatment of bronchial asthma, cannot, and will not, bring anything new or not known in the treatment of this illness. It was written to show that cases of long duration, complicated with other illnesses, can be cured [with hypnosis] and in this way encourage those with long standing complaints to undergo this treatment even when it seems that all is lost.

115

McFadden ER Jr, Luparello T, Lyons H, Bleecker E. **The mechanism of action of suggestion in the induction of acute asthma attacks.** Psychosom Med 31:134-143, 1969.

▶ suggestion, placebo

The effect of suggestion on the airway resistance of 29 asthmatic subjects was studied by whole-body plethysmography. The subjects were given physiologic saline to breathe although they were informed that they were inhaling different concentrations of an allergen which they indicated as the cause of their asthma attacks. Fifteen subjects developed bronchospasm, 14 did not. Repeat studies demonstrated that 13 of the 15 reactors remained responsive to suggestion, while all of the nonreactors remained unaffected. The intravenous administration of atropine sulfate abolished the bronchoconstrictor effect of suggestion. These observations demonstrate that a significant percentage of asthmatic subjects are able to alter their airway resistance in response to emotional stimuli through activation of efferent cholinergic pathways.

116

McFadyen C. **The respiratory nurse in action.** Can Nurse 74:30-31, 1978. (case report)

▶ hypnosis, suggestion

117

McLaren WR, Eisenberg BC. **Hypnosis in the treatment of asthma.** Acta Hipnol Lat Am 1:55-63, 1961. (in Spanish)

▶ hypnosis, psychotherapy

The author describes results and conclusions obtained with hypnotic trance in several cases, based on his experience in treating asthma, both from the clinical and allergicological aspect. He finds that symptomatic hypnotherapy is seldom sufficient and considers it necessary to investigate the underlying causes. This implies knowledge of elementary psychiatry as well as experience and capacity in psychotherapy. The allergist may use hypnotherapy as an interesting auxiliary method, if he has the time and skill to apply it.

118

Moraes Passos AC. **The value of hypnosis in the treatment of bronchial asthma.** Bol Brasil Soc Int Hipn Clin Exp 1:3-13, 1958. (in Portuguese)

▶ hypnosis

119

Moraes Passos AC. **Asthma treated with hypnosis.** Rev Brasil Tuberc 26:111-130, 1958. (in Portuguese)

▶ hypnosis, suggestion, relaxation

The author begins by presenting a short report of the evolution of hypnosis from mesmerism to actual hypnology. He quotes some articles in the field of hypnosis, particularly those of Crasilneck, Butler, Torres Norry and Chudnovsky, Kroger and DeLee, Faria, Ferreira Filho and Marmer. He points out the therapeutic applications of hypnosis in pulmonary diseases, particularly in asthma. He remembers Van Pelt's theory on asthma ("asthma is nothing more than a symptom: a symptom of underlying nervous disorder") and his original hynotherapeutic method. Prolonged suggested sleep, obtained and maintained exclusively by word (posthypnotic suggestion) without drug, is discussed. Hypnosis was induced by the author in 3 cases of asthma. One was treated by prolonged suggested sleep (19 hours a day) for 60 days, with very good result. The others were treated by direct suggestion (a half to one hour) of relaxation, with favorable results too.

120

Morwood JMB. **Relaxation by gramophone in asthma.** Practitioner 170:400-402, 1953.

▶ hypnosis, relaxation

A method is described of treating asthma by a relaxation technique using a gramophone record to induce a semi-hypnotic state. One neurotic patient was also greatly helped by this record.

121

Mun CT. **The value of hypnotherapy as an adjunct in the treatment of bronchial asthma.** Singapore Med J 10:182-186, 1969.

▶ hypnosis, family therapy, psychotherapy, doctor-patient relationship

Hypnotherapy is of value as an adjunct in the treatment of acute attacks of bronchial asthma. Hypnotherapy has been also shown to be a useful adjunct in obstetrics, surgery, and in the management of terminal cancer cases in which the need for narcotics and analgesics is markedly reduced. Hypnosis markedly potentiates the effectiveness of these drugs. Hypnotherapy is of value as an adjunct in the prevention of future attacks of bronchial asthma. It has also been shown to be a useful adjunct in other branches of medicine by the author elsewhere.

122

Mun CT. **The treatment of asthma by hypnotherapy.** Med J Malaya 18:232-233, 1964.

▶ hypnosis, suggestion

Extracted summary: First, an effort is made to regress the patient to the time of his first attack and to re-educate him to the effect that the cause of that first attack is no longer operative and that he need no longer have fears and tensions about the constantly recurring need to breathe. Posthypnotic suggestions are given that he will enjoy sound physiological sleep, and that should he awaken, there still will be no asthma, and that in the morning he will feel at ease and comfortable and will so continue. In many cases, in one or two sessions, despite long previous sufferings, lasting therapeutic results can be secured.

123

Napke E. **Hypnosis in infertility and allergy.** Can Med Assoc J 107:496, 1972. (letter)

▶ hypnosis

124

Neinstein LS, Dash J. **Hypnosis as an adjunct therapy for asthma: case report.** J Adolesc Health Care 3:45-48, 1982.

▶ hypnosis, psychotherapy

This study reports the effect of hypnotherapy in an asthmatic. The patient had moderately severe asthma with frequent attacks despite multiple medications. He received four weekly hypnosis sessions, and was then followed bimonthly for a year. The patient's course was followed by subjective daily scoring of wheezing severity, daily recording of peak expiratory flow rate by a Wright minispirometer, and once a month recording of his Forced Vital Capacity (FVC), Forced Expiratory Volume in one second/Forced Rate (MMRF). The severity rating showed improvement at one year when the start of therapy was compared to pretherapy (P less than .005). The daily peak flow rate averaged 486 liter/min before starting hypnotherapy and 502 liter/min after one year. There was no change in the FEV1/FVC and MMFR before and after therapy. School attendance and academic performance may be a helpful adjunct in asthma therapy during adolescence.

125

Philippus M, Dennis M. **Effect of suggestion on pulmonary function and induced asthma.** Ann Allergy 22:81-88, 1964.

▶ hypnosis, suggestion

The effect of hypnosis and posthypnotic suggestion was evaluated in a group of ten hospitalized asthmatic patients. Measurements of the first second forced expiratory volume were performed during attmepts to increase, with hypnosis, submaximal pulmonary function values, and to block the obstructive effect of inhaled acetyl-beta-methylcholine on the bronchial tree of these asthmatic subjects. No significant changes in measurement of airway function were produced. The method and results of this study were discussed.

126

Piscicelli U. **Hypnosis in medicine.** Minerva Med 60:1939-1949, 1969. (in Italian: no English abstract)

▶ hypnosis

127

Redondo D. **Hypnosis in the treatment of the asthmatic child.** Bull Tulane Univ Med Fac 20:307-313, 1961.

▶ hypnosis, suggestion

Five patients known to have repeated asthmatic attacks were treated with hypnotic suggestion. This suggestion consisted of "teaching" the asthmatic child to control the asthmatic attack first under hypnosis, and then after hypnosis with the aid of post-hypnotic suggestion. This method was used to demonstrate to the child that it was possible to control the asthmatic attacks, and either bring them on or stop them completely. The immediate results were encouraging in that 4 of the patients were markedly improved both in the frequency and severity of the attacks. A fifth patient needed psychotherapy after an initial short remission. These results cannot be interpreted as a proof of the value of hypnosis in the treatment of the asthmatic child. They do strongly suggest that many patients can benefit from this kind of therapy, and that a well-controlled clinical trial would be of tremendous value in determining its appliance in clinical practice.

128

Smith JM, Burns CLC. **The treatment of asthmatic children by hypnotic suggestion.** Br J Dis Chest 54:78-81, 1960.

▶ hypnosis, suggestion

Hypnotic suggestion on four occasions at weekly intervals failed to give any objective improvement, either immediate or delayed, in a series of 25 children of between 8 and 15 years of age, with chronic asthma.

129

Smith MM, Colebatch HJ, Clarke PS. **Increase and decrease in pulmonary resistance with hypnotic suggestion in asthma.** Am Rev Respir Dis 102:236-242, 1970.

▶ hypnosis, suggestion, relaxation

Pulmonary resistance measured during tidal breathing in 2 subjects with asthma before, during, and after hypnosis did not differ significantly. During hypnosis, coughing, suggestion of fear, anger, or of an attack of asthma increased pulmonary resistance and suggestion of relaxation decreased resistance. The changes in pulmonary resistance could not be explained by alterations in transpulmonary pressures secondary to different degrees of inflation of the lungs or by differences in gas flow. It appeared likely that the increases and decreases in pulmonary resistance represented constriction and dilatation of the bronchial tree. The findings indicated that cerebral centers directly influence the dimensions of the bronchial tree, and that suggestion and relaxation have a place in the treatment of patients with asthma.

130

Spector S, Luparello TJ, Kopetzky MT, Souhrada J, Kinsman RA. **Response of asthmatics to methacholine and suggestion.** Am Rev Resp Dis 113:43-50, 1976.

▶ suggestion

Effects of diluent, methacholine, and suggestion on pulmonary function were studied in 9 asthmatic subjects. On day 1, flavored diluent was given as a control preparation. On day 2, increasing concentrations of similarly flavored methacholine were administered. On day 3, the effect of flavored diluent plus suggestion was studied. Although all variables were affected, the dose-response relationships for methacholine were most pronounced for specific airway conductance and airway resistance, in contrast to maximal mid-expiratory flow, forced expiratory volume in 1 sec, and forced vital capacity. Suggestion toward bronchoconstriction significantly affected only the plethysmographic parameters, specific airway conductance, and airway resistance, and not the spirometric variables. Both airway resistance and 1-sec forced expiratory volume showed slight, but significant, changes as a result of bronchodilator suggestion, which was used to overcome the suggestion toward bronchoconstriction. Because suggestion had a greater effect on large airways than peripheral airways, a role for the vagus is implied. Thus, any protocol using body plethysmography must consider a possible effect of suggestion on results.

131
Stang RE, Luz A, Carr VB, Loune RS, Rieger R, Howard WA. **Grand rounds: self hypnosis in the treatment of asthma.** Clin Proc Child Hosp 19:199-205, 1963.

▶ autohypnosis, suggestion, relaxation, social casework

Extracted summary: The approach used in this case, the use of suggestion, not in terms of deep hypnosis, but in terms of the first stages of hypnosis which can be self-induced, is a device with which individuals can control their symptoms when they are on an emotional basis. This device might well be of use more often. It is well known that once an asthmatic process is established, once the pathways are established, it can be triggered not only by allergens but by intercurrent emotional factors. It would seem that recognition of the emotional factors gives us an additional therapeutic approach to the child with asthma. This has been shown to be of great help to physicians treating asthmatics.

132
Strupp HH, Levenson RW, Manuck SB. **Effects of suggestion on total respiratory resistance in mild asthmatics.** J Psychosom Res 18:337-346, 1974.

▶ placebo

Thirteen mild asthmatics were given inhalations of saline (described as either a neutral substance or a bronchoconstrictor) and Isuprel (described as either a bronchodilator or a bronchoconstrictor). Measurements of Total Respiratory Resistance (RT) were taken before and after each inhalation. Following inhalations of saline described as a bronchoconstrictor, four subjects evidenced increases in RT of 20 per cent or more (beyond their responses to saline described as a neutral substance). Some evidence was found of attenuation of the bronchodilative effect of Isuprel when it was described as a bronchoconstrictor. These data corroborate the findings obtained in other investigations, that one subgroup of the asthmatic population responds mainly to the pharmacological effect of the inhalant, while the other subgroup responds to its suggested effect. The observed bronchial changes could not be attributed to the stimulus value of the measurement technique.

133
Tashkin DP, Katz RM, Kerschnar H, Rachelevsky GS, Siegel SC. **Comparison of aerosolized atropine, isoproterenol, atropine plus isoproterenol, disodium cromoglycate and placebo in the prevention of exercise-induced asthma.** Ann Allergy 39:311-318, 1977.

▶ placebo

In 15 asthmatic children post-exercise bronchospasm was partially inhibited by placebo and by aerosolized atropine sulphate (1 mg) compared with no treatment, not significantly inhibited by atropine alone compared with placebo, partially blocked by disodium cromoglycate (20 mg) and by isoproterenol (0.625 mg) and completely blocked by the combination of isoproterenol and atropine. Pre-treatment with isoproterenol or atropine resulted in post-exercise values for specific conductance which were significantly greater than those following disodium cromoglycate by virtue of the bronchodilator effect of these drugs independent of or in addition to any specific inhibition of exercise-induced asthma. These results suggest that the bronchoconstrictor response to exercise is partially influenced by suggestion but is influenced to a significantly greater degree by mediator release and beta-adrenergic mechanisms and that bronchodilator drugs have therapeutic advantages over an inhibitor of mediator release in the prevention of exercise-induced asthma.

134
Uglov FG. **Symptomatic and pathogenetic therapy of bronchial asthma.** Klin Med (Mosk) 48:146-149, 1970. (in Russian: no English abstract)

▶ hypnosis

135
Van Pelt SJ. **Asthma Is there any such disease?** Br J Med Hypn 4:17-24, 1953.

▶ hypnosis, suggestion

Extracted summary: [H]undreds of similar cases show that there is a very real place for medical hypnotic suggestion as a means of manipulating the patient's imagination scientifically in order to free him of a complaint which has been brought about more often than not accidentally by the wrong use of that same imagination. Asthma is not a disease at all but merely a symptom—a symptom of an underlying nervous irritation—and the patient is far more likely to be sensitive to an irritating mother-in-law, an unfaithful spouse, a broken love affair or an impending bankruptcy than the usual substances such as feathers, house dust or various pollens which are invariably blamed by the orthodox believers in allergy. Even these will admit a fact, which has been often proved, that an asthmatic alleged to be sensitive or "allergic" to say, a rose, will have an attack if shown an artificial rose providing he thinks it is real. To what else then can asthma be due except suggestion?

136
Weiss JH, Martin C, Riley J. **Effects of suggestion on respiration in asthmatic children.** Psychosom Med 32:409-415, 1970.

▶ suggestion

Sixteen asthmatic children were studied in an attempt to replicate the findings of Luparello et al. on the effects of suggestion on airway reactivity. Maximum expiratory flow rates achieved in both forced and noneffort breathing, and expiratory duration were measured. S's were told that they would inhale potent allergens in a series of increasing concentrations until they began to wheeze. In fact, all S's inhaled physiologic saline. Of the 16 S's, one responded with decreased flow rate and wheezing in the suggestion session. In a control session involving saline and no suggestion, the same response occurred. All other S's failed to show any consistent response on any of the objective measures, although a number subjective sensations of tightness. Several reasons for the reported difference between our results and Luparello's are explored.

137
White HC. **Hypnosis in bronchial asthma.** J Psychosom Res 5:272-279, 1961.

▶ hypnosis

Ten patients with asthma, referred for psychiatric opinion, were treated by hypnosis and later observed for 6-11 months. Respiratory function tests were carried out before and after hypnosis, and during the review period. Although most patients reported improvement, hypnosis had no predictable effect upon respiratory function. Six patients became more active in work or social activities, and this was attributed to modification of neurotic attitudes.

138
Zamotaev IP, Sultanova A, Vorobeva ZV. **Effect of hypnotic suggestion in bronchial asthma.** Sov Med 2:7-10, 1983. (in Russian)

▶ hypnosis, suggestion

It has been found that as a result of hypnosuggestive therapy the bronchial choline receptor sensitivity diminished in all, and beta-blockade in 90% of patients with bronchial asthma. Disturbances (of various degree) of the choline receptor sensitivity were revealed in all, and beta-blockade in 52.6% of the patients examined.

139
Zeltzer L, LeBaron S, Barbour J, Kniker WT, Littlefield L. **Self-hypnosis for poorly controlled adolescent asthmatics.** Clin Res 28:862A, 1980. (abstract)

▶ autohypnosis

Self-hypnosis (SH) was taught to 6 adolescent asthmatics in poor control as defined by frequent attacks and ER visits, poor pulmonary function tests (PFT's), and noncompliance with medication. Following 2 months to stabilize doses of Alupent and Theodur and maintaining theophylline levels (TL's) in therapeutic range (= 15-17mg/ml), there was improvement in FEV_1 (p < .05), FMF (p < .03), and FEV_1/FVC (p < .05). After a 1-month baseline, patients learned SH for 5 months. In SH month 3, patients were asked to use their own imagery to improve their asthma. Structured self-reports, psychological tests, medical records, TL's, PFT's and skin tests (Multi-Test) were collected. Daily asthma severity was reduced (p < .05) by month 2 of SH, and attack frequency by month 3 (p < .03). Daily tension and attack severity were unchanged. Self-esteem was enhanced (p < .05). Frequency of ER visits was reduced as compared to the previous year (p < .02) and to the stabilization and baseline periods (p < 0.5) of the study year. PFT's did not significantly decrease from the gains made during stabilization phase, despite TL's decreasing (5.5mg/ml) by intervention month 3 and staying subtherapeutic. Response to skin tests was reduced by the end of the study (p < .005); response was totally absent for all antigens, including in 1 patient a negative response to the histamine control at retesting 2 weeks later under hypnosis. Follow-up 6 months after the study ended showed no significant worsening of symptom severity, attack frequency, daily tension, ER visits, or PFT's. These improvements in symptom control emphasize the need for a controlled study of hypnosis for asthmatics.

Meditation and Relaxation

140
Alexander AB. **Systematic relaxation and flow rates in asthmatic children: relationship to emotional precipitants and anxiety.** J Psychosom Res 16:405-410, 1972.

▶ relaxation

The present experiment was an attempt to replicate with better control, and to extend, previously reported work by the author and his colleagues. In that work, relaxation training, as compared to just sitting quietly, was found to result in an increase in PEFR over sessions in asthmatic children. In the present study, the relationship between the presence of emotional asthma precipitants and the amount of PEFR response, and the possibility that anxiety was mediating the effect were investigated. The previous findings were replicated in all important respects, while the results suggested that anxiety changes were probably not mediating the effect, and that the effect of relaxation on PEFR was generally greater for those subjects in whom emotional factors were prominent.

141
Alexander AB, Cropp GJ, Chai H. **Effects of relaxation training on pulmonary mechanics in children with asthma.** J Appl Behav Anal 12:27-35, 1979.

▶ relaxation, biofeedback

An experiment, designed to overcome shortcomings in previous work, was conducted to investigate the potential symptomatic benefits of relaxation training in the treatment of asthma in children. Fourteen chronic, severely asthmatic children received three sessions in which they rested quietly, followed by five sessions of relaxation training, and finally three sessions of relaxing as trained previously. Pulmonary function was assessed, in a manner far more definitive than in previous studies, before and after each session, and three additional times at 30-minute intervals thereafter. Tension in the frontalis muscles, heart and respiration rates, and skin temperature and conductance were also monitored. Heart rate and to some extent muscle tension results tended to confirm the attainment of relaxed states. However, the lung function results failed to substantiate the previous, preliminary findings of a clinically meaningful change in pulmonary function following relaxation. The status of relaxation in the treatment of asthma was discussed.

142
Alexander AB, Miklich DR, Hershkoff H. **The immediate effects of systematic relaxation training on peak expiratory flow rates in asthmatic children.** Psychosom Med 34:388-394, 1972.

▶ relaxation

Clinical experience has often suggested that having asthmatic patients sit quietly and/or relax during asthma attacks is helpful. The present study was an attempt to provide a controlled experimental demonstration of the effect of systematic relaxation on peak expiratory flow rate in asthmatic children. Eighteen male and 18 female asthmatic children were divided into two groups matched for mean age, sex composition and asthma severity. One group of subjects underwent three sessions of modified Jacobsonian systematic relaxation training, while the second group sat quietly for three sessions. Peak expiratory flow rate measures were obtained prior to and following each session. It was found that relaxation subjects manifested a significant mean increase in peak expiratory flow rate over sessions compared to a nonsignificant mean peak expiratory flow decrease for control subjects. It was suggested that these results have important implications both for the clinical treatment and the understanding of bronchial asthma.

143
Balluch H, Barolin GS, Rohrer T. **Autogenous training with asthma patient groups.** Wien Med Wochenschr 118:850-853, 1968. (in German: no English abstract)

▶ autogenic training

144
Bhole MV. **Treatment of bronchial asthma by yogic methods: a report.** Yoga Mimamsa 9:33-41, 1967.

▶ yoga

145
Darlas F. **10 asthmatic children treated by psychotherapeutic relaxation (Schultz-Sapiz method from adapted psychoanalytic inspiration).** Bronches 23:235-241, 1966. (in French)

▶ psychotherapy, relaxation

146
Erskine J, Schonell M. **Relaxation therapy in bronchial asthma.** J Psychosom Res 23:131-139, 1979.

▶ relaxation, autogenic training, meditation, imagery

Twelve patients with chronic bronchial asthma were matched in pairs and randomly assigned to two treatment groups. One group received mental and muscular relaxation; the second group received muscular relaxation alone. Treatment consisted of 4 weekly treatment sessions. Pre, post and follow-up phases each consisted of 3 weekly sessions. Respiratory function was measured by the forced expiratory volume in 1 second (FEV_1). Two self-report inventories were used to measure change in the symptoms and signs of the patient's asthma. Following factor analysis, 3 factors were used—psychological, physical and bronchoconstriction. Results showed that for each of these 3 factors and for FEV_1, there was no overall mean significant difference between results in either treatment group. In addition, patients showed no significant trend of improvement in respiratory function. No significant difference was shown between respiratory function recorded before and after relaxation treatment in each of the individual treatment sessions. There was a moderate correlation between objective recordings and the patient's subjective assessment of asthma severity.

147
Findeisen DG. **Kind, value and risks of known relaxation techniques in bronchial asthma.** Z Erkr Atmungsorgane 157:345-354, 1981. (in German)

▶ relaxation

Therapy and prophylaxis of bronchial asthma and cardiopulmonary consecutive diseases are commented upon with special reference to 1. indication and expected effectivity of scientifically based relaxation techniques, 2. some methods of treatment by gymnastics and breathing exercises as well by sports therapy, 3. nature, general risks and absolute contraindications by "modern" parascientific procedures.

148
Goyeche JR, Ago Y, Ikemi Y. **Asthma: the yoga perspective (I): The somatopsychic imbalance in asthma: towards a holistic therapy.** J Asthma Res 17:111-121, 1980.

▶ yoga, breathing exercises

While the standard physiological and even certain psychological characteristics of asthmatic patients are well known, the current diagnostic and therapeutic approach to asthma remains inadequate, as it neglects certain interrelated somatopsychic factors vital to an optimal diagnostic-therapeutic programme. These include the role of skeletal muscle tension and posture, the role of the "voluntary" respiratory musculature, especially the diaphragm, as well as anxiety, emotional suppression and excessive self-consciousness, all of which may be precipitants rather than the outcome of the onset of asthma. On the basis of these neglected factors and others, implications for an optimally effective therapy are discussed. The

physical medicine or physiotherapeutic, as well as other recent therapeutic approaches, are reviewed and evaluated. It is concluded that all of these therapies are too "specific," and that a more holistic approach is necessary (which is provided in "Asthma: The Yoga Perspective, Part II—Yoga Therapy in the Treatment of Asthma").

149
Goyeche JR, Ago Y, Ikemi Y. **Asthma: the yoga perspective (II): Yoga therapy in the treatment of asthma.** J Asthma 19:189-201, 1982.

▶ review: yoga, breathing exercises, relaxation

The integral yoga approach to asthma (and other psychosomatic disorders) is briefly outlined as meeting all of the requirements for an optimal, holistic, somatopsychic therapy (as outlined in Part I), including correction of distorted posture and faulty breathing habits, teaching a system of general muscle relaxation, techniques for the release of suppressed emotion and for reducing anxiety and self-conscious awareness, as well as special methods for the expectoration of mucus. Yoga practices are described in detail and the available psychophysiological research on yoga practice, as well as clinical-therapeutic studies on yoga as asthmatic therapy, are reviewed. It can therefore be concluded that yoga therapy is most effective with asthma.

150
Honsberger R, Wilson AF. **Transcendental meditation in treating asthma.** Respir Ther 3:79-81, 1973.

▶ meditation

During investigation of the physiological effects of transcendental meditation, health questionnaires answered by some practitioners of this easily learned and simple technique indicated benefit to asthma. Therefore, to evaluate such possible effects, a six-month study was conducted. Twenty-one patients kept daily diaries of symptoms and medications and answered questionnaires at the end of the study. Other measurements included physician evaluation, pulmonary function testing and skin resistance recordings. The results indicate that transcendental meditation is useful in the treatment of asthma by reducing airway resistance and severity of asthma symptoms over a period of months. Transcendental meditation has multiple immediate and long-term effects on a variety of physiological and psychological factors, and may be affecting asthma through a variety of avenues simultaneously.

151
Levendel L. **Treatment of bronchial asthma.** Orv Hetil 117:147-153, 1976. (in Hungarian)

▶ autogenic training

152

Levendel L, Lakatos M. **Treating asthmatic patients by relaxation.** Orv Hetil 121:1055-1057, 1980. (in Hungarian: no English abstract)

▶ relaxation

153

Polonsky WH, Knapp PH, Brown EL, Schwartz GE. **Psychological factors, immunological function, and bronchial asthma.** Psychosom Med 47:77, 1985. (also Advances 2:63, 1985.) (abstract)

▶ imagery

This study investigated the role of personality, imagery, and psychological treatment factors in the modification of immunological function and symptomatic indices associated with bronchial asthma. 32 subjects completed a six-week asthma treatment protocol: 11 subjects in an asthma imagery procedure, 13 subjects in a comparison imagery procedure, and 8 subjects in a waiting-list control condition. It was hypothesized that pre-post treatment improvement in histamine-sensitive, suppressor T cell function (used as an index of asthma-associated immunological overactivity) and symptomatic indices (specific airways conductance, bronchial reactivity, medication use, and symptomatic distress) would be associated with A) imagined asthma improvement over the treatment period, B) a procedure designed to promote imagined improvement (asthma imagery procedure), and C) pretreatment measures of "emotional inhibition." As predicted, actual improvement in asthma-related immunological function was associated with imagined improvement in asthma over the treatment period, ($r = .66$, $p = .01$). However, the asthma imagery procedure was not more effective than the other two conditions in the elicitation of imagined asthma improvement nor actual immunological improvement. As predicted, immunological improvement was also associated with pretreatment measures of "emotional inhibition" ($r = .67$, $p < .005$), suggesting that a non-restrictive approach towards unpleasant affect is related to the promotion of immunological improvement in bronchial asthma. It was also noted that immunological improvement was associated with a corresponding decrease in bronchial reactivity to a standard bronchodilating agent ($r = .49$, $p < .05$). These results suggest that changes in asthma-related immunological function may be associated with affective style and with changes in specific dimensions of somatic imagery.

154

Sauer J, Schnetzer M. **Personality profile of asthmatics and its changes in the course of various treatment methods.** Z Klin Psychol Psychother 26:171-180, 1978. (in German)

▶ autogenic training

Our study of 30 asthmatics showed an increase in the neurotic triangle (MMPI-Saarbrucken) and good agreement with the personality profile of neurotics with psychosomatic tendencies. To measure the effect of a 4-week-treatment-course on the personality structure of the patients, the FPI-scale was used, where only a slight change was found in the scale "Nervositat" (FPI 1 measures psychosomatic conflicts). In some of the patients who were also treated with autogenic training, the change was somewhat larger but not statistically significant, as compared to the group of patients without autogenic training. The treatment-course itself, judging only by the medical evaluations, was proved to be highly effective with statistical significance. A possible explanation for the discrepancy between the two findings could be the difference between the methods of investigation and/or the attitude of the patients to their asthma because many of them emphasize the somatic aspect of their illness, wishing to ignore or deny a possible psychosomatic explanation.

155

Schaeffer G, Freytag-Klinger H. **Objectifying the effect of autogenic training on disordered ventilation in bronchial asthma.** Psychiatr Neurol Med Psychol (Leipz) 27:400-408, 1975. (in German)

▶ autogenic training

Forty-one persons suffering from asthma (aged 20 to 55; duration of disease: greater than or equal to 2 years) were divided into 2 groups and participated in courses of instruction in autogenic training. The control group was comprised of 14 patients. The effects of autogenic training on the maximum rate of expiration as well as the limiting respiratory value were recorded. The control group showed a seasonal decrease in the maximum rate of expiration and the limiting respiratory value by 10 to 20% in the period extending from April through November. The autogenic-training patients showed a temporally similar increase in the maximum rate of expiration of 27 and 22%, respectively (the difference to the control group being 47 and 42%, respectively). In 35 patients the increase in the limiting respiratory value was equal to or greater than the effect produced by novodrine. Catamnesis after one year (n = 40): Absence from work in a twelve-month period was 663 days prior to autogenic training and 77 days (11.6%) subsequent to autogenic training. Accordingly, autogenic training may be considered to be an objectively effective component of a combination of therapeutical methods used in the treatment of bronchial asthma.

156

Schulte HJ, Abhyanker VV. **Yogic breathing and psychologic states.** Ariz Med 36:681-683, 1979.

▶ yoga, biofeedback, relaxation, imagery

Pranayama seems to create a biofeedback-like control of one's physiology. Until recently it was thought impossible to condition the autonomic nervous system, smooth muscles, and glands by other than Pavlovian techniques. Since 1960 there have been reports of learned control with instrumental conditions of a wide range of autonomic nervous system responses including the GSR, heart rate, blood pressure, vasomotor responses, salivation, and the relaxation of striated muscles. Yoga appears to be another option for attaining such physiologic control. Biofeedback and meditation states have also been investigated in the treatment of psychiatric illnesses. Perhaps our Western counterpart of Pranayama is biofeedback which brings with it many innovative approaches to treatment of stress-related disorders. As an adjunct to standard medical practice, Pranayama and other yogic procedures may warrant further investigation in emotional problems and in certain psychophysiologic disorders.

157

Sichel JP, Chevauche Baldauf A, Baldauf E. **Schultz's method of relaxation in asthma in children.** Rev Neuropsychiatr Infant 21:529-541, 1973. (in French)

▶ autogenic training, psychotherapy

With reference to a study of 14 cases of young asthmatics including one detailed case report, the authors examine the treatment of asthma by the method of relaxation. After some general considerations on the psychopathology of the asthmatic child, and on autogenous training and the advantages of its application to the child in whom it represents a true delegation of therapeutic power, the authors lay emphasis on the modes of application as shown by their experience. Their encouraging results with relief of the symptom lead them to recommend this method either on its own or in conjunction with classical treatments. It appears that the corporal experience of autogenous training in the child has been the basis of a verbal expression difficult to mobilize in any other way. It becomes substituted for the attack, favoured in this by the regular character of the technique which can be compared with the periodic nature of the attacks. The relationship, based on that of transference, permits the development of autonomy in relation to the mother. Finally, the Schultz technique may become the point of departure of a detailed psychotherapy which may be of prime importance.

158

Sirota AD, Mahoney M. **Relaxing on cue: the self-regulation of asthma.** J Behav Ther Exp Psychiatry 5:65-66, 1974.

▶ relaxation, desensitization

A 41-year-old woman with severe asthmatic difficulties was given brief training in muscular relaxation as a means of avoiding and reducing bronchospasm. A portable timer was used to cue naturalistic self-monitoring of muscle tension and self-relaxation. Client records of medication frequency indicated a dramatic improvement in respiratory functioning and excellent maintenance at a follow-up assessment. The encouraging results of this self-management strategy, when contrasted with years of unsuccessful medical treatment, suggest the need for more controlled research on applications of behavior therapy to respiratory disorders.

159

Tal A, Miklich DR. **Emotionally induced decreases in pulmonary flow rates in asthmatic children.** Psychosom Med 38:190-200, 1976.

▶ relaxation, behavior therapy

This study found that vividly remembered incidents of intense anger and similarly recalled fear decreased 1-sec forced expiratory flow rates (FEV_1) in 35 male and 25 female chronic asthmatic children who had no psychopathology. FEV_1 increased with relaxation. Changes in FEV_1 following anger correlated with changes following fear as highly as the reliabilities of the responses permitted, although anger produced a greater decrease than fear. FEV_1 decrease following anger and fear correlated with FEV_1 increase due to relaxation. The amount of change in each of the three conditions correlated with history of emotionally precipitated asthma. This pattern was interpreted to mean that the same phenomenon underlies emotional-bronchoconstriction, relaxation-bronchodilatation, and emotionally triggered asthma. No relationship was found between degree of allergic sensitivity (atopy) and FEV_1 changes in any of the three conditions nor did atopy correlate with history of emotionally triggered asthma. These results do not support the view that psychological and allergic factors are inversely related, alternative causes of asthma.

160

Wilson AF, Honsberger R, Chiu JT, Novey HS. **Transcendental meditation and asthma.** Respiration 32:74-80, 1975.

▶ meditation

A 6-month study with crossover at 3 months was designed to evaluate the possible beneficial effects of transcendental meditation upon bronchial asthma. 21 patients kept dialy dairies of symptoms and medications and answered questionnaires at the end of the study and 6 months later. Other measurements included physician evaluation, pulmonary function testing, and galvanic skin resistance. The results indicated that transcendental meditation is a useful adjunct in treating asthma.

Milieu Therapy

161

Bentley J. **Some thoughts on parentectomy.** J Asthma 12:125-128, 1975. (editorial)

▶ milieu therapy

162

Bernstein IL, Allen JE, Kreindler L, Ghory JE, Wohl TH. **A community approach to juvenile intractable asthma.** Pediatrics 26:586-595, 1960.

▶ milieu therapy, group therapy, psychotherapy

Rehabilitation of children with refractory asthma utilizing the existing facilities of a local institution has proven successful in Cincinnati. A complete description of the origins, aims and services of this program is presented. The local nature of such a program has some distinct advantages over a national institution doing the same kind of work, chief among which is the opportunity for long-term clinical observation and laboratory studies of discharged children. In general this preliminary presentation of our clinical results in 47 patients corroborates the good results previously reported by other centers involved in long-term rehabilitation of children with asthma. Specific factors which may influence or produce clinical remissions in these patients are under current investigation. In our opinion, it is not only feasible, but also highly desirable, for other urban areas to develop similar treatment centers. It is conceivable that some type of federation, either formal or informal, would be mutually beneficial to all who are involved in this gratifying work, in both local and national centers.

163

Blaha H. **Problems of the treatment of childhood bronchial asthma in health resorts.** Allerg Asthma (Leipz) 13:275-281, 1967. (in German: no English abstract)

▶ psychotherapy

164

Bloom FL, Spangler DL, McMichael JE, Wittig HJ, Upson P. **Sunshine station—Florida's first camp for children with asthma.** J Fla Med Assoc 63:710-713, 1976.

▶ milieu therapy

Forty-six children with asthma from throughout Florida participated in a camp experience for the first time in their lives. The camp was sponsored by the Florida Lung Association with the help of the University of Florida Department of Pediatrics. Because of the ready presence of nurses and physicians, there were no episodes of status asthmaticus in spite of there being 106 infirmary visits (about half for acute attacks of asthma) in the six days of the camp session. This initial camp session provided an otherwise unobtainable normal experience for these children with opportunity for personal growth in a safe setting, provided education for graduate nursing students, medical students, pediatric housestaff, pediatric allergy fellows, and an update in asthma therapy for some of the referring physicians.

165

Bukantz SC, Peshkin MM. **Institutional treatment of asthmatic children.** Pediatr Clin North Am 6:755-773, 1959.

▶ milieu therapy

Extracted summary: The foregoing description of the organization and principles of management of the child with intractable asthma in an institutional setting of the residential type should be considered only one example of the method of approach to this problem. There must be many other methods by which control measures are attempted, but, based upon an almost 20-year trial and error experimentation with several modifications of administrative control, these methods still seem to offer the most promise as a baseline upon which to develop the best program of institutional management of the intractable asthmatic child. Not enough emphasis can be placed upon the dominant concept of operation at the Jewish National Home for Asthmatic Children [Denver, Colorado], i.e., that everything which has been done is as a learning procedure which will suggest future modifications of our administration.

166

Chai H, Johnstone D, Falliers CJ. **Trieditorial: Specialized centers for asthma: use and misuse of institutions for residential care, rehabilitation, and research.** J Asthma 20:1-9, 1983. (3-part editorial)

▶ milieu therapy, psychotherapy, behavior therapy

167

Creer TL. **Psychologic aspects of asthma.** Respir Ther 7:15-18, 86, 88, 1977.

▶ milieu therapy, reinforcement, systematic desensitization, reciprocal inhibition, extinction

The role of psychological factors in the treatment and rehabilitation of children with asthma is discussed herein. Of particular interest is the manner in which goals of behavioral rehabilitation are achieved at the National Asthma Center, Denver, Colo. The general program of the center is described. In addition, the application of social learning principles to specific problems is chronicled.

168

Duchaine J. **Symposium on the treatment of allergic children in treatment institutions: introduction.** Acta Tuberc Pneumol Belg 57:8-12, 1966. (in French)

▶ milieu therapy

169

Falliers CJ. **Treatment of asthma in a residential center: a fifteen-year study.** Ann Allergy 28:513-520, 1970.

▶ milieu therapy

Clinical statistics at CARIH [Children's Asthma Research Institute and Hospital] reveal that the number of patients improving dramatically upon admission to this residential center for asthmatic children has dropped from a reported 98 percent of all admissions fifteen years ago to 38 percent in 1958-59 and to 12 percent in 1968-69. Demographic and environmental factors, as well as iatrogenic influences have been reviewed and selected data are presented. It appears that by the time most patients are referred to a specialized national center, such as CARIH, their daily requirement of bronchodilator and corticosteroid therapy is a reflection, a consequence rather than a cause, of the severity of their disease. This "dependence" on medication is promptly alleviated among those who experience a spontaneous improvement in asthma at CARIH, while primary reduction of drug therapy (restricted use of nebulizers) has not been found to result in secondary therapeutic gains such as lowering of steroid requirements or improvement in lung function. Prospective studies with meticulous and repeated assessment of immunologic, pulmonary physiologic, environmental and psychologic variables are needed to ascertain why chronicity and therapeutic refractoriness develop in a certain (still undetermined) number of cases of this otherwise intermittent respiratory disorder. It seems advisable, indeed necessary, to enhance the public awareness of the potential severity of asthma without creating further misconceptions and to promote the establishment of adequate local and regional facilities for the study and total care of all patients and especially those with frequent attacks or with chronic wheezing. Diagnostic laboratories, intensive care units, residential centers and family guidance programs ought to be available in any major community. National institutions, whether primarily investigational, residential or educational, could serve as coordinating units or as prototypes while attending to the medical needs of relatively few selected cases. They could conduct basic or applied research, and help to train specialists and to resolve theoretical or therapeutic controversies. They should not be expected to offer miraculous "cures" when, in most instances, the therapeutic team in the patient's own community, aided by modern specialized techniques, can offer adequate clinical services much sooner, more consistently and for a longer period of time.

170

Fialkov MJU, Miller JA. **Severe psychosomatic illness in children: effect on a pediatric ward's staff.** Clin Pediatr (Phila) 20:792-796, 1981.

▶ milieu therapy, psychiatry liaison

Observations of a pediatric ward's response to the repeated hospitalization of an asthmatic child revealed a close parallel to the transactional patterns described in families of children with psychosomatic illnesses. Characteristics of such families include enmeshment, overprotectiveness, rigidity and resistance to change, lack of conflict resolution, and use of the child's sick role to relieve tension and discomfort within the family. In this article we have attempted to demonstrate the similarity of responses between these families and groups of hospital ward personnel. Resolution of the ward personnel's internal conflict was followed by changes in the coping abilities of the staff, with a successful outcome for a second child with a similar clinical condition.

171

Ford RM. **The treatment of intractable childhood asthma by medium-term separation from home environment.** Med J Aust 1:653-656, 1968.

▶ milieu therapy

A review is presented of 163 children suffering from severe, intractable asthma, who were treated by removal from their family environment for a few months. It appears that this is a successful method of treatment, particularly for the child with a large emotional overlay to his disease. The condition of most of the children improved dramatically during their period away from their home environment, and many seemed to obtain a long-term benefit from such a separation. Possible reasons for this improvement are briefly discussed, and a plea is made for the more widespread establishment of such facilities in large communities, and for a trial period of this sort of separation treatment before corticosteroid therapy is prescribed for childhood asthma sufferers.

172

Freud E, Hurwich SB, Meijer A, Kagan H, Groen JJ. **Goals and methods of institutional treatment of asthmatic children in the Wizo pediatric clinic, Jerusalem.** Prax Kinderpsychol Kinderpsychiatr 19:98-109, 1970. (in German: no English abstract)

▶ milieu therapy

173
Ghory JE. **The short-term patient in a convalescent hospital asthma program.** J Asthma Res 3:243-247, 1966.

▶ milieu therapy, family therapy, group psychotherapy, psychotherapy, consultation-liaison

Extracted summary: Is there a place for a short-term patient in a convalescent hospital asthma program? The answer is "yes." It should be possible to admit a child to an asthma rehabilitation program, get him worked up completely, started on therapy, and dismissed in the scope of a few months. Within this period of time too, some inroads can be made toward readying the patient's home for his return, getting rid of both the allergic and emotional dust within the home.

174
Green M, Green E. **A tour of four residential centers for the care of asthmatic children in Europe.** J Asthma Res 3:299-304, 1966.

▶ milieu therapy

Extracted summary: Americans have always been prone to think that their scientific achievements surpass any similar efforts throughout the world. This illusion is applicable to allergy and asthma as well as to other fields of medicine. We visited four European residential centers for asthmatic children, and have been in intimate contact with a fifth. In the overall picture, particularly in the Netherlands and Switzerland, the medical care of these asthmatic children is equal and, in some aspects, superior to that in the United States.

175
Hallowitz D. **Residential treatment of chronic asthmatic children.** Am J Orthopsychiatry 24:576-587, 1954.

▶ milieu therapy, family therapy

In summary, there is a group of children suffering from severe, chronic, and intractable bronchial asthma who need a period of separation from the family and the home environment, in a residential treatment center which contains a program of medical treatment as well as a program for the treatment of emotional and psychological factors that contribute to the illness. I have discussed in this paper the effects of separation; the organic as well as the emotional and psychological factors in asthma; and the treatment approach to the problems involved that is in the process of being developed by the team of pediatricians, caseworkers, group workers, houseparents, psychiatrist, and a members of the administrative staff. The importance of casework with the parents during intake, while the child is under care, and in the aftercare period has also been

stressed. The combined teamwork approach is essential in the residential treatment of asthmatic children. The specific contributions of each of the professional disciplines woven together is the essence of residential treatment.

176
Isbister C, Mayer L, Hepburn S, Vaughan B. **Institutional care of intractable asthma in children: a pilot study.** Med J Aust 2:1217-1223, 1966.

▶ milieu therapy, family therapy

A treatment assessment and rehabilitation programme of institutional care for children with intractable asthma at home is described. It offered the following services: comprehensive medical assessment and supervision; schooling with specially qualified teachers; daily physiotherapy; regular exercise within the child's limitations; asthmatic attacks; a therapeutic group situation supervised by a recreational therapist; a controlled, relatively stable atmosphere that provided some relief from emotional problems. Parents visited children frequently and discussed their management and care with the doctors. The monthly follow-up provided supportive care and regular reassessment, and kept close contact with the general practitioner. A clinical research project planned in association with the programme is described, and preliminary results are presented. Twenty-three children who stayed for three months or longer and have been followed up after their discharge for the same period have been observed. A method of classification is presented as a possible basis for planning treatment. The response of the children to residential care is discussed, all having improved physically and emotionally and 18 having improved educationally. It is concluded that the programme so far appears to be beneficial, that it required skilled and understanding staff, and that it is essential that it be associated with a clinical research project and adequate follow-up to evaluate results. Some changes are forecast.

177
Jessner L, Long RT, Lamont JH, Whipple B, Bandler L, Blom GE, Burgin L. **A psychosomatic study of allergic and emotional factors in children with asthma.** Am J Psychiatry 114:890-899, 1958.

▶ milieu therapy

1. Eighteen children, hospitalized for asthma, when exposed to their own house dust showed no demonstrable change in their respiration irrespective of their skin sensitivities to house dust. 2. Our clinical studies describe a need for closeness in the asthmatic child which is expressed here as a regressive wish. This regressive wish is felt by the child's ego as obstructive to further growth and development, and therefore as dangerous. This psy-

chological conflict allows for an explanation of why hospitalizations lead to improvement of asthmatic symptoms. 3. We have described a methodology for validating clinical impressions. Our results are reported as trends which hold true only for this asthma group vs. this control group. We think that the analysis of our psychological test data shows that it is possible—though difficult—to devise objective ways of measuring dynamically meaningful hypotheses. We also feel there is good reason to believe that our particular choice of hypotheses has been fruitful in the study of asthma in children. 4. In a clinical study of the mothers of asthmatic children, we found evidence of the mother's wish to maintain the child in an infantile dependent state. Further, that this way of dealing with the asthmatic child stemmed from mothers' own early unresolved conflicts.

178
Kapotes C. **Emotional factors in chronic asthma.** J Asthma Res 15:5-14, 1977.

▶ milieu therapy, psychotherapy, family therapy

Extracted summary: During the years 1960-1965, 72 severely asthmatic children were hospitalized at St. Mary's Hospital for Children in Bayside, Queens [New York]. These children received psychotherapy and the standard medical treatments for the control of their asthma. Steroids were tapered off where they were in use, and they were not worked up allergenically. The study had a two-fold purpose: 1. The assessment of the effectiveness of a parentectomy approach, combined with and including psychotherapy. 2. The effects of a therapeutic milieu and psychotherapy upon the asthmatic child's personality in helping to reduce the severity of the asthmatic condition. The goal of the psychotherapy was to encourage free expression of feelings, to reduce tension and anxiety related to the asthma, and to increase ego strength and confidence. Data was collected continually between 1962-1965 by a graduate psychology student, a psychologist and the author through the use of a detailed questionnaire follow-up six months to a year after discharge. At this point, the author acknowledges his gratitude for a grant received from the Children's Asthma Foundation, and also thanks Drs. Peshkin and Abramson and Mr. Friedman. This grant helped fund the collection of the data. Of the 39 cases, 77% demonstrated moderate to considerable improvement. 23% failed to improve. Rapid improvement was noted in 73% of the improved cases in under 7 months of hospitalization. Forty-four per cent of the unimproved cases had failed to improve by 7 months. The single most significant factor related to improvement was the age upon admission—88% of the cases which failed to improve were between 7 and 12 years of age. The implication was that the younger the child, the better its chance to respond to a parentectomy approach.

179
Mascia AV. **Progress in the treatment of the asthmatic child in a convalescent setting.** J Asthma Res 3:239-241, 1966.

▶ milieu therapy, placebo

Treatment of the severe or intractable asthmatic continues to challenge us. I believe that the following factors have been helpful: a controlled, supervised situation; competent personnel who are aware of the nature of the illness; and the intelligent administration of drugs. It seems fitting that each organization grows and includes new ideas and equipment. Progress for us in the treatment of the severe asthmatic child may be briefly summarized as follows: management of the child without restrictions; attitude of the doctors, nurses and other personnel; simplicity of treatment; breathing excercises; and the proper use of cortico-steroids.

180
Mascia AV. **The role of a residential center in the care of the asthmatic child.** Ann Allergy 22:191-195, 1964.

▶ milieu therapy

In summary, I would like to review some of the factors that contribute to the improvement of the asthmatic child in a residential setting. Our facilities become a haven from difficult tense homes as is true in the experience of others in this field. We place the asthmatic children in a supervised, non-threatening atmosphere, with special care for the asthmatic, thus enabling them to be free from asthma. We attempt to do the following: (1) clear our environment of allergens and irritants, (2) concentrate on general good health, with constant re-evaluation, early treatment of asthma attacks, and early treatment of respiratory infections, and (3) offer careful and sympathetic supervision, reassurance and education by the staff. Supportive therapy is generally unplanned, given by physicians, nurses, house parents, teachers and older children. All of these factors in convalescence, whether environmental, medical, or emotional, have contributed toward the improvement of the asthmatic child resulting in the improvement of the scholastic standings, better understanding of their illnesses, and possibly, the ability to face the future a little better. We have not cured them. Our greatest handicap has been inadequate follow-up and inadequate data from the referring agencies. We are convinced that the asthmatic child does well in a residential setting and we would like to see more facilities of this kind available in the nation and in the world.

181

Mascia AV. **The goals and philosophy of a residential treatment center for asthmatic children.** J Asthma Res 8:43-50, 1970.

▶ milieu therapy, family therapy, social casework

In conclusion, the role of the residential treatment center is one of separation therapy. Its purpose is to prevent respiratory cripples by making tractable the intractable. The child is removed from an asthma-producing environment in which there is usually a disturbed parent-child relationship. The multidisciplinary approach of the residential center results in re-education and in instilling motivation in the child. The child is allowed to improve, developing some independence that all children require, with the asthmatic prevented from doing so unless suitable care is instituted.

182

Miroir R. **Treatment of asthma in children in a specialized institution.** Acta Tuberc Pneumol Belg 57:35-41, 1966. (in French: no English abstract)

▶ milieu therapy

183

Nitzberg H. **The social worker in an institution for asthmatic children.** Soc Casework 33:111-116, 1952.

▶ social casework, milieu therapy

Extracted summary: Casework treatment, operating on the level of ego development, can effect some basic changes in the child's personality. In one instance, a 10-year-old boy, through his relationship with a male social worker, was able to move from a dependent, passive attitude into a more active and aggressive role, finding pleasure in boasting of his prowess as a cowboy and soldier. The relationship provided opportunity for him to identify with a strong father-figure. The worker's attitude of warm interest and permissiveness, with encouragement to experiment with masculine activities, helped free him from the fears he had experienced in his own family relationships. It seems probable that the treatment will enable the child to meet future threats to himself without regression to an infantile level and without recourse to asthmatic illness.

184

Peshkin MM. **Role of environment in the treatment of a selected group of cases: a plea for a "home" as a restorative measure.** Am J Dis Child 39:744-787, 1930.

▶ milieu therapy

Extracted summary: 1. In a series of four hundred and twenty-five cases of asthma, it was found that in forty-one children, ranging in age from 2 to 14 years, or approximately 10 per cent, the asthma remained severe, persistent and of long duration, in spite of intensive modern treatment. 2. Twenty-five children (twenty-two children sensitive and three nonsensitive to protein) were treated by a change of environment. In spite of the fact that the inhalant and the dietetic restrictions were kept less rigid than at home, twenty-three children, or 92 per cent, were markedly improved or entirely relieved of asthma. Seventeen of these twenty-five children have been returned to their homes for periods varying from six months to five years or an average of two years per patient. Thirteen of these seventeen children, or 76 per cent, are now greatly improved or relieved from asthma. In some of these children appropriate treatment after change of environment was successful, whereas it had failed before. 3. Sixteen of these forty-one children were not treated by a change of environment because of lack of facilities and other reasons and so indirectly served as a control series. These children are still suffering from chronic asthma. 4. Allergy per se cannot be explained entirely on a basis of protein sensitization, because the sensitizing substances in themselves are merely exciting factors and not the basic cause of the symptoms. A patient in a state of "physicochemical equilibrium" enjoys freedom from symptoms in spite of exposure to etiologic substances. If any factor overthrows this governing mechanism, symptoms will appear. These factors may be specific or nonspecific or both. An appreciation of this fact will aid in establishing a clearer conception of asthma and will lay the foundation for a more intelligent management of the disease in childhood. 5. When the physicochemical imbalance was profoundly disturbed, the various specific and nonspecific factors always induced asthma, in spite of the fact that the patient was receiving appropriate treatment at the time. In these cases there is little that can be done to give relief until nature itself restores the physicochemical balance. In these cases it has been found that a change of environment, preferably to a "home" prepared to accommodate allergic patients, was of definite value in partially or completely restoring physicochemical balance. 6. Until newer methods of treatment are advanced which will successfully control or free this group of children from asthma, the establishment of a "home" where a child with chronic refractory asthma can be kept for at least six months is regarded as a humane, urgent and economic necessity as well as a therapeutic measure of definite value.

185

Peshkin MM. **The treatment of institutionalized children with intractable asthma.** Conn Med 24:766-770, 1960.

▶ milieu therapy, psychotherapy

Extracted summary: The function of the "Home" [Jewish National Home for Asthmatic Children, Denver, Colorado] in the rehabilitation of children with intractable asthma seems to comprise the following criteria: (1) It offers a haven for the desperately-ill child which allows him to be transferred from his emotionally adverse home environment to an emotionally favorable environment, thus aiding the child to lose those asthmatogenic patterns of psychological reactions which has made his bronchial asthma intractable; (2) It gives the carefully supervised child milieu therapy which allows him to make normal emotional adjustment to his illness, to his peers, and to his parent surrogates; (3) It gives the child whatever antiallergic, medical and specialized psychotherapy he may require to obtain optimal health; (4) It enables the child to respond favorably to specific antiallergic therapy which prior to Denver failed; and (5) It prepares the child emotionally for his eventual return to his own home in a manner which in many instances will prevent the recurrence of the state of intractable asthma. In my opinion, the Denver Home has been fulfilling these five functions admirably. The whole import of this study is that today we can approach the treatment of a child with intractable asthma with the knowledge that in the vast majority of instances we can help such a child recover from the state of intractable asthma and have him develop either complete freedom from asthma or substantial relief from his condition.

186
Peshkin MM. **Analysis of the role of residential centers for children with intractable asthma.** J Asthma Res 6:59-92, 1968.

▶ milieu therapy, family therapy

Extracted summary: In sum, the beneficial results obtained as a consequence of long-term residential care of intractable and chronic asthmatic children, if referred to in number only, substantiate the statement that the need for their rehabilitation in specialized residential treatment centers is no longer a contradictable or debatable question. The simple and constructive approach to this entire problem is to restore these children to healthy living, their rightful heritage, so that they may assume their place in their respective communities, grow up, and contribute their measure of usefulness for the total welfare of all.

187
Peshkin MM. **Intractable asthma of childhood: rehabilitation at the institutional level with a follow-up of 150 cases.** Int Arch Allergy 15:91-112, 1959.

▶ milieu therapy, psychotherapy

This paper considers the clinical course of 150 children ranging in age from 6 to 14 years who had intractable asthma. A child crippled with intractable asthma is one who, living for at least one year in his own home environment, fails to respond to the kind of conventional medical therapy which relieves or "cures" 90% of all children suffering from allergic bronchial asthma. Thus, about 10% of all asthmatic children suffer from intractable bronchial asthma . . . Optimal benefits resulted when the children with intractable asthma were treated in residence at the "Home" [Jewish National Home for Asthmatic Children, Denver, Colorado] for 18 to 24 months. In the "Home" 99% of the children with intractable asthma recovered substantially or completely from asthma. Ninety-seven per cent of the children maintained their improvement after returning home for 12 months—and 95% continued to be improved after residing at their own homes for an average period of three years.

188
Peshkin MM. **Management of the institutionalized child with intractable asthma.** Ann Allergy 18:75-79, 1960.

▶ milieu therapy, psychotherapy

Extracted summary: The function of the [Denver] Home in the rehabilitation of children with intractable asthma seems to comprise the following criteria: (1) It offers a haven for the desperately-ill child which allows him to be transferred from his emotionally adverse home environment to an emotionally favorable environment, thus aiding the child to lose those asthmatogenic patterns of psychological reactions which have made his bronchial asthma intractable; (2) It gives the carefully supervised child milieu therapy which allows him to make normal emotional adjustment to his illness, to his peers, and to his parent surrogates; (3) It gives the child whatever antiallergic, medical and specialized psychotherapy he may require to obtain optimal health; (4) It enables the child to respond favorably to specific antiallergic therapy which prior to Denver failed, and (5) It prepares the child emotionally for his eventual return to his own home in a manner which in many instances will prevent the recurrence of the state of intractable asthma. In my opinion, the Denver Home has been fulfilling these five functions admirably. The whole import of this study is that today we can approach the treatment of the child with intractable asthma with the knowledge that in the vast majority of instances we can help such a child recover from the state of intractable asthma and have him develop either complete freedom from asthma or substantial relief from his condition.

189
Peshkin MM. **The emotional aspects of asthma in children.** J Asthma Res 3:265-277, 1966.

▶ milieu therapy, group psychotherapy

Extracted summary: Many workers, in an effort to integrate and conceptualize the data regarding the interaction of etiological factors in asthma, conceived that an individual with asthma who utilizes an inappropriate, defensive or adaptive mechanism in an unsuccessful attempt to deal with stressful situations or unrealistic emotional conflicts, behaves as if his physiological defenses failed to defend or protect him psychologically. The unfortunate result is that he becomes ill because his own defenses have gone askew. Under such circumstances, when asthma persists over a prolonged period, actual tissue damage, or at least a susceptibility to infection, may occur. A state of severe or intractable asthma supervenes. A critical review of the world medical literature widely accepts the marked improvement in intractably asthmatic children as a consequence of long-term, residential treatment in convalescent asthma institutions. Climate is of no importance in the recovery of these children from intractable asthma. The psychodynamic explanation of maternal rejection advanced by Miller and Baruch was not validated by careful scrutiny of the data. Abramson contends that the reverse of maternal rejection occurs and that parents of allergic children suffering from severe allergic symptoms tend to engulf their children. This process ("Cronus complex") is one of introjection rather than rejection. The appropriate and logical treatment of asthma patients should be comprehensive; that is, both medical and psychological factors must be united to treat the patient as a whole.

190

Peshkin MM, Friedman I. **Residential asthma centers in the United States and problems in relation to them.** J Asthma Res 12:129-175, 1975.

▶ milieu therapy

Extracted summary: We would like to recommend that the Association of Convalescent Homes and Hospitals for Asthmatic Children should form a representative committee for the purpose of formulating standard requirements for admissions, standard data regarding the results of treatment during residential care, and follow-up studies. A successful application of these recommendations will, in the long run, make it possible to obtain statistics that will have meaning and value. It would be desirable that five years hence another comprehensive survey be conducted of the functioning residential asthma treatment centers.

191

Peshkin MM, Tuft HS. **Rehabilitation of the intractable asthmatic child by the institutional approach.** Q Rev Pediatr 2:7-9, 1956.

▶ milieu therapy, psychotherapy, consultation-liaison

Extracted summary: Psychotherapy is one of the most important phases of the rehabilitation program. This is accomplished by a staff psychiatrist as well as individuals specifically trained in the field, such as psychiatric- and medical-social workers and clinical psychologists. The psy-

chiatrist interviews every new patient. The clinical psychologist administers psychologic tests, including the Rorschach and Thematic Aperception tests. Each case is then reviewed by a team composed of the medical director, attending allergist, psychiatric personnel, houseparent, and recreation worker. Recommendations for further therapy and the goals of such therapy are established in these conferences. In this way, each worker gains a better understanding of the child, and all personnel can move in a positive direction in the handling of the patient. Patients not responding to this approach or those requiring more intensive therapy are treated individually by the staff psychiatrist.

192

Purcell K, Brady K, Chai H, Muser J, Molk L, Gordon N, Meurs J. **The effect on asthma in children of experimental separation from the family.** Psychosom Med 31:144-164, 1969.

▶ milieu therapy

This experiment evaluated the effects on asthma in children of altering their psychological environment. Twenty-five asthmatic children were studied medically and psychologically during periods in which they had no contact with their families but were cared for in their own homes by a substitute parent. It was predicted that 13 children would respond positively (show improvement) and that 12 would respond negatively (show no improvement in asthma) to separation. For the predicted positive group, all measurements of asthma indicated a statistically significant decrease in symptoms during the period of family separation followed by an increase in symptoms upon the family's return. For the group of 12 predicted negatives, only one (history of daily asthma) of four measurements suggested improvement during separation. It appears that a brief, specially designed, diagnostic interview may be useful in assessing the relevance of psychological variables to asthma.

193

Quarles van Ufford WJ, Van de Klashorst GO, Damme S, Abbink K. **Experiences with sending asthmatic children to so-called "therapeutic summer camps."** Allerg Asthma (Leipzig) 11:129-134, 1965. (in German)

▶ milieu therapy

The period of summer holidays means extra allergic and psychic contacts, causing more complaints. Special summer camps try to eliminate this factor and to give special therapy: therapia roborans, physiotherapy, development of hobbies, development of personality. Results of this therapy are discussed.

194

Richards W, Church JA, Roberts MJ, Newman LJ, Garon MR. **A self-help program for childhood asthma in a residential treatment center.** Clin Pediatr (Phila) 20:453-457, 1981.

▶ milieu therapy

A structured program designed to enhance self-treatment was successfully implemented in a residential center for asthmatic children. The ultimate objective of the program was to improve compliance with therapeutic regimens, which was felt to be a factor that had necessitated placement of many of the patients. The program was designed to educate the patient and the patient's family regarding the nature of asthma, its treatment and the importance of self-help. Efforts were also made to enhance the emotional maturity of the child. Patients remembered to take their medication over 90% of the time within 1 month of implementation of the program. A similar program was instituted for outpatient use.

195

Sadler JE Jr. **The long-term hospitalization of asthmatic children.** Pediatr Clin North Am 22:173-183, 1975.

▶ milieu therapy, psychotherapy

Extracted summary: To balance the types of services available to chronically severely ill asthmatic children, I propose that "medicoeducational" day treatment centers be established in regional areas. Such centers could offer special educational services by an educational staff trained regarding asthma and comfortable with the disease process. Properly staffed with nurses and "standby," i.e., child care staff experienced in the management of asthma and behavioral crises associated with asthma, such day treatment facilities could help correct educational lags inflicted by asthma-related school absences, prevent unnecessary hospitalization, and maintain close family ties. Such centers could form the research potential to study the difficult problems encountered between parents, teachers, and the asthmatic child. Until such centers are established, NJHRC [National Jewish Hospital and Research Center, Denver, Colorado] remains a viable, useful, therapeutic environment for the study and treatment of chronic intractable asthma, as well as for the training of personnel in multidisciplinary cooperation.

196

Scherr MS. **Role of summer camp in rehabilitation of the asthmatic patient.** Rev Allergy 22:169-175, 1968.

▶ review: milieu therapy

A review of rehabilitation programs for asthmatic patients is presented and a new treatment concept of summer camping has been developed from these existing programs. The criteria for this is presented as the concept of Bronco Junction. Bronco Junction evolved as an eight-week summer camp which provides rehabilitation recreation programs for children who have chronic bronchial asthma. The purpose of the camp is to prepare these children for normal physical and emotional development through medical/allergy treatment, physical conditioning and camping activities under constant medical supervision. The camp is situated near Charleston, West Virginia on 176 acres of rolling meadow and woodlands which form the backdrop for a rustic "Old-time Mountain Railroad Town." A narrow gauge operating railroad connects all major centers of camp activity and provides security in the event of an asthma attack by allowing transportation to be available at all times. The camp will add a fourth rehabilitation facility to the three current types of facilities in operation today. Rehabilitation has now become a permanent word in the vocabulary of the allergist. Today the allergist cannot think in terms of treatment of his patient without considering the role of rehabilitation which should be the first consideration in the process of restoring the patient to a normal life. Rehabilitation begins at the first visit of the patient to his physician and must be permeated with practical reality throughout the entire treatment course.

197

Scherr MS. **Camp Bronco Junction—second year of experience.** Ann Allergy 28:423-432, 1970.

▶ milieu therapy

Extracted summary: The institution of intensive allergy-medical care in a "normal environment" could be a great factor in the results obtained at Bronco Junction. Lenstrup et al, in Denmark reported that the atmosphere in most residential homes for disabled children is "so unlike normal conditions of life," that it has a restrictive influence on the patient's progress and on the possibility of improving their conditions. They emphasized that "the sterile, hospital-like atmosphere of residential homes for disabled children should be avoided, especially if the institution is too large and overcrowded." A plea was made for a normal environment for treatment in a small milieu where normal occupations and activities must be provided by a competent staff. Further studies of institutional facilities for the care of the chronically ill asthmatic must be carried out if their proper role is to be defined.

198

Schuller CF. **The asthma center, "Heidenheuvel".** Acta Tuberc Pneumol Belg 57:42-45, 1966. (in Dutch)

▶ milieu therapy

An outline is given of the medical, social and pedagogical organization of the centre for asthmatic children "Heideheuvel" at Hileversum.

199
Straker N, Tamerin J. **Aggression and childhood asthma: a study in a natural setting.** J Psychosom Res 18:131-135, 1974.

▶ milieu therapy

A study of 42 perennial childhood asthmatics in the natural setting of a summer camp revealed a statistically significant relationship between the severity of asthmatic symptomatology and aggressive behavioral expression. The treated, or symptomatic group of subjects whose bronchial function was signficantly more impaired than the untreated, or asymptomatic group were shown to be significantly less expressive of manifest aggression as measured by a modification of the Conner's Scale. Similar results were reported for high and low treatment groups for the entire summer. These findings support recent experimental studies which suggest the inhibition of aggressive impulses as playing a role in the etiology of bronchial asthma.

200
Suzuki I, Mitsubayashi T, Maruki K, Akasaka T, Maeda K, Nakayama Y, Asano T, Sannomiya A, Hirai M. **Long-term affects of residential care for asthmatic children.** Arerugi 33:396-402, 1984. (in Japanese)

▶ milieu therapy

201
Wohl TH. **Current concepts of the asthmatic child's adjustment and adaptation to institutional care.** J Asthma Res 7:41-45, 1969. (address)

▶ milieu therapy

202
Zivitz N. **Evaluation of intractable asthma of children in a new residential treatment center.** J Asthma Res 3:291-297, 1966.

▶ milieu therapy

So, to us, the program has already demonstrated its value for the intractable or the chronic asthmatic child. Some conclusion seems justified, but I am hesitant to do so in the presence of those who have had so many years of experience with this type of institution. However, one observation stands out clearly. These children seem to lose their fear of attacks of asthma. Help is immediately available from those who have the exclusive dedication to offer this help. Professionals do not panic as their parents did—they do not evidence anxiety by repeatedly questioning for the presence of symptoms. Patients are not engulfed, over-protected or used to fulfill the narcissistic needs of others. The patient has found a place where wheezing is

a common occurrence, and all, including his peers, are united in using total treatment procedures in an effort to make him well. There is, consequently, a series of constantly occurring corrective emotional experiences.

203
Zoller JE. **Ill and well, with or without doctors.** J Asthma 21:53-57, 1984.

▶ milieu therapy, psychotherapy

My recovery, to repeat, is attributable to doctors who treated the entire picture . . . allergy, physical, psychological, and emotional . . . simultaneously. I am convinced that my health has been maintained because I refuse to deal at any length with doctors who feel that my own symptomatic narrative is unimportant, or who regard their own field of specialization as unrelated to other fields. I always recall that my father once discontinued my visits with an allergist because he came to believe that if a child were brought to him with a compound fracture of both legs, he would first order scratch tests! Admittedly, not many fit that mold, but today's pressures at times force that trend.

Psychotherapy

204
Abramson HA. **Therapy of asthma with reference to its psychodynamic pharmacology.** Bull NY Acad Med 25:345-363, 1949.

▶ psychotherapy

Extracted summary: In order to avoid any misunderstanding in regard to the psychotherapy of the asthmatic patient, it should be noted that I believe that for the best results psychotherapy should be in charge of an allergist with suitable psychiatric training or of a psychiatrist with an understanding of the immunological aspects of asthma. It is not intended that the writer anywhere implies that unconscious material should be casually employed, or that the general practitioner should utilize techniques of deep psychotherapy. May I now summarize how the use of powerful sympathomimetic amines, antihistaminic drugs, sedatives and antibiotics in the treatment of bronchial asthma should be oriented. While it is generally agreed that therapy should not neglect the physiology and the immunology of the patient in the asthmatic state, the personality of the patient cannot be omitted in planning suitable therapeutic procedures. It is neither wise nor desirable for the patient suffering from severe asthma to be reminded of unconscious material that the doctor himself may be aware of. It is more than desirable in our present state of knowledge to use pharmacologically active drugs in connection with the total personality of the patient manifested during the acute asthmatic attack. Whether anxiety, phobia, depression, dependence, hostility, grief, or other pattern dominates the asthmatic attack, the physician should bring into the proper sphere the psychodynamic pharmacology of the drug employed in treating both the asthmatic spasm and the personality of the patient himself. In this way a better understanding of the action of the drugs on the personality of the patient will be obtained with much greater predictability in the therapy of bronchial asthma.

205
Abramson HA. **Psychic factors in allergy and their treatment.** Ann Allergy 14:145-151, 1956.

▶ psychotherapy, doctor-patient relationship, psychoanalysis

The psychotherapeutic potentialities practiced in ambulatory medicine are divided into two main types: I. Automatic psychotherapy. II. Purposeful or planned psychotherapy. The large majority of patients seen by the allergist can usually be treated by the allergist himself by all of the foregoing techniques except reconstructive psychotherapy, unless he is specially trained in this technique.

206
Abramson HA. **Psychodynamics of the intractably asthmatic state.** J Child Asthma Res Inst Hosp 1:18-22, 1961.

▶ psychotherapy, family therapy, milieu therapy

Extracted summary: The psychodynamic approach does not include measurable quantities, like skin tests and antigen-antibody reactions. It does not include x-rays. The psychodynamic approach differs from the foregoing immunological and "clinical" approach in the following way: It deals with quantities which are unmeasurable in the laboratory. It does not deal with Dr. Fremont-Smith's milliseconds. It does not deal with a shadow on an x-ray plate. It deals with feelings. It deals with techniques of value to allergic children who are sick. In what way do their feelings of anger, hate, love, frustration, and anxiety influence the disease, or possibly (as I believe in the case of hives) might cause the disease? Now, if we are going to get at the feelings of the sick child, we must know as much as possible about the emotionally significant events in the life of that child. In addition, we must know in what way that child's emotions were received by his parents during his psychosexual development. In other works, the psychodynamic approach is all-inclusive and, at first sight, almost impossible to attain. We should know, to a certain extent, how that child felt when he was born, during his early years, during his later years, and, in addition, know how his parents, his teachers, and his peers worked with him. It does not exclude, as I have mentioned, treating the child

physically. But it does focus on those unmeasurable qualities which we all have—feelings.

207
Ago Y. **Psychosomatic studies of so-called "intractable asthma".** Fukuoka Igaku Zasshi 70:340-359, 1979. (in Japanese)

▶ supportive psychotherapy, doctor-patient relationship

Extract of English summary: In conclusion, the psychosomatic approach has been proved to be of value in treating so-called "intractable asthma". It is the author's opinion that the aim of psychosomatic treatment is to facilitate the process of spontaneous remission by helping the patient modify his distorted perception, infantile or pathological defence mechanisms, and inadequate (superficially adaptive) behavior patterns in daily life in order to avoid falling into the so called "preparatory stage".

208
Aitken RCB, Zealley AK, Barrow CG. **The treatment of psychopathology in bronchial asthmatics.** Ciba Found Symp 8:375-380, 1972.

▶ psychotherapy, behavior therapy, consultation-liaison

Sixty-eight patients with bronchial asthma were selected at random from registers of diagnosed cases. These—and an additional 14 patients referred to psychiatrists (the authors) —were examined for psychopathology, along with control subjects. Investigations included the use of psychometric tests, clinical assessment of personality traits, and psychophysiological examination. There was virtually no evidence that the distribution of psychopathology in the randomly selected cases differed from that found in the general population; there was evidence of more psychopathology and more severe pulmonary disorder in the psychiatrically referred cases. No relationship could be discerned between the amount of psychopathology and the severity of pulmonary disorder in the randomly selected series. Forty of these cases were divided into four groups of similar severity of asthma. Two of the groups had higher scores than the median on combined psychometric tests and two of the groups had lower scores. The patients were assessed fortnightly during a three-month period. One group in each pair received intensive psychiatric treatment, based on behaviour therapy principles, for one hour on each of ten occasions during the second month. For those with higher psychometric morbidity scores, clinical ratings of "anxiety severity" and of "asthma severity" fell significantly more during the observation period, but this was irrespective of whether or not intensive psychiatric treatment was given. The rate of spontaneous fluctuations in skin resistance improved likewise. The psychiatric treatment allayed a tendency for ventilation volume to increase between successive occasions of measurement. At three-month follow up, more of the patients who were treated intensively felt improved, both with respect to anxiety and to asthma symptoms. It is concluded that anxious asthmatic patients benefit from regular contact with a psychiatrically orientated therapeutic team. It looks as if this contact need be a little more than minimal, i.e. sufficient only to make clinical observations.

209

Arnds HG, Hau TF, Studt HH. **Psychosomatics of bronchial asthma.** Med Klin 65:2267-2272, 1970. (in German: no English abstract)

▶ psychotherapy

210

Bacon CL. **The role of aggression in the asthmatic attack.** Psychoanal Q 25:309-324, 1956.

▶ psychoanalysis

Clinical evidence suggests that asthma and other forms of respiratory anxiety may be precipitated by nascent aggressive feelings involving anal, urethral, or sexual excretory impulses. Stimulation of the excretory mucous membranes by these fantasies sensitizes the respiratory mucous membrane, just as physical stimulation of the excretory membranes stimulates respiration. The nascent excretory aggression arouses fears of excretory aggression from the outside world. The persons whom the patient has felt to be "good" he now expects to be "bad" and to attack his respiratory apparatus in a talion manner, which responds physiologically as though it were really attacked by noxious substances.

211

Bakwin RM. **Essentials of psychosomatics in allergic children.** Pediatr Clin North Am 1:921-928, 1954.

▶ supportive psychotherapy, family therapy

There is no dividing line between the physical and emotional components. In all probability both factors should be appreciated and handled. As the allergist is the doctor to whom the child comes for treatment, he would appear to be the logical person to assume the responsibility. If he will take the time to get a good history, observe the parent and child in his office, and encourage them to discuss their difficulties, he can readily detect emotional tension if such exists. For optimal development children need support, security and strong acceptance. This holds true for all children, and should be the aim of the physician in his advice to parents. Attention to the emotional and situational problems of the child with allergy in no way precludes other forms of therapy.

212

Bangevits VV. **Psychotherapy in the complex treatment of bronchial asthma.** Klin Med (Mosk) 51:54-56, 1973. (in Russian)

▶ psychotherapy, autogenic training, hypnosis

213

Bentley J, Wilmerding JW. **Individual psychotherapy with asthmatic children as an adjunct to milieu therapy: two case studies.** J Asthma Res 15:163-169, 1978.

▶ milieu therapy, psychotherapy

Parentectomy stresses the physical separation of an intractable asthmatic child from his parents. In residential treatment the focus is on providing activities and opportunities for meaningful interactions and on the teaching of self-help skills, all primarily aimed at promoting greater autonomy in the child. For reasons not entirely understood, increased autonomy reduces the child's susceptibility to severe asthma. Although this is true, physically separating the child as a treatment modality assumes to a certain extent that the child is not in conflict about his wish to attain autonomy. To put this in another way, parentectomy seems to assume that severely ill asthmatic children are longing to be given opportunities to mature, and that as soon as these are offered the children will take them and use them to grow. In fact, asthmatic children are in great conflict about making an emotional separation from parents. On the one hand, they want to grow up; on the other hand (unconsciously) they want to be babied. Therefore, in certain cases, simply providing the new environment that promotes rather than stifles autonomy does not always succeed in making an emotional difference in the child's life. There are children who continue to act and feel as if they were still at home, still emotionally tied to and conflicted about parental figures. For such children, a period of individual psychotherapy focused on helping them understand how they feel towards others can be an extremely valuable adjunct to milieu therapy. The two patients discussed illustrate this. Prior to individual therapy, neither child was able to benefit from the new social milieu. In both cases, the therapist gave the child "center stage," an arena in which he could begin to explore his feelings and experience himself as a distinct and separate being.

214

Berman S. **The psychological implications of intractable asthma in childhood.** Clin Proc Child Hosp 23:210-218, 1967.

▶ psychotherapy, doctor-patient relationship, family therapy

The ability of the physician to establish a treatment alliance is not based solely on his skill to treat physical needs.

It also is related to his ability to listen, understand, and psychologically support the family through crisis after crisis. In this sense, his skill can do much to alleviate resentment and guilt, lessen despair, and encourage optimum physical and psychological development in the child.

215

Blaha H, Fischer E. **Psychological tasks in asthma therapy.** Z Physiother 23:145-150, 1971. (in German: no English abstract)

▶ psychotherapy

216

Bostock J. **Asthma: a synthesis involving primitive speech, organism and insecurity.** J Ment Sci 102:559-575, 1956.

▶ supportive psychotherapy

(1) A survey of 38 asthmatic children was undertaken to ascertain whether disturbed maturation involving co-ordination of respiration and speech is involved in the aetiology of asthma. This is substantiated. (2) Asthma is regarded as a synthesis involving the three factors of primitive speech maturation, organic involvement in respiration, and psychological insecurity. Two stages are involved. (1) Basic Stage: Orderly maturation of the respiratory system utilizes the primitive speech mechanism of "crying" as a basis for respiratory control in true speech. Insecurity of the child as in maternal rejection, psychological submergence, or prolonged discomfort as in dermatitis alters the infantile crying rhythm, thereby producing interference with maturation. A template is thus created for the eventual attack of asthma. This is the first or basic stage. Bottle feeding is often linked with rejection in the creation of insecurity. (2) Trigger Stage: Two factors are involved in a subsequent trigger stage. The first is an organic involvement of the respiratory system. Allergy is often contributory. The second depends on a psychological state evoked by feelings of insecurity. It would appear that the presence of both factors constitutes a trigger mechanism which evokes a modification of the unmaturated "cry." (3) There is evidence that the same aetiological factors which are involved in asthma of childhood occur in adults. (4) The psychological significance of rejection, submergence and breast or bottle feeding are surveyed. (5) The inability of certain asthmatic patients to "cry" is discussed. (6) The possibility of an inherited type of personality, being a predisposing factor, is under investigation. (7) The existence of objective and subjective phases in crying and asthma is considered. (8) Implications in therapy are reviewed.

217

Brown EA. **Combined allergic and psychosomatic treatment of bronchial asthma.** Ann Allergy 9:324-329, 367, 1951.

▶ psychoanalysis, psychotherapy, doctor-patient relationship

Extracted summary: Naturally enough, we do not and cannot completely adjust everybody to everything. In our patients who are, beyond cavil, allergic, and beyond argument, neurotic, we must combine the functions of internists, allergists, and psychiatrists. We do this by recognizing the causative factors in our fields. We accept as a working hypothesis the slogan that no one wheezes excepting for a cause and for a reason. We eliminate the direct cause, we immunize when we cannot eliminate, we medicate when elimination or immunization are impossible or incomplete. We operate when necessary. When all this has been done, we stop looking for causes and search for reasons. The recurrent pattern of the patient's responses gives us our cues.

218

Casey BD, Carson RN, Miller BD. **Consultation/liaison in the home environment: an extended family for the asthmatic child.** Psychosom Med 46:81, 1984. (abstract)

▶ consultation-liaison, family therapy, psychotherapy

On the Pediatric Psychosomatic Unit at National Jewish Hospital (NJH) a consultation/liaison model has been developed which addresses the needs of the asthmatic child and his family. Recent research done at NJH indicates that asthmatic children with significant psychological and family problems are at higher risk of dying from the illness than asthmatic children without these problems. The high-risk asthmatic child requires a well-coordinated effort between medical and psychosocial personnel. The consultation/liaison model implemented on the unit emphasizes the coordination of inpatient and community networks. As the inpatient multidisciplinary team of physicians, psychiatrists, psychologists, social workers, counselors, and nurses assesses the child and develops a treatment program, parallel resources within the community are identified. A specific advocate, often the referring physician or a mental health professional, is identified to lead and coordinate the community network. During the hospitalization, the unit staff helps the child and the family address difficult medical and psychological issues. The family issues are treated during ongoing conference calls and during intensive family sessions scheduled during therapeutic visits. This is concurrent with involving the parents in individual, marital, or family therapy in their own community. The community network is continually appraised of the child's progress. As discharge approaches, other resources which are indicated (i.e., social services, individual therapist, special recreational or educational persons) are contracted and aligned with the home treatment network. Discharge is scheduled when the child is "stable" and the community treatment is in place. This model was implemented in order to improve care for high-risk asthmatic children and in an effort to reduce the length of inpatient hospitalizations. The effectiveness of this model in stabilizing at-risk children is measured by improvement in self-care, reduction in the number of hospitalizations and emergency room visits post-discharge, improved school attendance, decreased family conflict, and referring physician satisfaction.

219
Chong TM. **The management of bronchial asthma.** J Asthma Res 14:73-89, 1977.

▶ review: psychotherapy, hypnosis, relaxation, family therapy, doctor-patient relationship

Shapiro (1956) shrewdly pointed out that the healing of illness in one person as a result of the activities or advice of another is always a complex process. The orthodox doctor would think that it is his medicine that makes the patient better. In all healing processes the motivation, confident hope, expectation and faith of the patients in the designated healer are more important factors. In the practice of medicine the wiser physician would deal with the problem involving the interrelation of biological, psychological and social factors in the production and treatment of illness. Understanding illness and curing sick people involve something more than a knowledge of disease.

220
Cobb S, Shands HC, Miles HHW. **A case of asthma treated with psychotherapy.** Am J Med 11:117-122, 1951. (psychiatric conference)

▶ psychotherapy

221
Condrau G. **On psychosomatic aspects of bronchial asthma.** Ther Umsch 24:352-355, 1967. (in German: no English abstract)

▶ psychotherapy

222
Creak M, Stephen JM. **The psychological aspects of asthma in children.** Pediatr Clin North Am 5:731-747, 1958.

▶ supportive psychotherapy, consultation-liaison, family therapy, group therapy

Extracted summary: Enough has been said to illustrate that this illness, perhaps more than any other, is not the exclusive therapeutic concern of any one group of doctors. Teamwork between the physician, the allergist, the pediatrician and the psychiatrist is essential, and is greatly facilitated by a clear evaluation of roles early in the treatment of case.

223
Detweiler HK. **The psychogenic factor in asthma.** Can Med Assoc J 62:128-130, 1950.

▶ psychotherapy

Attention is called to the importance of recognizing the psychosomatic element in asthma. Without wishing in any way to detract from the importance of studying the asthmatic patient from the conventional standpoint of allergy both atopic and bacterial, a plea is made to practitioners to pay special attention to the psychological background and the influence of emotional states upon the initiation of asthmatic attacks. Emphasis is placed upon the prime importance of a searching history from both the allergic and psychosomatic standpoints. Treatment based on a complete investigation of each individual case will of necessity include psychotherapy in its broad aspects, and will result in maximum benefit to the patient in this dread disease.

224
Deutsch F. **Thus speaks the body: some psychosomatic aspects of the respiratory disorder: asthma.** Acta Med Orient 10:67, 1951.

▶ psychotherapy

225
Dinard E, Charpin T. **Psychotherapy of the asthmatic child.** Acta Allerg (Kbh) 15 (Suppl 7):340, 1960. (in French: no English abstract)

▶ psychotherapy

226
Dirks JF, Paley A, Fross KH. **Panic-fear research in asthma and the nuclear conflict theory of asthma: similarities, differences and clinical implications.** Br J Med Psychol 52:71-76, 1979.

▶ psychotherapy, group therapy, couples therapy

Recent research with the MMPI panic-fear scale has identified personality traits implicated in the psychological maintenance of the medical intractability of asthma. Intensity of prescribed medication, length of hospitalization, and rates of rehospitalization have been found to relate to MMPI panic-fear scores independent of the objective medical severity of the illness as indexed by longitudinal pulmonary functions. In the present study, MMPI panic-fear scores are related to separation and protection conflicts arising in childhood. While the nuclear conflict theory of asthma maintains that such conflicts occur in nearly all asthmatics and form a genetic component of the asthma, the present study finds that childhood separation and protection conflicts occur in a minority of patients, but may be instrumental in maintaining the medical intractability of the illness.

227

Dogs W. **Psychogenesis and psychotherapy of bronchial asthma.** Hippokrates 20:386-388, 1949. (in German; no English abstract)

▶ psychotherapy

228

Edgell PG. **Psychiatric approach to the treatment of bronchial asthma.** Mod Treat 3:900-917, 1966.

▶ psychotherapy, group psychotherapy, consultation-liaison, social casework

From successful experiences in individual and group psychotherapy with bronchial asthmatics, one can draw conclusions relevant to all psychosomatic illness. It is my feeling that the human factor has been too long neglected in our clinic practice. Every clinic should have an active social worker and a volunteer assistant. These two individuals would try to get to know all the patients who attend the clinic. The first function of the social worker would be supportive psychotherapy—the lending of everyday human sympathy, perhaps advice, and practical help. The volunteer would help in a purely hospitable role. A second function would be case finding—the selection from the herd of the needful psychosomatic patients pointed out by the clinician, who would then be submitted to a streamlined screening process. The screening procedure would first bring the patient to the notice of the psychiatrist. Proposed patients would attend psychiatric movies in a group to be followed by a discussion period with a psychiatrist or psychologist, and on the basis of their participation or non-participation apparently suitable patients would be referred for a psychiatric interview. The unsuitable cases would carry on with the social worker and/or her volunteer assistant in group social therapy. Those selected by the psychiatrist would be appropriately indoctrinated in several individual interviews, given some reading material to explain the basis of group therapy, and fitted into a dynamic therapeutic group suitable to their personality and cultural characteristics. Psychotherapy would run concurrently with medical clinic attendance as long as symptoms necessitate. By this approach the total illness can be treated. A combined operation by physician, psychiatrist, psychologist, social worker and volunteer might be expected to diminish the burden of chronic psychosomatic illness, both to individuals and the community. Individual patients and individual doctors, the hospital community, and the community the hospital serves, all have good reason to feel dissatisfied with the partial, fragmented, symptomatic approach to illness that is now so usual in general hospitals.

229

Edgell PG. **The psychology of asthma.** Can Med Assoc J 67:121-125, 1952.

▶ psychotherapy

1. 20-25% of asthmas do not appear to be due to allergic causes. 2. Nearly all asthmatics present primary psychopathogenic patterns which may initiate or complicate the illness. 3. They have in common an underlying emotional insecurity and an intense need for parental protection which is masked by a variety of defense reactions. 4. Among these reactions is the asthma itself which may be solely or partly the expression of a repressed emotion. 5. Stripped of its defense, the underlying psychological state may be a mood, a psychoneurosis, or a psychosis. 6. Treatment for asthma must thus include treatment of the underlying state, and success will vary with the degree of the disturbance and the intensity of the treatment.

230

El-Kholy MK. **The mental factor in bronchial asthma: report on two cases.** Lancet 2:767-768, 1929. (case report)

▶ psychotherapy

231

Falliers CJ. **Psychosomatic study and treatment of asthmatic children.** Pediatr Clin North Am 16:271-286, 1969.

▶ review: psychoanalysis, psychotherapy, group psychotherapy, hypnosis, behavior therapy, desensitization, reciprocal inhibition, operant conditioning, milieu therapy, family therapy

Extracted summary: Attention to both the psychological aspects of asthma and to its potential clinical severity is evident in some of the earliest medical texts. The Hippocratic corpus, for example, contains advice for the asthmatic to avoid strong emotions, such as anger, but it also warns that "such as become hump-backed before puberty from asthma or cough die." Regrettably, this comprehensive view of both the disease and the patient is frequently lost through specialization. Correlations are attempted in which either the medical identification of the disease, or the objective assessment of psychological variables—or both!—are lacking. The psychosomatic approach to asthma can fulfill its purpose only if it examines certain basic psychophysiologic postulates, ascertains the value of modern psychodiagnostic tools, and defines the role of various therapeutic methods in the practice of pediatric allergy, without ever losing sight of the fact that we are not dealing simply with a disturbance in respiratory behavior, but with a seriously incapacitating disease.

232
Findeisen DG. **Indications of physiotherapeutic phases in bronchial asthma.** Arch Phys Ther (Leipz) 17:407-415, 1965. (in German: no English abstract)

▶ psychotherapy

233
French TM. **Psychogenic factors in asthma.** Am J Psychiatry 96:87-101, 1939.

▶ psychoanalysis

Extracted summary: All these observations would suggest that psychological and allergic factors probably stand in a somewhat complementary relationship to each other in the etiology of bronchial asthma, that in some cases asthma attacks may be precipitated by allergic factors alone, in others by emotional factors alone and that in still other cases cooperation of allergic and emotional factors may be necessary to produce the attacks.

234
French TM. **Emotional conflict and allergy.** Int Arch Allergy 1:28-40, 1949.

▶ review: psychoanalysis

Fear of estrangement from a mother and inhibition of crying play significant roles in the etiology of many cases of bronchial asthma. Such emotional factors and allergic factors complement each other in precipitating asthmatic attacks. For these statements there is ample evidence but the evidence concerning psychogenic factors in other allergic conditions is still fragmentary. We do not yet have adequate evidence to decide whether there is any more direct connection between allergy and emotional conflict.

235
Freour P, De Boucaud M. **Psychological aspects of asthma in children: phenomenological approach.** Allergol Immunopathol (Madr) Suppl 9:103-107, 1981. (in French: no English abstract)

▶ psychotherapy

236
Gardey F. **Contribution to the etiopathogenesis of the asthma crisis and its rational treatment by psychotherapy.** Semana Med 2:750-758, 1928. (in Spanish)

▶ psychotherapy

237
Garnett RW Jr. **The psychotherapeutic approach to asthma.** Va Med Monthly 82:61-63, 1955.

▶ psychotherapy

Extracted summary: The acutely ill patient must of course first be treated symptomatically. In addition to the usual medical procedures, the psychotherapeutic measures at this point should be conservative, supportive, cautious, permissive, indulgent; not probing, uncovering, disturbing. After the storm is weathered, the attention may be gradually focused on the basic difficulties, with the expectation that as significant areas of conflict are brought to light, symptoms will recur or increase, and the speed of treatment will have to be regulated accordingly. In most cases, medical management and psychotherapy can and should be carried on simultaneously. The aim in this type of psychotherapy is to re-expose the patient to his conflicts, bring up the repressed, unconscious, forbidden memories, attitudes, feelings; help him to desensitize himself to them, help him to discard immature, inappropriate reaction patterns; to accept himself and others more realistically, more rationally, and to learn to live more effectively, comfortably and productively. In asthma, the focus is usually on the unresolved, repressed, ambivalent dependency on the mother figure. This often includes a difficulty in handling emotions having to do with the desire for independence and, yet, a fear of it. Hence, attitudes such as aggression, self-assertiveness, hostility, give trouble. Also behavior associated with mature independent states, such as normal heterosexual activity, marriage, self-supporting work, etc.

238
Gaudet EL. **Dynamic interpretation and treatment of asthma in a child.** Am J Orthopsychiatry 20:328-345, 1950.

▶ psychotherapy, family therapy, consultation-liaison

Extracted summary: The role of the therapist was seen as one of acceptance of the child, helping him to gain a feeling of security so that he might become more mature and better able to handle the frustrations due to the parents' handling of him, and gradually revealing to him the nature of his defenses in the form of his asthmatic attacks, as well as how they constituted secondary adaptation to the symptom by means of which he had learned to utilize the attacks as a means of regaining the mother's love. In regard to the role of the therapist with the father, the essential thing seemed to be to make him aware of his part in producing the child's difficulties by his avoidance of responsibility for offering security to the child. The role of the therapist with the mother was similar to that with the father. However, it became evident early in the therapy that this goal would have to be modified. The therapist's role was one of acceptance of the mother and permitting her to release her feelings so that she would have less need to project on the child and the father. It is interesting that as the treatment progressed, the problem which began as a problem around the child's asthmatic attacks soon was seen as a personality problem in the child, and finally the severe marital problem which had not been evident in the beginning was revealed and handled in the work with the parents.

239
Gerard MW. **Bronchial asthma in children.** Nerv Child 5:327-331, 1946.

▶ review: psychoanalysis

Extracted summary: In many cases, asthma attacks did not occur in the beginning of the therapy after a satisfactory dependent transference relation to the analyst was established, but later, as impulses first became conscious and the fear of separation from the analyst emerged, and thus psychologically repeated in the analysis situations similar to those associated with the development of the emotional conflict in childhood. Cure of the condition in some cases and considerable decrease in the number and severity of the attacks in others occurred after resolution of the conflict, which allowed the patient to exert his own independence. With this new security in his own power he no longer needed the dependent relationship to a mother figure and consequently lost his fear of separation.

240
Gervais L. **Bronchial asthma and identification with the aggressor.** Can Psychiatr Assoc J 11:497-500, 1966.

▶ psychotherapy

A patient is described to exemplify the use of a specific defence mechanism in the production of bronchial asthma. This is not to deny the predisposition of the patient nor his maternal craving which no doubt played a part in the patient's illness; nevertheless, the important precipitating factor in the appearance of bronchial asthma seemed to have been the father's departure from home and the patient's use of a specific defence mechanism, that of identification with the aggressor.

241
Gillespie RD. **Psychological factors in asthma.** Br Med J 1:1285-1289, 1936.

▶ psychotherapy, hypnosis, suggestion

Extracted summary: We have therefore found asthma: (1) implanted in a psychoneurotic personality, as the expression of the cumulation of the anxiety; (2) equipotent with physical stimuli in precipitating individual attacks; (3) as

a conditioned response to a stimulus with psychological associations ("meaning"); (4) replaced by anxiety symptoms; (5) replaced by elation or depression in a manic-depressive psychosis, or by a schizophrenic psychosis; (6) expressing conflict—for example, a conflict of impulse with conscience; (7) as a protest against an unwelcome situation; (8) as a means of escape; (9) improved or removed by suggestion, either in the waking state or under hypnosis.

242
Grant IW. **The treatment of bronchial asthma.** BTTA Rev 1:43-52, 1971. (in French)

▶ review: psychotherapy

243
Gunnarson S. **Asthma in children as a psychosomatic disease.** Int Arch Allergy Appl Immunol 1:103-108, 1950.

▶ psychotherapy

As a summary, it may be said that asthmatic children display various neurolabile symptoms already before the onset of asthma. Repressed aggressions within the family and a pathologic fixation to the mother, may be especially important factors to consider on the arising of an asthmatic condition in neurolabile children. This seems to be true in children in whom a constitutional, somatic allergy can be shown as well as in children in whom somatic allergy tests show negative results. Attempts to liberate these psychic repressions should therefore constitute an important part of the treatment. Better treatment results are to be expected from combined somatic and psychic therapy. As yet, too little time has gone by in order to critically judge the results. They seem, however, especially promising.

244
Haiman JA. **Emotional factors in bronchial asthma.** J Med Soc NJ 39:80-83, 1942.

▶ psychotherapy, doctor-patient relationship

1. Bronchial asthma, vasomotor rhinitis and related states are often symptoms of vasomotor imbalance. 2. A "neuropathic constitution" predisposes the patient to functional disorders of which the asthmatic state is an example. Emotional upsets and unfavorable environmental factors are precipitating causes. 3. Successful treatment of asthma begins with the restoration of normal breathing and the giving of appropriate sedative medication to modify favorably or to stabilize the underlying "neuropathic terrain." 4. For lasting results, disturbed psychic states and unfavorable environmental factors must be corrected and improvement expected in diet, habits of rest, work and exercise. The physician must be sympathetic and able to

inspire the patient with confidence in his full recovery. 5. All physicians are not equally suited temperamentally for the treatment of these patients, hence some will secure better results by the method described than others.

245
Hajos MK. **Treatment of childhood asthma.** Allerg Asthma (Leipz) 13:286-290, 1967. (in German: no English abstract)

▶ psychotherapy

246
Halliday JL. **Approach to asthma.** Br J Med Psychol 17:1-53, 1937.

▶ psychotherapy

We must bear in mind how often asthma in an adult emerges out of emotional reaction. Because of this, treatment which is directed towards the "psyche" must be of primary importance. This does not mean that in Mrs. Eddy's words we have to "deny the physical," but rather that we must appreciate how psychological factors, through the mechanism of the triad of the diencephalon, autonomic nervous system and endocrine glands, can modify the physical, at first functionally, and later structurally. Moreover, consideration of this is necessary at the beginning of treatment and not as a reluctant and last shot. For practical purposes, therefore, asthmatic patients fall into two groups: first, "new" patients with asthma to whom this approach should be applied from the onset; secondly, the "old" patients who have been treated otherwise and who cannot now be expected to accept a volte face, and these must be referred to another practitioner so that they too may be rendered "new" patients.

247
Hamm J. **Long-term therapy of asthma bronchiale.** Dtsch Med Wochenschr 95:232-234, 1970. (in German)

▶ psychotherapy, psychoanalysis

248
Hansen K. **Allergic and psychical factors in asthma.** Proc R Soc Med 22:789-800, 1929.

▶ psychotherapy

Extracted summary: The aim of this paper is to show that such diseases, the incitement of which is manifestly subject to pathogenic physical components, are also absolutely dependent in their course, even in their origin, on special psychical influences acting on the patient. We are not yet able to give details as to what organic links the mind uses to prepare the body, and the question is, whether we shall ever be in a position to understand it in the sense of a

pure causal nervous system, that system over which our will has no control, and which is particularly determinable by psychical influences, as the physiological and pathological researches of the last few years have shown. The clinician cannot go too far in analysing all these threads, both psychic and organic, which have been shot into the finished web, and of which it is composed. But through this analysis the clinician will get only an incomplete view of the whole and of the meaning of its outward appearance, unless he recognizes, at the back of all analytically-gained data, the principle of a psycho-physical coordination by which alone the phenomenon of life is characterized; for in life, mind and body are not separated, but are always combined as the biological unity of the person.

249
Hau TF. **Stationary psychotherapy: indications and requirements on the psychoanalytic technic.** Z Psychosom Psychoanal 14:116-120, 1968. (in German: no English abstract)

▶ psychoanalysis, psychotherapy

250
Haynal A, Cramer B. **Bronchial asthma, a psychosomatic disease (medical psychology of the asthmatic).** Rev Med Suisse Romande 94:177-187, 1974. (in French: no English abstract)

▶ psychotherapy

251
Haynal A, Pariente R. **The effectiveness of psychotherapy for asthma.** Sem Hop Paris Ther 53: 253-254, 1977. (in French: no English abstract)

▶ psychotherapy

252
Henderson AT. **Psychogenic factors in bronchial asthma.** Can Med Assoc J 55:106-111, 1946.

▶ counseling

In conclusion, one cannot too emphatically repudiate the misleading suggestion that bronchial asthma should be considered as a psychical disorder. I believe that it should be conceived of primarily as an organic disease based on disturbed respiratory physiology—the result of allergic influences, in which psychic and emotional factors may indeed be important in precipitating, modifying or inhibiting attacks in patients already the subjects of asthma. Only in rare instances would the disease appear to be originally psychogenic, and even then careful search will usually reveal that a state of allergic equilibrium has been upset by the psychic trauma. There probably are some patients who consciously or unconsciously utilize their disease to excuse their deficiencies, and even to achieve their ends. In the case of children, the attitude of the mother is of real importance. Much wisdom and restraint is called for. Certainly overprotection and apprehension is most unwise and may serve as a "trigger mechanism" through suggestion. The physician should see to it that while important considerations are not lost sight of, neither should the idea be inculcated in the child that he is a potential invalid and therefore to be wrapped up in cotton-wool. A little healthy neglect may even be preferable to oversolicitude.

253

Hodek B, Skretova K, Skreta M. **On psychic factors in the development of bronchial asthma.** Allerg Asthma (Leipz) 11:178-202, 1965. (in German)

▶ psychotherapy

The connections between asthma and psychic factors can be quite complicated: Psychic factors may appear as predisposing factors of diseases and may, however, also be involved as releasing and influencing factors of the first visible symptoms by a mechanism of conditioned responses, or the repetitive allergic reactions influence the higher nerve functions so as to give rise to the known circulus vitiosus between the asthmatic complaints and the psychic phenomena. The simultaneous appearance of both psychic and allergic factors must not necessarily be due to an interdependence of cause and effect, and the coincidence between psychic and allergic moments may be quite accidental. There are also discussed the question of the specific type of personality, the problem of the particular conflict situation, and the practical evaluation of the part played by the psychic component. For the purpose of illustrating the overall situation, a case history is presented that shows the difficulty of discovering the psychic component which in the present case was not discovered until the employment of what we call narco-analysis.

254

Jackson M. **Psychopathology and psychotherapy in bronchial asthma.** Br J Med Psychol 49:249-255, 1976.

▶ psychotherapy, psychoanalysis, hypnotism, biofeedback, relaxation

The role of psychological factors in the genesis of bronchial asthma is much disputed, and hence the place of psychotherapy in its management is equally controversial. The opportunity to study a series of such patients and to attempt to provide psychotherapy for them has led the author to the view that significant psychopathology is more common in asthmatic subjects than is generally realized, and that psychotherapy has a vital part to play in management. Some case material is presented to support this

contention, and the application of psychoanalytic concepts, evaluation and treatment are discussed.

255

Jensen RA, Stoesser AV. **Emotional factor in bronchial asthma in children.** Am J Dis Child 62:80-91, 1941.

▶ psychotherapy

On the basis of our own observations and those reported by others, we should like to emphasize the importance of recognizing and dealing with emotional factors in every case of asthma, but more particularly in those cases in which the disease is refractory to the usual therapy. The early recognition of psychologic factors seems advisable if the possibility of a subsequent condition of semi-invalidism is to be prevented. It is ordinarily the rule to consider psychogenic and emotional factors only when everything else has failed. A more logical procedure would be to take cognizance of their importance and to make a conscious effort to deal with them early in the case of each individual patient suffering from bronchial asthma.

256

Jessner L, Lamont J, Long R, Rollins N, Whipple B, Prentice N. **Emotional impact of nearness and separation for the asthmatic child and his mother.** Psychoanal Study Child 10:353-375, 1955.

▶ psychotherapy

Those features which were striking in many, but not all, of the cases, such as passivity in the boys, or closeness to father in the girls, appear to be secondary to the more crucial issue of closeness and separation between mother and child. While such a conflict is to some extent universal, with the asthmatic child it seems to be of outstanding intensity and central significance. Mere physical separation brings only temporary relief. The aim of psychotherapy is to achieve a genuine differentiation between mother and child so that both can tolerate being together as well as apart and are free to establish true object love.

257

Jones NF, Dirks JF, Kinsman RA. **Assessment in the psychomaintenance of chronic physical illness.** J Psychiatr Treat Eval 2:303-312, 1980.

▶ psychotherapy, milieu therapy

Aspects of the psychomaintenance of chronic illness and an assessment battery which permits early identification of patients who are at risk for psychomaintenance of one illness (asthma) are presented. This assessment battery, the components of which have been presented in earlier papers, evaluates both general personality and illness-specific characteristics related to various maladaptive response styles which may defeat otherwise successful medical treatment of asthma. Its use helps to focus treatment strategies to counteract the role of psychological factors perpetuating illness. Three case studies are provided as illustrations of the application of assessment in a medical setting.

258
Julich H, Lachmann W. **Therapy of status asthmaticus (bronchial asthma).** Dtsch Gesundheitswes 27:1258-1261, 1972.

▶ psychotherapy

Introductorily, the authors briefly demonstrate diagnostic and differential-diagnostic characteristic features of bronchial asthma. The explanation of the relevant drugs—above all, xanthine derivatives, corticosteroids, sedatives and hypnotics, beta-stimulators, glycosides, anti-allergics, O_2-interval respiration—is centered mainly on therapeutic effectivity and side-effects. Special attention must be devoted to the patient's psychotherapeutic care. Finally, the authors critize that at present a great number of anti-asthmatic drugs (about 60 compounds, including asthma-cigarettes) are offered for sale in dispensaries without being liable to medical prescription by a physician.

259
Karol C. **The role of primal scene and masochism in asthma.** Int J Psychoanal Psychother 8:577-592, 1980.

▶ psychoanalysis

Early investigators, such as French, observed that asthma patients need to repress their sexual and aggressive impulses in an attempt to retain their mother's love. Early traumatic experiences, illness, primal scene, death in the family, miscarriage or birth of a sibling have all been mentioned as precursors of asthmatic attacks. These factors are also of considerable relevance in the case material presented here. Emphasized in this presentation, in addition to the above mentioned factors, are critical aspects of primal scene traumatic experiences and their role in the subsequent development of sadomasochistic character formation. This sadomasochism plays a considerable role in the later eruption of asthmatic symptomatology. The crucial factor in the asthmatic symptomatology arises from the effect of the traumatic experiences which are associatively linked to these sadomasochistic fantasies. Clinical material of an asthmatic girl with learning inhibitions and sleeping difficulties is presented. She demonstrates a clownish sadomasochistic type of behavior reflecting a disturbance in her object relationships. During the course of analysis, it was revealed that specific unconscious fantasies, associated with early traumatic experiences, played a predominant role in the development of her sadoma-

sochistic attitudes. These, in turn, were linked to her asthmatic attacks.

260
Kelly E, Zeller B. **Asthma and the psychiatrist.** J Psychosom Res 13:377-395, 1969.

▶ review

A number of comprehensive reviews of the literature concerning the psychiatric aspects of bronchial asthma figure amongst the 296 papers listed by Stokvis which have appeared up to and including 1959. The present review attempts to include and assess all available contributions since that date and is modelled on a previous survey made in 1953. A study such as this may prove useful as a source for those working on the psychiatric problems of bronchial asthma.

261
Kemper KA. **Brief therapy of a case of chronic bronchial asthma.** Prax Kinderpsychol Kinderpsychiatr 3:125-129, 1954. (in German)

▶ psychotherapy

262
Kersten W, Worth G. **Therapy in bronchial asthma.** Fortschr Med 95:2791-2794, 1977. (in German)

▶ psychotherapy

A division into two main groups is made: causal and symptomatic treatment. The first group includes elimination and avoidance of allergens and the specific hyposensitization according to own experiences. The second group is divided into medicamentous treatment (bronchodilatators, DNCG, corticosteroids, secretolytics, antibiotics, tranquilizers) and into a nonmedicamentous treatment like physiotherapy, climate therapy and psychotherapy.

263
Kinsman RA, Dirks JF, Schraa JC. **Psychomaintenance in asthma: personal styles affecting medical management.** Resp Ther 11:39-46, 1981.

▶ counseling, relaxation

"Psychomaintenance" refers to the perpetuation of illness or the defeat of medical treatment because of psychologic, as opposed to strictly physical, reasons. Nine personal styles, seven of which clearly are connected to the psychomaintenance of asthma, are described and discussed. They underscore the diversity of ways that people react during chronic asthma and its treatment and the need to consider these differences carefully in all aspects of management. Respiratory therapists can assume an active role in the resolution of specific problems.

264

Kleeman ST. **Psychiatric contributions in the treatment of asthma.** Ann Allergy 25:611-619, 1967.

▶ psychotherapy

Extracted summary: The all-important question which underlies this entire study is the following: Is a psychiatric approach to patients with asthma worthwhile? Although there is an insufficient number of patients in this group to allow for statistical analysis or firm conclusions it is quite apparent that many asthmatics have an emotional component to their illness. There is a definite indication from the cases studied that if one uses the psychiatric approach discriminately and differentiates between the neurotic and psychotic individuals with asthma and treats each appropriately, that the therapeutic results will bear out the value of adding psychiatric therapy to the rest of the armamentarium in asthma care.

265

Kleinsorge H. **Considerations of psychic factors in the prevention and therapy of bronchial asthma.** Deutsch Gesundheitswes 14:2353-2357, 1959. (in German)

▶ psychotherapy

266

Kleinsorge H. **Psychotherapy of bronchial asthma.** Ther Ggw 108:1744-1746, 1969. (in German: no English abstract)

▶ psychotherapy

267

Klumbies G. **Psychotherapy of bronchial asthma: an evaluation of the indication and chance of success.** Allerg Asthma (Leipz) 9:126-130, 1963. (in German: no English abstract)

▶ psychotherapy

268

Knapp PH. **Free association as a biopsychosocial probe.** Psychosom Med 42:197-219, 1980.

▶ psychoanalysis

Free association was used as an experimental approach in a pilot study of four healthy subjects. Physiologically simultaneous measurement of respiratory minute volume showed a wide range of moment-to-moment values, possibly reflecting shifts in emotional state. Psychologically, subjects manifested classical resistance and transference attitudes. These psychological findings were confirmed in a second study using seven mild asthmatics and six healthy comparison subjects. The asthmatics showed significant constriction of verbal associative productivity and also significantly greater "immaturity" in drawings of two humans and of an animal, serially administered before and after three free associative sessions. A third study of associative output after stressful stimulation, using 17 asthmatics and 16 controls, confirmed the verbal constriction of the asthmatics. Free association permits study of psychosocial context and, in particular, reconstruction of important self-other relationships. These factors are important in assessing the "strain" surrounding manifest expression of emotion. Verbatim associative productions from experimental subjects and from a patient in psychoanalysis are used to form a model of emotional processes in acute bronchial asthma. This is a special case of Engel's general biopsychosocial model of disease.

269

Knapp PH, Carr HE Jr, Mushatt C, Nemetz SJ. **Asthma, melancholia and death (II).** Psychosom Med 28:134-154, 1966.

▶ psychoanalysis

During two periods, serial 24-hr urine levels from a psychoanalytic patient with severe, ultimately fatal asthma were compared to "blind" ratings of four emotions (anxiety, anger, sadness, and erotic affect) and four complex, largely unconscious constellations of self-other fantasy ("Progressive" compliance; "Depleted" emptiness; "Somatized" bodily preoccupation; and "Perverse-pseudogratified" impulsivity). The 17-OHCS output fluctuated and, at times, was abnormally high, probably as a result of repeated ACTH treatment and possibly also as part of emotional turmoil, which may characterize asthmatic relapse. "Perverse pseudogratified" and "anxiety" ratings showed a significant inverse relationship to 17-OHCS output in the first period of study. An additional variable, "Loss of Defensive Control," rated during the second period, showed significantly positive correlation with 17-OHCS levels. Fragmentary data from five further asthmatic fatalities and from cases reported by others suggest that, although specific biologic factors may play a role, so may overt despair and hidden self-destructiveness. Autopsy in ours and other cases has generally shown diffuse bronchiolar obstruction by thick mucus. Explosive parasympathetic nervous influences, possibly leading to cardiac dysrhythmia, may act in concert with the inflammatory pulmonary process to produce a rapidly fatal course.

270

Knapp PH, Mushatt C, Nemetz SJ. **Asthma, melancholia, and death (I): Psychoanalytic considerations.** Psychosom Med 28:114-133, 1966.

▶ psychoanalysis

A 33-year-old male, severely ill with bronchial asthma, suddenly died on the day he was to resume psychoanalytic treatment after a summer interruption. Post-mortem examination showed diffuse bronchiolar obstruction. Prolonged psychoanalytic therapy had led to many gains but had resulted in a sort of "interminable treatment." Steroid medication, which he had also received, may palliate but not resolve this type of therapeutic dilemma. His psychological structure was melancholic. Manifest helpless and dependent attitudes were accompanied by secret craving for erotized excitement and explosive urges toward violence. His final remarks in psychoanalysis were about a murderer who had been detected by analysis of his painting of a beautiful woman. These associations suggested an attempt to solve intolerable conflict over loss by maintaining an idealized image of his mother, an effort jeopardized by hidden destructive impulses.

271
Knapp PH, Mushatt C, Nemetz SJ. **The context of reported asthma during psychoanalysis.** Psychosom Med 32:167-188, 1970.

▶ psychoanalysis

From the record of a man with moderately severe perennial asthma, psychoanalytic process notes just before 37 reported episodes of asthmatic exacerbation were compared with process notes from 44 periods when he was asthma-free. All were edited to remove medical cues. Two psychoanalyst judges had limited statistical success in separating "asthmatic" from "nonasthmatic" contexts, doing best when subjective confidence was high and after feedback. Two medical judges had less "training," examining only the last 50 occasions. They were not helped by feedback and followed a slightly different, less successful pattern of rating, mainly searching for contaminating medical information. Evidence of this was found in eight instances, although only three of these actually proved to be "asthmatic." Post hoc study of both successful and unsuccessful judgments helped refine the hypothesis that stress, emotional arousal, and failing defenses activate a postulated "primitive core" of unconscious conflict to form the psychological context of asthmatic exacerbations.

272
Knox SJ. **Psychiatric aspects of bronchial asthma: a critical review and case reports.** Ulster Med J 29:144-157, 1960.

▶ review: psychotherapy, consultation-liaison

Extracted summary: Psychotherapy, allied with medicinal measures as indicated, must remain the first and most important therapeutic measure. In assessing the patients's milieu social work is essential both as an exploratory and therapeutic measure. It is, of course, out of the question and unnecessary for a psychiatrist to see every case of asthma referred to hospital or seen by his practitioner.

On the other hand, psychiatric treatment can offer little in long-standing cases especially where irreversible secondary physical changes have occurred. Referral to a psychiatrist might be considered in the following instances: (i) where complex psychological factors become obvious to the clinician within the first few attendances, (ii) where there is an unexpected failure to respond to appropriate physical measures of known potency, (iii) where there is a discrepancy between the degree of physical incapacity and physical signs, (iv) where attacks consistently occur in certain circumstances; for example, if they clear up in hospital only to recur almost immediately on discharge, or again if they are noted to occur only when relatives are visiting. Experimental evidence on the part played by conditioning is an additional reason for early referral should emotional factors be considered important.

273
Leigh D. **Asthma and the psychiatrist: a critical review.** Int Arch Allergy Appl Immunol 4:227-246, 1953.

▶ review: psychotherapy

Whilst it is clear that the psychiatric aspects of asthma have attracted considerable attention, there yet exists no satisfying, authoritative paper on this subject. Speculation is rife and is nowhere substantiated by scientific study. The physician may remain as legitimately confused on this aspect of the problem as on other problems more related to his own field. The need, as it seems to this reviewer, is for the initiation of a long term (5, 10 and 15 years) project, using adequate control material, and methods subject to statistical analysis. What has already appeared in the psychiatric literature is stimulating, and fertile in ideas, but requires the test of experiment, of confirmation, and of time. Genetic psychiatric studies, and more research into psychophysical relationships in asthma are particularly needed. The treatment of asthma is a secondary problem at the moment. What is urgently required is careful study of the genesis of attacks, and of the psychophysical mechanisms which are concerned with their maintenance and prolongation. Finally, in spite of confident statements to the contrary, no specific psychological constellation has been proved to exist in asthmatics. It appears rather that the asthmatic attack may result from stimuli of varied provenance playing on an organism which is genetically and constitutionally "predisposed" toward such manifestations. To postulate a common personality and a common basic problem, is in this reviewer's opinion, quite contrary to the observable facts, and results from very special pleading.

274
Leigh D, Doust JWL. **Asthma and psychosis.** J Ment Sci 99:489-496, 1953.

▶ psychotherapy

(1) A clinical, radiological, psychiatric and physiological study has been made on 28 patients concurrently pre-

senting with bronchial asthma and a psychotic illness. (2) Sixteen were classified as suffering from an affective disorder (manic-depression), 11 from schizophrenia and 1 from a senile paranoid psychosis. (3) The incidence of asthma was 64 per cent in a mental hospital population, as contrasted with a 15-20 per cent incidence in the general population at risk outside it. (4) No significant deviation in the oxygen saturation of the arterial blood of the psychotic patient with asthma was found apart from that characteristic of the particular type of mental disorder from which he suffered. (5) No intimate relationship was found to exist between the psychosis and the asthmatic attack.

275

Leroy PE. **Notes on the role and modalities of psychotherapy in the treatment of asthma.** Therapie 23:899-902, 1968. (in French)

▶ psychotherapy, group psychotherapy, relaxation

114 asthmatic people were examined with a psychodynamic view for four years. The terms of the conflicts denoted by asthmatic attacks and the most frequent personality problems noted among these patients are described, as is the immediate psychotherapeutic care of the patient by the group or one of its members at at the time of the attack. Various psychotherapeutic treatments beyond the critical period are mentioned: individual brief psychotherapy, relaxation, breathing exercises. These therapies are used with the usual therapeutic care of asthma, at least at the beginning.

276

Lofgren LB. **A case of bronchial asthma with unusual dynamic factors, treated by psychotherapy and psychoanalysis.** Int J Psychoanal 42:414-423, 1961.

▶ psychotherapy, psychoanalysis

[T]he dramatic events leading up to the onset of the disease in the case to be described here, the theoretical implications, and the at least temporary cure of the asthma seem of sufficient interest to warrant a publication of this single case.

277

Long RT, Lamont JH, Whipple B, Bandler L, Blom GE, Burgin L, Jessner L. **A psychosomatic study of allergic and emotional factors in children with asthma.** Am J Psychiatry 114:890-899, 1958.

▶ psychotherapy

We would like to report some findings from a collaborative study on allergic and emotional factors in children with asthma. The point of departure for this investigation is a frequently recorded observation, namely that children with perennial, intractable asthma are often symptomatically relieved by admission to a hospital, even though maintained on the same medication in the hospital as they had received at home. Equally often they relapse upon return home on the same medication. Various explanations have been offered for this observation. Stated in the extreme, they are: 1. Allergists assume that the asthma is perpetuated by continuous exposure to an allergen, e.g., house dust. 2. Psychiatrists assume that there is excessive interpersonal tension within the home, especially between the mother and the asthmatic child. In both of these cases, hospitalization removes the irritant; be it allergenic or emotional. 3. Psychosomatic explanation regards the asthmatic symptoms as the result of a confluence of numerous factors—environmental, emotional, and allergic.

278

Loras O. **The psychotherapy of the asthmatic patient.** Clinique (Par) 56:521-532, 1961. (in French: no English abstract)

▶ psychotherapy

279

Lowenstein J. **Asthma and psychotherapy.** Med Klin 22:994-997, 1926. (in German: no English abstract)

▶ psychotherapy

280

Macedo de Queiroz A, Strauss A. **Some psychological contributions to the clinical treatment of the asthmatic child.** Acta Allergol 12:396-406, 1958.

▶ psychotherapy, family therapy

In the 40 children studied we encountered psychic components influencing asthma directly or indirectly. Also there were psychological problems of educational and emotional nature. The mental level was normal in this group. All children improved under associated medical and psychological orientation and treatment. Therefore psychological investigation seems absolutely justified. As an immediate suggestion we should like to mention that the facts considered above could constitute a starting point for the anamnesis and psycho-pedagogic orientation of the pediatrician and allergist. A specialized psychological examination would seem perfectly justifiable in cases with large psychological interference and when the family environment permits it.

281

Mandell AJ, Younger CB. **Asthma alternating with psychiatric symptomatology.** Calif Med 96:251-253, 1962.

▶ review: psychotherapy, consultation-liaison

Extracted summary: A group of cases and review of the literature is presented documenting the interesting clinical phenomenon of an inverse temporal relationship between asthmatic symptoms and clinical psychiatric symptoms in some patients. It is suggested that physicians treating asthmatic patients should be prepared to handle potential psychiatric complications that may be concomitants of the successful medical management of patients with asthma.

282
Mansmann JA. **Projective psychological tests applied to the study of bronchial asthma.** Ann Allergy 10:583-591, 1952.

▶ psychotherapy, hypnosis, suggestion

1. Projective technique should be used by physicians who wish to understand the psychosomatic problems of bronchial asthma. They can be compared to skin tests, a short cut to verify known personality factors and imbalances, and a help to quickly uncover the latent conflicts. Just as positive and negative skin tests sometimes are false, the degree of emotional imbalance necessary for asthma is not constant. Our studies indicate that when improvement is noted the psychic adjustment was not passive dependence but some degree of active striving to meet the life situation. Improvement also seemed to come when the personality imbalance was not fixed but in a state of confusion. 2. The intelligence scales of our patients were about average. Omitting one patient who died, improvement seemed to be associated with better than average intelligence. 3. The Rorschach tests definitely verified much that has been said about the emotional factors in bronchial asthma. When employed, these techniques will give much help. Additional study might indicate that these tests be used to determine what type of psychotherapy should be employed and how the patient might respond. They may also help in prognosis to determine whether the asthmatic attack is temporary or will be sustained.

283
Marx E. **The psychogenesis and psychotherapy of bronchial asthma.** Dtsch Med Wochenschr 49:477-478, 1923. (in German: no English abstract)

▶ psychotherapy

284
Mattsson A. **Emotional problems in asthmatic children.** Va Med Monthly 100:1024-1029, 1973.

▶ psychotherapy, relaxation

There is a need for psychiatric intervention in childhood asthma when psychologic factors may be of etiologic or aggravating importance, when symptoms are worsened by individual or family tensions, where behavior problems have appeared in the child or the family. Treatment may be directed toward prevention of emotionally triggered attacks, modification of attitudes toward the child's symptoms, and alleviation of concurrent behavior disorders.

285
Mattsson A. **Psychologic aspects of childhood asthma.** Pediatr Clin North Am 22:77-88, 1975.

▶ psychotherapy, family therapy, milieu therapy, relaxation, biofeedback, consultation-liaison

Extracted summary: Regarding the efforts to support as normal a personality development as possible for the child with asthma, there is general agreement that his psychologic environment, usually his biologic family, must be included in any counselling work. In many instances, the family tends to get overinvolved with the ill child, leading to overprotective, or, less frequently, nonaccepting, rejecting attitudes. Furthermore, many emotional conflicts between the parents, the siblings, etc., often get avoided or diffused due to everyone's overriding concern over the asthma situation; i.e., the patient may serve as a "conflict-avoidance tool" and a protection for other family members and their submerged problems of functioning well as a unit. Whenever significant family maladaptation complicates the course of childhood asthma, the pediatrician or allergist should consider a psychiatric consultation regarding the introduction of family psychotherapy into the total management of the patient. This technique, developed at the Philadelphia Child Guidance Clinic, seems to hold considerable promise with cooperative families who recognize the need to identify and change their faulty patterns of interaction that center around their child with asthma. There continues to be a need for placement in residential treatment centers for those children with severe asthma who are resistant to all available medical and psychological interventions in their community. In a majority of these situations, psychologic factors trigger or aggravate the situation significantly and marked family sociopathology has been present for a long time. As most parents and patients feel threatened by an extended separation, much time is usually required to explain its necessity and to assist the parents in coping with their sense of inadequacy and guilt and fears of losing their child emotionally. In addition, the child requires adequate preparation, which must include his understanding that the length of separation from his home has to be determined by the staff of the treatment center.

286
Mayer S. **Psychogenic asthma.** Northwest Med 43:287-289, 1944.

▶ psychotherapy, psychoanalysis, suggestion, doctor-patient relationship

An instance of psychogenic asthma has been presented. The implications of the psychiatric problem in asthma have been discussed.

287
Meijer A. **Psychotherapy of adolescent asthma patients.** Prax Kinderpsychol Kinderpsychiatr 34:49-54, 1985. (in German)

▶ psychotherapy

Amongst the frequent problems to be anticipated in the psychotherapy of asthmatic patients are ambiguous feelings on the part of both the treating physicians and the patients. Though psycho-physiological vulnerability varies, asthmatic patients like others are often highly sensitive to the loss of love and appreciation from meaningful figures. This hypersensitivity is generally associated with strong feelings of dependency and compliance, which may alternate with unregulated expression of anger. Initially, feelings of dissatisfaction or frustration are often inhibited or denied and diverted through preexisting somatic pathways instead of finding expression in the psychotherapeutic relationship. Increased awareness of pathogenic family and other interpersonal relationship patterns is an important step in the process of relieving anxiety, helplessness and depression with concomitant increase in self reliance and self esteem. The case vignettes illustrate that persistent improvement during psychotherapy in asthmatic patients is more likely in adolescence, a time when a developmental trend towards independence and strong innate hope for the future are powerful allies.

288
Mijatovic M. **Modern diagnosis and therapy of bronchial asthma.** Vojnosanit Pregl 27:406-408, 1970. (in Croatian: no English abstract)

▶ psychotherapy

289
Miklich DR. **Health psychology practice with asthmatics.** Prof Psychol 10:580-588, 1979.

▶ psychotherapy, behavior therapy, consultation-liaison

Behavioral and psychological problems associated with physical diseases can be most effectively and efficiently cared for by health psychologists—clinical psychologists who specialize in the care of such problems and who practice as independent professionals sharing responsibility for patient care with physicians treating the disease itself. If the optimum care of independent health psychology practice is to be realised, however, there must exist well-defined spheres of responsibility for each profession. These must be developed specifically for different diseases because each has particular problems. This article presents suggested divisions of responsibility in caring for asthmatics. I hope it will provide a model that can be appropriately modified for use in caring for patients with other diseases.

290
Miller H, Baruch DW. **The emotional problems of childhood and their relation to asthma.** J Dis Child 93:242-245, 1957.

▶ supportive psychotherapy, family therapy

Since 1946, we have systematically and consistently observed and treated allergic patients within the psychosomatic frame of reference. From this approach we have confirmed that not all occurrences of clinical allergy are caused by allergic reactions or other physical agents but may be set off and continued by emotional causes. We have also come to believe that in asthma there is a constitutional factor, a common denominator, which predetermines this clinical syndrome when it occurs whether from physical or emotional causes. In a group of 201 clinically allergic children studied, practically all at one time or another had had asthma. Allergy skin tests showed that the great majority were immunologically allergic as well as clinically allergic. In every instance the parents, sometimes the mother alone but in most instances the father also, were interviewed. The older children were also interviewed, and the younger ones were studied by means of diagnostic doll-play sessions, the "Draw Your Family" technique, and, where indicated, the Rorschach and other psychological tests.

291
Miller H, Baruch DW. **Psychotherapy in acute attacks of bronchial asthma.** Ann Allergy 11:438-444, 1953.

▶ psychotherapy

[A] regime for handling the acute attack of bronchial asthma has been outlined and described in terms of the psychodynamics of asthma by feeding the affect hunger, by lessening the fear of rejection, and when possible by lessening the patient's anxiety over his hostile components and helping him to release them. A few concrete techniques have been described. These are not all-inclusive. They are merely suggestive of the type of procedure which each physician can explore according to what his personality dictates and what he himself feels he can carry out.

292
Miller H, Baruch DW. **The psychosomatic aspects of management of asthmatic children.** Int Arch Allergy Appl Immunol 13:102-111, 1958.

▶ psychotherapy

Four cases histories of asthmatic children are presented in order to illustrate the accompanying emotional symptoms commonly seen in the physician's office. These were characteristic of a group of 60 asthmatic children in intensive psychotherapy for asthma, studied in comparison with a control group of 35 non-asthmatic and non-allergic children in intensive psychotherapy for behaviour problems. In all instances, the psychodynamic picture followed a consistent pattern. In all instances the emotional and somatic disturbances were set off in children with allergic constitutions who felt that they were not loved sufficiently by their mother. The need for further affection led to fear that such affection as had been offered might be at any moment withdrawn; that is, that the mother would leave either in reality or symbolically. The feeling of lack of affection invariably led to anger toward the mother which had to be repressed along with the expression of the need for more love. The somatic symptoms represented a repression of the feelings of longing for more affection, fear of losing the mother, and anger at the deprivation experienced and expected. Illustrations are given suggesting certain office practices directed toward supplying the need for love, assuaging the fear of desertion and releasing in safe channels the anger which had been generated.

293

Monsour KJ. **Asthma and the fear of death.** Psychoanal Q 29:56-71, 1960.

▶ psychoanalysis

Analytic treatment of asthma in adults is similar to the treatment of severe phobic states. The threat of dying is a major factor among these patients. As Grotjahn aptly said, "The analyst's unconscious must be prepared to face the terror of death in order successfully to treat the asthmatic patient." The classical parameter in treating phobic neurosis by exposing the patient to his actual feared situation in a later phase of analysis is as useless in bringing about a true resolution of the fear of death in asthma as it is in other phobias. The analyst cannot escape the dreaded situation in the transference by the device of accompanying the patient on a trip into a different and symbolic reality. In the analysis of adult patients, asthma will be relieved when the patient relinquishes the guilt-laden ambivalent response to the mother and accepts the analyst as a nonseductive parent who does not fascinate the patient by a seductive attraction into a mutually eroticized death experience. In many instances treatment of asthma in children requires separation from the mother. Since the symptoms of asthma often disappear under such circumstances, treatment requires a direct approach to the phobic core of the illness. Jessner, et al., have noted too that "the defensive system resembles that found in phobic children." Due regard must be given to the fact that children in our culture seem to pass through a phobic phase as a regular feature of their development. This requires keeping in mind that asthma may be replaced by phobic symptoms, may disappear as a manifestation of neurotic pathology during the latency period, or may alternate with other adaptive compromises, none of which mean reso-

lution of the major fear of death. The separated mother's own pathology awaits the forthcoming reunion with her asthmatic child. If this hope proves futile, she will shift the symbiosis to another sibling or develop further pathology of her own. Treatment of the mother seems inescapable in the cases of young asthmatic children.

294

Naber J. **Bronchial asthma and long-term healing through psychotherapy.** Zentralbl Inn Med 64:1, 1943. (in German)

▶ psychotherapy

295

Naber J. **Bronchial asthma: allergic treatment and psychotherapy.** Ther Ggw 70:437-442, 1929. (in German: no English abstract)

▶ psychotherapy

296

Nolte D, Schultis K. **Therapy of bronchial asthma.** Med Welt 24:1483-1485, 1968. (in German: no English abstract)

▶ psychotherapy

297

O'Neill D. **Asthma as a stress reaction: its diagnosis and treatment.** Practitioner 169:273-280, 1952.

▶ psychotherapy

The results of psychiatric investigation and treatment of 20 patients with asthma (13 adults and 7 chidren) are reported. The group is a selected one, being made up of patients referred for psychiatric appraisal. The asthma first appeared, in the children, either when the patient was the sole child in the family or shortly after the birth of the next sibling. In most of the adult patients the onset of asthma coincided with an intense emotional experience. In both adults and children emotional tension—mainly anxiety, resentment and guilt—was by far the most important precipitant of attacks. The results of psychiatric treatment were: Recovered or much improved, 9; improved, 4; improved and relapsed, 3; unchanged, 4. The reasons why treatment was effective in some cases and not in others are discussed.

298

Oberndorf CP. **The psychogenic factors in asthma.** NY State J Med 35:41-48, 1935.

▶ psychoanalysis

Extracted summary: In conclusion one may say that psychoanalytically the asthmatic attack represented the cry of the infant for the return of the mother only in a most superficial interpretation. At a deeper level of mentation it is a manifestation of a conflict concerning emission and reception, domination and submission, unconscious masculinity and conscious femininity. In its immediate form the conflict was one of conscious submissiveness to the mother and unconscious desire to dominate her; conscious reverence for the husband with an unconscious desire likewise to dominate him.

299
Parrow J. **Bronchial asthma—a curable psychoneurosis.** Dtsch Gesundheitswes 4:57-61, 1949.

▶ psychotherapy

The bronchial asthma is explained to be a psychoneurosis, all its symptoms originally having functional causes. Therefore it can be cured by psycho-therapy as well as—in the same way as stammering—by a specially developed breathing therapy. That therapy is based on a conception of the breathing mechanism which is explained in detail, emphazising the simultaneous antagonism of thorax-diaphragm and ascribing to the inner musculature of the thorax a supporting or adjusting function, to the region of the palate and the pharynx a reflectory, controlling part. Through systematic exercises based on that conception, the therapy reaches an intentionally relaxed abdominal respiration; according to the theory that kind of respiration is physiologically the only possible and correct one. It is always possible to bring about a normalized respiration mechanism, which, besides additional gymnastic excercises etc. and setting aside all remedies, can cure the asthma and will enable the patient to overcome the attacks by himself.

300
Pinkerton P. **The enigma of asthma.** Psychosom Med 35:461-462, 1973. (editorial)

▶ psychotherapy

301
Pinkerton P. **Correlating physiologic with psychodynamic data in the study and management of childhood asthma.** J Psychosom Res 11:11-25, 1967.

▶ psychotherapy, milieu therapy

(1) The equation of physiological "mildness" with the most commonly occurring form of psychodynamic aura (overprotection), poses the danger of dismissing such cases as insignificant, or "merely psychological." Even the mild case, so-called, is capable of sudden, severe episodic bronchoconstriction, such as characterized two of the fatalities; both of these had been judged overprotective. (2) It is equally misleading to dismiss the treatment of the "psy-

chological" case with the single prescription of parentectomy, a term devised by Peshkin to denote the therapeutic removal of the child from his "smothering" home environment. Parentectomy alone may prove effective where there is minimal over-investment, but our study demonstrates that the more intense the psychopathological aura, the greater the indication for definitive psychotherapy to be combined with temporary removal from home; not simply to secure emotional readjustment but also to promote the child's rehabilitation. Figure 13 shows that without positive intervention, relapse tends to occur soon after the patient's return home, through re-exposure to the original stressful stimuli. (3) If re-educative psychotherapy is indicated where there is positive over-investment, it is even more urgent where the affective aura is negative. Indeed, the more challenging or threatening the emotional climate within the home, the longer the child takes to settle down in hospital and respond physiologically, and the more intensive the psychotherapeutic approach called for. Since these are the cases which also show more serious impairment of ventilatory function, pharmacological and psychological considerations will be seen to be complementary rather than mutually exclusive. (4) Hitherto the more severely affected cases have been thought of as "genuine" or "organic," and therefore, by implication, "non-psychological". Thus these children are referred to as stoical and uncomplaining, while their parents are regarded as sensibly objective and unemotional in their management. This is in accord with their low neuroticism score on the M.P.I. scale. Therefore, the more serious the disability, the less it has tended to be linked with psychodynamic factors, and the less appropriate the considered need for psychotherapy. On the contrary, our study suggests that if it is misleading to dismiss the "psychological" case as insignificant, it is equally misleading to dismiss the severe case as "non-psychological." (5) In fact the term "psychological" as applied to juvenile asthma is altogether too diffuse and non-specific to be meaningful. Erroneously it has been restricted to the attitude of "fussing" overprotection and therefore "psychological" cases have come misleadingly to be regarded as universally mild. This study has shown that psycho-dynamic factors operate throughout the physiological spectrum, and since the more severely affected cases are those at greater risk, psychotherapeutic intervention with this group, to re-orientate the negative affect, may well be the more pressing indication.

302
Pinkerton P. **Childhood asthma.** Br J Hosp Med 6:331-338, 1971.

▶ psychotherapy, milieu therapy, consultation-liaison

Since we cannot eradicate the basic substrate of immunophysiological vulnerability, we should think in terms of providing a service rather than a cure. To this end, whatever the orientation of therapy prescribed, be it pharmacological, physiological, anti-allergic or psychotherapeutic, the object is to stabilize the labile bronchus. If this can be achieved in a setting of long-term support by physician, allergist and psychiatrist, working in concert to promote realistic acceptance, then the success of management is assured.

303

Pollnow H, Petow H, Wittkower E. **Psychotherapy for bronchial asthma.** Z Klin Med 110: 701-721, 1929. (in German: no English abstract)

▶ psychotherapy

304

Pozner H. **Short-term psychotherapy in the treatment of asthma.** J R Army Med Corps 98:15-21, 1952.

▶ psychotherapy

A very brief summary is made of the more important contributions to the literature of asthma and psychiatry. Two cases are described of long-standing asthmatic syndromes in military personnel, with comments on predisposing emotional stresses, treatment and progress. It is concluded that in certain selected cases of asthma, where psychological factors are predominant, short-term psychotherapy initiated in hospital and continued in an outpatient clinic may achieve immediately satisfactory results, shorten the periods of hospitalization and absence from duty, and restore valuable personnel to full and efficient military employment.

305

Prout CT. **Psychiatric aspects of asthma.** Psychiatr Q 25:237-250, 1951.

▶ review: psychotherapy

1. The literature on the emotional aspects of asthma has been reviewed. 2. The histories of five bronchial asthma patients hospitalized for mental illness have been presented. 3. The genesis of asthma is from allergy alone, from allergy and emotional factors, and in some cases is purely emotional. 4. Greater progress has been made in the understanding of asthmatic patients and their personalities than in relieving the invalidism of the asthma.

306

Rackemann FM. **Other factors besides allergy in asthma.** JAMA 142:534-538, 1950.

▶ doctor-patient relationship

1. The kind of asthma which begins after age 40 is not often due to allergy: the cause is something which the patient carries with him at all times. 2. Infections in the respiratory tract, primary or secondary, are important. 3. More general disturbances of the body as a whole are more important—they are called "psychosomatic." 4. Physical disturbances—focal infections, malnutrition or poor general health from any cause—must be recognized, for they make a vicious circle with the asthma. The clinical history will tell whether these disturbances are cause or effect. 5. Emotional factors are always present. Fear of the asthma must be controlled: the patient must be "protected" and given confidence. 6. Three observations support the theory of a psychosomatic disturbance as the basis of the asthma: (a) the good results of general treatment on that basis; (b) the good results obtained in many clinics which protect the patient and encourage him, and (c) the fact that death from asthma can occur from nothing more than emotional strain. 7. When the nature of the inherited factor, the nature of the common denominator and the mechanism of its release are understood, the treatment of asthma will be greatly simplified.

307

Raines GN. **Psychiatric aspects of asthma.** Med Ann DC 18:354-357, 1949.

▶ psychotherapy

In summary, asthma presents itself to the psychiatrist as a clear-cut psychoneurosis, characterized by the combination of a specifically determined somatic and psychic apparatus stimulated to pathologic response by an emotional disturbance arising in some interpersonal relation, manifesting itself clinically in psychiatric and somatic symptomatology, and yielding to properly applied therapy at any of the several levels of its development.

308

Reed JW. **Emotional factors in bronchial asthma.** Psychosomatics 3:57-66, 1962.

▶ psychotherapy

1. Historical data are presented from the time of Hippocrates, more than 2,000 years ago, to the present, regarding the experimental and clinical studies that have been done regarding the emotional and psychological factors in bronchial asthma. 2. On the basis of these data and his own clinical experience, the author presents a concept of the interaction of the etiological factors in asthma, i.e., allergic, infectious, endocrine, physical and emotional. He suggests that the emotional state of the patient (either vulnerable or non-vulnerable) plays a critical role in determining whether or not a susceptible individual will experience an asthma attack, when exposed to non-psychological etiological factors. 3. A discussion of some of the theories of the psychopathology of asthma is presented, with emphasis upon Wolff's concept that disease (asthma)

may well represent a symptom of man's unsuccessful attempt to deal with life's stresses. 4. A method of comprehensive, that is, medical and psychological treatment of asthma is discussed, with some specific recommendations regarding the pharmacotherapy of the condition. It is also suggested that psychotherapy for the asthmatic patient, although specifically indicated and necessary, is frequently overlooked or inappropriately given in many cases, for a variety of reasons. 5. Some techniques, types and objectives of individual and group psychotherapy in bronchial asthma are briefly discussed. 6. In conclusion, it is strongly recommended that a remarkable decrease in both the morbidity and the mortality of bronchial asthma will ensue if greater emphasis is placed on the significance and treatment of the emotional factors involved, rather than the continued overemphasis and concern regarding the infectious and allergic factors involved, which seems to be the principal approach of the majority of physicians treating this complex disorder today.

309

Rogerson CH. **Psychological factors in asthma.** Br Med J 1:406-407, 1943.

▶ family therapy, psychotherapy

Having formulated these general principles the treatment would appear clear enough. In many cases the person best able to modify and direct the child's personality development is the child's own parent, and the physician's role should be that of guide to the parents, and often their supporter in their efforts to follow his instructions. He should bear in mind that the relationship which he observes may not be entirely the fault of the parents, who are often not such fools as they may appear. Where the child's personality is very difficult psychiatric help may be required in modification, but the psychological problem is usually best dealt with by the physician who is looking after the case and who is in control of all the remedial agents. I do not believe there is any doubt that psychological treatment of the kind I have described can play a very important part in moderating the symptoms. Perhaps I may fittingly conclude with the remark of the mother of the child whose case I described at the beginning, who said after a period of guidance: "He used always to cling to me and wheeze so dreadfully; but now I have made him stand on his own bottom, and he does not have asthma any more."

310

Rogerson CH, Hardcastle DH, Duguid K. **A psychological approach to asthma and asthma-eczema-prurigo syndrome.** Guy's Hosp Rep 85:289-308, 1935.

▶ psychotherapy

In summarizing the practical aspects of our results we may say that in any case where "nervousness" is a prom-

inent complaint or where the personality of the patient appears to be abnormal, psychotherapy can contribute materially to the treatment of the case. The psychiatric problem presented can be approached in two ways. (1) Through attention to the personality difficulties of the patient. (2) Through attention to the environmental stresses. In the case of the adult the environment is a relatively fixed quantity and attention has therefore to be directed to the patient's own personality, its needs and strivings. In the case of the child, however, the environment is more easily adjusted. This may be done in various ways and it may prove valuable to direct attention to the personality of the parents along the lines just mentioned. The child himself may be treated in the same way as the adult, if sufficiently advanced in understanding, or a more indirect method may be employed in an endeavour to enable him to understand and express himself as fully as possible.

311

Sadler JE Jr. **Childhood asthma from the point of view of the liaison child psychiatrist.** Psychiatr Clin North Am 5:333-343, 1982.

▶ review: consultation-liaison, psychotherapy

Childhood asthma represents a significant pediatric illness that can be viewed as a specific example of Engle's biopsychosocial model. While recent medical pharmacologic advances in the treatment of the hyperreactive pulmonary tree have been exciting, the liaison child psychiatrist has a clear role in individual assessment, evaluation of family contributions to the precipitating and exacerbating events, as well as elaborating the factors causing maintenance of an illness posture by children and their families. The child psychiatrist can then play an effective role in developing hospital-based, school, and community programs to foster the developing child's autonomy in the mastery of his illness. These services are an adjunct to the unique role of the child psychiatrist in working with the child as his own person with his own unique struggle with his asthma, when individual child psychotherapy is diagnostically indicated.

312

Sadler JE Jr. **Coordinated pediatric care through a liaison team.** Pediatr Ann 1:72-78, 1972.

▶ consultation-liaison

History shows that collaborative relationships between child psychiatrists and pediatricians have not always been friendly. Development of the team concept in the child guidance movement provided the foundation for child psychiatrists working in team relationships in pediatric settings. The concept of the liaison team forms the basis for the emergence of a comprehensive picture of the child. At National Jewish Hospital [Denver, Colorado] such teams are continuing to try to deal with the whole child in spite of the problems involved.

313

Sampliner RB. **Psychic aspects of bronchial asthma: review and synthesis of the literature.** Psychiatr Q 13:521-533, 1939.

▶ review: psychotherapy, milieu therapy

Because asthma is a disease which leads, when allowed to run an unchecked course, to definite physical changes, it is important that it be successfully treated from its earliest stages. If allowed to continue under symptomatic treatment the patient will progress to outspoken emphysema, chronic bronchitis, or even status asthmaticus (which is apt to be fatal at any time), and then very little can be done for him. Because asthmatics usually receive the benefits of psychotherapy only after other means of treatment has failed, Gillespie pleads that every asthmatic be given a psychic workup by a competent psychiatrist, in addition to his medical examination. It is only in this fashion that we can decide early enough to prevent organic complications which patients come under the classification of psychogenic asthma. As to methods of therapy I have little to say. The wisest and most logical therapeutic method would seem to be a comprehensive one, aimed at both allergic and psychic factors. Actual desensitization may be of value. The one paramount consideration is that the patient is a personality and personalized treatment will be best for him. If this concept be embraced, the actual mode of treatment can be left to the clinical acumen of the physician.

314

Scalettar HE. **The holistic management of the adolescent asthmatic.** Acta Paediatr Scand (Suppl) 1: 256:27, 1975. (abstract)

▶ psychoanalysis, supportive psychotherapy

The difficulties encountered in the management of the adolescent asthmatic are presented. The overemphasis of the psychoanalytic view of asthma is scored. Theoretical concepts have been found wanting under statistical scrutiny. Asthma is briefly discussed with emphasis on recent definitions, classification, causes of status and the partial beta adrenergic blockade theory. The holistic view is stressed, with the main emphasis on environmental influences and supportive psychotherapy. A review of 70 cases of asthma in a special adolescent unit is reported. The approach to the adolescent in general and the specific influence of the incitant factor of animal dander are emphasized. The heterogeneous personalities and variable psychopathology of our young people is recorded. Many cases of recalcitrant asthma were modified and reversed by adhering to holistic principles. The primary physician should be the most important person in successful management of bronchial asthma. The psychiatric approach oft-times delays proper therapy. The recognition of a variety of environmental influences is of paramount importance in attaining the goal of reversibility. A disservice is rendered if one ignores the genetic, constitutional predisposition, the associated trigger mechanisms, and instead, indulges in the exclusivity of a primary psychiatric role in asthma.

315

Scherbel AB. **Treatment of bronchial asthma with psychotherapy.** US Armed Forces Med J 1:558-561, 1950.

▶ psychotherapy, family therapy

This patient presented a problem of severe bronchial asthma associated with a moderately severe personality disorder. His asthma appeared directly related to a combination of definite allergic diathesis, plus a disturbed emotional situation in the family environment, manifested primarily by poor parent-child relationships. Over a relatively short period of therapy in which the boy was seen once each week for 13 weeks by the psychiatrist, and the mother for half-hour periods at similar intervals by the psychiatric social worker, definite improvement occurred in family interpersonal relationships as well as in the boy's personality. The complete clinical remission of the patient's asthma, with the exception of one brief episode early in the pollen season, would seem to indicate that psychogenic factors were operating as an important trigger mechanism in setting off this patient's attacks of bronchial asthma.

316

Schultz JH. **Asthma as a psychotherapy problem.** Zentrabl Inn Med 50:344-361, 1929. (in German: no English abstract)

▶ psychotherapy

317

Schultz JH. **Psychotherapy for bronchial asthma.** Dtsch Med Wochenschr 54:964-965, 1928. (in German: no English abstract)

▶ psychotherapy

318

Schwobel G. **Psychosomatic therapy of bronchial asthma.** Arztl Forsch 2:481-487, 1948. (in German: no English abstract)

▶ autogenic training

319

Selesnick ST, Friedman DB, Augenbaum B. **Psychological management of asthma.** Calif Med 100:406-411, 1964.

▶ counseling, psychotherapy

Over-emphasis on physical factors in asthma probably has come about because psychological factors have seemed elusive, difficult to define and often misleading. Several concepts of classic causes of emotional disturbances that abet asthmatic attacks in children may be helpful in management of the patient and his environs. The first concept has to do with feelings of inadequacy in the mother which lead her to place the burden of decision-making upon the child. She is thus able to give the child very little support and communicates to him her anxiety. Often encouragement to the mother, through the physician's pointing out her very real capacities and achievements can be helpful to the child. The second concept has to do with the asthmatic child's character structure and his assumption of a pseudo-mature position. Among the things the physician can do is to advise the parents as to what is age-appropriate behavior for the child and instruct them in ways to make the child recognize his position of dependence. The third concept concerns threat of separation as a precipitant to the asthma attack. To deal with such a situation the physician may make a number of recommendations of methods for alleviating such a threat. In some families, the degree of disturbance is so great that the parents cannot respond to the physician's advice and may need psychiatric referral. Clues for recognizing such a situation are given along with recommendations on how to make a successful referral.

320

Sperling M. **Asthma in children: an evaluation of concepts and therapies.** J Am Acad Child Psychiatry 4:44-58, 1968.

▶ psychotherapy

It should be obvious by now that I do not regard the treatment of asthma as a simple matter. But then again even the rehabilitation of a neurosis requires expert handling and time. In a psychosomatic disease, such as asthma, the underlying personality disturbances and interrelated family dynamics are of a more severe pathological nature and one should anticipate and be prepared for the magnitude of the task. I am certainly not saying this in order to discourage doctors from treating asthmatic children. On the contrary, I rather hope that a fuller understanding and a more thorough approach by child psychiatrists to the problems involved in childhood asthma could be a stimulating and educational influence on pediatricians, allergists, and all those who see the child early enough to be able to spot the forerunners or earliest stages of asthma,

when by proper management the full course of events could still be prevented.

321

Stamm J, Drapkin A. **The successful treatment of a severe case of bronchial asthma: a manifestation of an abnormal mourning reaction and traumatic neurosis.** J Nerv Ment Dis 142:180-189, 1966.

▶ psychotherapy

A case of severe, nearly fatal, bronchial asthma has been presented. This syndrome developed for the first time a few weeks after the traumatic death of a seven-year-old son. It is our contention that the asthma was part of an abnormal mourning reaction based on a pathological narcissistic identification with the lost object and strongly resembled the picture of a traumatic neurosis. The asthma also expressed a need for punishment. The guilt complex in turn was related to his marked ambivalent feelings for his wife, to his pre-marital sexual indulgence with her and on a deeper level to his Oedipal guilt. The asthma permitted him to escape from an intolerable home situation and gratify his passive, homosexual yearnings. Although there was considerable secondary gain in the illness, it was not as great a factor as had been anticipated. Considerable improvement occurred after two years of treatment. This involved the close collaboration of both medical and psychiatric staffs; and the psychotherapy employed had to be considerably modified. The unequivocal importance of the psychic factor in this case is confirmed by the fact that on repeated occasions the patient would relapse upon returning home even while receiving the same medication he had had in the hospital. Six and one-half years after discharge medical examination indicated that the patient was asymptomatic, with only occasional minimal wheezing, and carrying on a full work schedule. Since July, 1959, there have been no hospitalizations and he has not missed a single day of work.

322

Steiner M, Elizur A, Davidson S. **A psychosomatic triad in a bipolar patient.** J Nerv Ment Dis 164:359-361, 1977.

▶ psychotherapy

A 56-year-old white male with a rare case of psychosomatic triad occurring during a single depressive episode is presented. The dynamics, course, and treatment are discussed. It is suggested that common psychosomatic mechanisms are interacting with the bipolar illness.

323

Steptoe A, Holmes R. **Mood and pulmonary function in adult asthmatics: a pilot self-monitoring study.** Br J Med Psychol 58:87-94, 1985.

▶ counseling

The relationship between mood and fluctuations in peak expiratory flow rate (PEF) was studied in seven mildly asthmatic adult men and seven non-asthmatic controls. Participants completed visual analogue mood scales and measured PEF four times per day for 24 days, and the Profile of Mood States was also filled in at the end of each day. Significant correlations between mood and PEF were found in six of the asthmatics. No specific asthma-related profile was identified, since each person showed idiosyncratic associations between mood and pulmonary function. The non-asthmatics did not show consistent correlations above a level expected by chance. Possible explanations of these results and their relevance to the management of asthma are discussed.

324
Straker N, Bieber J. **Asthma and the vicissitudes of aggression: two case reports of childhood asthma.** J Am Acad Child Psychiatry 16:132-139, 1977.

▶ review: psychotherapy

We report two children with childhood asthma who without prior evidence of psychosis manifested transient and completely reversible psychotic episodes in the course of psychotherapy. The dynamic conflicts which precipitated the transient psychosis would previously have precipitated an asthmatic episode had aggressive conflicts remained repressed. A brief review of the literature on the subjects of asthma and aggression and psychosis and asthma is presented. An attempt is made to explain the relationship between the observed psychotic episodes, the observed asthmatic episodes, and the vicissitudes of the aggression in these patients.

325
Strauss EB. **The psychogenic factor in asthma.** Guy's Hosp Rep 85:309-316, 1935.

▶ psychotherapy, play therapy

Extracted summary: It has long been known that psychic factors play a role in the determination of asthmatic attacks. Some observers prefer to talk about pseudo-asthma—i.e., the state in which asthma-like attacks occur in the absence of the asthmatic diathesis—and true asthma, which they would regard as a constitutional disease belonging to the allergic group of dyscrasias. On the other hand there are extremists who would like to consider asthma as a neurosis pure and simple—i.e., a form of conversion-hysteria with a constant semiology. Similarly certain people include Graves' disease, epilepsy, gastric and duodenal ulcers in the group of functional nervous disorders. There are certainly cases of asthma which for various reasons (i.e., the mode and age of onset, the inability to demonstrate sensitivity to any special allergens, and the like) appear to be predominantly psychogenic in the sense of "complex-determined." I described two cases of this kind

as long ago as 1927. Since then I have come across several more such cases.

326
Strauss EB. **The psychogenic factor in asthma (II): Asthma in adults.** Guy's Hospital Rep 87:273-286, 1937.

▶ psychotherapy, psychoanalysis, hypnosis, suggestion

What are the conclusions which can be legitimately drawn from these results? It would, perhaps, be wise if one were to point out a false inference, viz.: that asthma should be classified as a psychoneurosis. The furthest that one can go is to conclude that, even in the presence of the allergic diathesis, psychic factors contribute to the asthma syndrome in greater measure than has previously been thought likely. The study of detailed case-histories shows that this psychic participation takes various forms. 1. In its psychic aspects, asthma may in certain cases be complex-determined, i.e., included in the group of the conversion hysterias. 2. A person with the allergic diathesis, who is temperamentally a deviant from the conventional norm of his immediate social group, is likely to develop the asthma syndrome. 3. An asthmatic subject is liable to make his asthma the centre of his life, i.e., to develop and cultivate an asthmatic persona (to use one of Jung's terms). Such a person by the mechanism of what Kretschmer calls arbitrary reflex reinforcement can "turn on" his asthma on all possible occasions whenever it suits his unconscious or preconscious purposes. 4. Allergic subjects who live under conditions of extreme emotional strain and stress are liable to exhibit the asthma syndrome. 5. Asthma in an allergic subject may be part and parcel of a general anxiety state, the affect, when the anxiety-tension is very high, finding an autonomic reflex outlet. If these conclusions are justifiable, they suggest that psychotherapy, in the widest sense of the term, should reinforce physical methods of treatment (desensitisation, breathing exercises, and the like), the form of psychotherapy being determined by the case history. Analytical psychotherapy would appear to be indicated in groups 1 and 5. Patients who fall into group 2 should benefit by a personality analysis, as opposed to an experiential analysis (vide Kretschmer), and taught how to accept and adapt themselves to their own temperamental patterns. In the case of group 4, it will sometimes prove possible by means of active interference to modify the patient's environmental conditions. Patients who fall into group 3 should respond well to suggestive methods with or without hypnosis.

327
Studt HH. **Psychodynamics of the conflict provoking situation in bronchial asthma.** Z Psychosom Med Psychoanal 18:271-285, 1972. (in German: no English abstract)

▶ psychoanalysis

328

Theopold A. **Clinical contribution to the psychogenesis of bronchial asthma.** Z Psychosom Med 2:105, 1956. (in German)

▶ psychotherapy

329

Van Stegmann A. **Results of psychological treatment of some cases of asthma.** Zentralbl Psychoanal 1:377-382, 1911. (in German: no English abstract)

▶ psychotherapy

330

Von Leupold W. **Pathogenesis and therapy of bronchial asthma in children.** Kinderarztl Prax 42:391-401, 1974. (in German: no English abstract)

▶ psychotherapy

331

Weber A. **Psychosomatics of bronchial asthma in childhood.** Monatsschr Kinderheilkd 124:224-226, 1976. (in German: no English abstract)

▶ psychotherapy

332

Weiss E. **Psychoanalysis of a case of nervous asthma.** Int Z Psychoanal 8:440-455, 1922. (in German: no English abstract)

▶ psychoanalysis

333

Weiss E. **Emotional factors in allergy with special reference to asthma.** Arch Allergy 14:148-161, 1959.

▶ psychoanalysis

Psychosomatic study of an allergic problem utilizes separate techniques—physiological and psychological—applied simultaneously. This approach will frequently demonstrate that in a given case physical and emotional factors act in a complementary fashion to produce the disorder—in one instance specific physical factors may predominate, in another instance specific emotional factors. These are discussed. Personality disturbances both precede and follow bronchial asthma. The personality disturbances that antedate the asthma often have a causal relationship to the disorder while the emotional disturbances that follow often permit the patient to exploit the asthmatic symptoms for secondary gain. A case of chronic bronchial asthma is presented in which both sets of factors operate. Recovery, which has been maintained for eight years, followed successful psychoanalysis.

334

Wellisch E. **The Rorschach method as an aid to the psychotherapy of an asthmatic child.** Br J Med Psychol 22:72-87, 1949.

▶ psychotherapy, family therapy

Extracted summary: This study of the psychotherapy of a child suffering from bronchial asthma illustrates the value of the Rorschach method as a therapeutic aid. A case of asthma was particularly interesting to use as an example because an "asthmatic personality" has been described and the Rorschach method aims at exploring the structure of the personality.

335

Wilson CP. **Psychosomatic asthma and acting out: a case of bronchial asthma that developed de novo in the terminal phase of analysis.** Int J Psychoanal 49:330-335, 1968.

▶ psychoanalysis, psychotherapy

Extracted summary: Many years of experience with these and other asthmatic cases have led me to the following conclusions: the mothers in each case want their children to be sick and dependent; the basic dynamic structure is the same in asthma as in the phobias; omnipotence and magical thinking play a predominant role; one psychosomatic symptom is often exchanged for another—in the woman patient the weeping and psoriasis were replaced by asthma. There is no personality profile for the asthmatic and the unconscious fantasies behind the asthma vary from one patient to another. The psychosomatic disease can be termed a pregenital conversion neurosis; and an over-strict superego is present with the psychosomatic symptom. Sperling (1963) found similar dynamics in her work with asthmatic children. My experience with these and other psychosomatic problems indicate that classical analysis is the treatment of choice for patients with psychosomatic symptoms and that psychosomatic symptoms occurring during analysis are typical transference phenomena and can only be resolved in analysis.

336

Wilson CP. **Parental overstimulation in asthma.** Int J Psychoanal Psychother 8:601-621, 1980.

▶ psychoanalysis

A discussion of "The Role of Primal Scene and Masochism in Asthma," by Cecilia Karol, M.D. The author presents case material corroborating Dr. Karol's hypotheses about the role of primal scene exposure and sadomasochistic fantasies in asthma and which documents the thesis that primal scene is a part of a global pattern of parental overstimulation which in the pregenital maturational phases establishes the predisposition to develop asthma. He further confirms Melitta Sperling's hypothesis that unconscious conflicts of the mother or father predispose a child to the development of psychosomatic disease and that specific parental habits and fantasies involving the lungs determine the choice of the respiratory system for symptom formation.

337

Wittich GH. **Psychotherapy in bronchial asthma.** Prax Pneumol 28:327-332, 1974. (in German)

▶ psychotherapy

Realization that psychic factors play a part in the pathogenesis of bronchial asthma, i.e. recognition of bronchial asthma as a psychosomatic disease, has been helpful in the treatment of this condition. The benefits to be derived from psychotherapy alone should, however, not be overestimated.

338

Wittkower E, Petow H. **Reports on the clinical treatment of bronchial asthma and related conditions (V): On the psychogenesis of bronchial asthma.** Z Klin Med 119:293-306, 1932. (in German)

▶ psychotherapy

1) An allergic genesis of asthma without neurotic components is certainly valid for many cases of asthma. 2) A solely psychically influenced condition without somatic counterpart is also possible, in some cases actually probable, but not proven. 3) The vast majority of asthma cases are of dual nature.

339

Wolff HH. **Bronchial asthma, physical and psychological aspects.** J Irish Med Assoc 51:31-35, 1962.

▶ psychotherapy, doctor-patient relationship, suggestion, hypnosis

Extracted summary: When psychological factors are found to be of importance, and this will be the case in the majority of patients of all ages, simple psychotherapeutic interviews in which the patient is encouraged to talk freely and to express his emotions can be of very great benefit, as I have described. This can often be done by the patient's general practitioner, provided he has the time and interest to deal with the psychological problems involved. During such interviews it is essential to remain tolerant and sympathetic and to avoid being authoritative or disapproving, as asthmatic patients can easily be made worse and develop a severe attack if they feel themselves to be criticised, attacked or rejected. It is much more difficult to decide whether a patient needs more skilled psychoth-

erapeutic help from someone trained and experienced in analytical psychotherapy. In my experience such treatment, based on understanding of psychodynamics, can be of very real value in certain selected patients, particularly those who are intelligent enough to cooperate and who are aware of the fact that, quite apart from asthma, they have personal or psychoneurotic difficulties for which they would like help. Under such circumstances, prolonged psychotherapy, designed to give a patient psychological insight, can be of great benefit. It should be combined with the usual drug treatment required by asthmatics and, if necessary in a severe case, with steroids, but in my experience of psychotherapy of asthmatic patients, such drugs can gradually be reduced and often almost dispensed with as the patient gains understanding of the emotional basis of his asthma. This kind of treatment is of particular value from the point of view of research because it provides us with detailed understanding of the nature of the emotional disturbances which are of importance in the causation of asthma. Such understanding of the psychodynamic factors involved is, I find, of inestimable value when one is trying to help other patients in the course of a few interviews only. I should like to sound a word of warning, however, against the use of hypnosis, which is occasionally advised as a form of treatment for asthmatics. I have never used it personally, but I have seen cases which have been treated with hypnosis, some of whom, while their asthma has temporarily improved, have developed even more serious alternative illnesses as a substitute for asthma, including psychoses, severe anxiety states, or dermatitis.

340

Wright GL. **Asthma and the emotions: aetiology and treatment.** Med J Aust 1:961-967, 1965.

▶ counseling, supportive psychotherapy

A group of 233 asthmatics, adults and children, was studied with regard to the role played by emotional factors in their asthma. In 61% of cases, emotional factors appeared to affect the disease; acute emotional stress played a role in 47%, as did chronic emotional stress in 26%, and both were important in 12%. Patients with chronic emotional stress were not more likely to react to acute stress than the average. Continuous asthma was present in 55% of the cases studied. No relationship was found between (i) acute or chronic emotional stress and the likelihood of asthma becoming continuous, (ii) emotional stress and a history of infantile eczema, or (iii) infantile eczema and the likelihood of asthma becoming continuous. Chronic emotional stress was found to be (i) almost always (in 90% of cases) in interpersonal relationships, involving a member of the same household, (ii) mostly involving a relationship with a member of the opposite sex in that household (in 75% of cases), and (iii) mostly associated with an ineffective hostile reaction. The results of this study indicate that emotional stress (i) is very rarely the sole aetiological factor, (ii) may trigger off the development of asthma in a predisposed person, (iii) is no longer necessary for the continuance of asthma once it has developed, (iv) may affect the frequency and severity of episodes, but not the fundamental pattern of asthma in a given case, and (v) may mask changes occurring in the asthmatic state due to other factors, such as appear at adolescence. A study of patients with allergic rhinitis and of asthmatics who had emotional stress not related to their asthma suggests that, besides the presence of emotional stress, allergy and a general genetic predisposition, there is also required a state of potential "readiness" in the patient for the development of asthma at a particular time. General practitioners, because of access, specialized knowledge and experience, are in the best position to manage the emotional problems of their asthmatic patients. Other aetiological factors present need treatment at the same time as emotional stress.

341
Ziskind E. **Psychosomatic aspects of asthma: an eclectic therapeutic orientation for the non-psychiatrist physician.** Ann Allergy 24:153-161, 1966.

▶ psychotherapy, doctor-patient relationship, consultation-liaison

Two psychosomatic aspects for asthma have been considered, one of specific psychogenesis (chiefly espoused by psychoanalysts) and non-specific psychologic stresses leading to precipitation and/or aggravation of attacks. The former is unproven, the latter is well established. Primary psychogenicity calls for major psychotherapy by the psychiatrist, whereas secondary psychogenic stress effects call for minor psychotherapy. The latter should be carried out by the non-psychiatrist physician. The psychotherapeutic task, secondary to or associated with somatic therapies, is to care for the current situational stresses. The procedural guides for this type of therapy are presented in a number of tables with minimal discussion. The first task is to accept the responsibility of interpreting the psychogenicity of the patient; the second is to know the goals of psychotherapy, recognizing those within the sphere of the non-psychiatrist; the third is to acquire psychotherapeutic skills. These are best attained under supervision and should be added to the somatic therapeutic armamentarium of the family physician and allergist.

Combined Therapies

342
Ago Y, Ikemi Y, Sugita M, Takahashi N, Toyama N. **Treatment of bronchial asthma.** J Asthma Res 14:33-35, 1976.

▶ psychotherapy, autogenic training, behavior therapy, doctor-patient relationship

(1) To manage the patient's attacks so that we may establish a therapeutic trust relationship and thereby mo-

tivate him. (2) To help the patient understand that it is important for him to pay more careful attention to the factors composing the preparatory psychophysiological conditions (preasthmatic conditions) than to the precipitating factors. a) To help the patient be aware of the physiological conditions which may cause asthmatic attacks. (Autogenic training is effective at this stage). b) To help the patient be aware of relationship between the preasthmatic state and life situations or environmental conditions. c) To help the patient be aware of emotional states and interpersonal attitudes or behaviors in daily life situations and environment conditions. (Transactional analysis is effective at this stage.) (3) To help the patient modify his distorted perception, unnatural attitudes and maladaptive behaviors which he has acquired since childhood, and to help the patient manage the factors composing the preasthmatic conditions by learning a new mode of adaptation to apply to his daily life without much conscious effort.

343
Bentley J. **A psychotherapeutic approach to treating asthmatic children in a residential setting.** J Asthma Res 12:21-25, 1974.

▶ psychotherapy, milieu therapy

Extracted summary: No matter how amenable a child is to individual psychotherapy, however, the therapist's goals in a residential treatment center are more severely limited than they are in any other setting. The child will go home in a year or two, and whether or not he will continue to receive treatment with another therapist will depend largely on parental attitudes and economic circumstances. Therapists must be willing to face the possibility, too, that the child may be returning to a home situation which has not improved substantially since his leaving it. Under such circumstances, the permanent behavioral change which therapist and therapeutic personnel in the residence are able to effect may be less than one would hope for. The possibility for change, in any case, will be very much dependent on whether or not all those who work with the child can coordinate their efforts. Here again, the weekly staff meeting, with its discussions focusing on day-to-day interactions in the residence, is an essential.

344
Biermann G. **Bronchial asthma in childhood and adolescence from the psychosomatic point of view.** Z Allgemeinmed 46:494-498, 1970. (in German)

▶ autogenic training, milieu therapy, family therapy, psychotherapy, group therapy

345

Blumenthal MN, Cushing RT, Fashingbauer TJ. **A community program for the management of bronchial asthma.** Ann Allergy 30:391-398, 1972.

▶ milieu therapy, social casework, group therapy, family therapy

A community program for the management of bronchial asthma is described consisting of a school-year program which is made up of exercises, games, group discussions and instructional sessions for both the patient and family and a summer camp which is conducted as normally as possible without giving undue attention to the asthma. Results indicate that this program is achieving improvement in the physical condition of the patients, a better psychosocial adjustment to asthma and further education of the patient, his family and the community with regard to asthma and how to deal with it.

346

Burns KL. **Behavioral health care in asthma.** Public Health Rev 10:339-381, 1982.

▶ biofeedback, behavior therapy, relaxation

Asthma is a significant public health problem with regard to prevalence and cumulative costs to society and individual well-being. A biobehavioral framework is proposed wherein the central problem in asthma is viewed as the hyperreactive airway over which a degree of self-regulative control is attainable. Adaptive self-management practices are reviewed for (a) the prevention of symptoms and (b) their management upon occurrence. Emotional and cognitive influences, biofeedback and relaxation therapies and the psychosocial and developmental consequences of asthma are also reviewed from the standpoint of behavioral health care. The means whereby patients are enabled to attain greater health care knowledge and skills are discussed in terms of emerging trends in health psychology, professional training, health team composition and public health planning.

347

Carmona A, Leclerc C. **Respiratory psychosomatic changes: asthma.** Rev Med Chile 101:646-656, 1973. (in Spanish)

▶ review: psychoanalysis, milieu therapy

It is postulated as a hypothesis that some of the aetiological mechanisms of asthma may be explained as an instrumental apprenticeship of the autonomic response, which in its turn acts as a means to reduce some type of emotional stress. It is pointed out that in the present concepts of allergic asthma, and psychogenic asthma the differences between these two groups is not always clear and frequently it is impossible to separate the allergic factors from the emotional factors. According to experimental evidence, asthma may be learned. Reactions arising from Pavlovian conditioning may exist both in psychological and allergic asthma. The frequency of psychoneurotic upheavals or problems of character in the personality of the asthmatic is not sufficient for these to be classed as the personality of the asthmatic. Review of the literature shows clearly that the anguish, need for dependence, Oedipus complexes, castration fears, competitive impulses, envy, jealousy, repressed hostility, etc., which have been attributed as characteristics of the asthmatic personality, are also found in patients suffering from diseases which are frankly organic or who suffer from other psychological symptoms. These characteristics are also to be found in so called "normal" subjects. Aetiologies of psychoanalytic orientation claim that asthma surges from internal impulses that threaten the "linking of a person with his mother figure." Without doubt, well controlled clinical observations show that this affirmation is questionable, as many asthmatic children separated from their homes recover from their symptoms when separated from their parents and deteriorate when returned home. On the other hand, analytic therapy given over several years does not appear to give positive results in the treatment of this alteration. The authors emphasize the necessity to consider the problem from new aetiological standpoints and present evidence as to the voluntary modification of the respiratory responses and the apprenticeship to "present" the symptoms. It is supposed that there exists the possibility to learn to exaggerate the intensity of the state of equilibrium of the bronchial response and to diminish its latency; by earlier experiences, exteroceptive stimuli will have been associated with emotionally conflictive experiences that the patient "does not wish" to record again or will have learned to not agree with.

348

Cernelc D, Skuber P, Kos S. **The medical and psychological study of children with asthma—controled study of allergic and psychological background of asthmatic children.** Allerg Asthma (Leipz) 14:33-43, 1968.

▶ milieu therapy, psychotherapy, family therapy, group therapy, play therapy, art therapy

278 children with asthma were compared medically and psychologically with 27 rheumatic children as a control of the same sex, age and socio-economical situation and similar psychological family relationships. All statistical explorations showed significant higher disturbances in asthmatic children and their mothers than in control group. The results of psychotherapy in asthmatic children and emotionally disturbed mothers were most satisfactory.

349
Cohen SI. **Psychological factors in asthma.** Postgrad Med J 47:533-540, 1971.

▶ couples therapy, supportive psychotherapy, behavior therapy, hypnosis, placebo

Extracted summary: This illustration of the summation of emotional factors and of the way simple psychotherapy may proceed in asthma, while not an everyday experience, is by no means uncommon. Many patients, however, present more complex problems, and may then have to be dealt with much more intensively, although the particular method of psychotherapy used will depend more upon the nature of the patient's problems than upon the fact that he has asthma. Psychotherapy acts principally by helping to reduce anxiety and tension; it does this by helping the patient to deal with his problems, by interrupting the vicious circle involving anxiety which is so often present, and sometimes more directly by encouragement, support and suggestion. Clinical evidence would indicate that the effect on the trachea and main bronchi, as described by the Dutch workers, may be of considerable importance in a substantial number of asthmatics, especially in the sort of patient whose wheezing stops extremely quickly once he is put at his ease, and it is a frequent observation that there are patients in whom the wheezing can be, as it were, switched on and switched off during an interview according to the topic under discussion. Using this model, one could argue that one is more likely to be successful in treatment if one sees the patient before changes dependent upon autonomic responses, such as increased secretion into the bronchi, have become established. It is general experience that a substantial number of asthmatic attacks will subside in response to simple psychological measures which may amount to no more than the presence of a doctor who inspires both confidence and tranquility. This type of management, which I have characterized as "the hand-holding technique in the treatment of asthma," may operate through reduction of anxiety, through suggestion, and through the interruption of the conditioned responses, while the pharmacalogical effects of any drugs given may at times be less important than their placebo effects.

350
Conners CK. **Psychological management of the asthmatic child.** Clin Rev Allergy 1:163-177, 1983.

▶ review: relaxation, autogenic training, hypnosis, suggestion, placebo, biofeedback, psychotherapy, psychoanalysis, family therapy, group therapy

Based upon a thorough assessment of the asthmatic child and his or her family, one should devise an individual treatment plan that includes provision for operationally defining target symptoms (including measurement of both pulmonary function and the behavioral symptoms of interest); gathering a baseline with enough repeated measurements to ensure stability; careful specification of an intervention procedure, with appropriate methods to ensure compliance; a treatment phase during which data are collected regarding response to treatment; and regular follow-up and maintenance treatments as required. The practitioner who wishes to apply one of the many available treatment modalities where previous research has been insufficient or equivocal faces a dilemma. He or she must act despite the lack of sound information. There is a strong tendency in the face of the psychological complexities to develop a therapeutic nihilism and to rely solely upon pharmacologic or immunologic treatment. Consequently it is desirable to employ procedures that are operational, give continuous feedback regarding progress, and are limited enough in scope that they have some chance of being implemented within the immediate future. Too many treatable children have had the severe complications and precipitants of their disease ignored or have been left to languish in interminable, poorly defined treatment programs whose components are either unspecified or so vague as to be useless. Many of the behavioral programs described above have shown promising results, and choosing among them becomes a problem. One solution is to implement the least expensive and most direct approaches first, followed by others in succession or combination. For example, verbal suggestion produces relaxation and behavioral change, and so does biofeedback. The two together might be more effective than either alone, or simple suggestion might do as well as both. This has been found for example in the comparison of relaxation and assertive training for asthmatics. Although the combination is best, assertiveness training by itself adds very little to the results.

351
Coodley A. **Psychosomatic aspects of asthma.** Western Med 7:334-338, 1966.

▶ psychotherapy, milieu therapy, family therapy, group psychotherapy, hypnosis, doctor-patient relationship

The precipitating event or context in which bronchial asthma occurs is the crucial key to understanding the relevant psychosomatic implications. Asthma has been variously interpreted as a protective adaptive reaction, a learned response, a cry for mother's love, or a substitute for neurosis or psychosis. It is most often linked with allergic, atopic heredity. Treatment of the asthmatic reflects the diverse etiological theories as well as the orientation or bias of the physician. It may be that the reciprocal doctor-patient relationship is the medium in which all psychological and to some extent physical therapy occurs. Of particular treatment relevance is the value of confession or emotional catharsis.

352

Creer TL. **Asthma.** J Consult Clin Psychol 50:912-921, 1982.

▶ behavior therapy, psychotherapy

This article focuses on the assessment and treatment of the asthmatic patient. Problems that arise in the assessment process are illustrated by describing three areas of concern to medicine and psychology: diagnosis, characteristics of asthma, and classification. Psychological and behavioral approaches to treatment are also described. It is concluded that behavioral scientists have a role in the assessment and treatment of the asthmatic patient, particularly in respect to the management of asthma-related behaviors. To fulfill this promise, however, we need to become more familiar with the course of the disorder and to learn how to medically investigate and control asthma.

353

De Boucaud M, Darquey J, Gachie JP. **Psychosomatic outlooks of asthma.** Sem Hop Paris 44:2953-2957, 1968. (in French: no English abstract)

▶ psychotherapy, group therapy

354

De Vicente P, Posada JL. **Medical sophrology and yoga respiration in the physiotherapy of bronchial asthma.** Allergol Immunopathol (Madr) 6:297-310, 1978. (in Spanish)

▶ relaxation, yoga, breathing exercises

[T]he authors made a study, as described in their monograph, of experiments carried out with the aid of twenty volunteers. Their ages ranged from seven to 72 years, and they had all received some training in a technique combining Caycedo's dynamic relaxation Grade II with that method of breathing which is basic to the practice of yoga. Their training in relaxation was carried out according to the rules of the International School of Medical Sophrology. Their breathing exercises followed those of the Yoga Research Institute of Kaivalyadhama, India. The technique can be summarized as follows: The abdominal muscles and the diaphragm must be used in breathing. The duration of exhalation must be double that of the inhalation. Resistance must be made to the free passage of air when breathing in and out, by contracting the larynx or by pursing the lips. The patient must let his mind follow the process of exhalation, and then the doctor must induce relaxation by Caycedo's dynamic relaxation (the methods of Schultz or Jacobson, are similar). In making the experiments the authors used a Collins spirometer. The oxygen consumption was registered twice. The first time for ten minutes with the subject resting and using normal breathing; the second time also for ten minutes, but using the technique summarized above, and in which the subject had been trained. The reading of the spirometer showed an average reduction of 54% of oxygen consumed when the breathing technique was used, compared with normal breathing. The greatest deviation obtained was 73% less oxygen consumed, and the least 43% less. The authors also recorded an improvement in the maximal voluntary ventilation rate per minute, of an average of 40% with the technique, over normal breathing. The reduction in the consumption of oxygen is found to be due to several factors brought into play by the combination of the two techniques: I—Caycedo's dynamic relaxation, Grade II: Causes a decrease in muscular tension and results in a lower oxygen consumption. Lessens distress and anxiety and increases emotional control. Facilitates the practice of yogic breathing. II—Breathing according to the practice of yoga: Increases pulmonary perfusion, by an increase in negative thoracic pressure made by resistance to free flow of air when breathing in (similar to Muller's manoeuvre). The same resistance when breathing out avoids a tendency to bronchial collapse. Increases alveolar ventilation because of a reduction of volume of dead space gas, and improves diaphragmatic mobility. Reduces the consumption of oxygen. Finally, the authors conclude that if the mean reduction of passage of air in an obstructive respiratory disease, is less than 54%, a patient trained in these techniques will be able to overcome an attack by himself, without the need of medication.

355

Deenstra H. **The treatment of asthma in children and adults.** Ned Tidjschr Geneeskd 117:1094-1095, 1973. (in Dutch: no English abstract)

▶ autogenic training, relaxation, deconditioning

356

Devine JE. **Relaxation and parent training in the treatment of bronchial asthma: a clinical study.** Diss Abstr Int 40:1887, 1979.

▶ relaxation, family therapy

Bronchial asthma is characterized by episodes of breathlessness caused by constriction of the smooth muscles of the bronchiole tubes. In the past two decades the principles of learning have been applied to the treatment of bronchial asthma in children. Two behavioral treatments were chosen for the present study: relaxation training and parent training. Relaxation training has been shown to be effective in increasing pulmonary functioning as measured by Forced Expiratory Volume/First Second (FEV_1) in both inpatient and outpatient treatment facilities. Parent training has been shown to be effective in reducing the frequency of asthma in the home. The purpose of the present study was to determine whether the treatments could be combined in an outpatient treatment facility to both increase pulmonary functioning and decrease the frequency of asthma attacks in the home. This purpose was accomplished in an experiment which compared the effects of relaxation training and parent training on pulmonary functioning and parental reports of asthma in the home. Twenty-two asthmatic children were paired and then randomly assigned to one of two treatment sequences after being matched in FEV_1 scores. Twelve subjects actually completed the program. The first treatment sequence was eight sessions of relaxation training followed by six sessions of parent training. The second treatment sequence was six sessions of parent training followed by eight sessions of relaxation training. Six subjects who dropped out of the program during the initial measures agreed to act as a medical control group. Subjects in the two treatment sequences were seen two times per week for ten weeks. The medical control group was seen during the three baseline periods in order to obtain FEV_1 scores. Analysis of the data indicated that both treatment sequences significantly increased the FEV_1 scores and decreased parental reports of asthma in the home. The medical control subjects did not significantly improve their FEV_1 scores over the same time period. However, because of the small number of subjects completing the program and the unequal initial baseline measures which occurred because of a differential dropout rate in the two treatment sequences, no differences were found between relaxation training and parent training on the two dependent measures. The results suggest that a combination of relaxation training and parent training can significantly increase FEV_1 scores and decrease parental reports of asthma in the home. In addition there is a need for further research in the area to identify the specific effects of the two treatments using a design which will not be confounded by temporal or carryover variables.

357

Erskine-Milliss J, Schonell M. **Relaxation therapy in asthma: a critical review.** Psychosom Med 43:365-372, 1981.

▶ relaxation, systematic desensitization, biofeedback, autogenic training, transcendental meditation

This review discusses the relationship between the psychological and physiological factors responsible for airways in asthma and indicates the mechanisms by which psychological methods of treatment may influence airway caliber. The effects of mental and muscular relaxation therapy, systematic desensitization, and biofeedback-assisted relaxation are evaluated in children and adults with asthma. The methodology and results of studies are analyzed critically to present a balanced opinion of the subjective and objective effects of these methods of treatment. Muscular relaxation therapy alone appears to have no effect. Certain mental relaxation techniques, such as autogenic training and transcendental meditation, system-

atic desensitization, and biofeedback-assisted relaxation, can produce subjective improvement as well as clinically significant improvement in respiratory function and other objective parameters. As with any therapy the response is variable and is influenced by factors such as age and severity of asthma.

358

Eyermann C. **Emotional component of bronchial asthma.** J Allergy 9:565-571, 1938.

▶ hypnosis, suggestion, behavior therapy, psychotherapy

In summary, if the asthma is unassociated with personality problems, one should treat it as such, having due thought of the probability of inducing unfavorable emotional influences by inept emphasis upon diagnostic procedures and by unconsidered insistence upon therapeutic measures of indeterminate outcome. If the asthma is associated with emotional instability, one must treat the patient with all his problems as well as the local complaint. I will conclude with the following quotation: "There are moments, of course, in cases of serious illness when you will think solely of the disease and its treatment, but when the corner is turned and the immediate crisis is passed you must give your attention to the patient. Disease in man is never the same as disease in the experimental animal, for in man the disease at once affects and is affected by what we call the emotional life. Thus the physician who attempts to take care of a patient while he neglects this factor is as unscientific as the investigator who neglects to control all the conditions that may affect his experiment."

359

Ferguson RG, Webb A. **Childhood asthma: an outpatient approach to treatment.** Can Nurse 75:36-39, 1979.

▶ family therapy, group therapy, biofeedback, behavior therapy, hypnosis, social casework, milieu therapy

Asthma is a condition that involves a large number of children. In fact, the prevalence of asthma in recent years appears to be increasing. The asthmatic process is a complex one usually involving all members of the family. In view of the multiplicity of factors and complexity usually involved with asthma the resources of an interdisciplinary team are often required. The Asthma Program at the Alberta Children's Hospital in Calgary has developed this sort of treatment model and has found that, over time, significantly less inpatient treatment is necessary for the 350 families involved in the program. In addition to being considerably less costly, an outpatient focus to the management of asthma allows for more activity in the area of prevention.

360

Garfinkel R. **Treatment of a psychosomatic ailment in an elderly woman.** Psychosomatics 21:1015-1016, 1980.

▶ psychotherapy, relaxation

As is generally true of psychotherapy with the elderly, there was a great deal of communication between the therapist and the other important persons in the patient's life. When a psychotherapist works with an elderly person, he or she must assume more active responsibility for the patient's life than is usual with younger patients. To summarize briefly, it appears that within a context of a safe, dependent, and warm psycotherapeutic relationship, this elderly patient learned a coping strategy that allowed her to feel some sense of mastery over her own body and, by generalization, over her own life. This case illustrates the common phenomenon of the physical vulnerability of older people in highly stressful psychosocial situations. Even if they are reasonably healthy, the aged are more vulnerable and fragile than younger adults. Perhaps with increasing age, the risk of developing psychosomatic symptoms rises. And certainly the elderly are in greater danger from those symptoms than are younger, more robust persons. We are all familiar with the phenomenon of increased morbidity and mortality among the recently widowed. That illustrates the physical vulnerability of the elderly who are under psychological stress. Hypnosis, relaxation, and other noninvasive psychological techniques can be of value in helping this high-risk population.

361

Graham DT. **Psychology, behavior, and the treatment of asthma.** J Allergy Clin Immunol 60:273-275, 1977. (editorial)

▶ behavior therapy, systematic desensitisation, reciprocal inhibition, biofeedback

362

Hindi-Alexander M. **The team approach in asthma.** J Asthma Res 12:79-85, 1974.

▶ review: psychotherapy, group therapy, milieu therapy, reciprocal inhibition, consultation-liaison

Extracted summary: Whether pathological emotional aspects of asthma are a "cause" or an "effect" of this disease is yet to be answered; but the fact that this question cannot now be answered is no reason to ignore the basic problem or pretend it does not exist. While some are trying to answer it, the rest should at least try to deal with it and treat it. Physicians are usually quite willing to send their patients to specialists either for corroboration or because they feel their colleagues are more competent in a particular matter. This has not happened with the allergist. The allergist, having had minimal training in psychiatry or psychology, could not adequately treat the emotional aspects of asthma unless medical schools revamp their curriculum to include such training. As emphasized by Stoeckle and Zola "... There is need not only for upgrading traditional medical teaching in some schools but for greater recognition of their responsibility to the community and of the need for newer programs in the social study of illness and disease."

363

Hock RA, Bramble J, Kennard DW. **A comparison between relaxation and assertive training with asthmatic male children.** Biol Psychiatry 12:593-596, 1977.

▶ relaxation, assertiveness training

This study showed that relaxation training has a beneficial effect upon the respiration of male asthmatic children in an outpatient clinic. The magnitude of improvement reached 17.7% by the end of the training and was statistically significant from both a medical control group and an assertive-training group by the posttreatment session 1 month after training was terminated. The relaxation group was found to be functioning as well respiratorily at posttreatment as a normative group of nonasthmatic patients matched for sex, age, and socioeconomic status. Relaxation training is an economical, easily taught technique that children can practice at home. There was a high (88%) attendance rate in this program, suggesting that the boys enjoyed the training and were not threatened by it. Assertive training produced no respiratory improvement in this study. There was however, an increase in the self-ratings of Vigor of the assertive group compared to the other two groups. This finding suggests that assertive training makes the asthmatic feel more energetic but concurrently increases his respiratory resistance. This is an important finding, indicating that some dangers may exist in an assertive, activating mode of treatment for asthmatics; and close monitoring of physiological responses is indicated for such treatments or research programs. Two explanations were considered for the failure of assertive training to improve respiration in asthmatics. It is possible that increased vigor produces sympathetic nervous system activation for the asthmatic child which induces the bronchiole constriction peculiar to the asthmatic. An alternative explanation is that the mood changes produced behavioral changes that increased anxiety for the asthmatic's family, and they reacted toward the child in a manner increasing his conflict, tension, and asthmatic symptoms.

364

Hock RA, Rodgers CH, Reddi C, Kennard DW. **Medico-psychological interventions in male asthmatic children: an evaluation of physiological change.** Psychosom Med 40:210-215, 1978.

▶ relaxation, assertiveness training

The purpose of this study was systematically to evaluate the effectiveness of several modes of psychological intervention used with male asthmatic children being treated in the Allergy Outpatient Clinic. Therapeutic effectiveness was measured by large airway changes in respiratory function, and the number of recurrent asthmatic attacks. The psychotherapeutic modes used were relaxation training, assertive training, and combined relaxation plus assertive training. All patients were administered medication by the responsible physician. The group psychotherapy experiences were controlled by using patients who received medication alone and by patients who received medication and met in a leaderless group. The effectiveness of the therapeutic interventions was determined by comparisons between pretreatment measures and measurements taken during and after the eight-week treatment program. Both relaxation training by itself and combined relaxation plus assertive training increased respiratory functioning and reduced the number of attacks. Assertive training alone failed to improve respiratory function and had a tendency to increase the frequency of asthmatic attacks. It was concluded that the most effective management in male asthmatic children was achieved by the combination of medical and psychological treatments.

365

Kaminski Z. **Case report: an asthmatic adolescent and his "repressed cry" for his mother.** Br J Med Psychol 48:185-188, 1975.

▶ psychotherapy, family therapy, group therapy

A case of asthma in an adolescent male is presented. Involvement of the patient in individual, group and family psychotherapy is discussed in detail and particular emphasis placed on the use of family sessions as a therapeutic tool. Alexander's concept of the "repressed cry for the lost mother" is suggested as of aetiological importance.

366

Kellner K. **The psychosomatic viewpoint of bronchial asthma.** Med Klin 71:300-304, 1976. (in German: no English abstract)

▶ behavior therapy, psychoanalysis

367

Khan AU. **Present status of psychosomatic aspects of asthma.** Psychosomatics 14:195-200, 1973.

▶ review: biofeedback, psychoanalysis, psychotherapy, family therapy, milieu therapy, behavior modification, desensitization, conditioning

Except for a few psychiatrists working in the context of a general hospital, interest of practicing psychotherapists in the treatment of psychosomatic illnesses appears to be decreasing. One deterring factor for most busy clinicians is the difficulty of keeping up with the great amount of

research in the areas of immunology, allergy, neurology, and biochemistry. On the other hand, it has been the systemic observation of many clinicians which has led to the development of various theories and hypotheses about the psychosomatic nature of asthma. It is hoped that this review will generate some interest in the much needed psychiatric care of asthmatic children.

368

Khan AU. **Effectiveness of biofeedback and counterconditioning in the treatment of bronchial asthma.** J Psychosom Res 21:97-104, 1977.

▶ biofeedback, counterconditioning

Extracted summary: Attempts to desensitize asthmatics to multiple conditioned stimuli have been only mildly successful because of an infinite number of possible precipitants and the difficulty in determining them from the reports of the patients. The approach combining the principles of biofeedback and counter-conditioning deals directly with the acquired hypersensitivity of the airways and appears to be more successful in extinguishing the conditioned asthmatic response. Autonomically active drugs such as Isoproterenol are especially useful in shaping up the desired response during the preliminary biofeedback training. Counter-conditioning was involved during the linking training to promote an antagonistic response to bronchoconstriction, that is, to train asthmatic patients to control bronchoconstriction and substitute bronchodilation when faced with previously conditioned stimuli. Initial induction of bronchospasm and subsequent bronchodilation during the linking training, with or without the assistance of Isoproterenol, also provided the children with a sense of confidence in their ability to control mild asthmatic attacks and lessened their fear and apprehension which are frequently induced by the onset of a natural asthmatic attack.

369

King NJ. **The behavioral management of asthma and asthma-related problems in children: a critical review of the literature.** J Behav Med 3:169-189, 1980.

▶ review: relaxation, desensitization, assertiveness training, biofeedback, deconditioning

This review focuses upon the behavioral approach to childhood asthma. Asthma is defined as intermittent, variable, and reversible airways obstruction with a complex multidimensional etiology. The major measures of asthma include physiological, symptomatic, and collateral measures. The behavioral management of childhood asthma has been restricted to relaxation training, systematic desensitization, assertive training, biofeedback, and deconditioning of exercise-induced asthma. The efficacy of such intervention strategies for asthmatic children is in doubt, although the management of asthma-related problems in children appears to be a more promising area of research. The author suggests that the power of intervention programs for asthmatic children may be strengthened by the development of multifaceted treatment programs contingent upon the antecedents and consequences of the individual case. Also, behavior therapy may be of assistance to mild asthmatic children.

370

Kinsman RA, Dirks JF, Jones NF, Dahlem NW. **Anxiety reduction in asthma: four catches to general application.** Psychosom Med 42:397-405, 1980.

▶ biofeedback, relaxation

Anxiety reduction procedures as adjuncts to medical treatment have almost invariably been reported to benefit asthmatic patients in individual case studies. However, the results of more systematically controlled studies are clearly inconsistent. This discrepancy is understandable in view of what is now known about anxiety in asthma. Four catches, each based on what has been reported about the roles and forms of anxiety in asthma, are presented. Each catch argues against general, across-the-board application of anxiety reduction procedures in asthma. Careful evaluation leading to more problem-oriented treatment is needed in view of the different roles of anxiety in asthma.

371

Kotses H, Glaus KD, Bricel SK, Edwards JE, Crawford PL. **Operant muscular relaxation and peak expiratory flow rate in asthmatic children.** J Psychosom Res 22:17-23, 1978.

▶ operant conditioning, biofeedback, relaxation

The effects of two types of operant muscular relaxation, frontalis relaxation and brachioradialis relaxation, on peak expiratory flow rate were studied in a group of 40 asthmatic children. Using a yoked control design, conditioned frontalis relaxation was shown to occur in one group of asthmatic children. These individuals exhibited increases in PEFR, whereas children in the frontalis conditioning control group showed no improvement in this variable. Conditioned brachioradialis relaxation could not be demonstrated with the training procedures currently employed. Also, in this case, neither the brachioradialis conditioning nor its yoked control group experienced PEFR changes as a result of training. The results of the present study provided support for the previous finding that frontalis muscle relaxation effects PEFR increases in asthmatic children.

372

Kotses H, Glaust KD, Crawford PL, Edwards JE, Scherr MS. **Operant reduction of frontalis EMG-activity in the treatment of asthma in children.** J Psychosom Res 20:453-459, 1976.

▶ operant conditioning, relaxation, biofeedback

The effect of operantly produced frontalis muscle relaxation on peak expiratory flow rates in asthmatic children was studied in an investigation incorporating a Contingent Feedback group and two control groups, one a Noncontingent Feedback group yoked to the experimental group and the second, a No Treatment group. Thirty-six asthmatic children, ranging in age from 8 to 16 yr, were assigned equally to the three groups in a manner designed to balance the groups along a variety of subject variables. The evaluation of frontalis muscle activity revealed the presence of a strong conditioned effect with the Contingent group exhibiting reliably lower values than the Noncontingent group over the course of the experiment. Group peak expiratory flow rates, measured prior to the initiation of muscle relaxation training and subsequent to training, improved substantially in the Contingent group but not in the Noncontingent or No Treatment groups. Also, more children in the Contingent group showed improvement in peak expiratory flow rate than in either of the control groups. It was concluded that operantly produced frontalis muscle relaxation may be of potential significance in the development of asthma therapies based on conditioning.

373

Landau LI. **Outpatient evaluation and management of asthma.** Pediatr Clin North Am 26:581-601, 1979.

▶ family therapy, psychotherapy, milieu therapy,
  behavior therapy, relaxation, doctor-patient
  relationship

Family therapy, psychotherapy, residential therapy, and other types of behavioral therapy have been used in the management of asthma. In the majority of children with asthma, the physician plays a major role in the psychotherapeutic relationship by allaying anxiety within the family, since most of the emotional problems are a result of the asthma rather than a cause of it. There is a very small group of children with severe social and emotional upheaval in whom psychiatric and institutional care may be necessary. It is important to recognize these children, who often have severe chronic asthma with severe abnormalities of pulmonary function. They are frequently absent from school and may have been hospitalized repeatedly.

374
Leigh D. **Psychological aspects of bronchial asthma.** Med Press 136:153-156, 1956.

▶ psychotherapy, psychoanalysis, group therapy, hypnosis, suggestion, relaxation, milieu therapy

Extracted summary: So many treatments exist that only one fact stands out—so far no specific therapy has been discovered. Ranging from what is grandiloquently called thalasso-therapy, to the latest product of the suprarenal-cortex, the physician need never be at a loss to prescribe for his asthmatic patient. Yet all physicians know what an unsatisfactory condition asthma is to treat in practice. The results of psychiatric treatment in isolation are probably no better and no worse than any other treatment. But it is probable, although no satisfactory evidence as yet exists, that if the comprehensive view which I have expressed is the theoretical basis for treatment, then results will inevitably be better. Due attention to physical factors must accompany all attempts at psychotherapy, for psychotherapy is without doubt the most commonly employed psychiatric treatment in cases of asthma . . . In conclusion, it cannot be denied that the psychiatrist has an important contribution to make toward the understanding and treatment of bronchial asthma. He is no more, nor less, important than the physician, the allergist, or the general practitioner, but forms one of the team which is so necessary for the care and well being of the asthmatic patient.

375
Menger W. **Possibilities of rehabilitation in children with bronchial asthma.** Rehabilitation (Stuttg) 11:199-208, 1972. (in German)

▶ milieu therapy, psychotherapy

Nearly 1% of the total child population suffers from bronchial asthma, for which only the earliest possible treatment promises good prospects of success. For the outbreak of the disease, frequently in the first or second year of life, bronchial infections are mainly responsible, and at later ages also allergies and psychic factors. Too, weather conditions and air pollution may trigger attacks. Treatment of acute attacks is given by the family doctor or in a hospital, but intermediate treatment without administration of cortisone is also very important: physiotherapy, allergen tests and deallergisation as well as elimination of allergens, if necessary a change of place or residence and psychotherapy. For climatotherapy a six-week cure in a sanatorium for children is not enough; the financing of fully adequate treatment is still a problem. There is yet an urgent need for residential care facilities in areas with a favourable climate and within reach of an ordinary school, having boarding facilities and a hospital to secure also vocational rehabilitation as well as for asthma counseling centres.

376
Moorefield CW. **The use of hypnosis and behavior therapy in asthma.** Am J Clin Hypn 13:162-168, 1971.

▶ hypnosis, desensitization

Nine patients with asthma were treated with hypnosis and behavior therapy. All of these patients showed subjective improvement to a rather marked degree, except for one patient who has had three slight attacks of asthma since the onset of her treatment. These patients have been followed from eight to approximately 24 months. The results so far have been rather encouraging and the author believes that this form of treatment will prove to be of benefit in the treatment of asthma and possibly many other related conditions.

377
Panzani R. **Neuropsychological factors in bronchial asthma.** Med Psicosom 5:67, 1960. (in Italian)

▶ psychotherapy, conditioning, placebo

378
Peper E. **Hope for asthmatics—biofeedback systems teaching: the combination of self-regulation strategies and family therapy in the self-healing of asthma.** Somatics 2:56-62, 1985.

▶ biofeedback, behavior therapy, family therapy

The biofeedback systems intervention avoids blaming either the parents or the child for inducing asthma. Instead it restructures the family interactions with the child and simultaneously teaches him non-asthma breathing patterns.

379
Peshkin MM. **The role of emotions in children with intractable bronchial asthma.** J Asthma Res 2:143-146, 1964. (address)

▶ milieu therapy, family therapy, psychotherapy

380
Phillip RL, Wilde GJS, Day JH. **Suggestion and relaxation in asthmatics.** J Psychosom Res 16:193-204, 1972.

▶ review: suggestion, relaxation, behavior therapy

This investigation is concerned with the differential effects of suggestion and relaxation on asthma. The literature is critically examined in terms of personality studies, experimental techniques, learning theory, behaviour therapy, suggestion and physiological responses. Asthmatic subjects were divided into those who had an allergic basis to their symptoms (EX) and those who did not (IN). Ten extrinsic (EX) and ten intrinsic (IN) asthmatics were studied using changes in vital capacity and FEV_1 as the dependent variables. Pulmonary challenge with nebulized

Mecholyl and a neutral saline solution were coupled with correct (control) or false information (suggestion), regarding the nature of the inhalants, thus providing 4 possible experimental combinations. Relaxation training was given to 5 EXs and 5 INs, the remaining serving as controls. As predicted, INs reacted more than EXs to suggestion in the absence of Mecholyl. Both groups reacted less to Mecholyl when told that it was the neutral solution, thus demonstrating cognitive-mediation of the breathing response. For EXs Mecholyl was a necessary and sufficient stimulus, whereas for INs Mecholyl was not necessary; suggestion being sufficient. Relaxation training improved respiratory efficiency on a short-term basis, and also the patients' tolerance for Mecholyl. There were indications that INs benefited more than EXs from relaxation training. The results are discussed in terms of non-verbal response differences, anxiety, shifts in autonomic arousal, a hypothetical psychophysiological model of respiration and the use of behaviour therapy with asthmatics.

381
Piazza EU. **Comprehensive therapy of chronic asthma on a psychosomatic unit.** Adolescence 16:139-144, 1981.

▶ desensitization, psychotherapy, milieu therapy, family therapy

There are different approaches for the treatment of the chronic intractable asthmatic child. Emphasis may be placed on de-sensitization, corticosteroids, broncho dilation, psychotherapy, or separation from parents. We propose a comprehensive use of all the above methods including intensive work with parents. This study includes 32 patients who were hospitalized on the Psychosomatic Unit from September 1970 to June 1976 and were followed from 6 months to 6 years.

382
Richter R, Dahme B. **Bronchial asthma in adults: there is little evidence for the effectiveness of behavioral therapy and relaxation.** J Psychosom Res 26:533-540, 1982.

▶ review: behavior therapy, relaxation, meditation, autogenic training, desensitization, biofeedback

A review of the literature currently available suggests there is little evidence for the effectiveness of behavioral therapy and relaxation in adult bronchial asthma. The results of our review are rather disappointing: although there is some evidence that meditation and autogenic training bring about an improvement, neither relaxation nor systematic desensitization yield general beneficial effects. Operant control via biofeedback of the oscillatory resistance seems to be possible, but nothing is known about the long-term therapeutic effects of this expensive technique. Our conclusions contradict those drawn by other authors. The explanation for this discrepancy is that most investigators fail to satisfy methodological and statistical requirements. They also fail to distinguish asthma in children from adult asthma.

383
Sandler N. **Working with families of chronic asthmatics.** J Asthma Res 15:15-21, 1977.

▶ family therapy, milieu therapy

Extracted summary: I have identified four phases in our work with the family with specific foci related to each phase. The preadmission phase has its focus on establishing a working contract with both family and child, spelling out the problem areas and those areas to be worked. The six-week to two-month evaluation and beginning phase focuses on separation problems, sensitive to the consequences of improvement in or separation of one family member leading to possible decompensation in others, and a more accurate diagnosis and evaluation of the family dynamics. In the middle phase, the family problems are worked through either at Blythedale [Valhalla, New York] or within a family agency in the community. This is a time when we attempt to nurture the family as we nurture the child, so that the child is not perceived as receiving all the goodies at the expense of the family. We thus encourage family involvement and continued commitment to the child. The final, or separation, phase is one where the family is helped either to reintegrate the child into the home or consider the alternative of placement. Particularly where there is a young child, the family may be unable to provide an emotionally healthy environment, or they may be unable to tolerate a more normally functioning child with a healthier ego adaptation. In view of the child's dependency on the family, alternative care may be a medical necessity. An older child who has learned to depend on himself may be in less medical jeopardy and able to tolerate a more pathological home environment. A fifth phase, which is post-discharge, might be included. In this phase many of the original problems resurface after the child returns home. It has been my experience that by and large a relatively time-limited crisis intervention restores the family to a new homeostasis. It is our goal in working with the family to help them establish a different equilibrium on a more effectively adaptive level, so that there is less family impoverishment and less need to use maladaptive and destructive methods for attaining satisfaction; where the family need-response pattern is altered to minimize emotional neglect and there is no positive value attached to not asking for help. "Families, like combat teams and other collectivities, have a morale and an esprit de corps to maintain if they are to be effective."

384

Scherr MS, Crawford PL. **Three-year evaluation of biofeedback techniques in the treatment of children with chronic asthma in a summer camp environment.** Ann Allergy 41:288-292, 1978.

▶ biofeedback, milieu therapy, relaxation

Systematic biofeedback techniques were applied and evaluated in the treatment of chronic bronchial asthma in a summer camp environment during three consecutive summers—1974, 1975 and 1976. From this three-year study the investigators have concluded that biofeedback mediated muscle relaxation training can be a valuable adjunct in the treatment of bronchial asthma.

385

Sporkel H. **Combined somatic and behavioral therapeutic assessment for the treatment of bronchial asthma.** Krankenpflege (Frankfurt) 37:391-394, 1983. (in German: no English abstract)

▶ biofeedback, behavior therapy, systematic desensitization, family therapy

386

Steiner H, Fritz GK, Hilliard J, Lewiston NJ. **A psychosomatic approach to childhood asthma.** J Asthma 19:111-121, 1982.

▶ review: psychotherapy, family therapy, milieu therapy

Extracted summary: While the concept of the psychosomatic unit may not be practical for every children's hospital, we suggest serious consideration of this modality for the treatment of those disorders that do not pigeonhole nicely into either pediatric or psychiatric units. We also think that a period of intensive acute assessment should precede any kind of recommendation for longer-term residential treatment of asthmatic children. In terms of funding for this kind of approach, we have been most impressed by the 90% reimbursement rate from third-party payers.

387

Steinhausen HC. **On the psychosomatic theory of bronchial asthma: a review.** Monatsschr Kinderheilkd 125:129-136, 1977. (in German)

▶ review: behavior modification, family therapy

Following a review of classical psychosomatic theory on bronchial asthma new research findings leading to a revised formulation of an actual psychosomatic concept of this disease are reviewed. Furthermore results of different research studies in the literature using behavior modification methods and structural family therapy are pre-

sented. Finally, clinical implications of the findings reviewed are proposed.

388

Stokvis B, Welman AJ. **Group therapy and sociotherapy as adjuvants in treating asthma.** Ned Tijdschr Geneeskd 99:693-703, 1955. (in Dutch)

▶ psychotherapy, group therapy

The authors survey their opinion of the application of group psychotherapy, and indicate the significance of group therapy and sociotherapy as a resource for the somatic treatment and individual psychotherapy. The course of the group therapy combined with sociotreatment in a group of male asthma patients is communicated. The results were favourable. The importance of group treatment as an adjuvant of the individual psychotherapy is indicated.

389

Strauss EB. **Psychogenic asthma.** Lancet 1:962, 1927.

▶ psychotherapy, hypnosis

These two cases show that it is always worth while to consider the psychological side of asthma. In Case 1 there was no obvious cause for the condition. In Case 2 there were three factors: (a) bronchitis; (b) enlarged tonsils; (c) a deflected nasal septum, which might have been regarded as causal and to the elimination of which treatment might have been exclusively—and fruitlessly—directed.

390

Swanton C. **Asthma and other psycho-physical interrelations.** Med J Aust 1:138-145, 1947.

▶ family therapy, milieu therapy

Extracted summary: Whatever treatment is instituted for an asthmatic, I feel that it must be inadequate unless the patient is viewed as an identity or person, an identity who is reacting as a whole to his environment in an abnormal fashion. Even if we accept the fact that he has an inherited handicap of diathesis or autonomic stigmatization, we do know that he reacts abnormally with his personality to certain external factors and internal demands. We should therefore in all cases attempt to alter his attitude to himself, and secondly, attempt to alter the external which, is the case of children at any rate, produce the inhibitions which retard his normal growth and maturation and prevent him from developing into an independent and adequate person.

391
Treuting TF, Ripley HS. **Life situations, emotions and bronchial asthma.** J Nerv Ment Dis 108:380-398, 1948.

▶ hypnosis, suggestion, psychotherapy

Extracted summary: In one instance, hypnosis was used as a means both of obtaining relaxation and of implanting the suggestion that the patient would feel better thereafter. In this particularly suitable subject these results were obtained, and the effect persisted and was discernible in the change in the patient's attitude toward his illness. Thirteen of the patients received sodium amytal in amounts ranging from 0.1 to 0.5 Gm., intravenously. This technique was used in cases where it seemed desirable to obtain further information about the dynamics of the personality reactions. When it was given to patients during an attack of asthma, it was found that by inducing feelings of security signs and symptoms could be ameliorated or dispelled. When it was given to patients who were asymptomatic at the time, wheezing and difficult breathing appeared when topics to which they were emotionally sensitive were introduced into the interview. Therapy was directed toward allowing the patient to ventilate freely with full support and reassurance from the physician, with the aid of the usual medications which are used for the symptomatic relief of asthmatic attacks generally. The patient who acquired a capacity to tolerate or deal with difficult life situations showed the greatest improvement. In those who developed self-confidence and emancipation from excessive childlike dependency there was a coincident amelioration of attacks.

392
Tunsater A. **Emotions and asthma (II).** Eur J Respir Dis (Suppl) 136:131-137, 1984.

▶ psychotherapy, hypnosis

Factors such as the patient's coping mechanisms and their prognostic value are discussed. Different psychotherapeutic methods as a complement to conservative treatment are reviewed, especially hypnosis. The author stresses the multifactorial etiology of asthma. He points out the need for controlled studies of psychotherapeutic methods of treatment and objective verification of their efficacy.

393
Vachon L, Rich E. **Visceral learning in asthma.** Psychosom Med 38:122-130, 1976.

▶ biofeedback, reinforcement

The hypothesis of visceral learning has opened a new avenue in the search for a pathway between psychosocial stimuli and physiological changes. To apply this approach to asthma required a technique for the measurement of the airways' patency, which could be interfaced with the strategy of visceral learning. The method of forced oscillations was shown to correlate highly with whole body plethysmography. The rapid output of the instrument was used on line to control a visual reinforcement signal. Forty-six mild asthmatics, blind to the effect sought in order to minimize the role of suggestion, were tested in a series of evolving experiments. In the first series, two groups of subjects (N = 15,13) were able, with this sensory feedback, to decrease (p < 0.01) their total respiratory resistance; subsequently a smaller group of subjects (N`), who received reinforcement signals unrelated to the state of their airways, showed no such change. Similar results were obtained in the second series of tests:in A-B-B-A order, the subjects (N = 13) received either contingent or noncontingent reinforcement; furthermore, the reinforcement was available only if their lung volume was within the range observed during baseline.

394
Zamotaev IP, Rozhnov VE, Sultanova A. **Role of psychotherapy in the treatment of bronchial asthma taking into account the "internal picture of the disease."** Ter Arkh 55:34-37, 1983. (in Russian)

▶ psychotherapy, hypnosis, suggestion, autogenic training

Drug and psychotherapeutic treatment was received by 85 patients with bronchial asthma of varying severity. These patients had failed to respond to other treatment methods. The treatment was performed with regard to the "internal disease picture." The main types of the disease survival that determined the internal disease picture background were divided into astheno-depressive, hystero-hypochondriac, hypochondriac, phobic, anosognosic, and apathetic. The psychotherapeutic exposures involved hypnosuggestive therapy, autogenic training and explanatory conversations. As a result of such a treatment 30 patients were discharged in a state of a significant improvement, 53 in a state of improvement and 2 did not respond to the treatment.

395
Zelesnik C. **Some implications of concepts of multicausality in the etiology and treatment of chronic intractable bronchial asthma.** J Asthma Res 5:123-128, 1967.

▶ milieu therapy, psychotherapy, family therapy, placebo

There is a final implication which we may draw from the principle of multiple causality of importance to us. We have seen, I hope, the need for continuous and increasingly sophisticated research whereby we may educate ourselves with regard to our task. Research, however, in complex fields, is a joint effort. Research thereby implies continued communication. We need to tell each other what we are doing and what our results have been. We need to communicate with all of the personnel involved, with the children, and with their parents, and with the community as a whole as to what our problems are and how far we have come in their solution. Communication is not an individual function; it is a group function. The final word rests with no one. Dr. Peshkin has had the honor of saying the first word, but I trust he would not presume to say the last word, nor would I. Nevertheless there is a constant danger of premature closure. When any one of us dares to assert that we have the final answer, that others must do things in our way because our way is not only correct, but the only correct way, we return to the simplistic scheme which science has given up and which produced so little. We must constantly learn, therefore, from one another, from the children, from those farthest down the totem pole. This requires some kind of uniformity in our operational concepts, but it calls for great variability in what we do. And, I think, most especially we must be sensitive to our failures. When one has a fixed idea about a situation, and the situation fails to conform as it is thought it should, there is an invitation to anger. I have seen us get angry at children who did not get well as we wanted them to and expected that they might. These are the children who present the real challenge to our existing outlook and from whom we may learn the most.

Asthma and Eczema

396
Abramson HA. **The father-son relationship in eczema and asthma (II).** J Asthma Res 1:173-206, 1963.

▶ psychoanalysis

In this second paper of the series (Bill's progress from the fifteenth to forty-eighth psychoanalytic session) his dreams essentially disclosed his violent inner life through his obsessional references to his complicated relationship with his father. We shall see that all of this turmoil was not in vain.

397
Abramson HA. **The father-son relationship in eczema and asthma (III).** J Asthma Res 1:317-349, 1964.

▶ psychoanalysis

This paper continues the series of verbatim recordings of psychotherapeutic interviews in a case of intractable eczema and asthma. In the case to be presented, the patient, Bill, had 140 therapeutic interviews during a little more than one year of psychotherapy. The preceding papers dealt primarily with those psychotherapeutic interviews which were based on the patient's first dreams of violence. Thus the fragment of the analysis that has been published and will be published gives us important glimpses into the nature of his conflicts.

398
Abramson HA. **The father-son relationship in eczema and asthma (IV).** J Asthma Res 2:65-94, 1964.

▶ psychoanalysis

The transference dream to be presented in this chapter gave Bill an opportunity, so to speak, to reconstruct the anxieties developed in the relationship with his own father, in a setting with a father figure that was much less threatening. In other words, he tested himself out, and found that he could face marriage and leaving home because of the reconstruction in the therapeutic situation, of his relatiionship with his father.

399
Abramson HA. **The father-son relationship in eczema and asthma (V).** J Asthma Res 2:147-174, 1964.

▶ psychoanalysis

In this chapter Bill is faced with the task of cutting the umbilical cord and dealing with the intricacies of the web of marriage. His dreams, and his feelings connected with his dreams as well as the interpretation of the dreams, all point up the complexity of the problem that he had to face in connection with marriage and the dangers of marriage. The reader can best be taken through Bill's travail by reading the material in this chapter.

400
Abramson HA. **The father-son relationship in eczema and asthma (VI).** J Asthma Res 5:29-81, 1967.

▶ psychoanalysis

In this paper, the way in which Bill's physical symptoms changed with the progress of his analysis will be documented by means of a content analysis of all the recordings. A comparison of his progress will be made with the symptomatic (somatic) progress made by Alice (another case of eczema and asthma) in "The Patient Speaks." Again I wish to emphasize that data of this type validate the mechanisms involved in the improvement produced by psychotherapy. Those who claim that improvement would have occurred anyway without psychotherapy neglect the long years during which symptoms have unfailingly persisted. They also neglect the ego reconstruction usually engendered by the learning process of psychotherapy. Any statistical survey comparing untreated with treated neurotics must include a psychodynamic appraisal in terms of the ability to deal with stress, as well as the disappearance of specific symptoms.

401
Abramson HA. **Reassociation of dreams (I): Repetitive analysis of the first dream to induce regression, resolve a negative transference, and assess improvement.** J Asthma Res 8:115-150, 1971.

▶ psychoanalysis

Discusses data from psychoanalytic interviews with a female patient with severe eczema and asthma. The 1st dream of the patient entering psychoanalytic therapy is considered the chief complaint of the unconscious. Relating the 1st dream is a tacit acknowledgment by the patient of the analysand state. A verbatim recording of the patient's 1st dream was reassociated during 3 yr. of analysis. Verbatim recordings of interviews 4, 81, 292, and 410 are presented and discussed from the viewpoints of chief complaint of the unconscious, regression, negative transference, and termination of the analysis. An assessment index of improvement is presented based on the material available in all 4 interviews. The patient, 15 yr. after the termination of therapy, still retains the improvement in adaptive ego revealed in interview 410.

402
Abramson HA. **Reassociation of dreams (II): An LSD study of sexual conflicts in eczema and asthma.** J Asthma Res 13:193-233, 1976.

▶ psychoanalysis

Presents a case history of a 40-yr-old mother who entered psychoanalysis for the treatment of depression complicating severe eczema and asthma, and illustrates the use of LSD as part of the treatment. Verbatim recordings of therapy sessions in which a dream about sexual conflicts was reassociated with and without LSD are presented to provide data for assessing the value of the drug as an adjunct to dream analysis. Brief data on the safety of using LSD during therapeutic interviews are also included.

403
Abramson HA. **Reassociation of dreams (III): LSD analysis of a threatening male-female dog dream and its relation to fear of lesbianism.** J Asthma Res 14:131-158, 1977.

▶ psychoanalysis

Following the reassociative analysis of the "Beetle Bug" dream (Interviews 235 and 236) in the preceding paper of this series, improvement occurred and nearly all of [the patient's] psychosomatic complaints such as eczema,

asthma, hay fever and headaches were eliminated. Problems connected with her sex life were mobilized by a dream about two dogs preparing for the sex act. Analysis of the dream was unsuccessful because the patient's anxieties overcame her usual interest in ascertaining the nature of the symbolic meaning of the dream. Under LSD-25 the nature of the anxieties connected with the dog dream were, in part, successfully analyzed. However, out of this interview a fear of homosexuality within herself, previously rather latent, became intense. The verbatim recordings outline the patient's psychosexual development which led her to confusing her childhood manner of relieving anxiety through masturbatory channels with later aspects of clitoral stimulation without the male. This led to the patient's believing that she was using a lesbian technic and to a fear of lesbianism. In a follow-up interview the partial fantasy of lesbianism was instrumental in developing a new feeling, that of love for her husband. This feeling of love was clouded by the conflict provided by the residues of the ever present need of the introjected phallic mother's drive to establish the dominating position in the marriage and thus assume a "masculine" or in the patient's view a lesbian role. Although insight was gained and new feelings arose, with partial elimination of the guilty fears of childhood associated with the introjected phallic mother, important sexual conflicts still persisted. These will be presented in Interviews 382 and 383 in the next paper. Rather than discussing some broad aspects of the analytic material here, the next paper in this series will attempt to tie together some cultural and psychological aspects of the problem.

404
Abramson HA. **Reassociation of dreams (IV): A second LSD analysis of the beetle bug dream: its relation to a shark dream and fear of lesbianism.** J Asthma Res 15:23-62, 1977.

▶ psychoanalysis, hypnosis

Summarizes verbatim records of psychoanalytic treatment of a woman with asthma, eczema, and depression who is treated with the use of hypnosis or LSD at times to aid in the recall and understanding of dreams. The basis of her fears of lesbianism and dreams related to this are discussed in detail. Follow-up over 20 yrs showed that the improvement achieved during analysis had been maintained both physically and emotionally.

405
Abramson HA. **The father-son relationship in eczema and asthma.** J Child Asthma Res Inst Hosp 1:349-399, 1961.

▶ psychoanalysis

Extracted summary: This is the last chapter, so to speak, in the story of Bill's psychoanalysis, but it is the first to be told. I hope that telling the end of the story in the first of this series of papers will enhance rather than diminish the interest of the reader. In the study of the mind during psychotherapy, the final action is often less interesting than the psychological forces which led there. This conclusion is not valid here, because these last visits represent an illuminating incident in the termination of a series of therapeutic processes specifically designed to relieve Bill's incapacitating eczema and asthma.

406

Abramson HA, Gettner HH, Sklarofsky AB. **Content analysis of somatic symptoms in 314 verbatim psychotherapeutic interviews in an allergic patient.** J Child Asthma Res Inst Hosp 1:165-171, 1961.

▶ psychoanalysis

This is a study of the somatic symptoms revealed in the verbatim recordings of the psychoanalysis of a 30-year old married woman with eczema and asthma. The basis of the study is the transcribed verbatim recordings of the first 314 of 400 sessions of this patient's approximately 50-minute interviews covering a period of 5 years from 1949 to 1953, inclusive. From the 1,327 single-spaced type-written pages, the following data was complied: (1) the number of interviews; (2) the total number of pages in all interviews; (3) the total number of lines in all interviews; and (4) the total number of lines devoted to somatic symptoms. The symptomatology of the patient is traced in this way to a permanent cure through psychotherapy. The significance of the data is stressed in connection with the future program of the Children's Asthma Research Institute and Hospital in Denver [Colorado].

407

Altschulova HG. **Psychotherapy of the asthma-prurigo syndrome in children.** A Crianca Port 17:683-687, 1958.

▶ psychotherapy

Extracted summary: the results may be summarised as follows: It was interesting that in all cases the asthma responded to psychotherapy sooner than the eczema. Of the 23 patients: 11 patients have been discharged well and 10 have been followed up for up to 4 years. 4 of them had also been suffering from asthma. 4 still attend for follow-up 4 times a year, usually during school holidays. This includes one free from asthma. 1 attends at 6-weekly intervals and her skin is not clear. 5 stopped attending after a time and their eczema, according to reports, varies in severity from time to time, except in one boy who is reported to have continued improving steadily, 2 of the 4 in this sub-group who also had asthma had overcome it when they left us. 2 patients had completely uncooperative mothers. These patients are reported to be still disabled. One now aged 9 is in hospital where he has been for most

of his life and the other one, now aged 15, is at home receiving home tuition and his mother writes "He is still a long way from being cured but I hope his troubles will be cleared up this year."

408

Bentley J. **Psychotherapeutic treatment of a boy with eczema and asthma.** J Asthma Res 12:207-214, 1975.

▶ psychotherapy, play therapy, milieu therapy

Presents a case history in which individual play therapy was used to treat eczema and asthma in a 9-yr-old boy in a residential treatment center for asthmatic children. Therapist helped him work out his fears of his own aggression which dated from severe environmental deprivation in infancy. While the patient remained on some steroids when discharged after over a year of residential treatment, including weekly psychotherapy, his asthma had decreased and his condition seemed stabilized.

409

Bryan WJ. **Sexual problems encountered with patients suffering from asthma and eczema.** J Am Inst Hypn 13:26-34, 1972.

▶ hypnosis, psychotherapy

Considers that asthma may be a suppressed cry for help or an expression of reassurance on being alive. It is suggested that eczema may represent the repressed desire for pre- or extramarital relationships, anger over sexual frustration, or a punishment for sexual desires. The cases and treatment of 2 women with eczema and 2 women and 1 man with asthma are described to illustrate the applications of these theories.

410

Friedman DB, Silesnick ST. **Clinical notes on the management of asthma and eczema: when to call the psychiatrist.** Clin Pediatr 4:735-738, 1965.

▶ psychotherapy, psychiatry liaison

Understanding of some of the special psychodynamic features of allergic illnesses such as asthma and eczema provides the physician with guide lines and general concepts of good mental health which can be emphasized when counselling families with a chronically ill child. Families unresponsive to instruction or direction from the physician may need psychiatric referral. Discussed here are major situations in which a psychiatric referral is indicated and some suggestions for making the referral successful.

411

Mohr GJ, Tausend H, Selesnick S, Augenbraun B. **Studies of eczema and asthma in the preschool child.** J Am Acad Child Psychiatry 2:271-291, 1963.

▶ family therapy, psychotherapy

Extracted summary: The procedure was as follows: a complete psychiatric diagnostic study was done on each case. This included the social worker's interviews with both parents for the purpose of eliciting detailed case history information; psychiatric interviews with the parents and the child; psychological testing of the mother and the child; and a home visit by the nursery school teacher to observe the child in his familial setting. The child was then enrolled at the nursery school and the mother assigned to a caseworker or a psychiatrist for therapy. Seven of the fathers were also seen in therapy. Once the child had become adjusted to the nursery school, he was also assigned to an individual therapist. The mothers attended weekly meetings of a discussion group which included mothers of other nursery school children. An observation team was trained to collect data on the children's behavior in the nursery school. The project pediatrician periodically inspected the children's physical condition, and records of symptom exacerbations and remissions were kept by the parents. The small number of cases studied, the extended period of contact with each family, and the variety of data-collection procedures used allowed us to develop intimate and detailed knowledge of our subjects and their interactions. Repeated conferences were held on each family in an attempt to organize accumulating information, and to develop explanatory hypotheses in relation to the issues under consideration.

412

Portnoy ME. **A case of asthma and eczema treated by hypnosis.** Acta Hipnol Lat Am 1:71-76, 1961. (in Spanish: no English abstract)

▶ hypnosis

413

Woodhead B. **The eczema-asthma syndrome: psychiatric considerations.** Br J Dermatol 67:50-52, 1955.

▶ psychotherapy

Extracted Summary: I agree with MacAlpine when she says that the psychological basis of the disorder is psychotic not neurotic. By that I do not mean that the patients are insane but that their mental mechanisms are psychotic. One boy of 16 years who was asthmatic had eczema as a baby; he said, "Asthma is my friend, I shall be lonely without my asthma." When the asthma subsided he had to stay for a time in a mental hospital. It may sound as if he was made worse by treatment but it was his road to

recovery. It has been my experience not to find patients with eczema in mental hospitals, for once they have become frankly psychotic the eczema is not needed.

Urticaria

414

Czubalski K. **Psychotherapy and psychopharmacotherapy in the treatment of chronic urticaria.** Psychiatr Pol 5:65-68, 1971. (in Polish)

▶ psychotherapy

Psychotherapy and psychopharmacotherapy are valuable in the treatment of chronic urticaria, particularly if applied concomitantly. These methods are especially beneficial where psychogenic factors have played a part in the etiology of an allergic illness. The presence of such factors may be a criterion for the use of both psychotherapy and psychopharmacotherapy.

415

Daniels DK. **Treatment of urticaria and severe headache by behavior therapy.** Psychosomatics 14:347-351, 1973.

▶ behavior therapy, relaxation, desensitization, reinforcement, hypnosis

The success of the treatment program may have been due to the effects of combined behavior therapy techniques and it is conjectured that magnitude and speed of anxiety reduction may be increased by combining two behavior therapy techniques, although such an assumption can only be verified by experimental test. Nevertheless, it may have wide application in the treatment of the neurodermatoses since the symptoms accompanying these disorders are physiological as well as psychological and often are so uncomfortable and incapacitating that patients seek immediate relief. When symptom reduction is rapid, rapport and confidence in the entire therapeutic process is enhanced and can be maintained. Such a strategy and rationale is also offered for the treatment of patients suffering from other psychosomatic disorders.

416

Graf-Best AM. **Psychological treatment of urticaria.** Psychoanal Prax 2:40-44, 1932. (in German: no English abstract)

▶ psychotherapy

417

Gruber L. **Urticaria from cold cured by psychotherapy.** Hautarzt 3:182-183, 1952. (in German)

▶ psychotherapy

418

Kaneko Z, Takaishi N. **Psychosomatic studies on chronic urticaria.** Folia Psychiatr Neurol Jpn 17:16-24, 1963.

▶ hypnosis, suggestion

1) 26 patients suffering from chronic urticaria were interviewed and given projective techniques (Rorshach Test and TAT) in order to find basic personality traits common among the patients, whereby the psychodynamics of the disease may be inferred. As a result, one of the important psychodynamics of the disease was inferred as following: The frustrations often experienced in childhood led the patients to have excessive need for affection and poor ability to have the need gratified by establishing warm relationship with their superiors. Consequently, the patients are prone to be easily frustrated and harbor aggressiveness, be it oriented outward or inward. 2) 27 patients suffering from chronic urticaria were treated with hypnosis with considerably good results. 3) In four patients urticaria was artificially produced by directly suggesting urticaria or by suggesting emotional conflicts of repressed aggression. The results are considered as a positive evidence of the relation of emotional factors to the disease.

419

Kaywin L. **Emotional factors in urticaria: a report of three cases.** Psychosom Med 9:131-136, 1947.

▶ psychotherapy

Three cases of urticaria were presented and the emotional factors in each indicated and discussed. Some factors were outlined which may aid in the emotional recognition and evaluation of the role the emotions play in urticaria. These are: 1. A history of an unhappy and rather anxiety-provoking existence for a period preceding the onset of symptoms. 2. Usually a sudden onset of symptoms, precipitated by a frustrating experience. 3. Frequently no previous allergic history or manifestations. 4. The presence of subjective and objective signs of anxiety. 5. The chronicity of symptoms. 6. A personality type who is shy, easily embarrassed, prone to blushing, relatively passive-dependent and immature, and with, perhaps, a tendency toward exhibitionism.

420

Keegan DL. **Chronic urticaria: clinical psychophysiological and therapeutic aspects.** Psychosomatics 17:160-163, 1976.

▶ psychotherapy, relaxation, hypnosis, behavior therapy, counseling

The paper will present an overview of the literature, emphasize an etiological assessment and treatment which is broadly based and summarize four case examples from a study group of nine patients. A multifactorial and dynamic approach to the problem of chronic urticaria has been used to describe a prototype for other psychophysiologic disorders. Four clinical cases, of nine studied, were examined in relationship to the present literature. Physicians must no longer deal with problems as though physical aspects of life occur in a psychosocial vacuum and must recognize the effect of the mileu on illness and the resultant effect of illness on the mileu in their clinical practice. The family physician is key to this type of approach.

421

Kraft BK, Blumenthal DL. **Psychological components in chronic urticaria.** Acta Allergol 13:469-475, 1959.

▶ psychotherapy, hypnosis

The patients presented found it difficult to express anger—a problem common in many other psychosomatic diseases. The feature particular to these patients, however, was a failure to recognize hostile feelings to any significant extent, even though they felt trapped, hurt, frustrated and helpless.

422

Moan ER. **GSR biofeedback assisted relaxation training and psychosomatic hives.** J Behav Ther Exp Psychiatry 10:157-158, 1979.

▶ biofeedback, relaxation

Auditory GSR feedback has been shown to be effective in the treatment of phobic reactions. The case of a 28-yr-old female who had experienced outbreaks of hives daily over a 3-yr period indicates that the technique may be of clinical value in the treatment of nonspecific anxiety and the psychosomatic disorders that may stem from it.

423

Musaph H. **Psychiatric study of chronic urticaria patients.** Ned Tijdschr Geneeskd 100:3169-3174, 1956. (in Dutch)

▶ psychotherapy

Psychiatric study of chronic urticaria patients.—Report on a psychiatric study of 30 chronic urticaria patients (21 women and 9 men), all of whom were neurotics. Their passive attitude during contact was obvious; there was also considerable anxiety tolerance. Intense feelings of rage and resentment were strongly warded off. The affective relation to key persons is ambivalent and quite vulnerable; it is attended with great uncertainty, closely related to a lack of security, of "belonging." The infantile structure of object relations shows qualities reminiscent of the mechanisms of melancholy and depression, as described by Freud and Abraham. It appeared that in most cases the patients had been intensely annoyed just before the urticaria eruption, but had not shown this to their surroundings, and had greatly resented their own annoyance. All of this is connected with their infantile personality structure. Various forms of psychotherapy may be used in treating chronic urticaria.

424
Rudzki E, Borkowski W, Czubalski K. **The suggestive effect of placebo on the intensity of chronic urticaria.** Acta Allergol 25:70-73, 1970.

▶ suggestion, placebo

1. Suggestion associated with the administration of placebos for antihistaminics produced improvement in 94 per cent of patients with chronic urticaria. 2. The duration and degree of improvement vary between patients and do not seem to depend on occasionally coexisting neurotic manifestations.

425
Saul LJ, Bernstein C Jr. **The emotional settings of some attacks of urticaria.** Psychosom Med 3:349-369, 1941.

▶ psychotherapy

Extracted summary: It is needless to state that nothing in this discussion is meant to imply that all allergic symptoms are psychogenic, or that the emotional state is of any importance in certain cases. Moreover, the converse question of the possible effects upon the psychological state of allergic responses has not been considered. This paper has focused exclusively upon the emotional factor in cases selected because of the prominence of this factor. It may be, of course, that all allergic individuals show, in varying degrees, a common peculiarity in their personalities as some authors believe. If so, it may be that this peculiarity is largely a reflection of an underlying, unsatisfied longing in a certain status, or of reactions to it. But thus far, only a beginning has been made toward the answer of this fundamental question.

426
Schowalter JM. **A case of allergy cured by hypnotic suggestion the modern way.** Br J Med Hypn 10:29-30, 1959.

▶ hypnosis, suggestion

It is not the fact that the [patient's] entire allergy was due to his hatred and guilt complex that makes the case outstanding . . . but rather the "short" cut to the underlying cause through Doctor Van Pelt's "thought" suggestion method.

427
Shertzer CL. **Hypnosis in the treatment of urticaria.** Diss Abstr Int 42:3003, 1982.

▶ hypnosis, suggestion

The present study tested the hypothesis that patients with chronic urticaria (hives) would respond to hypnosis with diminished signs and symptoms. Responsivity to such treatment was predicted only for patients who were hypnotizable according to the Barber Creative Imagination Scale. The experimental treatment suggested to patients that wheals, itching and discomfort would decrease and then disappear. The dependent variables selected were number of wheals, self-reported itch severity and itch duration. A control condition was included in the design in order to separate treatment effects from time or placebo effects. All subjects received both experimental and control conditions. Results show that hypnosis was followed by a statistically significant reduction in itch severity and duration but not by a reduction in number of wheals. However, these changes were not related to hypnotizability. Hypnotizability was related to symptom exacerbation following the control condition.

428
Shoemaker RJ, Levine MI, Shipman WG, Mally MA. **A search for the affective determinants of chronic urticaria.** Am J Psychiatry 119:358-359, 1962.

▶ psychotherapy

1. Medical study of 40 patients failed to produce evidence of an allergic mechanism or a causative physical agent in the etiology of their chronic urticaria. 2. Chronic urticaria may be viewed as a regressive, physiological expression of unconscious conflict when previously operating mechanisms of defense have become inadequate to bind strong affect. Anxiety is the dominant affect in this disorder. 3. Regression from a predominate action level of tension discharge to an organ level of expression is dynamically crucial to the formation of chronic urticaria. 4. The prime affective force in chronic urticaria stems from a revival of abandonment fear and companion rage, called up in a

state of helplessness engendered by a particular set of life circumstances. 5. The conversion process offers the most satisfactory explanation for the physical reaction of chronic urticaria among the patients in this series.

429
Stokes JH, Kulchar GV, Pillsbury DM. **Effect on the skin of emotional and nervous states: etiologic background of urticaria with special reference to the psychoneurogenous factor.** Arch Dermatol Syph 31:470-499, 1935.

▶ psychotherapy, relaxation, desensitization

Urticaria is presented as a disease of complex rather than single causation, with groups of predisposing and exciting causes and with special consideration of the psychogenous component ... The urticariogenic psychoneurogenous background lies in a personality type rather than in external impinging circumstance. Illustrative cases are cited, with description of the response to adjustment and a relaxation technic. The therapeutic methods employed were the use of an acid-calcium regimen, nonspecific desensitizations, psychotherapy, actinotherapy, dietotherapy and occasionally the administration of atropine and ephedrine. Sixty per cent of the known outcomes were good ("cures"); improvement occurred in 34 per cent of the patients and failures in 6 per cent. The significance of these results is discussed. The exclusion of substances to which the patient gave a positive reaction (scratch tests) and an elimination diet were conspicuously unsuccessful as therapeutic measures. A comparison of two groups of published therapeutic results, different methods and emphasis being used with our own, seems to support the view that attention to several factors in a case rather than to one alone increases the proportion of good results; that a variety of quite different methods, this hypothesis being taken into account, may be effective, and that in an unknown proportion of cases urticaria is self-cured. Dogmatic assertion as to sole causes is, therefore, to be deprecated.

430
Teshima H, Kubo C, Kihara H, Imado Y, Nagata S, Ago Y, Ikemi Y. **Psychosomatic aspects of skin diseases from the standpoint of immunology.** Psychother Psychosom 37:165-175, 1982.

▶ autogenic training, relaxation

Analyzed changes in the allergic responses of 53 Japanese patients with urticaria, following psychosomatic treatment. Findings indicate that emotional stress had a great influence on the immune system, manifested in skin disease. Skin tests in Ss significantly improved with autogenic training and relaxation. For clarification of the effects of autogenic training and relaxation, various parameters were simultaneously assessed during the treatment. Serum lev-els of histamine and dopamine-beta-hydroxylase fluctuated; levels of serum immunoglobulin E and findings on the Prausnitz-Kuestner test varied only slightly. Before the onset of urticaria, there were changes in life-style and considerable stress in daily life, as well as exposure to an allergen. Using AKR and C3H mice subjected to stress, the functions of T cells and macrophages were also evaluated. Stress appeared to have a definite influence on the functions of these cells, as related to the roles of the immune system and skin. Thus, the role of stress in clinical disease must always be given consideration.

Combined Allergic Disorders

431
Abramson HA. **Technique for screening verbatim psychotherapeutic recordings and its application to allergy.** Ann Allergy 9:19-30, 1951.

▶ psychotherapy

Extracted summary: Although verbatim recordings result in an unusually large volume of transcribed psychological material, using the technique described in the foregoing, it is believed that the records will provide a rich source of data readily accessible to psychodynamic investigation and interpretation for the formulation of psychodynamic theory. It will also serve as an aid to the therapist in treating the patient.

432
Abramson HA. **Psychosomatic allergy and its management.** Q Rev Allergy 7:197-219, 1953.

▶ review: psychotherapy

1. The literature of psychosomatic allergy covering approximately the past five years is reviewed. 2. It appears evident, irrespective of what antigen-antibody mechanism may account for in the syndrome of hypersensitivity, that the management of patients with various syndromes of allergy requires consideration of the total family constellation. 3. The relationship of laboratory findings to the symptoms and the management of these symptoms in relation to the parents, marital partner, and the community is a complicated problem requiring skill in both physical and psychologic aspects. 4. Evidence through verbatim recordings is presented showing how a conflict situation with authoritative figures led to itching and scratching independent of known antigen-antibody sensitivities. 5. It is the function of the specialist in allergy to manage the patient as a whole and to embody in the management, whether by himself or by the aid of specialists in related fields, the integration of mind-body functions of the patients.

433

Abramson HA. **Evaluation of maternal rejection theory in allergy.** Ann Allergy 12:129-140, 1954.

▶ psychotherapy

Although the treatment of the allergic patient should begin with the study of his allergic hypersensitiveness from the point of view of specific antigens, it should not end at that point. This beginning, especially in cases where the therapeutic results are unsatisfactory, should be supplemented by instruction of the patient in matters other than antigenic sensitivity. He should be instructed to look for personal sensitiveness, that is, to emotional tensions within himself in response to people—not only to chemicals; to feelings—not only to unknown or ill-defined allergens. These sources of emotional conflicts within him may be sought in the home, at work, and in his goals focused in the community at large. The physician who by nature and interest is willing to deal with certain of elementary aspects of psychotherapy should bear in mind that the allergic individual may either have had a childhood in which parental domination and engulfment prevented his growth of independence or where in adult life this dependency upon a demanding, engulfing parent has not been replaced by mature relationships. Parental rejection may occur when the parent becomes enraged at the failure to form the character of the allergic child in a pattern based upon the parent's own narcissistic needs. The physician who includes this methodology in his therapeutic program of the allergic patient will probably find himself richly rewarded not only by better therapeutic results but by himself gaining more insight and more appreciation of the dramatic emotional episodes occurring within the inner life of the patient and the relationship of these episodes within the patient to his allergic symptomatology.

434

Abramson HA. **Psychosomatic aspects of hay fever and asthma prior to 1900.** Ann Allergy 6:110-147, 1948.

▶ psychotherapy

The early recognition that anger and hostility influences the asthmatic paroxysm goes back at least to the time of Hippocrates. This concept persisted through the Middle Ages without correlation with known physical causes. Emotional aspects were still emphasized in the 18th century. The relationship to infection and pathologic residues was pointed out, and the notion of superimposed emotional disturbances was introduced. By the beginning of the 19th century, the notion of repressed emotions entered into the discussion of the causation of asthma. However, these early observations were soon brought into line with the immunologic information accumulating in connection with pollen studies on hay fever. On the one hand, the rise of modern immunology, and on the other hand, the accept-

ance of psychoanalytic psychology, led to the more modern points of view which have developed primarily in the last one-half century. These two fields now remain to be synthesized by the clinician in theory and in therapy.

435

Alexander F. **The allergic child in a seaside preventorium.** Acta Tuberc Pneumol Belg 57:28-34, 1966. (in French)

▶ milieu therapy

436

Aston EE. **Treatment of allergy by suggestion: an experiment.** Am J Clin Hypn 1:163-164, 1959.

▶ hypnosis, suggestion

(Journal) editor's note: This clinical note is published for several reasons. First of all, it demonstrates clearly how a symptom-complex [food allergies] may persist long after the personality needs that engendered it have passed, and how it may continue indefinitely to dominate seriously the daily life of the patient. Next, it illustrates the remarkable ease, simplicity, and effectiveness, as judged by actual results and their duration, with which the use of hypnosis can sometimes correct a long-established distressing handicap to the personality. Finally, it discloses that problems in psychotherapy need not always be intricate, involved, and time-consuming. Instead, it is sometimes possible, using hypnosis, to correct a symptomatic manifestation of major proportions in the patient's everyday functioning by a brief, simple, forthright, unassuming approach. The fact that neither participant in this successful experimental psychotherapy was medically qualified is not actually a pertinent issue. Two people, professionally trained and in a combined medical-dental teaching situation, posed and answered a scientific question.

437

Baruch DW, Miller H. **Group and individual psychotherapy as an adjunct in the treatment of allergy.** J Consult Psychol 10:281-284, 1946.

▶ group therapy, psychotherapy

From these cases it would appear that both group and individual therapy were of value in relation to both the emotional adjustments and the allergic exacerbations. They seemed to supplement one another. Summarizing quickly: 1. Individual therapy went deeper more rapidly. 2. The group stimulated ideas that could then be brought into individual sessions. 3. Hearing other people talk about the same difficulties helped people feel easier about their own problems. 4. The group furnished a supportive sense of belongingness. 5. It gave real and concrete evidence that good relationships can be maintained even when resentments are openly expressed. As one patient put it, "We get mad at each other and uncomfortable and then we accept. We get mad and uncomfortable and then we accept each other all over." She had come to know that acceptance and supportiveness can prevail in spite of the expression of few differences. And this is an enormously strengthening thing.

438
Deutsch F, Nadell R. **Psychosomatic aspects of dermatology with special consideration of allergic phenomena.** Nerv Child 5:339-363, 1946.

▶ psychoanalysis

In this paper an attempt is made to illustrate the psychosomatic factors which are the presuppositions for the development of chronic allergic and related skin conditions. They can be formulated as follows: 1. Skin symptoms in earliest childhood, probably originating on a genetic basis. 2. Deviation or fixation of instinctual drives during the earliest psychic development, and fusion of these with the different sense perceptions related to the skin. 3. Complementary neurotic traits of the environment favoring the amalgamation of the psychosomatic entity. 4. Development of a narcissistic and exhibitionistic personality pattern tinged with compulsive neurotic traits.

439
Fischer L. **Psychosomatic management in the respiratory allergic patient.** J Med Soc NJ 46:516-519, 1949.

▶ psychotherapy

The message of this paper is this: In chronic "organic" illness, there is almost always a psychologic or emotional component. Whether the emotional component preceded the somatic one or vice versa is not the issue. The physician must be equipped to handle both. This should be obvious to the doctor who has tried to refer patients to psychiatrists when the former come to him with organic complaints for which he can find no basis. By mastery of the tool, psychiatry, which includes the administration of insight into the patient, the doctor may defeat the basic reluctance of the patient to improve. When this tool is used, in combination with a case contract agreement regarding the fee (a maneuver which is necessary to control an unwittingly unwilling patient) it is a step forward in combatting disease.

440
Freeman EH, Feingold BF, Schlesinger K, Gorman FJ. **Psychological variables in allergic disorders: a review.** Psychosom Med 26:543-575, 1964.

▶ review: psychotherapy, hypnosis, group therapy

Experimental and clinical studies relating psychological variables and allergic illness are summarized and critically reviewed. Special emphasis is given to methodological issues. The review, embracing principally English-language reports since 1950, focuses on respiratory allergy—asthma, rhinitis, hay fever.

441
French TM. **Emotional conflict and allergy.** Arch Allergy Appl Immunol 1:28-39, 1950.

▶ review: psychoanalysis

Fear of estrangement from a mother and inhibition of crying play significant roles in the etiology of many cases of bronchial asthma. Such emotional factors and allergic factors complement each other in precipitating asthmatic attacks. For these statements there is ample evidence but the evidence concerning psychogenic factors in other allergic conditions is still fragmentary. We do not yet have adequate evidence to decide whether there is any more direct connection between allergy and emotional conflict.

442
Friend MR, Pollak O. **Psychosocial aspects in the preparation for treatment of an allergic child.** Am J Orthopsychiatry 24:63-72, 1954.

▶ psychotherapy, family therapy

Extracted summary: Most of us child analysts or psychiatric social workers do not weigh the various factors in the early phases of treatment relationship. Too often we term as "resistance" multiple factors operating in our pateints' environment which could easily be clarified at the start. Very often, as with this allergic child, we need extensive preparation of the family for their assured support of the child's treatment. We, furthermore, believe that our experiences only corroborate what has long been known in the analyses of psychosomatic conditions of children; i.e., a severely disturbed family-child equilibrium needs support before the direct treatment of the child can proceed. As Emmy Sylvester states: "In many cases, the preparation for analytic work" (speaking of child analysis) "is longer than the analysis proper." We would like to see the same attitude continually carried out to include family in the beginning phases of psychoanalytically oriented psychotherapy by the caseworker, and by this we do not mean necessarily deep insight therapy for the parents. We recognize that this is by no means novel, but do feel that therapy by the caseworker continually involves greater areas for help than the traditional ones, for example, in psychosomatic conditions. There is a tendency even in the most experienced to forsake the total situational approach and to minimize the extensive role of preparation. The utilization of a social scientist can be of great value in the teaching of the therapeutic process.

443

Groen JJ. **The clinical-scientific examination technic in psychosomatic medicine.** Verh Dtsch Ges Inn Med 73:17-27, 1967. (in German: no English abstract)

▶ psychotherapy

444

Haiman JA. **The psychosomatic approach to the treatment of allergy, bronchial asthma, and systemic disorders.** Med Rec 161:467-473, 1949.

▶ supportive psychotherapy, doctor-patient relationship, milieu therapy, spiritual healing

Like improvements in asthma can be obtained where the physician thoroughly understands the psychogenic background of the patient and treats the psyche as well as the soma. Some physicians become confused when they try to trace these sympathetic stimulations from their origin to their effect, while others accept these statements given us by physiologists or neurologists as facts. Some will dispute the fact that there are "trigger centers," sympathetic and parasympathetic nerves, and secretory glands, which are stimulated and inhibited by many emotional disturbances. Those who investigate and treat these distressing manifestations which are produced by irritating influences find that the so-called pathological conditions disappear when these irritative influences are removed. The physician who is only interested in observing pathological changes will state that, "these facts are merely theoretical," playing an unimportant role in the cause of pathological change. Unless he has been trained early to study the psychological and emotional effects upon tissue, the doctor will find it difficult to appreciate the overall picture of psyche and soma as one entity. A large number of physicians still criticize unfavorably the small number of confreres who practise psychosomatic medicine, stating that they are not in accord with this method of treatment. It is too bad for the patients that more doctors are not in accord with it. The psychosomatic approach is becoming more and more incorporated into the practice of medicine today, than it was fifteen years ago. Dr. Anthony Bassler, in discussing an early presentation of the writer's, stated that in bringing up a subject of this type the first five years would bring years of condemnation, the second five years, toleration, and the third five years, conciliation. He continued, "After that, they will remark, "Why harp on the same subject. Everyone has known these facts for the past fifteen to twenty years."

445

Ikemi Y, Nakagawa S. **Psychosomatic study of so-called allergic disorders.** Jpn J Med Progr 50:451-474, 1963.

▶ desensitization

We made a psychosomatic experiment on 81 subjects with so-called food allergy and were able to prove that in the majority of the cases conditioning by auto-suggestion exerted a significant influence upon the occurrence of their symptoms. Also we obtained demonstrative data on the relationship between constitutions confirmed by skin reaction and psychological factors. Our next experiment was concerned with psychosomatic aspects of contagious dermatitis. We were able to confirm that conditioning by auto-suggestion played a dominant role in 51% of 51 subjects. Also our histological finding proved that the dermatitis induced by touching noxious trees and the dermatitis elicited by conditioning had a striking resemblance. Lastly, psychosomatic observations were also made on rhinitis, urticaria and bronchial asthma mainly from the clinical standpoint. Psychological desensitization of our own origin was applied to the cases of food allergy, contagious dermatitis and urticaria, all of which were influenced strongly by psychological factors, and we were able to obtain noticeable results.

446

Kaufman W. **A commonsense approach to psychotherapy in allergic practice.** Ann Allergy ll:291-296, 1953.

▶ psychotherapy, doctor-patient relationship

Each allergist must decide for himself how much psychotherapy he wants to use in his practice. Even the allergist who limits himself to the psychotherapy inherent in the patient-doctor relationship is in a position to give many patients the aid they need. Only patients with complex emotional and psychological problems require more formal types of psychotherapy. The most important aspect of the treatment of an allergic patient is a thoroughgoing search for the nature of allergens which cause his allergic disease. When this is discovered, it is often possible to ameliorate not only his allergic illness, but also secondary disturbances in his emotional and psychological behavior caused by his primary allergic illness. Psychotherapy is often a useful aid in the management of allergic illness. But it is never a substitute for careful allergic workup and treatment. Nor, for that matter, are allergic study and therapy a substitute for the much-needed psychotherapy of a patient who has both primary allergic and concomitant primary psychiatric disorders. A master allergist will always blend allergic therapy and psychotherapy to meet the realistic needs of his sick patient. This may mean that some allergic patients will receive mainly psychotherapy, and others, mainly allergic therapy. But above all it means that allergists will try to give their allergic patients whatever modalities of treatment they need to get well.

447

Kraft B, Blumenthal D. **The psycho-physiologic approach in the management of the allergic patient.** Ann Allergy 19:897-902, 1961.

▶ psychotherapy, doctor-patient relationship

When emotions exist, which cannot be expressed by words, actions, or thoughts, they may find expression through some organ or organ system. The organ which speaks is most likely the one which is constitutionally predisposed or has in some other way become invested with feeling when environmental conditions were stressful. The major adjustment the doctor using the psycho-physiologic approach needs to make, is to get the emotional life of the patient into a biological frame of reference along with the organic data. He has to become accustomed to considering significant emotional responses as being just as real and as pertinent to the clinical picture as an eosinophilia or a wheeze in the chest. The interpretation of the psychogenic mechanism to patients with psycho-physiologic components requires the same professional matter-of-factness, the same sympathetic interest and understanding with which any other medical advice is given. Simultaneous allergic and psychotherapeutic management is possible. Some physicians do not have the time, the training or the inclination to treat the patient psychotherapeutically as well as allergically. Even in these cases, however, the patient's emotional relationship to the doctor can have a psychotherapeutic function. If the doctor continues to emphasize during visit after visit that he understands how emotional tension is keeping the patient upset and his allergies active, and if he points out that the immunologic and pharmacologic therapies also have their value, then the patient benefits emotionally from the relationship. Physicians who have had training in psychotherapy may go even further than this. While they continue their immunologic and pharmacologic therapies, they also discuss emotional problems with the patient. By using the psycho-physiologic approach, one will touch the lives of very many people more constructively than one might otherwise have done. We not only help the patient who comes to us but all the members of his family and other people with whom he is connected.

448
Kraft B, Howell JD, Blumenthal D. **A psychotherapist's integration into an allergic practice.** Ann Allergy 15:168-171, 1957.

▶ psychotherapy, consultation-liaison

There is a constant change in all scientific thinking today away from states and entities in the direction of dynamics and processes. We have tried to show that illness can be treated more effectively by shifting the approach from a disease-focused concept to an "organismic" concept. The team work we have described has more often than not provided these patients with relatively effective means of relieving their symptoms. In many cases it has provided them with psychologic improvement also. Many of the patients who have been helped have been able to make changes in their life situations so as to protect and fortify themselves against a return of the same conditions that aggravated their physical symptoms in the first place. Psychotherapy was facilitated by the fact that most of the

patients had already established rapport with the office, had confidence in the physicians and nurses and transferred this confidence quickly to the psychotherapist. This enhanced the value of the psychologically supportive interviews and this support was extended to the patient even after he had terminated the interview. We believe that further improvement in our therapeutic methods can only result from a persistent re-examination of our theories and experimentation with new techniques.

449
Kroger WS. **Current status of hypnosis in allergy.** Ann Allergy 22:123-129, 1964.

▶ hypnosis, autohypnosis, psychiatry-liaison, group psychotherapy, placebo, imagery

Psychogenic factors in the production of symptoms in allergy are reviewed, and the use of hypnotherapy in their control is discussed. Hypnosis, as part of a multi-dimensional approach, can be effective, but it is not a panacea or a substitute for proven immunological methods. It can, in selected cases, potentiate standard methods and often save considerable time or even referral to a psychiatrist. Asthmatic attacks in individuals susceptible to certain allergens have been prevented by hypnosis despite the appearance of positive skin tests. Attacks have been precipitated and then terminated by posthypnotic suggestions in patients who have been "exposed" to offending allergens. Reinforcement of helpful suggestions is necessary to maintain good results. Several case histories are cited which present patients who were refractory to usual therapeutic procedures. There are no dangers in hypnosis per se, but the physician must guard against the use of words which may have a traumatic effect on the patient. Proper diagnosis is essential and seriously disturbed or psychotic patients should be referred to a psychiatrist. Physicians who fear substitute symptoms may use a "trading down" technic. Dramatic successes as well as dramatic failures do occur. Nevertheless, allergists should be conversant with recently developed hypnotic technics that are patient centered rather than doctor directed.

450
Levine MI, Geer JH, Kost PF. **Hypnotic suggestion and the histamine wheal.** J Allergy Clin Immunol 37:246-250, 1966.

▶ hypnosis, suggestion

Recent articles by several British investigators report that the responses to skin test reactions in immediate and delayed hypersensitivity can be inhibited by direct suggestion under hypnosis. With the use of a standardized hypnotic technique, groups of normal, allergic, and urticarial subjects were given skin tests with histamine and ragweed, in an attempt to alter the whealing response. However, under the conditions of this experiment no significant change was observed.

451

Lubens HM. **Self analysis: a practical method of psychotherapy for allergic patients.** J Asthma Res 9:87-97, 1971.

▶ psychotherapy, doctor-patient relationship, autohypnosis

The psychodynamic aspect of chronic allergic diseases should be given adequate consideration in a therapeutic regimen. The psychodynamic factor in patients with allergic diseases seems to be very closely related to nervous tension, psychoneurosis, anxiety, and other similar entities. This psychodynamic tension is viewed as an actual imbalance resulting from an excess loading of negative, disturbing, emotional thoughts in the mind. Psychodynamic tension increases the sensitivity of the allergic shock organs and tissues and enhances the intensity of the allergen-antibody reactivity. It is believed that an imbalance in the autonomic nervous system is one factor in this process. The self analysis psychotherapeutic method, a form of self analysis by the patient under physician's guidance and motivation, is intended to correct the imbalance. In conjunction with other essential anti-allergenic therapy, psychotherapy aims at a concentrated effort to correct and eradicate the causes of negative emotional imbalance. The preponderance of the positive aspect of the mind (peace of mind, security, etc.) are reasserted to promote total well being.

452

Lubens HM. **A psychotherapeutic technique for allergic patients.** J Asthma Res 1:167-171, 1963.

▶ psychotherapy

The psychodynamic aspect of allergic diseases should be given adequate consideration in any therapeutic regimen. The psychodynamic factor in patients with chronic allergic disease is very closely related to nervous tension, psychoneurosis, anxiety, and other similar entities. This psychodynamic tension is viewed as an actual imbalance resulting from an excess load of negative emotional forces in the mind. The psychodynamic nervous tension increases the sensitivity of the allergic shock organ tissues and enhances the intensity of allergen-antibody allergic reactivity. This psychotherapeutic method, a form of self analysis by the patient under the physician's guidance, is intended to correct the imbalance. In conjunction with other essential anti-allergenic therapy, the psychotherapy aims at a concentrated effort to correct and eradicate the causes of negative emotion. The preponderance of the positive aspect of the mind (peace of mind, security, etc.) are reasserted to promote well-being.

453

Macaulay B. **Treatment of asthma and hayfever by hypnosis.** Lancet 1:1129, 1958. (letter)

▶ hypnosis

454

Mason AA, Black S. **Treatment of asthma and hayfever by hypnosis.** Lancet 1:1129-1130, 1958. (letter)

▶ hypnosis

455

Mason AA, Black S. **Allergic skin responses abolished under treatment of asthma and hayfever by hypnosis.** Lancet 1:877-879, 1958.

▶ hypnosis

A patient with a long history of allergic asthma and hayfever was relieved of her symptoms by hypnotic treatment. Weekly skin tests showed her decreasing sensitivity to the known allergens. When finally the patient had no symptoms or skin reactions, intradermal injection of her serum into a non-allergic volunteer made it possible to demonstrate the passive transfer of the skin sensitivity to the original allergens. (Prausnitz-Kustner reaction.)

456

Metzger FC. **Allergy and psychoneurosis.** J Nerv Ment Dis 109:240-245, 1949.

▶ supportive psychotherapy

The clinical picture presented by the allergic individual is clouded by psychoneurotic manifestations in a great number of patients. Many reactions from medicines and hyposensitization treatments are on a fear basis, and not an allergic one. Many allergic seizures which cannot be explained on a basis of increased exposure to allergens can be explained on the basis of a complicating emotional experience. A neurosis complicating allergy requires recognition and treatment.

457

Miller H, Baruch DW. **Psychotherapy of parents of allergic children.** Ann Allergy 18:990-997, 1960.

▶ family psychotherapy

When a parent can give up the child as part of himself, when a parent can give up the child in the image of his own parent, when the parent has become able to love the child maturely, then he can let the child be himself and grow as himself and speak for himself, as he feels in all honesty, then the allergic symptoms no longer are needed to serve mutual purposes. The child can then make better use of his allergy treatment to get well.

458
Miller H, Baruch DW. **Psychological dynamics in allergic patients as shown in group and individual psychotherapy.** J Consult Psychol 12:111-115, 1948.

▶ group therapy, psychotherapy, play therapy

1. Psychogenic factors produce far-reaching biological changes. 2. In individuals with allergic constitution these factors are expressed as allergic symptoms. 3. The underlying psychogenic factors in 22 allergic individuals were brought out by group and individual psychotherapy and by play-therapy, each method being described. 4. Protocols of sessions utilizing these three methods showed that allergics use their symptoms to express emotions which have been blocked from conscious outlet. 5. Allergic symptoms were shown to represent attempts to gain sympathy, to express hostility and to mask a feeling of guilt or anxiety. 6. The release of emotions in psychotherapy is paralleled by a decrease in symptoms. 7. Twenty-one of the twenty-two patients showed improvement. One remained unchanged.

459
Miller H, Baruch DW. **Some paintings by allergic patients in group psychotherapy and their dynamic implications in the practice of allergy.** Int Arch Allergy Appl Immunol 1:60-71, 1950.

▶ group psychotherapy

Twenty men and women, half of them allergic, have been observed in group therapy under the guidance of the authors. Spontaneously some of these brought in paintings of their fantasies and dreams. Associating to these the allergic patients consistently manifested a characteristic emotional syndrome of hunger for affection, hostility to the parents and blocking i.e., repression or inhibition of the expression of emotion. Several patients came to the realization that their allergic symptoms represented the expression of emotions which they could not otherwise bring out by word or deed.

460
Miller H, Baruch DW. **Marital adjustments in the parents of allergic children.** Ann Allergy 8:754-760, 1950.

▶ family therapy

1. In this, as in previous studies, maternal rejection is seen as an important item in the emotional climate of the allergic child's environment. 2. In its etiology, maternal rejection is found to be related to the mother's emotional immaturity, a product of her own life history. 3. Of primary importance are the mother's rejection by her own mother, the unresolved Oedipal attachment to her father, and the hostility to her mother derived from both. 4. As a result of childhood conflict, sexual adjustment in the marriage of these women is poor. 5. Statistically, poor sexual adjustment is significantly related to maternal rejection. 6. The influence on father-child relationship is discussed.

461
Miller ML. **Allergy and emotions: a review.** Int Arch Allergy Appl Immunol 1:40-49, 1950.

▶ review: psychoanalysis, psychotherapy

Treatment by fostering independence (not pseudo-independence) and emotional maturity, whether by psychoanalysis or other treatment, particularly in children, seems to be able to diminish the effectiveness of allergens in producing allergic responses in many cases.

462
Mitchell AJ, Frost L, Marx JR. **Emotional aspects of pediatric allergy—the role of the mother-child relationship.** Ann Allergy 11:744-751, 1953.

▶ supportive psychotherapy, family therapy, consultation-liaison

1. We found the mothers of our allergic children to be relatively and absolutely rather strong, active, and anxious, with a great need to be in control. By relatively, we mean in comparison with a psychologically weak father. 2. The position of the child in the family was "special"; he was either on an "exposed" spot among his siblings, or for other reasons occupied a role of particular importance to the mother. These children were born outstandingly in the beginning or towards the end of the mothers' childbearing period. This has been statistically the most striking data of our series. 3. There was a periodic oscillation of the mother's attitude towards the child, changing from extreme concern and overprotection to one of intolerant and impatient annoyance. 4. The children of both sexes showed much stronger identification with the mother than with the father. Younger children showed a noteworthy inhibition of motor activity; while older children, particularly girls, showed symptoms of emotional depression and hysterical manifestations. 5. Throughout, the children showed great ungratified dependency needs, and at the same time unconsciously portrayed their parents and other family members as equally frustrated persons from whom they could expect and receive little gratification. 6. It is our belief that in general the allergist or pediatrician is in a much more advantageous position to supply emotional support and insight with his therapy. Only the exceptional case in which psychologic problems are overwhelming may require the handling by a psychiatric specialist. 7. Much anxiety of the mother can be

alleviated by the allergist, during initial and subsequent visits, by understandingly inquiring into and accepting the mother's concern and problems in relation to the child. Such an interest in itself is reassuring, but more so if combined with an attitude and a conveyed impression that these factors are often found in connection with and related to allergies. The allergist may profitably show a personal interest in the child and become a counter-balancing factor when mothers' need to control becomes excessive. Wherever feasible, a joint approach with a psychiatrically oriented social worker, a psychologist, or a psychiatrist may be an interesting and mutually rewarding experience.

463
Mitchell JH, Curran CA. **A method of approach to psychosomatic problems in allergy.** W Va J Med 42:271-279, 1946.

▶ psychotherapy, doctor-patient relationship

Extracted summary: We question now our natural tendency to blame all the patient's symptoms on some minor pathological change which we may be able to demonstrate, or to feel that we have solved the problem if some minor deviations from the normal are indicated either in the physical examination, laboratory tests or the skin tests. Actually these findings do not solve the problem but usually complicate the picture all the more. On the other hand, when we approach these patients from the psychological point of view, we find that a large number prove to be maladjusted and may receive noticeable help from psychotherapy.

464
Mullins A. **Asthmatic children take the waters.** Lancet 2:440-441, 1960. (letter)

▶ milieu therapy

465
Perloff MA, Spiegelman J. **Hypnosis in the treatment of a child's allergy to dogs.** Am J Clin Hypn 15:269-272, 1973.

▶ hypnosis, imagery

Extracted summary: There would appear to be no method available at this time to conclusively establish the mechanism effective in eliminating this patient's allergic manifestations to the causative allergen. To evaluate the effectiveness of hypnotherapy in relationship to hyposensitization therapy in allergic individuals would require a study involving random selection of patients, with allergic manifestations to the same allergen, into two groups. One group would be treated with hypnotherapeutic techniques, and the other with hyposensitization techniques. Improvement statistics in each group could then

be compared. This is a formidable undertaking, but worthwhile. It would require a protocol involving a cooperative, collaborative group of allergists and physicians experienced in hypnotherapy. Although this report concerns a successful result, it may be of greater long range value if it stimulates a larger and more scientific investigation into the mechanisms underlying the effectiveness of hypnotherapy.

466
Prior HJ. **Emotional factors in allergy.** Med J Aust 2:556-559, 1951.

▶ psychotherapy, psychoanalysis, family therapy, play therapy

Extracted summary: 1. The relationship of emotional factors to allergic sensitivity has not yet received a completely final answer. 2. It seems certain that emotional factors can precipitate, prolong, modify or prevent the allergic attack. (In certain patients no attack will occur, even in the presence of allergens, if emotional factors are removed or controlled.) 3. The complete psychopathology of the individual case may cover a wide field and present an intricate superstructure of secondary reactions and manifestations as well as more basic psychopathology. But in any case psychiatric assessment would often appear desirable for complete understanding of the patient and his situation, and psychotherapy necessary if the process is to be arrested and possible complications, both physical and psychic, prevented. 4. In just what proportion of the total allergic population these emotional factors are sufficiently important to warrant more detailed investigation is not very clear. My impression is that the figure would be at least 20% and quite possibly nearer 40% or 50%.

467
Rapaport HG. **Scope of the problems of pediatric allergy.** Ann Allergy 30:352-358, 1972.

▶ supportive psychotherapy, doctor-patient relationship, milieu therapy

Extracted summary: Most physicians today are neither trained for nor accustomed to dealing with chronic disease. We have come to expect quick solutions in this age of the so-called wonder drugs, and as a consequence we may be losing touch with some of the more fundamental qualities of our profession. Qualities such as patience, careful observation, understanding, periodic reassessment of problems, and involvement with our patients as sympathetic and caring human beings. Coping with allergy makes these demands on us; if we are to cope successfully, it will bring out the best we have to offer.

468
Rogerson CH. **The psychological factors in asthma-prurigo.** Q J Med 6:367-394, 1937.

▶ psychotherapy

A certain group of children with asthma-prurigo has been studied. In many of them are found special personality features and special environmental difficulties which are closely related to the attacks. In those which have been studied some have followed very closely the typical findings, others have done so to a less extent. It is believed that the facts as they have been presented may help to clarify the psychological understanding of asthma and particularly to co-ordinate the physical and psychological aspects of treatment.

469
Salazar Mallen M. **Psychologic factors in allergic disease.** Gac Med Mexico 79:238, 1949. (in Spanish: no English abstract)

▶ psychotherapy

470
Sanger MD. **Psychosomatic allergy.** Psychosomatics 11:473-476, 1970.

▶ supportive psychotherapy, doctor-patient relationship

The allergist must recognize that the treatment of the patient including the emotional factors belong in his province and not necessarily in the psychiatrist's domain. The allergist has a unique opportunity to observe and treat the immunologic and psychologic aspects of the allergic patient. This can be accomplished when the patient has a rapport with his physician; he can then be "reached" and a meaningful interpersonal relationship takes place. This technique will bring to the awareness of the physician and the patient, the emotional problems which are the "triggering mechanism" of allergic attacks. When these are adequately handled by both the physician and patient, a return to homeostasis may rapidly occur.

471
Saul LJ. **The relation to the mother as seen in cases of allergy.** Nerv Child 5:332-338, 1946.

▶ psychotherapy

Extracted summary: The dermal and respiratory mechanisms, trends, and relations to the mother are analogous to the oral ones. They are fundamental to an understanding of psychobiological functioning. Preliminary observations strongly suggest that they play a role in the skin and respiratory allergies similar to that of the oral ones in the gastro-intestinal disorders.

472
Schatia V. **The role of emotions in allergic disorders.** Int Arch Allergy Appl Immunol 1:93-102, 1950.

▶ psychoanalysis, psychotherapy

Literature on the role of emotions in allergic diseases was reviewed and divided into four schools of thought: 1. Personality problems are caused by allergy. 2. Emotional upsets may precipitate individual attacks in allergic individuals. 3. Allergic constitution parallels an allergic personality structure. 4. Allergic diseases are entirely psychogenic. Detailed case material illustrating the third school of thought was presented. The need of the allergic patient for psychotherapy directed toward mature integration of total personality rather than to relief of individual allergic attacks was emphasized.

473
Selinsky H. **Emotional factors relating to perennial allergy.** Ann Allergy 18:886-893, 1960.

▶ psychoanalysis, psychotherapy, doctor-patient relationship

It is the aim of psychotherapy to relieve symptoms by reducing tensions which have accompanied the patient's burden of anger, rage, hate and anxiety. It is also to the patient's advantage to understand his hunger for warm attention and interest. Helpful attention from the physician or nurse is unconsciously interpreted as loving attention from a parent figure. It is gratifying to observe that a number of allergists have come to recognize the need of an atmosphere in the office which is of a friendly and personal character, rather than the coldly impersonal one where patients are attended to as so many animate objects. It is strongly urged that the ingenuity of the physician be employed to develop devices to enhance the friendly atmosphere in the office where a great many patients are being treated. It would be advantageous for the physician to be mindful of how important the interrelationship is between physical processes and the emotional stress of tension and anxiety. Just as the individual may be hypersensitive to physico-chemical irritants, so is he also inwardly hypersensitive to emotional stimuli. The feeling that he is being given personal attention helps in counteracting the feelings of rejection which he endured earlier in life. We know that while there may be occasional remarkable and sudden disappearances of symptoms, it is more usual for treatment of the allergic disorder to be a "long term" process. There is a gradual diminution of attacks as the threshold of vulnerability is raised; psychologically the patient gains increasing awareness of the deeply repressed or stoutly denied feelings involving conflict about significant persons in his life. There is a need to respect his psychic as well as physical vulnerability. One can reasonably expect therapeutic results from pscyhotherapy to range from mild improvement to cure, depending upon the accessibility of the patient to insightful work. The psychotherapeutic approach must be geared to the capacity of the patient at the given moment to respond to investigative or insightful techniques. Considerable difficulty may be experienced in the therapist-patient relationship if the patient needs his symptoms as a defense against a conflict which is causing great anxiety; breaching such a defense might threaten total collapse of the patient's precarious hold on the appearance of sanity. He prefers to be sick rather than to appear very unhappy. It will be recalled that earlier in this communication what Groddeck said was given great weight: that psychosomatic illness serves to postpone solution of inner conflicts. The art of approaching some patients who can accept symptoms of physical illness, but who cannot accept symptoms reflecting emotional ill-health, is one that requires patient tact and skill. It is admittedly difficult. Finally, may I recall the enigmatic statement with its hint of profound truth that Thomas Mann made in a tribute to Freud a number of years ago: "All heightened healthiness must be achieved by the route of illness."

474
Sirmay EA. **The role of psychotherapy in allergy: credits and debits.** Calif Med 78:456-458, 1953.

▶ psychotherapy

Psychological problems play an important role in the production and exacerbation of allergic disease, just as they do in other illnesses, especially those of a chronic nature entailing economic and social problems. Some psychotherapy is implicit in the practice of all physicians. While most patients make satisfactory progress with whatever treatment is outlined, a few do not, and they may be helped if a little extra time is taken to investigate and rebalance their mental environment. In the treatment of patients with allergic disease, dealing with emotional problems is considered as adjunctive to specific desensitization.

475
Sontag LW. **A psychiatrist's view of allergy.** Int Arch Allergy Appl Immunol 1:50-60, 1950.

▶ psychotherapy

In speaking of allergy as a psychosomatic disease, psychiatrists do not mean to minimize the part of inheritance of a predisposition to develop a hypersensitivity to allergens. Neither do they feel that psychotherapy is a substitute for elimination of allergens or for desensitization. They believe that, in addition to the individual's capacity to develop hypersensitivity in certain body cells, emotions through their modification of autonomic system function play a substantial part in many cases of allergy. Emotional stress may be the deciding factor as to whether hyper-

sensitive cells function normally or go into an allergic state. A careful psychiatric history is in order whenever the allergist finds that his usual method of handling a case is not adequate to relieve the patient. The psychiatrist, both in the role of a consultant for the appraisal of emotional factors and as a therapist in many allergy cases which are resistant to the usual measures, can be of real help to the allergist.

476
Sperling M. **Psychologic desensitization of allergy.** Bull NY Acad Med 44:587-591, 1968.

▶ psychoanalysis

Extracted summary: In conclusion I want to say that it appears that somatic patterns of behavior, such as allergies, are established in childhood and, further, that emotional attitudes of the parents, such as unconscious needs and anxieties relating to instinctual activities of the child—in the case of allergies particularly to anal activities—by promoting or intensifying the child's own conflicts, anxieties, and guilt feelings can become the "triggers" to set off the allergic reactions. Psychologic (self) desensitization operates by rendering harmless these psychological triggers. This would seem to me a vast and fruitful area for research, especially for those who are trained in both child and adult analysis.

477
Squier TL. **Emotional factors in allergic states.** Wis Med J 40:793-796, 1941.

▶ psychotherapy

In the literature of psychosomatic medicine psychic factors are stressed as the primary or even exclusive cause of asthma or other allergic diseases. Allergists on the other hand are often inclined to dismiss emotional factors with scant consideration. Truth probably lies somewhere between these two diametrically opposed viewpoints. The allergic patient has acquired hypersensitivity to a specific foreign substance and has developed antibodies against that substance. Some of these antibodies (reagins) circulate in the blood stream and some are attached to the tissue cells of various organs of the body. When the sensitized tissue cells again encounter the specific foreign substance, an explosive union occurs between that substance (antigen) and the reagin in or on the tissue cells of the shock organ. This results in increased capillary permeability, edema, spasm of smooth muscle and, in the more severe reactions, a marked fall in blood pressure, shock and collapse. It is difficult to conceive how the union of antigen and antibody could be prevented through psychogenic means any more than the chemical reaction of acid and base could be prevented in a test tube. Emotional factors, however, conceivably can alter the clinical response from the antibody-antigen union. Administration of epinephrine immediately before testing will obliterate or markedly diminish cutaneous reactions. Similarly, it is not improbable that in a person with a labile vegetative nervous system emotional factors may lower the threshold of reaction so that allergic equilibrium is upset and symptoms result. An unstable vegetative nervous system will accentuate and may at times, through stimulation of the parasympathetic system, even counterfeit true allergic reactions. When a stage of partial tolerance has been reached, allergic balance can be upset by many non-allergic factors, among which emotional stress may be of major importance. The aggravating effects of psychic trauma should be recognized and reduced to a minimum. However, it must be realized that if permanent equilibrium is to be achieved the primary allergic offenders must be eliminated or controlled.

478

Stokvis B. **Psychotherapeutic questions, methods and outcome for allergic patients.** Hippokrates 28:496-500, 1957. (in German)

▶ psychotherapy

479

Stokvis B. **Allergy as a psychosomatic problem.** Acta Psychother 9: 368-378, 1961.

▶ psychotherapy

The author finds it entirely justifiable to look upon allergy as on a psychosomatic problem. The discussion is open to a great number of different opinions, according to the origin and the "Weltanschauung" of the research worker. The time should come when the difficulties which still stand in the way of reciprocal understanding between research workers in the whole world will be removed, clearing away all obstacles which are still preventing the re-creation of the old commonwealth of scientists. He quotes the words of Loeb Baruch: "The constant friendship and eternal peace between all scholars, are they but dreams? May we soon awake out of those dreams."

480

Szyrynski V. **Psychotherapy with families of allergic patients.** Ann Allergy 22:165-172, 1964.

▶ family psychotherapy, psychotherapy, group therapy

In this paper, we have reviewed the basic principles, psychodynamic mechanisms, and some fundamental techniques of the psychotherapeutic approach to family members of allergic patients. It has been assumed that intrafamilial emotional tension states are based on the mutual influence of various family members, which is communicated in a verbal and non-verbal manner. In some individuals, such an intrafamilial climate may produce or aggravate allergic reaction patterns. Psychodynamic treatment of significant family members may produce for an allergic patient a markedly changed environment resulting in improvement of his allergic condition.

481

Wahl CW. **Psychodynamics of the allergic patient.** Ann Allergy 18:1138-1143, 1960.

▶ psychotherapy, doctor-patient relationship, consultation-liaison

As Dr. Edward Weiss is fond of saying, "The psychosomatic approach means not that you study the soma less, but that you study the psyche more." It means to be more the physician and less the doctor. It means to include in our histories an interest and concern for the psychological events of the patient's life as well as the medical ones, and to know reasonably well the kinds of life situations which in human existence induce and foster conflict. It means that as physicians we are committed to the scrutiny of and treatment of the whole person. None of us can exempt ourselves from the responsibility of learning the interview techniques and the techniques of simple psychotherapy which will enable us to ameliorate the patient's physical and psychical ills and to identify his more serious psychological problems. We should be able to refer patients without undue conflict for the more necessary intensive help. If this capability of ministering to both kinds of the patient's needs, somatic and psychic, is a desideratum for most specialists, it is surely a necessity for the successful practice of allergy. I have been surprised to note how often the allergists who, I find, do good work resemble the "old family doctor." Like him, they are masters of that fine art of fostering and encouraging warm, reassuring relationships with their patients. They know how to communicate and to encourage communication with others. They know much about life and its vicissitudes, deviations and complexities, and are skillful in helping their patients to see the relationships between stress, worry and physical illness. They can assist them to identify and remove exogenous sources of stress. They foster and encourage confidence and scrupulously keep a patient's confidences. When referral for any medical or psychological reason is indicated, they do this without frightening the patient, without punishing him, or without abandoning him. In short, some of the finest all-round medicine I have seen has been practiced by allergists. I hope that the years ahead result in an ever closer interaction and cooperation between our two specialties.

482

Weiss E. **Psychosomatic aspects of allergic disorders.** Bull NY Acad Med 23:604-630, 1947.

▶ psychotherapy, group psychotherapy

The allergic and the neurotic populations are so large that they must overlap. If for no other reason, therefore, these disorders will exist in the same individual. But, in addition, personality studies suggest a more intimate connection—a specific relationship between neurotic character structure and allergic disorder—possibly representing parallel manifestations of the same basic fault, the one discharging on the level of psychic representation through thoughts and feelings and the other on the physiological level by means of disturbances in organ functioning. Just as we try to establish certain postulates for an allergic problem, hay fever for example, 1) heredity, 2) seasonal history, 3) skin tests, 4) antibodies, 5) induction of an attack with pollen, 6) hyposensitization or avoidance of offending substance in controlling attacks; so in the psychosomatic problem we try to establish 1) a family history of a background for psychopathology, 2) evidence for a childhood neurosis, 3) sensitivity to specific emotional factors (temporal relationship of present illness and emotionally disturbing event), especially at epochal or crucial life periods (puberty, marriage, childbirth, climacteric, etc.), 4) a specific personality structure (other evidence of neurosis or character disturbance), 5) demonstration of specific behavior on taking the history (artificial exposure to a conflict situation), 6) hyposensitization by psychotherapy or the avoidance of the provocative situation. Psychosomatic study of an allergic problem, therefore, utilizes separate technics—psychologic and physiologic—applied simultaneously; and the diagnosis must be established not simply by exclusion or evaluation of physical factors but with additional positive evidence of personality disorder meeting certain psychosomatic postulates. This will demonstrate that in a given case physical and psychologic factors act in a complementary fashion to produce the disorder—in one instance specific physical factors may predominate, in another instance specific emotional factors. The latter seem to be determined by certain trends within the personality—just as oral attachments seem to determine gastrointestinal disorders so do respiratory and dermal attachments (to the mother) apparently help to determine respiratory and dermal allergic manifestations. A study of 24 patients with migraine suggests that it is more closely related to the character structure and personality trends observed in patients with essential hypertension, having to do with the amount and disposition of hostile impulses. The allergic disorders seem to fall into the group of organ neuroses that can be termed vegetative, representing early and profound deviations of personality development. What role the constitution may play cannot be determined—no methods are available to delimit constitutional and acquired factors. One can, however, evaluate physical and psychologic factors and proper management depends on such evaluation. Then psychotherapy plus the allergic approach will mean better treatment for the individual with an allergic disorder.

483
Wittkower E. **Psyche and allergy.** J Allergy 23:76-86, 1952.

▶ psychotherapy

Extracted summary: [N]either the allergic nor the psychiatric aspects of the disease should be neglected in treatment. The physician should treat the patient and not his allergy alone. On examination an assessment of the relative degree and relative significance of allergic and emotional factors should be made and the patient should be treated accordingly. In some patients emotional factors are of minor importance, in others they deserve consideration, in still others they are all-important.

484
Ziwar M. **Allergy and psyche: a psychosomatic study.** Egypt Yearbook Psychol 1:7-22, 1954.

▶ psychotherapy

Other Allergic Disorders

485
Anderson EL. **Effect of hypnotic instructions on the nasal congestion of 24 hayfever sufferers.** Diss Abstr Int 44:1050, 1983.

▶ hypnosis, placebo

During 1981 over 17 million people suffered from hayfever and the associated side effects of medication used to relieve hayfever attacks. The need to analyze the behavioral effect of hypnosis on these attacks stems from complaints of headaches, drowsiness and inability to concentrate after taking hayfever medication. Section one of this study examined the hypnotizability of hayfever sufferers. A Hypnotic Induction Profile and Stanford Hypnotic Clinical Scale for Adults were used to measure hypnotic responsivity. The significant correlation between these measures indicates subjects performed similarly between both measures. Moreover, subjects were also capable of significantly judging their ability to experience hypnosis. The second section examined what effect hypnotic responsivity had on phenylephrine, placebo and hypnosis nasal congestion treatments. Five minute post-treatment and fifteen minute post-treatment effects across all three treatments indicate that the greatest reduction in nasal airways resistance was produced by high hypnotizable subjects during hypnosis treatment and placebo treatment responses. Across all three nasal airways resistance treatments high hypnotizable subjects produced the greatest reduction in nasal airways resistance. Furthermore, during the subjective period high hypnotizable subjects perceived a greater increase in nasal patency within the significant hypnosis treatment. Rhinoscopy findings revealed high hypnotizabel subjects significantly reduced nasal edema and closely approached a significant reduction in blood pressure during the hypnosis treatment. Responses from a follow-up survey one month after the treatment study showed high hypnotizable subjects reporting the greatest reduction in hayfever attacks and medication use. Recommendations include a need to: (1) revise hypnosis training skills for low hypnotizable subjects to help them "reap" the benefit of hypnotherapy; (2) further assess the interaction of hypnotic responsivity with chemotherapeutic treatments; and (3) explore the biological relationship between hypnotic responsivity and stress by comparing neurotransmitter blood levels within a hayfever population.

486
Beselin O. **The management of hay fever during office visits.** HNO 15:281, 1967. (in German)

▶ psychotherapy

487
Brodsky CM. **'Allergic to everything': a medical subculture.** Psychosomatics 24:731-742, 1983.

▶ behavior modification

With the emerging subculture called "clinical ecology," patients are diagnosed as "allergic" or "environmentally ill" and treated with special techniques and avoidance of whole environments. In reviewing a group of eight persons who had filed worker's compensation claims for injury ostensibly caused by allergic response to substances in the workplace yet who showed no physical evidence of injury, the author found withdrawal from work, a life-style engineered to avoid exposure to putative noxious substances, and an identity as a disabled person.

488
De River JP. **Psychology of hay fever.** NY Med J Med Rec 117:730-731, 1923.

▶ psychotherapy

Extracted summary: What are we to do for these patients? Assuming that the primary condition is hay fever, and acknowledging that it is in itself due to some disturbance in the vasomotor system, as a rule ingrafted upon a psychoneurotic diathesis. This leads one to ask, first, are we to treat the condition locally? Second, if local treatment is used alone, can we expect to gain results by ridding the patient of an element which is psychoneurotic? And third, shall we use a combination of both methods, viz., the treatment of a local condition furnishing symptomatic relief

together with the intelligent use of psychotherapy? The last method I am indeed partial to, and we, as otolaryngologists, find it our duty to attack nasal pathology, correcting all deviations from the normal in order to restore the physiological functions as near as possible. The application of pollen antigens when indicated, local applications of medicinal substances, the surgical correction of all anatomical defects of the nose and throat, and the proper use of psychotherapeutic measures are indispensable adjuncts. Only by recognizing the psyche, which is the directing force, and realizing that the spirit, soul and body are inseparable are we able to treat the whole human being scientifically, with the hopes of gaining results.

489
Kaufman W. **Some psychological aspects of the treatment of patients who have food allergies.** Ann Allergy 9:660-664, 1951.

▶ psychotherapy

Untoward reactions to the ingestion of wholesome foods may be caused by psychogenic or allergic mechanisms, or combinations of the two. Sometimes it is important to evaluate the role that psychogenic and allergic factors play in untoward reactions of a patient. Food becomes associated symbolically with diverse emotional meanings very early in life, so that for each individual scarcely a food is emotionally neutral. Psychogenic food reactions may include anxiety, guilt, depression, hostility, passive dependent attitudes, euphoria, relaxation. The most common somatization of psychological reactions to food is to the gastrointestinal tract, including nausea and vomiting, epigastric discomfort or pain, intestinal cramps, aerophagia, belching, and rarely diarrhea, all being part of the riddance reaction. Primary allergenic food reactions are followed by secondary psychogenic reactions which may be more incapacitating than the initiating noxious stimulus. A person with a steady state of allergic reaction resulting from daily ingestion of offending foods may make reasonably good adjustments to his illness and life problems, although his over-all efficiency is lowered by his allergic illness. But often an individual with unpredictable intermittent allergic food reactions such as headache, fatigue, and mental syndromes develops severe frustration reactions, since he can never predict how he will feel. He develops non-problem-solving behavior and becomes intensely concerned with minutiae in an obsessive compulsive manner, and often neglects to do necessary goal-directed work. Psychotherapy can help patients to overcome incapacitating secondary conditioned-behavior patterns. Elimination of allergenic foods removes the etiologic agent, thereby relieving the patient of primary allergenic and secondary psychogenic reaction patterns. Combined allergic therapy and psychotherapy usually yield the best results.

490

Mackenzie JN. **The production of the so-called "rose cold" by means of an artificial rose: with remarks and historical notes.** Am J Med Sci 91:45-57, 1886.

▶ behavior therapy, desensitization, suggestion, confrontation

A case of a woman with recurrent seasonal allergic rhinitis induced by roses is presented. The symptoms were elicited by exposure to an artificial rose. Following a confrontation in which the patient was shown that the "rose" was only a facsimile, her symptoms improved dramatically.

491

Wilson GW. **A study of structural and instinctual conflicts in cases of hay fever.** Psychosom Med 3:51-65, 1941.

▶ psychoanalysis

An attempt has been made to demonstrate certain psychological similarities with particular emphasis upon the persistence of preoccupation with olfactory stimuli in seven cases of hay fever that were psychoanalytically studied. Significant unconscious material reported by one patient who suffered from severe seasonal hay fever preceding the advent of an attack of severe acute rhinitis is presented and discussed.

492

Winkler WT. **Psychosomatic contribution to vasomotor rhinitis.** Z Psychosom Med 3:7, 1956. (in German)

▶ psychoanalysis, autogenic training

Autoimmune, Rheumatic, and Connective Tissue Disorders

Rheumatoid Arthritis

493

Achterberg J. **The psychological dimensions of arthritis.** J Consult Clin Psychol 50:984-992, 1982.

▶ review: psychotherapy, behavior therapy, group therapy

Reviews the literature on the psychological assessment and therapy of persons with arthritis, focusing primarily on the diagnostic category of rheumatoid arthritis. Assessment has involved attempts to define an arthritic personality using psychoanalytic concepts, but more recently it has included the identification of stressors as precursive and exacerbative of disease and the measurement of the impact of arthritis on psychosocial and functional variables. Psychological or behavioral therapy strategies for pain and stress management, psychotherapy in group settings, and attention to medical compliance are among the sparsely reported treatment techniques. It is concluded that therapies that initially address the physical condition, as opposed to mental health needs, are likely to be most acceptable to the patient and most successful in outcome.

494

Achterberg J, Mcgraw P, Lawlis GF. **Rheumatoid arthritis: a study of relaxation and temperature biofeedback training as an adjunctive therapy.** Biofeedback Self Regul 6:207-223, 1981.

▶ relaxation, biofeedback

Relaxation and biofeedback strategies have demonstrated utility in alleviating both pain and stress-related symptomatology and were tested for efficacy with rheumatoid arthritis in a 2-phase study with 32 patients. Results of exp I indicate significant and positive changes following treatment that were primarily related to pain, tension, and sleep patterns in the relaxation/biofeedback and physiotherapy groups. Results of exp II consistently favored the relaxation and biofeedback over the physiotherapy group on the physical/functional indices.

495

Anonymous. **Emotional factors in rheumatoid arthritis.** South Med J 47:795-796, 1954. (editorial)

▶ supportive psychotherapy

496

Antonelli F. **The rheumatic neurosis.** Z Psychosom Med 3:1, 1956. (in German)

▶ psychotherapy

497

Blom GE, Nicholls G. **Emotional factors in children with rheumatoid arthritis.** Am J Orthopsychiatry 24:588-601, 1954.

▶ psychotherapy

Extracted summary: It is difficult to state how emotional factors are dynamically related to the onset of arthritis. The emotionally charged event prior to onset seems to be more a precipitant than the cause. Basically we believe we are dealing with an infantile personality structure, growing out of a long sustained conflict situation, where the outstanding element is the inability of the child to achieve separateness from the mother. It does not seem to us to grow out of the specific conflict of a critical phase of development. Instead we feel that at these periods the struggle of the child to move apart from the mother is accentuated.

498

Booth GC. **Personality and chronic arthritis.** J Nerv Ment Dis 85:637-662, 1937.

▶ psychotherapy

1. The results of the personality studies in both rheumatoid and osteoarthritis reveal that there is no essential difference between these two diseases, thus concurring with the results of the studies of the organic pathological changes. 2. The dynamic predisposition to acquire chronic arthritis rests upon the following factors: (a) an urge to

be active, manifested chiefly in the extrapyramidal motor system; (b) low general vitality; (c) inadequate response of the vasomotor system in making adjustments to the environment, the response being physically inadequate to temperature changes, and psychologically inadequate to emotional contacts; (d) an urge to remain independent of environmental influences, due to circumstances in childhood conducive to a neurotic defensive attitude. 3. The predisposition to become a chronic arthritic can be ascertained from an investigation of the psychological makeup. 4. Chronic arthritis attacks persons so predisposed, when it becomes impossible for them to pursue their original life plan, as a result of the fact that the pre-existing equilibrium between their vitality and the demands of the environment is upset. This disturbance may be consequent upon either a decrease in vitality, or increase in environmental difficulties. 5. The pathological changes of chronic arthritis appear to constitute a regressive method of pursuing the original life plan; once the individual has proved too weak to maintain his security from external interference by activity, the muscles are relieved of their burden by the passive stiffening of the joints. 6. The original personality make-up in chronic arthritis is not affected by the pathological changes; it provides the mould for the outcome of the endogenous and exogenous processes which together constitute the disease of chronic arthritis. 7. The prophylaxis and therapy of chronic arthritis must be based on an appraisal of the dynamic relationship between the individual and his environment. They can succeed only insofar as the necessary equilibrium can be restored, and the biological cause for regressive response removed.

499

Booth GC. **The psychological approach in therapy of chronic arthritis.** Rheumatism 1:48-59, 1939.

▶ psychotherapy, doctor-patient relationship

Therapy of arthritis should meet the following requirements: a) The psychological situation of the patient within his environment must be carefully appraised and be relieved from strain as far as possible. b) The emotional relationship between the patient and the physician calls for particular attention because arthritics feel frustrated very easily. c) The physical part of the therapy should be explained to the patient as dealing with his pathogenic vicious circle. The following methods bear directly on this task: general building up of health, elimination of pain, and re-education of the motoric habits through massage and gymnastics. d) Psychotherapy by a specialist should be used in cases where other methods have failed to produce satisfactory results.

500

Bradley LA, Young LD, Anderson KO, McDaniel LK, Turner RA, Agudelo CA. **Psychological approaches to the management of arthritis pain.** Soc Sci Med 19:1353-1360, 1984.

▶ review: biofeedback, behavior therapy, group psychotherapy, relaxation, imagery

The present review examines the literature regarding the efficacy of cognitive-behavioral and other self-control interventions in helping arthritis patients reduce their pain and functional disabilities. The evidence indicates that self-control interventions have produced significant and positive changes in the pain and functional disabilities of patients with rheumatoid arthritis and arthritis secondary to hemophilia. However, the literature suffers from deficiencies with regard to the use of small subject samples; inadequate control procedures and follow-up assessments; failure to demonstrate that positive outcomes are related to changes in subjects' covert experiences or control of physiological variables; and reliance upon self-report measures of outcome. The review is followed by a description of a multidisciplinary study of the efficacy of a biofeedback-assisted, cognitive-behavioral group therapy program for rheumatoid arthritis patients that features several methodological improvements relative to previous investigations. The preliminary outcome data show that the cognitive-behavioral intervention is associated with reductions in pain behavior and self-reports of pain and disability. It is concluded that, although the self-control interventions have shown promising results, psychologists must demonstrate positive and reliable outcomes among large numbers of arthritis patients over extended periods of time if the interventions are to be viewed as credible by rheumatologists.

501

Cioppa FJ, Thal AB. **Rheumatoid arthritis, spontaneous remission, and hypnotherapy.** JAMA 230:1388-1389, 1974. (letter)

▶ hypnosis, autohypnosis

502

Cioppa FJ, Thal AD. **Hypnotherapy in a case of juvenile rheumatoid arthritis.** Am J Clin Hypn 8:105-110, 1975.

▶ hypnosis, psychotherapy

A 10-yr-old old girl with a diagnosis of juvenile rheumatoid arthritis responded minimally to large doses of salicylates and physical therapy over 7 wks. 3 sessions of hypnotherapy were given. Despite resistance to the 1st session, questionable improvement ensued. At the time of the 2nd session, the patient still had to be carried frequently by her mother. 4 hrs after the 2nd session, she rode her bicycle and was without pain for the 1st time in 12 wks. 2 reinforcing hypnotherapy sessions were added. School work and social adjustment improved markedly. The child remained well for the ensuing 31 mo. Hypnotherapy appears to have initiated an attitudinal change at a level sufficiently deep to accelerate remission.

503

Clark CC. **Women and arthritis: holistic/wellness perspectives.** Top Clin Nurs 4:45-55, 1983.

▶ imagery, relaxation, biofeedback, yoga

Extracted summary: Combined with visualization, progressive relaxation can be used as a way to reduce rage and heal inflamed joints. Directions for combining progressive relaxation with visualization and suggestion are presented in the box. The nurse can read the directions to the clients or ask the clients to tape record the words and replay them for self-practice at home. Sessions two or three times per day and a quiet, restful environment are recommended. The vasodilation that occurs during biofeedback exercises of this type can ward off the reduction of muscle blood flow that occurs in arthritis and the subsequent muscle atrophy, as well as place responsibility for care in the hands of the client. In one study, both biofeedback-relaxation and client groups receiving physiotherapy significantly improved in walking time and in activities of daily living. In addition, the biofeedback-relaxation group members were more involved in their treatment and reported less pain. All the biofeedback-relaxation clients experienced either stable or improved erythrocyte sedimentation rates (a measure of disease or infectious activity) while two of the three physiotherapy clients showed improvement. Although the sample is small, this study shows that biofeedback-relaxation is equal or superior to physiotherapy in terms of the outcomes measured.

504

Cobb S, Miles HHW. **Psychiatric conference.** Am Pract 3:407-411, 1949.

▶ psychotherapy, doctor-patient relationship

The final impression was that of a true psychosomatic illness. The patient seemed in the balance between a frank neurosis and clearcut arthritis, with the arthritic process still at a reversible stage (no objective findings of joint disease). It was interesting that the opinions of psychiatric staff members differed a good deal in regard to diagnosis and dynamic formulations, whereas ordinarily there would be considerable agreement in discussing a patient with a psychoneurosis. Interviews uncovered important conflicts in a number of areas. The more obvious problems were in connection with eating, heterosexuality, relationship to the mother and racial discrimination, but for the purposes

of treatment it seemed wise to avoid disturbing interpretations and to stick to the present complaints. The temporal relationship between symptoms and situations was developed, and it seemed that the significant feeling was one of rejection. Interpretations were not carried further than the pointing out of this relationship, i.e., it was in situations where she felt rejected and angry that her joint pains occurred. It was believed that the therapy was helpful essentially on the basis of support (of a good doctor-patient relationship) and ventilation. In cases where the patient finds it so difficult to bring out her strong emotions and disturbing fantasies it is usually wise to avoid interpretations which will intensify the anxiety.

505

Cormier BM, Wittkower EO, Marcotte Y, Forget F. **Psychological aspects of rheumatoid arthritis.** Can Med Assoc J 77:539-541, 1957.

▶ review: psychotherapy

1. The motor activity of 18 patients with rheumatoid arthritis (r.a.) has been compared with the motor activity of their nearest siblings free of the illness. The comparison shows that the r.a. patients are overactive as children but inhibited later in life (before their illness), whereas their siblings who are free of the illness start life with normal or inhibited motor activity and seem to be able to use their motor apparatus successfully for instinctual discharge later on in life. 2. Motor overactivity early in life in the r.a. patients seem to serve as an outlet for aggressive drives in a socially acceptable or unacceptable form. After puberty, overactivity is progressively abandoned as an inadequate means of expression of instinctual drives as well as a psychological defence against them. Deprived of discharge of instinctual tension in movement and impulsive action, the r.a. patients take recourse to aggressive fantasies which give rise to feelings of guilt and anxiety. 3. The intensification of these incompletely recognized, intolerable, aggressive fantasies (and the concomitant guilt and anxiety) by disturbing events in the patient's life history often precedes and probably precipitates the onset of rheumatoid arthritis. 4. The comparison of the Rorschach findings in 13 r.a. patients with the findings in the 13 nearest siblings free of the disease corroborated closely the clinical assessment. 5. The severity of the illness seems to be proportionate to the severity of the impairment in the capacity to express aggression. 6. The psychotherapeutic implications of these findings are discussed with clinical examples.

506

Czirr R, Gallagher D. **Case report: behavioral treatment of depression and somatic complaints in rheumatoid arthritis.** Clin Gerontol 2:63-66, 1983.

▶ behavior therapy

Contends that medical and psychological practitioners can cooperate to assess and treat both sets of symptoms in elderly depressed patients with somatic complaints related to rheumatoid arthritis (RA). The case of a 62-yr-old man is presented to illustrate the interconnection of daily events, mood, and RA symptoms and to demonstrate how techniques to control depression can also increase the patient's control over somatic symptoms of RA.

507
Dogs W. **Hypnotic analgesia in patients with rheumatism.** Psychother Psychosom 14:96-99, 1968.

▶ hypnosis, autogenic training

508
Ellman P, Mitchell SD. **The psychological aspects of chronic rheumatic joint disease.** Rep Chron Rheumat Dis 2:109-119, 1936.

▶ counseling, psychotherapy, consultation-liaison

We conclude with a short reference to the important subject of treatment of the mental aspects of arthritis. To treat one must first recognise. It does not require a trained psychiatrist to realize how largely the mental factor bulks in these cases, as in all chronic diseases. For the average patient, whether at hospital or in private practice, suggestion and persuasion are all that will be possible. Certain selected cases might, however, with benefit be referred to a psychiatrist for more intensive psychotherapy.

509
Haydu GG. **Integrative psychotherapy in rheumatoid arthritis and allied states.** Adv Psychosom Med 3:196-202, 1963.

▶ psychotherapy

Integrative psychotherapy endeavors to help the person create an integrated system of drive deflections. The patient without such integration has difficulty in the process of his vital need fulfilment. The force-complexes of the rheumatoid patient maintain a rigid and energy consuming stance. It is a variety of pre-depressive state. The aim of integrative psychotherapy is to bring together the integrable aspects of the incongruent or antagonistic self structure forces, and to facilitate thereby whole-making by the patient himself.

510
Hoffman AL. **Psychological factors associated with rheumatoid arthritis: review of the literature.** Nurs Res 23:218-234, 1974.

▶ review: psychotherapy

Investigations of psychological factors relevant to individuals with rheumatoid arthritis are reviewed. The research projects, classified according to methodological procedures, include case and impressionistic, actuarial, factor analytic, correlational, and natural process studies. Results of investigations are compared, their findings are related to a proposed grouping of psychological hypotheses, and directions for future research are recommended.

511
Johnson A, Shapiro LB, Alexander F. **Preliminary report on a psychosomatic study of rheumatoid arthritis.** Psychosom Med 9:295-300, 1947.

▶ psychotherapy

This presentation will be restricted to the psychodynamic findings in a study of 33 cases of rheumatoid arthritis; 18 of these were seen in therapeutic sessions; 15 in anamnestic interviews. There were 4 male and 29 female patients. The psychodynamic formulations pertaining to women have accordingly a greater validity at this point.

512
Katzenelbogen S. **The psychosomatic aspect of rheumatism.** Bol Assoc Med Puerto Rico 40:190-194, 1948.

▶ psychotherapy

In the etiology of the two forms of chronic arthritis with organic changes in the joints, several factors are at work: special predisposition; metabolic disorders, faulty assimilation, both leading to auto-intoxication; infection in one area also causing intoxication to which the joints, given a certain predisposition, react specifically; emotional factors, in causing circulatory disturbances through the autonomic nervous system and increased tension and spasms of the muscular system through the voluntary nervous system, contribute importantly to the onset and development of arthritis. This is illustrated by our two cases. And I should like to make it clear that when I speak of emotional disorders I mean both, those of which the patient is fully aware and which are obvious to others; and those of which the patient is not aware at all or not fully aware; the hidden emotions act as stimuli of the apparent emotional reaction and also of the physiological reactions. The second case, moreover, clearly brings to the fore the role of emotional factors in maintaining the rheumatoid condition, apparently as long as no attempt is made to treat the emotional condition.

513
Lefer J. **Fusion and rheumatoid arthritis.** Contemp Psychoanal 9:63-78, 1972.

▶ psychoanalysis

Describes 2 patients suffering from rheumatoid arthritis, depression, and obsessive-paranoid disorders. Their histories, courses, and analyses are presented to examine the physiology, familial, interpersonal and intrapsychic aspects of the disease, particularly in view of the fact that the etiology is unknown. Silences, fusion, separation, etc., as expressed in dreams and behavior, and the changes of the somatic symptoms, are described and interpreted. It is noted that during their nearly 4 yrs of analysis the analgesics and steroids could be diminished or were no longer necessary. It is suggested that there exists a correlation between the fusion with "bad" internalized significant persons or family networks and the conflictual movements of muscle groups. The somatization, viewed in terms of a system field, becomes an appeal for relief and a signal for significant others. Both patients simultaneously appealed for relief and to be taken care of in the course of the somatic symptoms.

514
Lincoln PJ. **Serological investigation of a faith healer's patient.** Nurs Times 71:2011-2012, 1975.

▶ faith healing

The case referred to our laboratory involved a patient who had just returned from a visit to the Philippines where he had been seeking treatment from the faith healers. According to his general practitioner, the patient had been suffering from a generalised rheumatoid arthritis affecting his spine, hips and hands. Before visiting the faith healers he was unable to walk upright. But when he returned home he was walking erect and experienced no pain. While in the Philippines he underwent several operations which were claimed by healers to involve incisions and bleeding which led to staining of some clothing he was wearing at the time. We carried out a blood grouping investigation on this clothing and on a fresh blood sample taken from the patient. The object was to determine whether the stains were the patient's own blood. More details of the investigative methods are given later. The results of chemical and species tests showed that the staining was indeed blood but was not of human origin!

515
Lindquist I. **Therapeutic use of play.** Paediatrician 9:203-209, 1980.

▶ play therapy

Extracted summary: In Sweden, a special governmental commission on Child Care started working in 1973. One of their issues was the situation of the child in hospital. In their proposal to the government the commission listed a number of measures. The principal and most important one was that every child in hospital should be entitled to play therapy. Parliament complied with this recommendation and the new child care law promulgated in April 1976 and valid as of January 1977 imposes on the bodies in charge of organizing hospital care to make play therapy available to every child in hospital.

516
Ludwig AO. **Psychogenic factors in rheumatoid arthritis.** Bull Rheum Dis 2:33-34, 1952.

▶ counseling, doctor-patient relationship

Extracted summary: The therapeutic implications are important. One should look for and evaluate emotional disturbances associated with the onset of exacerbations in each case. Since loss of security and underlying dependency of many of these patients appears to be significant the physician should provide or restore as much security as possible in the treatment situation. This can be done by interest in the patient as a human being, and by allowing and encouraging him to air his problems. It is vital for these patients to have one person, especially if there are consultants, who is his doctor and in charge to interpret the opinions of the others and to advise the patient with authority. If the relationship is successful, the patient establishes a dependence upon the physician, which can have important bearing on the treatment as long as the patient continues to trust the doctor and to feel that he will be available when needed. The precipitate flights into passive dependence may have to be dealt with by gentle encouragement in the direction of increased activity. Those patients who attempt to negate their dependent attitudes by overactivity may need to be curbed, but it is well to remember that the overactivity in itself serves to release aggressive impulses and if improperly handled, may lead to exacerbation. Some patients with rheumatoid arthritis need the added care of a psychiatrist, but most of these cases can be treated by the internist who understands and is willing to take the time to practice the art of medicine.

517
Ludwig AO. **Psychiatric considerations in rheumatoid arthritis.** Med Clin North Am 39:447-458, 1955.

▶ doctor-patient relationship, psychotherapy, psychoanalysis

Extracted summary: Since it is apparent that disruption of a meaningful relationship with resulting emotional trauma frequently precedes an attack of arthritis, the first task of therapy from the psychiatric point of view will be to restore the patient's sense of security. This can be done by establishing a positive contact with him, which may follow easily as a corollary of the usual medical treatment, especially if the disease is acute and hospitalization is necessary. This contact does much to gratify dependent needs by attention to the patient's comfort through medication and nursing care. It is possible that some of the spontaneous remissions of the disease, so characteristic in the early stages, have some bearing on the patient's ability, with the aid of his contact with the doctor, or through other means, to restore his sense of security by replacing the disrupted relationship with another … Such a substitution for the lost relationship cannot be considered in any sense to constitute a "cure," from the psychologic standpoint. In carefully chosen cases it is feasible to attempt by means of psychotherapy to resolve this peculiar dependent relationship in the physician. In view of the depth of the psychopathology, which has its roots in the very early life experiences of the patient, this will be a lengthy process. Efforts of this sort would seem to carry a possible favorable prognosis in those patients who are treated early in the course of the disease before extensive, irreversible joint damage has occurred. However, the remissions that are observed in rheumatoid arthritis late in the disease give a clue that psychotherapy may occasionally be useful in such cases as well. At any rate it is logical in patients highly vulnerable to stress, to resolve psychic conflicts as fully as one attempts to treat physical and dietary defects.

518
Luparello TJ, McFadden ER, Lyons HA, Bleecker ER. **Psychologic factors and bronchial asthma.** NY State J Med 71:2161-2165, 1971.

▶ placebo

Among those factors playing a significant part in the etiology and pathophysiology of bronchial asthma, the role of psychologic variables has been one of the most difficult to evaluate. The problem in assessing these variables stems primarily from the complexity and the difficulty in providing meaningful controls for them in most experimental situations. By using the experimental model described, it is possible to induce significant changes in the airway reactivity in a number of asthmatic patients in a laboratory setting by means of psychologic stimuli. The airway changes so induced can be in the direction of both increasing Ra or decreasing Ra, depending on the expectation of the patients. These studies further indicate that such phenomena are probably mediated by vagal efferents, since such airway responses can be blocked by atropine.

519
McGraw PC. **Rheumatoid arthritis: a psychological intervention.** Diss Abstr Int 40:1377, 1979.

▶ relaxation, biofeedback

A psychological intervention involving relaxation training and biofeedback training for the control of peripheral skin temperature was investigated in this study with 27 female rheumatoid arthritics as participants. A two-group design was used with the only difference being the direction in which participants were instructed to alter their peripheral skin temperature. A temperature increase group was to use biofeedback to achieve an increase in peripheral skin temperature, while a temperature decrease group was to achieve a decrease. Both groups received identical relaxation training. Based on analysis of the temperature data, it was concluded that the biofeedback response was not learned. From electromyographic data, it was concluded that participants did learn to relax. The hypothesis that the two treatment components would have beneficial affects on the physical, functional, and psychological aspects of rheumatoid arthritis was answered partially. No differential effects as a function of biofeedback training were found as the data for the temperature increase and temperature decrease groups were statistically combined in multiple analyses of variance for repeated measures. Although no differential effects were obtained, numerous positive changes were found. Correlated with the relaxation training were decreases in reported subjective units of discomfort, percentage of time hurting, percentage of body hurting, and general severity of pain. Improved sleep patterns were reported as was increased performance of activities of daily living. Reductions were also found in psychological tension, and in the amount of time mood was influenced by the disease. Shifts were not found in imagery, locus of control, and other psychological dimensions. Constitutional improvements were also absent. Relaxation training was recommended as an adjunctive therapy and its implications were discussed. Future research is suggested.

520
McGregor HG. **The psychological factor in rheumatic disease.** Practitioner 143:627-636, 1939.

▶ psychotherapy

Extracted summary: Although it must be remembered that any patient in a psychopathic state tends to seek justification for his morbid mental or physical disabilities in external misfortunes, yet the investigations contain enough carefully analysed material to warrant much closer study. The whole subject is one of undoubted difficulty, and nothing approaching finality has yet been reached. Much of the work is rendered uncertain by the difficulty of establishing control groups for the type of disease investigated. There is nothing conclusive in establishing a relation between emotional events and attacks of rheumatism unless it can be shown that such a relation is peculiar to the disease in question. At present this has not been done, and there is room for further research here on the lines of that which has recently been done by Wilson at the Tavistock Clinic in the case of peptic ulcer. In these investigations the emotional difficulties and personality types of persons suffering from peptic ulcer was carefully compared with a group of patients suffering from an entirely unrelated complaint. When the two groups were contrasted from a constitutional and personality point of view, the characteristics of the ulcer group stood out in clear relief against the featureless background of the control group. If this kind of study were to be carried out in the case of rheumatoid arthritis it would be easier to speak with conviction about the psychological factor in this disease. At present all that can be said is that rheumatism without structural change is nearly always psychogenic; whereas in certain classes of rheumatism in which structural change is evident psychological factors are found with great frequency, and appear to be closely related to the onset and exacerbations of the malady. It remains for the future to decide the exact part played by these factors.

521
Nissen HA. **Chronic arthritis and its treatment.** N Engl J Med 210: 1109-1115, 1934.

▶ psychotherapy

Extracted summary: Of what use is it to cure a body if a mind is left ill? Certainly it is not enough to arrest or cure body disease if the motivation for living is ignored. Psychotherapy is stressed because in many arthritics, particularly in the so-called rheumatoid, or the patient showing proliferative joint changes, the physio-chemical changes in the body appear to follow psychical changes; endocrinal dysfunction ensues, and subsequently the body systems so controlled are affected insidiously. Hence if one undertakes the treatment of chronic disease he must be prepared to give the time and patience necessary to this form of treatment.

522
Nissen HA, Spencer KA. **The psychogenic problem in chronic arthritis.** N Engl J Med 214:576-587, 1936.

▶ consultation-liaison, psychotherapy

This paper was arranged primarily to present to a group of trained psychopathologists a problem of internal medicine, in which the internist realized his limitation in the treatment of rheumatism, or chronic joint disturbances. To any man in practice, specialist or general practitioner, similar observations of marked changes in motivation of living and emotional reaction in many patients must be apparent. To date, the authors have yet to interview any man interested in rheumatism and allied rheumatic conditions, who did not admit to a certain percentage of failures, patients who had progressed steadily to complete destruction of all joints in spite of every effort. This paper offers a therapeutic aid to the man who will give sufficient attention to the psychical aspects of the chronic arthritic, particularly in the early stages. It is a measure which has been neglected. One of the most recent publications on arthritis does not contain in its index the words psyche, psychiatry or psychogenic. The physician who wishes to utilize psychotherapy has two alternatives, first, to apply it himself, or secondly, to call in a consultant. The first

means he must know enough of the function of the thalamus and hypothalamus, the endocrines, body metabolism and psychogenic manifestations, to apply this knowledge in his practice. If he does not know, he must learn. The second alternative is to recognize his emotionally unstable patient (his potential arthritic) and to call in consultation, and work with, a psychiatrist if one is available. He must select, however, a man broad-minded enough to be interested in applying his specialty (psychopathology), and no more, to one group of patients (arthritics in this instance) over a period of years.

523
Noda HH. **An exploratory study of the effects of EMG and temperature biofeedback on rheumatoid arthritis.** Diss Abstr Int 39:3532-3533, 1979.

▶ biofeedback

Rheumatoid arthritis is a chronic, painful, and frequently disabling illness which is characterized by swelling and destruction of the joints. There is no cure and the mechanism of its action is presently unknown. Rheumatoid arthritis patients experience fluctuating levels of disease activity and often have to contend with pain and both localized and systemic manifestations of disease activity. A study was conducted to investigate the effects of electromyogram and temperature feedback training on symptom and disease activity in rheumatoid arthritic subjects. Subjects were volunteers recruited from the rheumatology clinic of a general hospital. All subjects were females, ranging in age from 45 to 68 years, and having histories of rheumatoid arthritis ranging from 1 to 18 years duration. A total of six subjects were used in the study. Two subjects were randomly assigned to each treatment group. Three treatments were used: electromyogram feedback training, temperature feedback training, and combined electromyogram and temperature feedback training. The design of the study was a single-case design with single-modality feedback subjects assigned an A-B-A-B sequence, and EMG + temperature feedback subjects an A-BC-B-BC sequence. This design was modified slightly based on the subject's progress in learning feedback. The study was conducted over a ten-week period, with subjects receiving twice-weekly training sessions, each of which entailed 12 two-minute training periods. Symptomatic joints and muscles were used as feedback loci. Grip strength was used as the primary measure of change, although subjective measures were also used, such as onset of arthritic fatigue, duration of morning stiffness, and ratings of pain. Preliminary data analyses used an intra-subject graphical presentation to assess changes in EMG and temperature across the sessions of the experiment. These were augmented by an analysis using Fisher's r to z transformation to assess the significance of the correlation between physiological variables and session number. A similar analysis was completed using grip strength. Results indicated that one subject in the EMG feedback group and one subject in the temperature feedback group were able to alter EMG and temperature, respectively. However, none of the subjects who received just one form of feedback training demonstrated an increase in grip strength. One subject in the combined feedback group was able to significantly decrease EMG, increase temperature, and increase grip strength. Subjective measures did not change significantly over the course of the study. Results were confounded by the lack of control over the locus of feedback. It appears probable that the placement of electrodes and thermistors on the cervical muscle could also account for the results achieved by the combined feedback subject. Additional findings indicate that symptomatic muscles located on the body periphery often demonstrated spontaneous low-level activity which was not controllable through feedback methods. Suggestions for further research using additional feedback modalities, multivariate analyses, and group comparisons of treatment are also made.

524

Nolan M. **A combination of hypnotherapy, megavitamins and "folk" medicine in the treatment of arthritis.** Aust J Clin Hypnother Hypn 4:21-25, 1983.

▶ hypnosis, autohypnosis, relaxation, imagery

Administered a treatment program that combined hypnotherapy, megavitamin therapy, and folk medicine to 53 ss treated over 14 mo and suffering from varying degrees of rheumatoid arthritis. Hypnotherapy included relaxation, self-hypnosis, and imagery. Within 4-8 wks of commencement, 49 ss reported freedom from pain and symptoms of the disease to the point where they resumed normal activities. Among the 40 cases followed up over 3-4 yrs, the remission continued for 36 ss who remained on a maintenance program, while 5 who ceased the program also became symptom free.

525

Orme GC. **Hypnosis, pain control and personality change in rheumatoid arthritic patients.** Diss Abstr Int 41:3192, 1981.

▶ hypnosis

The purpose of this project was to examine the effect of hypnosis as a treatment in the control of pain in a population of rheumatoid arthritic patients and further to examine any associated change in emotionality. Three groups of patients suffering from the pain of rheumatoid arthritis were selected. One group served as a control group. The other two groups served as a modified control group and as a treatment group, respectively. All three groups were pre, mid, and post-tested using the McGill Pain Questionnaire, the Minnesota Multiphasic Personality Inventory, the California Personality Inventory Well-Being scale items,

and a check of their medication intake. The testing periods were before any treatment procedures were introduced, after a 6-week therapy involvement period for the modified control group and treatment group, and after another 6 week period with no further interaction of the patients with the therapists. The treatment group received hypnosis instruction for the treatment of pain, the modified control group received a ventilation or talk therapy, and the control group was not seen by any therapist. It was found that self-hypnosis offers a viable and practical treatment technique to individuals in the control of their pain. Individuals were not only able to reduce their perception of pain and its effect on their lives, but they were also able to be the ones in control of the process. Both the treatment group and the modified control group were able to achieve positive change in several emotional factors. The treatment group were able to achieve a more significant change and one that persisted after the therapy sessions were terminated. The members of the treatment group were thus able to increase their emotional functioning and decrease their dependency on medications. The treatment group was the only group able to decrease medication intake significantly thus again indicating the importance of learning a self-help procedure for controlling pain. It would seem from the results of this study that using self-hypnosis for pain control is useful and practical.

526

Otop J. **Psychotherapy in the rehabilitation of patients with rheumatoid arthritis.** Wiad Lek 31:135-137, 1978. (in Polish)

▶ psychotherapy

527

Pipineli-Potamianou A. **The mother-child relationship in a case of rheumatoid arthritis.** Rev Neuropsychiatr Infant 20:199-205, 1972. (in French)

▶ psychoanalysis

The analytic data derived from this patient suffering from rheumatoid arthritis is interesting because of the opportunities given for the exploration of her inner world and the type of relationship that she establishes with her child. The author believes that the data reveal a body image constructed with all the resentment of a binder bound; a body that lives in a phallic image, unable to accept the unthinkable implication of an approach towards the feared and forbidden (Oedipus). The hypothesis is advanced that the excess of aggressivity encountered in these women when they attempt to move towards a conceived goal is matched by a superego which at these times effectively presents realization. The somatization of the conflict fixes the patient physically and psychologically at a certain level of dependence and gives a truly destructive realization of the aggressivity to herself as well as to others, particularly to her son whom she refuses to regard as the child of a father.

528
Prick JJG. **The problems of chronic rheumatism in its psychological, psychiatrical and psychosomatic aspects.** Folia Psychiatr Neurol Neurochir Med 57:121-161, 1954.

▶ psychotherapy

When finally the chronic rheumatism appears then there is a close interweaving of the neurotic state with the chronic rheumatism. The neurosis then proceeds to influence unfavourably the rheumatism and vice versa the rheumatism worsens the neurosis. The pathological totality neurosis-chronic rheumatism should be regarded as being a disorder of the whole personality, that is to say, one meets it expressed in all of life's provinces, in the rational volitional, in the sensitory, and in the vegetative corporality. The personality structure of the rheumatic patients investigated, was further analysed from the following standpoints: genetic psychological, depth analytical, and test psychological. In view of the nature of the chronic rheumatism as this is enunciated above a combined therapy is indicated—medical and physical therapy and at the same time psychotherapy.

529
Randich SR. **Evaluation of stress inoculation training as a pain management program for rheumatoid arthritis.** Diss Abstr Int 43:1625, 1982.

▶ relaxation, behavior modification, imagery, attention-comparison

In recent years there has been a growing interest in pain management by psychological means. Stress Inoculation Training (SIT) is a comprehensive treatment package which aims to combine the effective elements of many pain management approaches. It has been shown to be effective with experimentally induced pain and with clinical pain in case study reports and a small number of experimental studies. The current study evaluated the effectiveness of SIT with 44 rheumatoid arthritis patients. In the SIT condition, patients were taught systematic relaxation, cognitive modification, and the use of imagery and other cognitive strategies in 6 weekly group sessions. In an "attention control" condition patients participated in unstructured group discussions about coping with pain. A group of patients who received no psychological intervention comprised a second control condition. Subjects were assessed pre- and post-treatment and at 8 week follow-up. Measures included the McGill Pain Questionnaire, daily home pain ratings, a log of daily work, leisure, and social activities, and a checklist of daily activities adapted from the Disability Index Questionnaire, a mea-

sure of functional ability and activity. A factor analysis reduced the number of outcome variables to two source variables, pain perception and activity level. Medication intake was analyzed separately. Repeated measures analyses of variance were performed on the resultant factor scores for pain and activity, and on medication intake. It was found that the activity levels of the subjects receiving SIT increased significantly relative to the two control groups, with gains maintained at follow-up. No differences were found between groups as a result of treatment for pain perception. No differences between groups attributable to treatment were found for medication intake, but methodological problems with this variable suggest that no meaningful conclusions can be drawn from this result. These findings indicate that training in pain management skills, although not modifying pain perception, seemed to enable patients to cope more effectively with pain as evidenced by their increased activity levels. Thus, this study lends support to the utility of Stress Inoculation Training as a pain managment program for patients with a chronic painful disease. As such, this treatment may provide a worthwhile adjunct to drug and physical therapy.

530
Rimon R. **Depression in rheumatoid arthritis.** Ann Clin Res 6:171-175, 1974.

▶ supportive psychotherapy

37 depressed female inpatients with definite or classical rheumatoid arthritis were treated with antidepressant drugs and supportive psychotherapy for a period of 3-8 wks. Rheumatological recovery was significantly more marked in those patients in whom clinical depression disappeared (as measured by the Beck Depression Inventory) than in patients with persistent depression throughout the relatively short therapy period. In most of the persistently depressed patients the clinical rheumatological state deteriorated or remained unchanged. The therapeutic regime proved beneficial in 57% of the patients, and both chlorimipramine and sulpiride seemed to be of comparable value in the treatment. The role of psychiatric consultations and therapy methods in the treatment of rheumatoid arthritis is discussed and evaluated.

531
Robinson EG. **Emotional factors and rheumatoid arthritis.** Can Med Assoc J 77:344-345, 1957.

▶ psychotherapy, social casework

Extracted summary: In a group of 43 patients with chronic rheumatoid arthritis under my observation during the past five years, it is thought that a few generalizations can be made regarding emotional stress coincident with or preceding their illness. The onset of arthritis in many instances was associated with loss of support, such as: (a) death of husband or wife; (b) separation from husband or wife; (c) prolonged separation from family; (d) leaving home to become established. It will be noted that these situations could produce acute and short periods of emotional stress on the one hand, or chronic prolonged stress on the other. Regarding the individual personalities it is rather difficult to generalize. However, many of these patients tended to be immature and dependent; they usually tried overly hard to please both in professional and social contacts, and either concealed hostility or expressed it indirectly. Many of them were rather perfectionistic and ambitious. This trait is actually an asset in the treatment program, if controlled, as they are often more zealous and productive in a rehabilitation program than might be expected, considering their physical disability. . . . Most of the psychological problems can and should be dealt with by the family doctor or internist, rather than by the psychiatrist. In exceptional circumstances where close cooperation and team work are possible it is rewarding to have psychiatric treatment as part of the combined teamwork approach to the disease. We have also been impressed by the value of casework as provided by social workers trained in the special techniques of professional social casework in a medical setting. As is probably generally known, the successful practice of casework, as in medicine, implies an acceptance of the patient as a person—his interests, desires, strivings and failings; a recognition of his problems; a respect for emotionally determined attitudes towards his illness and the physician; and a willingness to work with the patient in terms of his own way of looking at the world and other people. By decreasing the individual's emotional burdens and increasing his capacity to meet life's frustrations, casework attempts to help the patient make use of his own strengths and the environmental resources. He is thus able to cope with these difficulties more adequately as well as to participate more constructively in the general treatment program.

532
Ruiz KN. **An experiment using an imaging method based on Senoi-Dreamwork with rheumatoid arthritics.** Diss Abstr Int 44:324, 1983.

▶ imagery

The purpose of the study was to introduce an imaging method based on Senoi-Dreamwork as a possible treatment package for use in the treatment of rheumatoid arthritics. A rationale was developed based upon existing findings in the literature of rheumatoid arthritis, pain and imaging which established the basis to explore the use of this imaging method with rheumatoid arthritis patients. The method used was single case experimental design with six diagnosed rheumatoid arthritis subjects. Self-reported pain was measured on a 100 mm analog scale and individual functionality was measured on behavioral checklists. The design used was an AA'BA'B where the A phase

was a baseline measurement, the A' phase was placebo treatment and B phase was the imaging method based on Senoi-Dreamwork. The results were measured by visual inspection of the data plotted on a graph and by statistical analysis. The statistical method used was a regression analysis using a linear model for a split plot (repeated measures) design. The results of the regression analysis indicated that response to treatment was quite individual with no overall effect of treatment found. A negative correlation significant at the .01 level was found between pain and functionality. A patient effect did exist for functionality which indicated that individual patients responded to the treatment differently due to some patient variable. Therefore, the results are discussed on an individual basis. A discussion of qualitative and clinical data is given which raises questions that lead to future research.

533
Schwartz LH, Marcus R, Condon R. **Multidisciplinary group therapy for rheumatoid arthritis.** Psychosomatics 19:289-293, 1978.

▶ group therapy, consultation-liaison

A group therapy approach to the psychosocial treatment of rheumatoid arthritis, with co-leaders from the disciplines of psychiatry, internal medicine, and physical medicine, is described. This group experience offers innovative treatment as well as a learning experience in psychosomatic medicine for the physicians involved. This type of group approach could become a valuable instrument for teaching psychiatry to residents and medical students.

534
Sharp OB. **Psychological factors in rheumatism.** Br Med J 1:419-420, 1937. (letter)

▶ psychotherapy

535
Shern MA, Fireman BH. **Stress management and mutual support groups in rheumatoid arthritis.** Am J Med 78:771-775, 1985.

▶ group therapy

Stress management and mutual support groups are employed widely in chronic illness, although their efficacy has not been established. To determine the effect of these measures on morbidity and psychologic health in rheumatoid arthritis, 105 patients meeting diagnostic criteria for rheumatoid arthritis were evaluated for depression, life satisfaction, functional disability, and indicators of disease activity. Patients were randomly assigned to one of three groups: (1) stress management; (2) mutual support; (3) no intervention (control). After completion of 10 weekly sessions, identical tests were performed for all patients in the intervention and control groups. Patients in the intervention groups showed greater improvement in joint tenderness than did the control patients but did not differ significantly from the patients in the control group in any of the other outcome measures.

536
Shocket BR, Lisansky ET, Shubard AF, Fiocco V, Kurland S, Pope M. **A medical psychiatric study of patients with rheumatoid arthritis.** Psychosomatics 10:271-279, 1969.

▶ psychotherapy

A small group of patients with documented rheumatoid arthritis was studied extensively—medically, psychiatrically, and socially—to examine how life circumstances affected the course of this illness and to determine if there were discernible precipitating psychological factors in exacerbations of the illness. This group of patients was found to be specifically vulnerable to separation, real or threatened. Onset or exacerbation of symptoms of rheumatoid arthritis was temporally related to a major life crisis involving separation in this group of patients.

537
Straube W. **Experience with psychotropic drugs, autogenic training and psychologic dialogs with the physician in rheumatic diseases.** Verh Dtsch Ges Rheumatol 5:37-39, 1978. (in German)

▶ autogenic training, group therapy

Autogenic training in small groups can play an important role in treating disturbances of a psychosomatic nature, by alleviating pain and promoting general relaxation. It is important that the patient can and should continue the treatment by himself—actively structuring his own therapy. In connection with autogenic training, after exercises in small groups, patients themselves eagerly entered into a medical discussion.

538
Struthers GR, Scott DL, Scott DG. **The use of "alternative treatments" by patients with rheumatoid arthritis.** Rheumatol Int 3:151-152, 1983.

▶ faith healing

In a study of 199 patients with rheumatoid arthritis, 68% were found to have tried "alternative treatments." Some treatments (acupuncture and faith healing) gave subjective benefit in nearly half those who tried them and were considered to be better than others (such as copper bracelets). No adverse reactions were reported. "Alternative treatments" play an important role as self prescribed therapy in rheumatoid arthritis and their use should not be ignored nor underestimated.

539
Udelman HD, Udelman DL. **Emotions and rheumatologic disorders.** Am J Psychother 35:576-587, 1981.

▶ psychotherapy, group therapy, patient education, couples therapy

Reviews the literature on the emotional components of rheumatologic disorders, and presents 2 case studies (a 45-yr-old female and a couple in their 40's). Varied psychotherapeutic approaches are suggested, including individual and group psychotherapy, didactic sessions, and husband-wife co-therapy. The importance of family relationships is stressed.

540
Udelman HD, Udelman DL. **Rheumatology reaction pattern survey.** Psychosomatics 19:776-780, 1978.

▶ group therapy

Preliminary findings of the survey included an older age at onset of illness for men; greater severity of rheumatoid disease in rheumatoid factor-positive patients; higher hope scores in women; and greater use of steroids and/or psychotropics by women. A family history of rheumatoid arthritis was found more frequently in women. The authors suggest that appropriate channeling of aggression may help to lessen the progression of rheumatoid disease. They also speculate on the anticipation of loss of status relative to the older age at onset of illness in men.

541
Udelman HD, Udelman DL. **Group therapy with rheumatoid arthritic patients.** Am J Psychother 32:288-299, 1978.

▶ group therapy, psychotherapy

Describes a brief group-psychotherapy program instituted on an inpatient arthritis unit by a husband-wife co-therapist team working in clinical collaboration with the rheumatologists. Methods of organizing and managing the program are described. Staff and patient resistance required constant attention and education. Accounts of the results achieved by the group are given, highlighted by descriptions of the progress of 4 patients. Four levels of group interaction are identified, ranging from educative through exploratory-dynamic. Areas of exploration have included body-image, job status, family relationships, and coping mechanisms. Preliminary findings and research possibilities are discussed.

542
Warter P. **Emotional factors in rheumatic diseases: their role and treatment.** Bull Tufts N Engl Med Center:44-49, 1957.

▶ psychotherapy, hypnosis

Extracted summary: The response of the patient to a tried and true therapeutic program will be more profitable if he can be conditioned to positive thinking. The patient's desire to get well is the crux of a successful therapeutic program. There have been innumerable approaches to aid in treating the emotional factors of the rheumatic problem. Treatment by psychotherapy must be divided into two groups. In one, the patient is morose with an impending depressive psychosis; in the second, the emotional states are readily discernible and their conflicts not too deep. Most all rheumatics are in the second group. The first group of patients must be recognized early and treatment by a psychiatrist instituted. Patients in the second group must first be made acquainted with their problem by a realistic and reassuring approach. Such a patient must be impressed with the fact that no therapeutic program will be of lasting value unless he allows it to be, and that no drug will work beneficially unless he allows it to do so. He must accept every phase of the treatment as an essential and integral part of his desired recovery. Many of the so-called "dramatic" cures are the result of a conquered frustration or inhibition. The improvement continues if the psychic overlay does not return. When the patient and the physician are fortified with this knowledge, it is safe to embark upon other phases of treatment. Hypnotherapy has been of definite aid in determining the degree of function possible in questionable cases. It has aided a few arthritics to overcome some of the inhibitions and fears which have plagued them. I use the word "few" justifiably because this procedure should be used only when the patient has been thoroughly appraised by a psychiatrist. The treatment by hypnosis should be given only by a psychiatrist trained in this art.

Other Autoimmune Disorders and Raynaud's Disease or Phenomenon

543
Adair JR, Theobald DE. **Raynaud's phenomenon: treatment of a severe case with biofeedback.** J Indiana State Med Assoc 71:990-993, 1978.

▶ biofeedback

Raynaud's phenomenon is a combination of vasospastic disease and an accompanying pathologic process. Medical and surgical treatments have proven to be unsatisfactory in the long-term management of these patients. A case is presented of a 66-year-old white female with Raynaud's symptoms of 35 years duration and scleroderma. She was admitted to the hospital with multiple small ulcerations on her fingers. She received 10 temperature biofeedback treatments in eight days. She was followed for six months post discharge. Objectively, she significantly increased her baseline and maximum finger temperature during her training and, although these temperatures diminished in the six months of follow-up, they stayed above the pretreatment baseline. Her ulcerations began to heal and she used fewer analgesics. The patient reported that her fingernails were growing for the first time in 10 years and her finger mobility was still improved.

544
Kirkpatrick RA. **Witchcraft and lupus erythematosus.** JAMA 245:1937, 1981. (case report)

▶ folk medicine

545
Kirkpatrick RA. **Witchcraft and lupus.** JAMA 247:176, 1982. (letter)

▶ folk medicine

546
Millikin LA. **Arthritis and Raynaud's syndrome—as psychosomatic problems successfully treated with hypnotherapy.** Br J Med Hypn 15:37-44, 1963.

▶ hypnosis

The entire gamut of rheumatic treatments, including local counter-irritants, such as red pepper rubs, salt rubs, whirlpool baths, sprays, mud baths, hot and cold packs following various rituals, religious or voo-doo magic meetings, have been in vogue for many years. Societies and clubs for treatment of arthritis are using some forms of the above with about the same average of failures, their only success being in the financial gain for themselves. It is becoming more evident that every non-septic arthritis is the result of pathological tension which is developed from one or more emotional conflicts. These usually produce a symptom pattern which can easily be recognized and the proper treatment can be instituted. There is marked progressive improvement in cases of acute rheumatic fever, rheumatoid and hypertrophic or osteoarthritis and Raynaud's syndromes, when treated with hypnotherapy.

547
Taub E, Stroebel CF. **Biofeedback in the treatment of vasoconstrictive syndromes.** Biofeedback Self Regul 3:363-373, 1978.

▶ biofeedback, autogenic training

In summary, thermal biofeedback and associated techniques have been shown to be very promising as a therapeutic approach to Raynaud's disease and allied vaso-constrictive disorders. Treatments currently available for this disease are generally unsatisfactory, because of either minimal effect, unpleasant side effects, or radical nature. In contrast, temperature self-regulation has two major advantages. First, long-term use has not been observed to have any secondary consequences, and certainly no un-desirable side effects, in either normal subjects or Ray-naud's disease patients. Second, since the vasospastic at-tacks are episodic, the patient need employ the technique only when attacks threaten to occur; no continuous reg-imen is necessary. Consequently, thermal biofeedback can appropriately be considered a useful alternative therapy for Raynaud's disease and related vasoconstrictive syn-dromes.

548
Yocum DE, Hodes R, Sundstrom WR, Cleeland CS. **Use of biofeedback training in treatment of Raynaud's disease and phenomenon.** J Rheumatol 12:90-93, 1985.

▶ biofeedback

To assess biofeedback training in Raynaud's, we retro-spectively reviewed 23 patients' records. Eleven had Ray-naud's disease and 12 had Raynaud's phenomenon; 9 had recurrent digital ulcers. Patients demonstrated lower baseline digital temperatures than controls (p less than or equal to 0.001), patients with Raynaud's and scleroderma manifesting the lowest. After biofeedback training all pa-tients elevated baseline temperatures. Patients with scler-oderma and systemic lupus erythematosus had the great-est elevations. Improvement, both subjective (57%) and ulcers (44%), persisted one year after treatment. Four of 7 patients were capable of elevating digital temperatures within 5 min, 18 months after their last training session. These findings support biofeedback training as beneficial therapy in Raynaud's.

549
Cousins N. **Anatomy of an illness (as perceived by the patient).** N Engl J Med 295:1458-1463, 1976.

▶ doctor-patient relationship, laughter, placebo, faith healing

The author relates an account of his recovery from an-kylosing spondylitis having been told by specialists that he had one chance in 500 of recovering fully. Even before diagnosis, the patient was discontent with the approach that the hospital had towards a seriously ill individual. Using his own active coping efforts and positive emotions to strengthen his endocrine system—in particular, the ad-renal glands, the author started on his road to recovery by leaving the hospital environment. Ascorbic acid was substituted for anti-inflammatory drugs. As he had a strong belief that laughter is good medicine, he used amusing

films to induce laughter. The conclusions he draws from his entire experience are that the will to live is not a theoretical abstraction, but a physiologic reality with ther-apeutic characteristics. Also he felt incredibly fortunate to have an understanding doctor who encouraged him to believe that he was a respected partner in the total un-dertaking. The doctor also acted in the best tradition of medicine in recognizing that he had to reach out beyond the usual verifiable modalities in this case.

550
Elitzur B, Caspi D, Yaron M. **Hypnosis for acute emo-tional reactions in Sjogren's syndrome.** Harefuah 104:230-231, 1983. (in Hebrew: no English abstract)

▶ hypnosis

551
Emery H, Schaller JG, Fowler RS. **Biofeedback in the management of primary and secondary Raynaud's phenomenon.** Arthritis Rheum 19:795, 1976. (abstract)

▶ biofeedback

Twelve patients with Raynaud's phenomenon were stud-ied. Seven had underlying diseases including scleroderma (5 patients), mixed connective tissue disease (1 patient), and systemic lupus erythematosus (1 patient): 5 had no detectable related disease. Three had received vasodilator medications without improvement. Pulse patterns and presence or absence of digital artery occlusions were de-termined by plethysmography and Doppler technique. Baseline records were kept of discomfort, color changes and coldness experienced by each patient prior to therapy. During biofeedback training sessions a temperature probe was taped to one finger, and changes in digital tempera-ture were registered on a dial and a printed recording. Patients were instructed to concentrate on warming their hands. After ten half-hour training periods, all patients learned to raise their digital temperatures voluntarily at least 4 degrees C, and some as much as 10 degrees C. The raised digital temperatures were shown to correlate with increased pulse heights on plethysmography. Digital ulcers healed in 1 patient who had extensive ulcerative changes. No patients have developed new ulcers since starting therapy. All patients have noted subjective im-provement: many are able to participate in previously in-tolerable activities such as swimming and skiing. Biofeed-back appears to be a useful, noninvasive technique in the management of Raynaud's phenomenon.

552
Freedman R, Ianni P, Hale P, Lynn S. **Treatment of Ray-naud's phenomenon with biofeedback and cold sen-sitization.** Psychophysiology 16:182, 1979. (abstract)

▶ biofeedback

STUDY 1. Ten subjects with primary or secondary Ray-naud's phenomenon of 2-10 yrs duration were given 12 sessions of finger temperature biofeedback consisting of a 16-min stabilization period, a 16-min baseline, 24 min of feedback, and a final 16-min baseline. After subtracting baseline drift from feedback temperatures, a 2-way repeated measures ANOVA showed a significant effect for sessions ($F (11/749) = 1.88$, $p < .05$). Primary Raynaud's patients had significantly higher overall finger temperatures than secondary patients ($T = 2.95$, $p < .005$) but were significantly poorer temperature controllers during biofeedback ($T = 6.99$, $p < .001$). Frontalis EMG was generally negatively correlated with finger temperature while pulse volume in the two hands was always positively and significantly related. The number of reported Raynaud's attacks decreased significantly between pretreatment (2-28/week) and 1-yr follow-up (0-2/week) measures. Three of 4 subjects tested were able to control finger temperature outdoors at 19 degrees C when monitored by radiotelemetry. STUDY 2. To facilitate transfer of temperature training to the natural environment, a second group of 8 patients received 6 biofeedback sessions as described above and 6 sessions in which the finger being monitored for feedback was subjected to mild cold stress. The temperature of a thermoelectric module was dropped from 30 degrees C to 20 degrees C at a rate of 1 degree/min, then held at 20 degrees C for 10 min. Subjects reported the 20 degrees to be moderately cold. Of 7 subjects trained in this procedure so far, 5 have shown significant finger temperature control during exposure to the 20 degree stimulus. All subjects have reported substantial improvements in frequency of vasoconstrictive attacks.

553
Freedman RR, Ianni P, Wenig P. **Behavioral treatment of Raynaud's phenomenon in scleroderma.** J Behav Med 7:343-353, 1984.

▶ biofeedback, autogenic training

Twenty-four patients with Raynaud's phenomenon and scleroderma were randomly assigned to receive finger temperature biofeedback, frontalis EMG biofeedback, or autogenic training. Only those receiving temperature feedback showed significant increases in finger temperature during training and during a posttraining test of voluntary control, effects not attributable to general relaxation. However, no group demonstrated significant clinical improvement, assessed by symptom reports and by ambulatory monitoring of finger temperature. The need for careful classification of patients with Raynaud's disease and Raynaud's phenomenon in scleroderma is emphasized.

554
Freedman RR, Lynn SJ, Ianni P, Hale PA. **Biofeedback of Raynaud's disease and phenomenon.** Biofeedback Self Regul 6:355-365, 1981.

▶ biofeedback

Six Raynaud's disease and four Raynaud's phenomenon patients were treated with 12 sessions of finger temper-

ature biofeedback. The mean frequency of vasospastic attacks was reduced to 7.5% of that reported during the pretreatment baseline and was maintained for a 1 year follow-up period. Significant control of digital temperature was demonstrated during laboratory training sessions. Raynaud's phenomenon patients showed significantly greater temperature increases during feedback periods than Raynaud's disease patients. Correlations between finger temperature and other physiological measures suggested that results could not be attributed to general physical relaxation. The role of imagery in self-control of digital temperature is considered.

555
Gerber L. **From the NIH: training of patients with Raynaud's phenomenon normalizes responses to drops in temperature.** JAMA 242:509-510, 1979. (Research Findings)

▶ biofeedback

556
Hartmann von Monakow K. **Therapy of vegetative peripheral circulatory disorders.** Bibl Psychiatr Neurol 139:514-515, 1969. (in German)

▶ psychotherapy

557
Huebschmann H. **On transference in the treatment of organic diseases.** Psychother Psychosom 31:288-293, 1979.

▶ psychotherapy

Discusses a case study of transference in a 39-yr-old suicidal female with hepatitis. Analytic therapy, aimed at converting transference as repetition of behavior into recollection, can be useful in cases of this type.

558
Jacobson AM, Hackett TP, Surman OS, Silverberg EL. **Raynaud phenomenon: treatment with hypnotic and operant technique.** JAMA 225:739-740, 1973.

▶ biofeedback, autohypnosis

Trained a 31-yr-old male with Raynaud phenomenon to increase the temperature in his hands bilaterally, using autohypnosis and biofeedback. An increase in temperature of as much as 4.3 C was observed in both hands, along with marked symptomatic improvement that was still in effect 7 1/2 mo after the last treatment.

559

Keefe FJ, Surwit RS, Pilon RN. **Collagen vascular disease: can behavior therapy help?** J Behav Ther Exp Psychiatry 12:171-175, 1981.

▶ autogenic training, biofeedback

This study examined the efficacy of a simple autogenic and biofeedback treatment package in the management of Raynaud's phenomenon secondary to diagnosed collagen vascular disease. The patient, diagnosed as suffering from mixed connective tissue disease, had an average of 6.3 vasospastic attacks per day during a 2 week baseline period. The frequency of daily attacks dropped to 4.2 after 10 weeks and 2.5 attacks after 1 yr of training. In addition, the patient displayed a gradual improvement in the ability to maintain digital skin temperature in the presence of ambient cold stress.

560

Mufson I. **An etiology of scleroderma.** Ann Intern Med 39:1219-1227, 1953.

▶ psychotherapy

Evidence collated from a clinical and psychologic study of several patients supports the belief that scleroderma, like Raynaud's disease, is a manifestation and the result of a psychosomatic disturbance with a definite pattern. The patient's sense of security always depends upon a commensalistic type of existence. When by force of circumstances this is destroyed, the inflexible nature of his personality does not permit readjustment. The dread fear initiates a generalized spasm of the minute vessels and the evolution of cutaneous and visceral scleroderma. While this life situation is operative the process persists and is cumulative in its self-destruction. If and when security is reestablished by chance or design, the process is reversed and the complicating thrombotic manifestations become amenable to vasodilating therapy. To attempt such therapy without first reestablishing security is to court failure and disappointment which, in turn, aggravate the disease. Though the problem was presented from the medical viewpoint of one interested in peripheral vascular disease we required the cooperative help of the psychiatrist, the surgeon, the psychologist and the social worker to gain this insight, which frequently prevented the evolution of simple vasospasm to scleroderma.

561

Norris A, Huston P. **Raynaud's disease studied by hypnosis.** Dis Nerv Syst 17:163-165, 1956.

▶ psychotherapy, hypnosis

Extracted summary: We wish to report the case of a patient with Raynaud's disease with scleroderma ... We

have studied a person with the narcissistic, dependent type of personality so often reported in Raynaud's disease. However, the illness did not follow closely the loss of a love object, nor was there any other stress which could be designated as a precipitating cause. As the disease progressed it became apparent that emotional factors such as anger and fear could precipitate individual attacks during a period of exacerbation of the disease, but no evidence that these factors could produce an exacerbation. There was the suggestion that as the patient acquired more responsibility and fulfilled a more important role, her illness abated. This differs from most reports where exacerbations seem to occur with frustration of dependency needs. Hypnosis proved valuable in the investigation of possible psychological factors and provided extremely clear memory pictures with appropriate emotions associated with attacks of spasm. However, under these conditions spasm did not occur; nor was there any significant change in skin color, skin temperature or heart rate. This report suggests that the psychodynamics of Raynaud's disease as heretofore reported are not adequate or specific. Against this suggestion it could be argued that the hypnotically relived emotions were different from "natural" emotions; or perhaps the patient could not be expected to have spasms since she was in a state of remission. Emotion, however, may precipitate attacks when the disease is active.

562

Peterson LL, Vorhies C. **Raynaud's syndrome: treatment with sublingual administration of nitroglycerin, swinging arm maneuver, and biofeedback training.** Arch Dermatol 119:396-399, 1983.

▶ biofeedback

Sublingual (SL) administration of nitroglycerin, a swinging arm maneuver, and biofeedback were evaluated for their effectiveness in decreasing hand rewarming time after ice immersion in six patients with Raynaud's disease and four patients with Raynaud's phenomenon. After ice immersion of their hands, ten normal patients showed rewarming to baseline temperatures in less than six minutes, while in nine of ten patients with Raynaud's syndrome, rewarming took more than 40 minutes. Two of ten patients with Raynaud's syndrome showed rewarming in less than six minutes after SL administration of nitroglycerin, while eight of ten patients with Raynaud's syndrome showed rewarming in less than 20 minutes after biofeedback training sessions. Six of the ten still showed rewarming in 20 minutes or less eight weeks afer the sessions were over. A swinging arm maneuver provided no objective improvement. Sublingual administration of nitroglycerin provides a new alternative therapy for certain individuals. Effective biofeedback training can be learned in a relatively short time but should be reserved for the well-motivated patient.

563

Richardson HB. **Raynaud's phenomenon and scleroderma: a case report and psychodynamic formulation.** Psychoanal Rev 42:24-38, 1955.

▶ psychoanalysis

This is the report of the case of a patient who suffered from Raynaud's phenomenon and scleroderma. The vascular changes in Raynaud's phenomenon provide an excellent opportunity for observing the relationship between emotions and bodily changes. The patient described (in this case report), who suffered from Raynaud's phenomenon and scleroderma, provides a clear instance of a disease in which the affected portion of the body is the focus of powerful and fundamental emotions. Her disability affects her hands, and the emotions concerned are mainly love, fear and rage. Her illness recapitulated the death of a relative in the form of a slow destruction of her own body, as if to expiate her guilt.

564

Schild R. **Possibilities and limitations of psychosomatic research in rheumatology.** Hippokrates 38:955-960, 1967. (in German: no English abstract)

▶ doctor-patient relationship, psychotherapy

565

Smith SJ. **A multidimensional approach to pain relief: case report of a patient with systemic lupus erythematosus.** Int J Clin Exp Hypn 31:72-81, 1983.

▶ relaxation, behavior therapy, systematic desensitization, hypnosis autohypnosis, imagery, psychotherapy

Used techniques associated with behavioral therapy (deep muscle relaxation, systematic desensitization), hypnosis (trance states, guided imagery, age regression, anesthetic induction and transfer, and auto-hypnosis), and psychodynamic psychotherapy (dyadic interchange, suggestion, encouragement, interpretation of resistance, and the transference/countertransference relationship) to help a 41-yr-old female with systemic lupus erythematosus obtain virtual freedom from disabling pain and the necessity for analgesic and tranquilizing medications. Follow-up over a 3-yr period demonstrated the utility of the approach.

566

Surwit RS. **Biofeedback: a possible treatment for Raynaud's disease.** Semin Psychiatry 5:483-490, 1973.

▶ biofeedback

The physiology of Raynaud's disease and the efficacy of biofeedback in controlling various physiologic functions are reviewed. Five case studies are presented in which biofeedback was used as the primary mode of treatment of Raynaud's disease or Raynaud's phenomenon. The outcome of these studies is discussed in terms of the questions they raise for future research. It is suggested that although biofeedback cannot, at present, be considered a reliable treatment of Raynaud's disease, it might be preferable to more drastic surgical procedures.

567

Surwit RS. **Behavioral treatment of Raynaud's syndrome in peripheral vascular disease.** J Consult Clin Psychol 50:922-932, 1982.

▶ behavior therapy, relaxation, biofeedback

Raynaud's syndrome is a vasospastic phenomenon that occurs in numerous peripheral vascular diseases. Because these vasospasms are sympathetically mediated, they are, in theory, treatable behaviorally. Research conducted over the past 10 years has demonstrated that biofeedback, autogenic training, and progressive relaxation can all be used to treat even severe Raynaud's syndrome. However, there is no distinct advantage of one technique over the other. These techniques can be combined with sympathetic blocking agents to produce an additive effect. It is concluded that behavioral procedures have much to add to the treatment of Raynaud's syndrome.

568

Surwit RS, Allen LM III, Gilgor RS, Duvic M. **The combined effect of prazosin and autogenic training on cold reactivity in Raynaud's phenomenon.** Biofeedback Self Regul 7:537-544, 1982.

▶ autogenic training

Prazosin and autogenic training had an additive effect in attenuating vasomotor tone during an ambient cold challenge in patients with Raynaud's phenomenon. The combination of these two treatments significantly elevated finger temperature during a 16° ambient exposure, while neither treatment alone was found to produce this effect. This suggests that autogenic training and prazosin had an additive effect on reducing peripheral vasomotor activity.

569

Thulesius O. **Psychiatric treatment of Raynaud's phenomenon.** Lakartidningen 76:4234, 1979. (letter: in Swedish)

▶ psychotherapy

570

Wilson E, Belar CD, Panush RS, Ettinger MP. **Marked digital skin temperature increase mediated by thermal biofeedback in advanced scleroderma.** J Rheumatol 10:167-168, 1983. (letter)

▶ biofeedback

571

Zander W. **Psychodynamic factors in some rheumatoid factor negative arthritic diseases.** Munch Med Wochenschr117:1475-1478, 1975. (in German)

▶ psychotherapy

A total of 32 patients with rheumatoid factor negative diseases were investigated by depth psychology: patients with palindromic rheumatism, Reiter's disease and psoriatic arthritis. In each case a typical psychosyndrome could be found correlative with the somatic syndrome, in which the specific form of working out of aggression was at the focal point. An association of psychic factors in the etio-pathogenesis of these arthritic diseases is consequently very probable.

Books and Book Chapters on Immunologic Disorders

572
Abramson HA. **Psychodynamics and the Allergic Patient.** Minneapolis: Bruce, 1948.

573
Abramson HA. **Psychodynamic pharmacology in the therapy of asthma.** In: HA Abramson (ed.), Somatic and Psychiatric Treatment of Asthma. Baltimore: Williams & Wilkins, 1951.

574
Abramson HA. **The Patient Speaks.** New York: Vantage Press, 1956.

575
Abramson HA. **Psychological Problems in the Father-Son Relationship; A Case of Eczema and Asthma.** New York: October House, 1969.

576
Achterberg J, Lawlis GF. **Rheumatoid arthritis: a psychological perspective.** In: J Achterberg, GF Lawlis, Bridges of the Body Mind: Behavioral Approaches to Health Care. Champaign, Illinois: Institute for Personality and Ability Testing, Inc., 1980.

577
Aitken RCB, Zealley AK, Barrow CG. **The treatment of psychopathology in bronchial asthmatics.** In: R Porter, J Knight (eds.), Physiology, Emotion and Psychosomatic Illness. New York: Associated Scientific Publishers, 1972.

578
Alexander AB. **Asthma.** In: SN Haynes, L Gannon (eds.), Psychosomatic Disorders: A Psychophysiological Approach to Etiology and Treatment. New York: Praeger, 1981.

579
Alexander AB. **The treatment of psychosomatic disorders: bronchial asthma in children.** In: BB Lahey, AE Kazdin (eds.), Advances in Clinical Child Psychology. Vol. 3. New York: Plenum, 1980.

580
Alexander AB. **Behavioral medicine in asthma.** In: RB Stuart (ed.), Adherence, Compliance and Generalization in Behavioral Medicine. New York: Brunner/Mazel, 1982.

581
Alexander AB, Solanch LS. **Psychological aspects in the understanding and treatment of bronchial asthma.** In: JM Ferguson, CB Taylor (eds.), The Comprehensive Handbook of Behavioral Medicine. Vol. 2. New York: SP Medical and Scientific Books, 1981.

582
Baruch DW. **One Little Boy.** New York: Julian Press, 1952.

583
Baruch DW, Miller H. **Interview group psychotherapy with allergy patients.** In: SR Slavson (ed.), The Practice of Group Therapy. New York: International Universities Press, 1947.

584
Bastiaans J, Groen J. **Psychogenesis and psychotherapy of bronchial asthma.** In: D O'Neill (ed.), Modern Trends in Psychosomatic Medicine. London: Butterworth, 1955.

585
Bhole MV. **Rationale of treatment and rehabilitation of asthmatics by yogic methods.** In: Swami Digambarji (ed.), Collected Papers on Yoga. 1st ed. Varanasi, India: Kaivalyadhama Lonavla, 1975.

586
Bull II. **Use of hypnotherapy in a case of bronchial asthma.** In: RB Winn (ed.), Psychotherapy in the Soviet Union. New York: Philosophical Library, 1961.

587
Cohen SI, Lask B. **Psychologic factors.** In: TJH Clark, S Godfrey (eds.), Asthma. Philadelphia: Saunders, 1977.

588
Collison DR. **Hypnosis and respiratory disease.** In: GD Burrows, L Dennerstein (eds.), Handbook of Hypnosis and Psychosomatic Medicine. New York: Elsevier, 1980.

589

Collison DR. **Hypnotherapy in asthmatic patients and the importance of trance depth.** In: FH Frankel, HS Zamansky (eds.), Hypnosis at its Bicentennial. New York: Plenum, 1978.

590

Cousins N. **Anatomy of an Illness as Perceived by the Patient: Reflections on Healing and Regeneration.** New York: Norton, 1979.

591

Creer TL. **Asthma: psychologic aspects and management.** In: E Middleton, CE Reed, EF Ellis (eds.), Allergy: Principles and Practice. Vol. 2. St. Louis, Missouri: Mosby, 1978.

592

Creer TL. **Asthma Therapy: A Behavioral Health Care System for Respiratory Disorders.** New York: Springer, 1979.

593

Creer TL, Renne CM, Chai H. **The application of behavioral techniques to childhood asthma.** In: DC Russo, JW Varni (eds.), Behavioral Pediatrics. Research and Practice. New York: Plenum, 1982.

594

Davis MH, Saunders DR, Creer TL, Chai H. **Relaxation training facilitated by biofeedback apparatus as a supplemental treatment in bronchial asthma.** In: T Barber, LV DiCara, J Kamiya, NE Miller, D Shapiro, J Stoyva (eds.), Biofeedback and Self-Control. Chicago: Aldine, 1971.

595

Dennis M, Hirt M. **Treatment of the asthmatic patient.** In: M Hirt, Psychological and Allergic Aspects of Asthma. Springfield, Illinois: Thomas, 1965.

596

Derner GF. **Aspects of the Psychology of the Tuberculous.** New York: Hoeber, 1953.

597

Dilley JW. **Treatment interventions and approaches to care of patients with acquired immune deficiency syndrome.** In: SE Nichols, DG Ostrow (eds.), Psychiatric Implications of Acquired Immune Deficiency Syndrome. Washington: American Psychiatric Press, 1984.

598

Dudley DL. **Medical management of diffuse obstructive pulmonary syndromes.** In: DL Dudley, Psychophysiology of Respiration in Health and Disease. New York: Appleton-Century-Crofts, 1969.

599

Dudley DL. **Life situations, emotions, and reversible DOPS.** In: DL Dudley, Psychophysiology of Respiration in Health and Disease. New York: Appleton-Century-Crofts, 1969.

600

Dunbar F. **Rheumatic fever and rheumatoid arthritis.** In: F Dunbar, Psychosomatic Diagnosis. New York: Hoeber, 1953.

601

Edwards G. **The hypnotic treatment of asthma.** In: HJ Eysenck (ed.), Experiments in Behavior Therapy. New York: Macmillan, 1964.

602

Freedman R, Wenig P. **Pathophysiology and behavioral treatment of scleroderma.** In: RS Surwit, RB Williams, A Steptoe, R Biersner (eds.), Behavioral Treatment of Disease. New York: Plenum, 1984.

603

Freeman J. **Emotions, moods and tensions.** In: J Freeman, Hay Fever: A Key to the Allergic Disorders. London: Heinemann, 1950.

604

French TM. **Psychogenic factors in bronchial asthma.** In: VJ Derbes, HT Engelhardt (eds.), Treatment of Bronchial Asthma. Philadelphia: Lippincott, 1946.

605

French TM. **Brief psychotherapy in bronchial asthma.** In: Proceedings of the Second Brief Psychotherapy Council. Chicago: Institute for Psychoanalysis, 1944.

606

French TM, Alexander F (eds.). **Psychogenic factors in bronchial asthma.** In: Psychosomatic Medicine Monographs. Part 1: No 4, Part 2: Nos 1,2. Washington, DC: National Research Council, 1941.

607

French TM, Johnson AM. **Psychotherapy in bronchial asthma.** In: F Alexander, TM French (eds.), Studies in Psychosomatic Medicine: an Approach to the Cause and Treatment of Vegetative Disturbances. New York: Ronald, 1948.

608

Gerard MW. **Bronchial asthma in children.** In: F Alexander, TM French (eds.), Studies in Psychosomatic Medicine; an Approach to the Cause and Treatment of Vegetative Disturbances. New York: Ronald, 1948.

609

Godfrey S. **Childhood asthma.** In: TJH Clark, S Godfrey (eds.), Asthma. Philadelphia: Saunders, 1977.

610

Groen JJ. **Psychosocial influences in bronchial asthma.** In: L Levi (ed.), Society, Stress and Disease. New York: Oxford University Press, 1971.

611

Groen JJ. **Present status of the psychosomatic approach to asthma.** In: JJ Groen (ed.), Clinical Research in Psychosomatic Medicine: A Collection of Papers. The Netherlands: Van Gorcum, 1982.

612

Groen JJ. **Present status of the psychosomatic approach to bronchial asthma.** In: OW Hill (ed.), Modern Trends in Psychosomatic Medicine. Vol. 3. London: Butterworth, 1976.

613

Haas A, Castillo R, Lustig F. **The application of rehabilitation medicine to bronchial asthma.** In: EB Weiss, MS Segal (eds.), Bronchial Asthma: Mechanisms and Therapeutics. Boston: Little, Brown, 1976.

614

Harms E. **Somatic and Psychiatric Aspects of Childhood Allergies.** New York: Macmillan, 1963.

615

Ikemi Y. **Psychological Desensitisation in Allergic Disorders, Hypnosis and Psychosomatic Medicine.** New York: Springer, 1967.

616

Ikemi Y, Nakagawa S, Kusano T, Sugita M. **The application of autogenic training to "psychological desensitization" of allergic disorders.** In: W Luthe (ed.), Autogenic Training: Correlationes Psychosomatiqae. International Edition. Orlando, Florida: Grune & Stratton, 1965.

617

Jores A, Kerekjarto V. **The Asthmatic Patient: Etiology and Therapy of Bronchial Asthma from a Psychological Point of View.** Bern: Huber, 1967.

618

Knapp PH. **The asthmatic child and the psychosomatic problem of asthma: toward a general theory.** In: SI Harrison, JF McDermott (eds.), Childhood Psychopathology. New York: International Universities Press, 1972.

619

Knapp PH. **Psychotherapeutic management of bronchial asthma.** In: ED Wittkower, H Warnes (eds.), Psychosomatic Medicine: Its Clinical Applications. Hagerstown, Maryland: Harper & Row, 1977.

620

Knapp PH. **Psychosomatic aspects of bronchial asthma.** In: S Arieti (ed.), American Handbook of Psychiatry. Vol. 4, 2nd ed. New York: Basic Books, 1975.

621

Knapp PH, Mathe AA, Vachon L. **Psychosomatic aspects of bronchial asthma.** In: EB Weiss, MS Segal (eds.), Bronchial Asthma: Mechanisms and Therapeutics. Boston: Little, Brown, 1976.

622

Knapp PH, Mushatt C, Nemetz SJ. **Collection and utilization of data in a psychoanalytic psychosomatic study.** In: A Auerbach, L Gottschalk (eds.), Methods of Research in Psychotherapy. New York: Appleton-Century-Crofts, 1966.

623

Kraepelien S. **Children's homes for asthmatics.** In: WJ Quarles van Ufford (ed.), The Therapy of Bronchial Asthma. Leiden, The Netherlands: Stenfert Kroese, 1956.

624

Kroger WS, Fezler WD. **Asthma and allergy.** In: WS Kroger, WD Fezler, Hypnosis and Behavior Modification: Imagery Conditioning. Philadelphia: Lippincott, 1976.

625

Lachman SJ. **Psychotherapy for psychosomatic disorders.** In: SJ Lachman, Psychosomatic Disorders: A Behavioristic Interpretation. New York: Wiley, 1972.

626

Lachman SJ. **Psychosomatic respiratory disorders.** In: SJ Lachman, Psychosomatic Disorders: A Behavioristic Interpretation. New York: Wiley, 1972.

627

Lask A. **Asthma: Attitude and Milieu.** Philadelphia: Lippincott, 1966.

628

Leffert F. **Management of the emotional consequences of chronic childhood asthma.** In: BA Berman, KF MacDonnell (eds.), Differential Diagnosis and Treatment of Pediatric Allergy. Boston: Little, Brown, 1980.

629

Leigh D. **Asthma and the psychiatrist: a critical review.** In: ML Hirt, Psychological and Allergic Aspects of Asthma. Springfield, Illinois: Thomas, 1965.

630

Leigh D, Marley E. **Psychiatric contributions to the study of bronchial asthma.** In: D Leigh, E Marley, Bronchial Asthma: A Genetic Population and Psychiatric Study. Oxford: Pergamon, 1967.

631

Ludwig AO. **Rheumatoid arthritis.** In: ED Wittkower, RA Cleghorn (eds.), Recent Developments in Psychosomatic Medicine. Philadelphia: Lippincott, 1954.

632

Ludwig AO. **Psychiatric studies of patients with rheumatoid arthritis.** In: CH Slocum (ed.), Rheumatic Diseases. Philadelphia: Saunders, 1952.

633

Magonet AP. **Hypnosis in Asthma.** London: Heinemann, 1955.

634

Maher-Loughnan GP. **Hypnosis in bronchial asthma.** In: EB Weiss, MS Segal (eds.), Bronchial Asthma: Mechanisms and Therapeutics. Boston: Little, Brown, 1976.

635

Maher-Loughnan GP. **Hypno-autohypnosis in treating psychosomatic illness.** In: OW Hill (ed.), Modern Trends in Psychosomatic Medicine. Vol. 3. London: Butterworth, 1976.

636

Margolis H. **Psychosocial factors in rheumatoid arthritis: considerations for their clinical management.** In: JH Talbott, LM Lockie (eds.), Progress in Arthritis. Orlando, Florida: Grune & Stratton, 1958.

637

Mascia AV. **Rehabilitation of the child with chronic asthma.** In: JA Downey, NL Low (eds.), The Child with Disabling Illness: Principles of Rehabilitation. New York: Raven, 1982.

638

Mason AA. **Suggestion and hypnosis in the treatment of asthma.** In: Bronchial Asthma: A Symposium. London: The Chest and Heart Association, 1959.

639

McGovern JP, Knight JA. **Treatment.** In: JP McGovern, JA Knight, Allergy and Emotions. Springfield, Illinois: Thomas, 1967.

640

Melamed BG, Johnson SB. **Treatment and assessment of chronic illness: asthma and juvenile diabetes.** In: EJ Mash, LG Terdal (eds.), Behavioral Assessment of Childhood Disorders. New York: Guilford, 1981.

641

Miller H, Baruch DW. **The Practice of Psychosomatic Medicine as Illustrated in Allergy.** New York: Blakiston, 1956.

642

Miller H, Baruch DW. **Maternal rejection in the treatment of bronchial asthma.** In: HA Abramson (ed.), Somatic and Psychiatric Treatment of Asthma. Baltimore: Williams & Wilkins, 1951.

643

Miller H, Baruch DW. **Allergies.** In: SR Slavson (ed.), The Fields of Group Psychotherapy. New York: McGraw Hill, 1956.

644

Nolte D. **Asthma.** Baltimore: Urban & Schwarzenberg, 1980.

645

Olton DS, Noonberg AR. **Asthma.** In: DS Olton, AR Noonberg, Biofeedback: Clinical Applications in Behavioral Medicine. Englewood Cliffs, New Jersey: Prentice-Hall, 1980.

646

Peshkin MM. **Intractable asthma in children.** In: EB Weiss, MS Segal (eds.), Bronchial Asthma: Mechanisms and Therapeutics. Boston: Little, Brown, 1976.

647

Pinkerton P, Weaver CM. **Childhood asthma.** In: OW Hill (ed.), Modern Trends in Psychosomatic Medicine. Vol. 2. London: Butterworth, 1970.

648

Rainwater N, Alexander AB. **Respiratory disorders: asthma.** In: DM Doleys, RL Meredith, AR Ciminero (eds.), Behavioral Medicine: Assessment and Treatment Strategies. New York: Plenum, 1982.

649

Reed JMW. **Breathing exercises and relaxation.** In: Bronchial Asthma: A Symposium. London: The Chest and Heart Association, 1959.

650

Rosman B. **The role of the family in the treatment of chronic asthma.** In: TJ Guerin (ed.), Family Therapy Theory and Practice. New York: Gardner, 1976.

651

Ross IM, Wilson CP. **Psychotherapy in bronchial asthma.** In: HA Abramson (ed.), Somatic and Psychiatric Treatment of Asthma. Baltimore: Williams & Wilkins, 1951.

652

Saul LJ, Lyons JW. **The psychodynamics of respiration.** In: HA Abramson (ed.), Somatic and Psychiatric Treatment of Asthma. Baltimore: Williams & Wilkins, 1951.

653

Schaefer CE, Millman HL, Levine GF. **Asthma.** In: CE Schaefer, HL Millman, GF Levine (eds.), Therapies for Psychosomatic Disorders in Children. San Francisco: Jossey-Bass, 1979.

654

Scherr MS. **Special camp treatment of asthmatic children.** In: BA Berman, KF MacDonnell (eds.), Differential Diagnosis and Treatment of Pediatric Allergy. Boston: Little, Brown, 1980.

655

Schneer HI (ed.). **The Asthmatic Child.** New York: Hoeber, 1963.

656

Scott A. **Woman with Arthritis.** New York: Abelard Shuman, 1957.

657

Selesnick S, Sperber Z. **The problem of the eczema-asthma complex: a developmental approach.** In: N Greenfield, WC Lewis (eds.), Psychoanalysis and Current Biologic Thought. Madison, Wisconsin: University of Wisconsin Press, 1965.

658

Sirota AD. **Assessment of asthma.** In: FJ Keefe, JA Blumenthal (eds.), Assessment Strategies in Behavioral Medicine. Orlando, Florida: Grune & Stratton, 1982.

659

Speer F. **Psychologic factors in pediatric allergy.** In: F Speer (ed.), The Allergic Child. New York: Hoeber, 1963.

660

Stern A. **Asthma and Emotion.** New York: Gardner Press, 1981.

661

Stokvis B. **Psychosomatic and psychotherapy aspects in allergic diseases.** In: JM Jamar (ed.), International Textbook of Allergy. Oxford: Blackwell, 1959.

662

Stokvis B, Welman AJ. **Psychotherapy in allergic patients.** In: WJ Quarles van Ufford (ed.), The Therapy of Bronchial Asthma. Leiden, The Netherlands: Stenfert Kroese, 1956.

663

Tredgold AF. **Bronchial asthma.** In: AF Tredgold, Manual of Psychologic Medicine for Practitioners and Students. Baltimore: Williams & Wilkins, 1943.

664

Tuft HS. **The institutional rehabilitation of the intractable asthmatic child.** In: WJ Quarles van Ufford (ed.), The Therapy of Bronchial Asthma. Leiden, The Netherlands: Stenfert Kroese, 1956.

665

Udupa KN. **Stress and arthritis.** In: KN Udupa, Disorders of Stress and their Management by Yoga. Varanasi, India: Banaras Hindu University Press, 1978.

666

Udupa KN. **Bronchial asthma.** In: KN Udupa, Disorders of Stress and Their Management by Yoga. Varanasi, India: Banaras Hindu University Press, 1978.

667

Wahl CW. **The psychodynamics of the allergic patient.** In: CW Wahl (ed.), New Dimensions in Psychosomatic Medicine. Boston: Little, Brown, 1964.

668

Walton D. **The application of learning theory to the treatment of a case of bronchial asthma.** In: HJ Eysenck (ed.), Behavior Therapy and the Neuroses. New York: Pergamon, 1960.

669

Weiner H. **Bronchial asthma.** In: H Weiner, Psychobiology and Human Disease. New York: Elsevier, 1977.

670

Weintraub A. **Psychorheumatologie.** Zurich: Karger, 1983.

671

Weiss E, English OS. **The respiratory system.** In: E Weiss, OS English, Psychosomatic Medicine: A Clinical Study of Psychophysiologic Reactions. 3rd ed. Philadelphia: Saunders, 1957.

672

Yorkston NJ. **Behavior therapy in the treatment of bronchial asthma.** In: T Thompson, WS Dockens (eds.), Applications of Behavior Modification. New York: Academic, 1975.

673

Young SH, Rubin JM, Daman HR (eds.). **Psychobiological Aspects of Allergic Disorders.** New York: Praeger. (in press)

Hematologic
Disorders

Hemophilia

674

Agle DP. **Psychiatric studies of patients with hemophilia and related states.** Arch Intern Med 114:76-82, 1964.

▶ psychotherapy

A psychiatric study is reported, emphasizing the importance of the mind-body relationship in bleeding disorders. Findings from this study suggest that psychological factors often may influence the course of the illness. For example, the neurotic response, counterphobia, may occur and result in increased risk-taking behavior and injury. Furthermore, a psychophysiological mechanism of bleeding superimposed upon the organic defect is suggested by reports of spontaneous bleeding at times of emotional stress. In addition an improved clinical state has been reported by some hemophiliacs to accompany a reversal of behavior from a passive-dependent state to an aggressive independence. These findings suggest some re-evaluation of previous therapeutic concepts regarding bleeding disorders with greater emphasis given to encouragement of healthful activity and reasonable aggressive pursuits.

675

Chilcote RR, Baehner RL. **Atypical bleeding in hemophilia: application of the conversion model to the case study of a child.** Psychosom Med 42:221-230, 1980.

▶ family therapy

Although it has been suggested that psychosocial events may trigger bleeding in patients with hemophilia, few specific instances have been described. In this report we interpret a series of atypical bleeding episodes in a child with a factor VIII deficiency. Although the specific pathophysiologic events that led to bleeding into the elbow are unknown in this child, they are probably similar to those of "psychogenic purpura." It is likely that these episodes of atypical bleeding can be interpreted in terms of conversion model and that conversion reactions in children required involvement by at least one parent.

676

Crodel HW. **Organ diseases treated as neuroses—a psychotherapeutic task.** Z Gesamte Inn Med 31:293-294, 1976.

▶ psychotherapy

On the basis of experiences with haemophilics the significance and possible neurotic basis of organic diseases is reported on. In 60 outpatients the reasons of the verbal causes evoking the false treatment are described. Insufficient and exaggerated information can be maldigested in the same way. Test examples are given and the therapeutic implications are discussed.

677

Dubin LL, Shapiro SS. **Use of hypnosis to facilitate dental extraction and hemostasis in a classic hemophiliac with a high antibody titer to factor VIII.** Am J Clin Hypn 17:79-83, 1974.

▶ hypnosis, suggestion, imagery

A 21-year-old class A, very severely affected hemophiliac patient required the extraction of an upper molar. Because of the known tendency of all hemophiliacs to bleed excessively after dental extraction, and because this patient also had a potent antibody titer to factor VIII, the usual replacement techniques, including antihemophilic globulin (AHG) were not expected to be sufficient to prevent hemorrhage. Thus, hypnosis was used as an adjunct to both anesthesia and hemostasis. The procedure was extremely successful. No bleeding occurred at any time and minimal oozing was permanently stopped on the fourth postoperative day without the use of the transfusions that had been previously required of this patient.

678

Dufour J, D'Auteuil, Dionne P. **Dental extractions under hypnosis of a hemophiliac.** Rev Fr Odontostomatol 15:955-960, 1968. (in French: no English abstract)

▶ hypnosis

679
Fredericks LE. **The use of hypnosis in hemophilia.** Am J Clin Hypn 10:52-55, 1967.

▶ hypnosis

In conclusion, let me say that hemophilia is a disease showing a coagulation defect and that emotional stress is important in creating spontaneous bleeding as well as massive operative and post-operative hemorrhages. The use of hypnosis in controlling these emotional factors is discussed and it is pointed out that massive transfusions are not required during or after surgery in hemophiliacs treated with hypnosis. A case of severe post-gastrectomy hemorrhage is presented, in which hypnosis was used to successfully stop the hemorrhage.

680
Fung EH, Lazar BS. **Hypnosis as an adjunct in the treatment of von Willebrand's disease.** Int J Clin Exp Hypn 31:256-265, 1983.

▶ hypnosis

Hypnosis has been used to control bleeding, both in normals and hemophiliacs. Case material is presented to demonstrate how hypnosis was used as an adjunct to standard medical treatment of a boy and his mother with von Willebrand's disease, initially to reduce anxiety and improve self-esteem and the parent-child relationship, and later, to reduce bleeding. This use of hypnosis illustrates the relationship between hemostatic control and psychological adaptation.

681
Handford AH, Charney D, Ackerman L, Eyster ME, Bixler EO. **Effect of psychiatric intervention on the use of antihemophilic factor concentrate.** Am J Psychiatry 137:1254-1256, 1980.

▶ psychotherapy, family therapy, autohypnosis

Extracted summary: The purpose of our study was to evaluate the effects of emotional status on a patient's use of Factor VIII concentrate by assessing the relationship between psychiatric intervention and a patient's use of Factor VIII concentrate over a given time period. In the following case report we describe an adolescent with severe hemophilia, and we compare the levels of Factor VIII concentrate he used during three 15-month periods of time—before, during, and after psychiatric intervention.

682
Jonas DL. **Psychiatric aspects of hemophilia.** Mt Sinai J Med 44:457-463, 1977.

▶ psychotherapy, group therapy, family therapy, couples therapy

Hemophilia, as a chronic disease, challenges the full adaptational capabilities of the patient and his family through all stages of development. Adequate early and lifelong psychiatric intervention, as indicated, may help the hemophiliac achieve maximal adaptation; this has been aptly described by Agle (referring to Poinsard) as "overcoming overdependence, avoiding excessive revolt, and considering the limitations of his illness as a challenge to be accepted."

683
LaBaw WL. **Self-hypnosis and hemophilia: the Colorado experience (1968-1980).** Hemophilia Lett 2, 1980.

▶ hypnosis

684
LaBaw WL. **Auto-hypnosis in haemophilia.** Haematologia (Budap) 9:103-110, 1975.

▶ autohypnosis, suggestion, group therapy

A pilot study to determine the use of adjunctive trance therapy in the treatment of haemophiliacs has been carried out. Over a period of forty months, twenty randomly selected males were assigned to a control and an experimental group. All received due haematologic care. The ten patients in the experimental group utilized medical hypnosis as well, in group suggestive sessions to train and sustain them, but primarily in self-induced trance states. Results were compared at intervals on the basis of the amount of transfused blood and blood products. This provided an objective measure of the efficacy of trance therapy. Statistical analysis of the data confirmed the clinical observation of a greater improvement among patients in the experimental group.

685
LaBaw WL. **Regular use of suggestibility by pediatric bleedings.** Haematologia (Budap) 4:419-425, 1970.

▶ suggestion, autohypnosis, group therapy

The usefulness of suggestive therapy with bleeders has been long recognized. This pilot study documents the validity of encouraging the use of their suggestibility by these children more routinely than is documented, rather than reserving it only for urgent problems. The employment of trance by patients by themselves to achieve diminished morbidity was the end desired and realized. While the primary clotting defect is not modified by the mobilization of his suggestibility by a bleeder, other additives to it are minimized with resulting lower total morbidity.

686

LeBaron S, Zeltzer LK. **Research on hypnosis in hemophilia—preliminary success and problems: a brief communication.** Int J Clin Exp Hypn 32:290-295, 1984.

▶ review: hypnosis, suggestion, relaxation, psychotherapy

Although little is known about physiological effects of hypnosis on hemophilia, hypnosis for reduction of pain and/or bleeding in hemophilia has attracted increasing attention. Literature on this topic is reviewed, and important problems in conducting clinical research on hypnosis for hemophilia are discussed.

687

Lucas ON. **The use of hypnosis in hemophilia dental care.** Ann NY Acad Sci 240:263-266, 1975.

▶ hypnosis, suggestion

In 1959 we first started using hypnosis in hemophiliacs undergoing oral surgical procedures. The purposes for using hypnosis were to establish rapport, control anxiety, and obtain a relaxed, confident and cooperative patient during the preoperative, operative, and postoperative periods. Different types of emotional states have been suggested as agents capable of initiating and/or complicating hemorrhagic episodes in hemophiliacs. Anxiety is common in hemophiliacs scheduled for any type of dental treatment. Block and/or infiltrative anesthesia, by themselves, can produce severe hematomas with sometimes life-threatening possibilities. This presentation does not imply that hypnosis alone stops bleeding in hemophiliacs following exodontia. Hypnosis is an adjunct utilized to control anxiety. Combined with excellent surgical technique, proper cosmetic of the surgical areas, proper packing of the socket with local hemostats, and proper protection of the area, hypnosis can render dental extraction nonhemorrhagic. Besides control of fear in surgical patients, hypnosis has many other important applications in dentistry. Hypnosis can be used to instill proper behavior patterns in preventive dentistry. This is especially useful in children, and it can be of great help in adults.

688

Lucas ON. **Dental extractions in the hemophiliac: control of the emotional factors by hypnosis.** Am J Clin Hypn 7:301-307, 1965.

▶ hypnosis, psychotherapy, group psychotherapy

Details of a technique that basically consists of three principles, 1) Hypnosis, 2) Packing of the sockets, and 3) Pro-

tection of the extraction area, used in the management of dental extraction in hemophiliacs are explained. The importance of emotional factors as a cause of spontaneous hemorrhage as well as the control of the emotional factors by hypnosis are stressed. A good surgical technique, careful packing of the socket and protection of the surgical area play a very important role in the success of nonhemorrhagic dental extraction in hemophilia. Further research is necessary to establish a more scientific basis in the relationship between emotional factors and spontaneous bleeding in hemophiliacs and to determine by which neuro-physiological mechanism emotional stress might be triggering spontaneous hemorrhage. Further investigations should be considered into the psychological problem of the patient with hemophilia and the use of psychotherapy either individually or in a group to help the hemophiliac to adjust to his condition.

689

Lucas ON. **Hypnosis and stress in hemophilia.** Bibl Haemotol 34:73-82, 1970.

▶ hypnosis

Extracted summary: In summary, it has been found that through hypnosis it is possible to establish a good relationship, obtain confidence and cooperation from the hemophiliac and most of all dispel fear of pain and bleeding that may be involved during or after the surgical procedure. It is well known that bleeding engenders fear and fear of bleeding is considerably greater in the hemophiliac than in a normal individual. It is not known what forces are brought into play to help control bleeding by hypnosis; however, it may well be that some neuroendocrine mechanism is the trigger that influences the vascular factor of hemostasis and therefore favors the control of hemorrhage.

690

Lucas ON, Carroll RT, Finkelmann A, Tocantins LM. **Tooth extractions in hemophilia: control of bleeding without use of blood, plasma or plasma fractions.** Thromb Diath Haem 8:209-220, 1962.

▶ hypnosis, suggestion

Hypnotic suggestion, loose packing of sockets and protection of the extractions area when properly done make it possible to carry out virtually painless tooth extractions in even the most severe hemophilics, with a minimum of hemorrhage and of physical or psychic trauma. Following the principles outlined 91 teeth were extracted from 20 hemophilic patients, 17 of whom had classical hemophilia "A" ranging in severity from mild to very severe (75 extractions), while 3 had hemophilia "B" (16 extractions). Fifty extractions were carried out without hospitalization. None of the extractions required pre- or postoperative bleeding in any of the patients. A successful non-hemorrhagic extraction depends on effective cooperation between oral surgeon and haematologist and the scrupulous execution of all three principles stated and not any single one in particular.

691

Lucas ON, Tocantins LM. **Problems in hemostasis in hemophilic patients undergoing dental extractions.** Ann NY Acad Sci 115:470-480, 1964.

▶ hypnosis, suggestion

It is evident that much emphasis is given to transfusion therapy and that the importance of good psychological preparation of the patient has been neglected. The importance of having a confident and emotionally stable patient prior to, during, and after surgery has, historically, either been minimized or not considered. A careful surgical technique is also very important, as is the packing of the sockets with hemostatic material and the continuous protection of the original clot. Our system is designed to assure and protect the natural hemostatic forces of the body in terms of the influence of vascular and extravascular factors; they prove that even in the most severe type of hemophilia, hemostasis can be effected without attempting to correct the coagulation time by transfusion. However, we must emphasize that we do not reject the importance of transfusion therapy when indicated. Finally, a successful nonhemorrhagic postoperative course even after removal of up to six teeth in a severe hemophilic depends on the careful execution of all of the principles mentioned above and not any one in particular. An attempt to use hypnosis alone will most certainly lead to disappointing results. Following these principles, 110 dental extractions were done in 17 patients with hemophilia A and four hemophilia B; not one of them presented abnormal postoperative bleeding. No transfusions were necessary to effect hemostasis in any of the patients. It must be emphasized that close association between the hematologist and the oral surgeon is essential for the scrupulous execution of this technique.

692

Lucas ON, Tocantins LM. **Management of tooth extractions in hemophiliacs by the combined use of hypnotic suggestion, protective splints and packing of sockets.** J Oral Surg Anesth Hosp Dent Serv 20:488-500, 1962.

▶ hypnosis

1. A combination of hypnosis, protective splints and critical packing of sockets with absorbable hemostatic material was used to obtain hemostasis after extraction of teeth in 12 patients with hemophilia "A" without the use of plasma, plasma fractions, blood transfusions, or local

coagulants. 2. A successful nonhemorrhagic extraction depended on the coordination of these three methods and not on any single one in particular. Postoperative complications have not been noted. 3. Detailed preparation of the field and preoperative prophylaxis of the total oral cavity are essential. When the patient had come for extraction and had had no previous local bleeding, effective hemostasis was uniformly obtained after the extraction. When the patient was already bleeding when first seen, hemostasis was much more difficult to accomplish. 4. The technics employed permit the removal of teeth in patients with hemophilia "A" with a minimum of trauma, a short period of hospitalization and no attempts at preliminary systemic correction of the defect in blood coagulation.

693

Martin J. **Hypnosis may reduce hemophiliacs' blood needs.** JAMA 250:1814-1815, 1983. (News)

▶ autohypnosis

694

Newman M. **Hypnosis and hemophiliacs.** J Am Dent Assoc 88:273, 275, 1975. (letter)

▶ hypnosis

695

Ritterman MK. **Hemophilia in context: adjunctive hypnosis for families with a hemophiliac member.** Fam Process 21:469-476, 1982.

▶ hypnosis, family therapy

This is a report of preliminary findings of a pilot study conducted at the Philadelphia Child Guidance Clinic and Children's Hospital of Philadelphia. The study examined the use of adjunctive hypnotic techniques with families in which at least one member was a hemophiliac. It is suggested that hypnotic approaches may be more effective if they take into consideration patient-family and family-hospital relationships. Advantages of an open-systems, clinical-research model of hemophilia are presented.

696

Sanders S. **Hypnotic self control strategies in hemophilic children.** J Am Soc Psychosom Dent Med 28:11-21, 1981.

▶ autohypnosis

This paper reviews some basic issues related to pain perception in hemophilia and describes the use of self hypnosis training and metaphoric communication to help the child to learn new patterns of behavior in order to cope with and to control pain perception. Two hemophilic boys were trained in these techniques for four consecutive weeks and were then seen for a follow-up visit three months later. Both children showed a marked reduction in the frequency and duration of the bleeds.

697

Varni JW. **Behavioral treatment of disease-related chronic insomnia in a hemophiliac.** Behav Ther Exp Psychiatry 11:143-145, 1980.

▶ relaxation, meditation, behavior therapy

Hemophilia represents a congenital chronic disorder characterized by recurrent unpredictable internal hemorrhages with accompanying acute bleeding pain. The medical management od a 38-year-old hemophiliac with severe classic hemophilia was further complicated by a high titer factor VIII antibody, increasing the life-threatening status of a severe hemorrhage. The patient had a one-year history of less than 2 hours of sleep per night as a result of daily chronic tension and intrusive cognitions about the dangers of his illness. A treatment package consisting of progressive muscle relaxation, meditative breathing, cognitive refocusing, and stimulus control procedures resulted in an average of 6 hours per night of uninterrupted sleep; improvement was maintained over a 27-week follow-up period. The treatment is discussed within the context of the behavioral medicine approach in hemophilia comprehensive care.

698

Varni JW. **Behavioral medicine in hemophilia arthritic pain management: two case studies.** Arch Phys Med Rehabil 62:183-187, 1981.

▶ relaxation, meditation, imagery, biofeedback

Hemophilia represents a congenital hereditary disorder of blood coagulation characterized by recurrent unpredictable bleeding episodes affecting any body part, especially the joints and extremities. Repeated hemarthrosis eventually results in degenerative arthritis accompanied by severe chronic pain. As contrast to acute bleeding pain, which serves as a functional signal, chronic arthritic pain is a debilitating condition often resulting in analgesic abuse and/or addiction. Two adult hemophiliacs with severe chronic arthritis received training in progressive muscle relaxation exercise, meditative breathing, and imagery associated with past experiences of pain reduction. Imagery training resulted in clinically significant reductions in arthritic pain perception for both patients, maintained over an 8-month follow-up period. Concomitant measures also demonstrated significant therapeutic gains. Thermal biofeedback assessment of the arthritic joint provided a biophysiological measure of learned temperature control through the imagery techniques. The findings are discussed in relationship to medical observations on the therapeutic value of warming and heat application in the management of arthritic joints, as well as other potential mechanisms which might have contributed in the reduction of arthritic pain perception. Finally, the importance of differentiating between acute bleeding pain management and chronic arthritic pain is emphasized, as well as the necessity of the application of the techniques within an interdisciplinary team setting.

699

Varni JW, Gilbert A. **Self-regulation of chronic arthritic pain and long-term analgesic dependence in a haemophiliac.** Rheumatol Rehabil 21:171-174, 1982.

▶ relaxation, meditation, imagery

Haemophilia is characterized by recurrent internal bleeding episodes, with repeated haemorrhages into the joint areas eventually resulting in a chronic condition similar to osteoarthritis. A 31-year-old haemophiliac, with a nine-year history of narcotic analgesic dependence secondary to chronic arthritis pain, learned self-regulation techniques consisting of progressive muscle relaxation exercises, meditative breathing, and guided imagery. Long-term follow-up evidenced clinically significant decreases in arthritic pain intensity and analgesic intake subsequent to self-regulation training.

700

Varni JW, Gilbert A, Dietrich SL. **Behavioral medicine in pain and analgesia management for the hemophilic child with factor VIII inhibitor.** Pain 11:121-126, 1981.

▶ relaxation, meditation, imagery

The present report describes the application of self-regulation techniques (progressive muscle relaxation, meditative breathing, and guided imagery) to the management of bleeding and arthritic pain and analgesic dependence in a 9-year-old hemophilic child with factor VIII inhibitor. Self-regulation training was effective in decreasing pain intensity and analgesic dependence, with 1-year follow-up demonstrating substantial improvements across both medical and psychosocial parameters.

Purpura

701

Agle DP, Ratnoff OD. **Purpura as a psychosomatic entity: a psychiatric study of autoerythrocyte sensitization.** Arch Intern Med 109:685-694, 1962.

▶ psychotherapy

The result of a psychiatric study of patients with a chronic purpuric state, autoerythrocyte sensitization, has been described. The findings suggest the propensity of these patients to express emotional problems in a physical form through both hysterical mechanisms and psychophysiological reaction. Another common feature appears to be a prominent element of masochism in their character. The study further suggests that purpuric bouts occur at times of emotional stress. Whether the emotional stress causes the hemorrhagic bouts or alters the threshold at which these patients react to otherwise subliminal stimuli is not determined. The relationship between emotional disorders and cutaneous purpura has been described earlier by other workers. The emotional background of patients with autoerythrocyte sensitization displays similarities to that previously described in some individuals with bleeding stigmata. Investigators using psychoanalytic techniques believe that the bleeding lesions in these earlier cases represent in a symbolic manner the physical expression of psychic influences upon the vascular beds. Finally, it is tempting to inquire about the specific symbolism of purpura for our patients. For example, are these abreactions of previous real trauma or the beating fantasies of masochists? Data to answer these questions accurately are not yet available. Autoerythrocyte sensitization, then, may be a psychophysiological entity, that is, a reaction involving organs or viscera innervated by the autonomic nervous system. Such a reaction does not necessarily result in the relief of anxiety, it can produce structural change and the reaction would appear to be physiologic rather than symbolic in the origin of symptoms. Perhaps, however, further studies may indeed clarify such symbolism. These findings suggest that psychiatric treatment for certain purpuric states should be explored.

702

Klein RF, Gonen JY, Smith CM. **Psychogenic purpura in a man.** Psychosom Med 37:41-49, 1975.

▶ psychotherapy

A 53-year-old man with chronic back and leg pain developed recurrent painful ecchymoses after lumbar laminectomy. No hematologic abnormality could be detected, but an ecchymosis developed after subcutaneous injection of his blood into the region of pain. A detailed study of the psychological setting of the illness and his personality revealed this to be an example of psychogenic purpura. This is the third report of the syndrome in a male.

703

Kremer WB, Mengel CE, Nowlin JB, Nagaya H. **Recurrent ecchymoses and cutaneous hyperreactivity to hemoglobin: a form of autoerythrocyte sensitization.** Blood 30:62-73, 1967.

▶ psychotherapy

Our patient shows once again that psychological disturbances play an important role in autoerythrocyte sensitization. Her emotional makeup and the course of her illness are so strikingly similar to those of other patients with this illness that her case history might well serve for all of them. Like others, our patient showed masochistic character traits, hysterical conversion reactions, a close relationship between emotional stress and the appearance of ecchymoses, and an apparent addiction to surgical procedures. Most impressive were her total involvement with pain and her covert anger. Although factitious bruising in our patient was a means of introducing red cells intradermally, this does not account for the enormity of the skin reaction that followed. It was amply demonstrated that this reaction was not dependent upon factitious bruising but rather on the intradermal placement of red cells. The fact that our patient bruised herself is merely one manifestation of her disturbed personality. It has been suggested that patients with autoerythrocyte sensitization express emotions or feeling states in the physical form of ecchymoses. Even though psychologic factors are closely associated with the abnormal skin reactivity to erythrocytes, the pharmacologic or physiologic explanation of this syndrome is far from clear.

704

Lindahl MW. **Psychogenic purpura: report of a case.** Psychosom Med 39:358-368, 1977.

▶ psychotherapy

Autoerythrocyte sensitization, a disease characterized by recurrent and painful ecchymoses, was renamed psychogenic purpura by Agle and Ratnoff in 1968. The patients, usually female, share certain described personality characteristics. The case is reported of a 20-year-old woman who had suffered from the disease since age 12. She was treated for 3 years in intensive psychotherapy resulting in a complete remission of her symptoms of bleeding.

705

Ogston D, Ogston WD, Bennett NB. **Psychogenic purpura.** Br Med J 1:30, 1971. (case report)

▶ psychotherapy

706

Ratnoff OD, Agle DP. **Psychogenic purpura: a re-evaluation of the syndrome of autoerythrocyte sensitization.** Medicine 47:475-500, 1968.

▶ psychotherapy

The clinical features of autoerythrocyte sensitization, as observed in 27 of our own cases and 17 others recorded in the literature, have been summarized. This disorder, first delineated by Gardner and Diamond, is characterized by the occurrence of repeated crops of painful ecchymoses which often have an inflammatory component. The syndrome appears to be confined to adult women who usually have multiple systemic complaints. Prominent among the many symptoms described are severe headaches, transient paresthesias, transient paresis, repeated syncope, diplopia, abdominal pain or distress, bouts of nausea, vom-

iting or diarrhea, chest pain or distress, dyspnea, dysuria or frequency, joint, muscle or back aches and remarkable fluctuations of body weight. Consonant with Gardner and Diamond's original description, the initial symptoms of autoerythrocyte sensitization began after physical injury or surgery in 19 of the 27 patients, and the typical bruise could be reproduced by the intracutaneous injection of blood in 18. A closer correlation could be obtained between severe emotional distress and the onset or exacerbation of symptoms. Five psychologic components were almost always present in our patients, hysterical and masochistic character traits, problems in dealing with their own hostility, and overt symptoms of depression and anxiety. These features suggested that a relationship existed between the patient's emotional problems and the development of lesions. Supporting this, the skin test for autoerythrocyte sensitization could be influenced by hypnotic suggestion, and new bruises appeared at sites suggested under hypnosis. Our studies are consistent with the hypothesis that in patients with autoerythrocyte sensitization the purpuric lesions are related to emotional stresses. The mechanisms through which these stresses are translated to cutaneous bruising are unknown. A factitious origin for the patients' ecchymoses could not be rigidly excluded, but this possibility seems inadequate to explain the symptom complex observed. We propose, therefore, that the term psychogenic purpura may be more appropriate than autoerythrocyte sensitization.

707

Roden RG. **Psychoanalytically oriented hypnotic treatment of autoerythrocytic sensitization and blindness.** Am J Clin Hypn 21:278-281, 1979.

▶ psychoanalysis, hypnosis, psychotherapy

A patient with petechial rash and purpura on the lower extremities and hysterical blindness did not respond to conventional medical treatment or to initial courses of psychotherapy, including hypnosis. However, a psychoanalytically oriented hypnotic method was able to elicit the sources of the illness and enabled the design of a successful therapeutic approach.

Other Hematologic Disorders

708

Diespecker D. **Applied imagery.** Int J Eclectic Psychother 1:1-10, 1982.

▶ imagery, relaxation

Discusses the increasing usage by therapists of visual imagery. It is proposed that techniques of applied visual imagery, when used with positive volition and responsibility, enable the visualizer to improve his/her health through healing and by repairing the consequences of trauma. A case history is provided of a 25-yr-old man suffering from thalassemia who used imagery to regain his health. The therapist monitored S's relaxation sessions in which S imagined a bird of friendship that helped to direct the training sessions. During the relaxation sessions, the client and therapist mentally explored the parts of S's body that caused him suffering. After these sessions, client and therapist discussed these healing voyages.

709

Lucas ON. **Hypnosis in the treatment of blood dyscrasias.** Acta Hipnol Latino Tomo 3:127, 1962. (in Spanish)

▶ hypnosis

710

McElroy SR. **Psychoanalgesic remediation of sickle cell anemia painful crisis.** Diss Abstr Int 41:1118, 1980.

▶ autogenic training

The Problem. The study researched the psychological effects of sickle cell disease. Based on a set of phenotypic categories as a function of chronic pain patterns psychometrically assessed, the objectives of the study were to administer psychometric procedures in an effort to define pain perception patterns in sickle cell anemia patients, and, based on the attributes of the aforementioned categories, it was postulated that sickle cell patients experiencing painful crisis would psychometrically segregate into the pain coping pattern of the neurotic triad. Autogenic training, a psychophysiological method of self-hypnosis to promote adequate and healthy reactions of body and mind, was used with the defined patients. Method. Principal methodological operations were the enumeration of individuals with sickle cell disease entering a clinical center's emergency room experiencing painful crisis; the placement of the patient psychometrically into a psychodiagnostic category, and the correlation of detailed information relating to socioeconomic level, age at discovery of disease, predisposing factors that trigger painful crisis, analgesic history, clinical course of treatment during the study period. The MMPI, Emotions Profile Index (EPI), the Pain Apperception Test (PAT) and clinical interviews using the Psychological Profile composed the psychometric test battery. Autogenic training was started after interviewing and testing. Benefits of autogenic training were to induce rest, recuperation, self-relaxation, self-regulation of autonomic functions, increased physical output, and pain relief. Results. Effects of autogenic training noticed by patients within the final two weeks of training were greater relaxation, reduced anxiety, better sleep, an improved memory, and greater motivation, thereby increasing the ability of the patient to handle stress and develop greater muscle relaxation. Autogenics appeared to end pain caused by the tension and anxiety related to the characteristics of the chronic pain patient personality. Two-thirds of the patients experienced painful crisis which occurred following life events, to which they responded with intense psychological effects. The highest identified effect was hypochondriacal, the second was depressive, and third was hysteria. Feelings of sadness, guilt, hopelessness and helplessness were described by the patients. Autogenics appeared to remediate all of these feelings. Hypochondriasis and depressive effects appeared to be important factors contributing to painful crisis. Conceptualizing the relationship between events and hypochondriasis, depressive effects and sickle cell crisis seem to be linked to biologic changes associated with the "giving up" complex which may contribute to the physical illness through biologic interaction. It is hypothesized that unknown biochemical changes accompanying the hypochondriasis and depressive effects provide an environment for the erythrocytes containing SS hemoglobin conducive to massive sickling causing painful crises triggered by tension.

711
Merenstein A, Schenkman M. **Pernicious anemia: the disease and physical therapy management: a case report.** Phys Ther 64:1076-1077, 1984.

▶ biofeedback

This case demonstrated the physical and cognitive losses that can occur as a result of untreated pernicious anemia. We summarized the role of physical therapy in treating a patient with this disease. Biofeedback therapy played an important role, provided the patient with sensory awareness of the lower extremities, and facilitated strengthening and functional training. In addition, this mode of treatment challenged and motivated the patient during a long and tedious rehabilitation. Finally, this case demonstrated the level of return that can occur despite an apparently severe neurologic insult and complete functional dependence.

712
Thomas JE, Koshy M, Patterson L, Dorn L, Thomas K. **Management of pain in sickle cell disease using biofeedback therapy: a preliminary study.** Biofeedback Self Regul 9:413-420, 1984.

▶ biofeedback, relaxation, behavior therapy, autohypnosis

Fifteen patients with a history of painful episodes of sickle cell disease were given training in progressive relaxation, thermal biofeedback, cognitive strategies, and self-hypnosis to help them develop self-management skills to relieve pain. Results show a 38.5% reduction in the number of emergency room visits, a 31% reduction in the number of hospitalizations, and a 50% reduction in the inpatient stay during the 6 months since the beginning of therapy compared to 6 months prior to therapy. Analgesic intake was reduced by 29% for those who were using it regularly. This is a preliminary study, and the results are considered only as suggestive of the potential use of biofeedback therapy and behavioral management in alleviating painful episodes in sickle cell disease.

713
Zeltzer L, Dash J, Holland JP. **Hypnotically induced pain control in sickle cell anemia.** Pediatrics 64:533-536, 1979.

▶ autohypnosis

Recurrent painful vaso-occlusive crises often represent sources of frustration and debilitation to those afflicted with sickle cell disease. We present two adolescents with sickle cell disease who have been able to gain control over the frequency and intensity of these crises by utilizing self-hypnosis. We feel that the utilization of similar technique(s) may allow many ill children and adolescents to obtain mastery over abnormal physiologic processes concomitant with their particular disease status.

Books and Book Chapters on Hematologic Disorders

714
Luthe W, Schultz JH. **Hemophilia.** In: W Luthe, JH Schultz, Autogenic Therapy: Medical Applications. Vol. 2. Orlando, Florida: Grune & Stratton, 1969.

715
Varni JW, Russo DC. **Behavioral-medicine approach to health care: hemophilia as an exemplary model.** In: M Jospe, J Nieberding, BD Cohen (eds.), Psychological Factors in Health Care. Lexington, Massachusetts: Lexington Books, 1980.

Infectious

Disorders

Tuberculosis

716

Anderson AS. **Psychogenic factors in chest diseases.** Dis Chest 19:570-576, 1951.

▶ psychotherapy, doctor-patient relationship

Without enlarging further upon the need for psychosomatic treatment for our chest patients, let us consider briefly the value of this step to our specialty. If every chest physician made a special effort to deal with his patient not only as a case of organic disease, but as an emotionally sick, fearful and anxious individual, he would find such a grateful response as would indeed warm his heart. The widespread practice of this art would soon label the chest physician as outstanding in his understanding of the care of the sick individual. Could we ask for a finer compliment? Let me implore that we hold fast to those agents, in the combating of tuberculosis, that have passed the test of time and science. We are today emphasizing the psychosomatic angle in order that we may add to the effectiveness of our therapeutic agents and not detract from their value.

717

Begoin J. **Pulmonary tuberculosis and psychosomatic problems.** Rev Med Psychosom 7:159-195, 1965. (in French)

▶ psychoanalysis

The author describes a situation of crisis in the actual treatment of pulmonary tuberculosis. Since the introduction of antibiotic and chemotherapy, the increasing difficulties for the patients to accept their treatment and the increasing frequency of troubles of behavior and of psychiatric reactions among patients (40% of all cases, upon an average) have led chest physicians to ask help from psychiatrists. The psychoanalytical examination of these cases, illustrated by clinical examples, leads to appreciation of the appearance of P.T. under the aspect of a process of somatisation which constitutes the ultimate defense mechanism against depression. This defense depends on mechanisms of omnipotence and denial of psychic reality, with reintrojection of a very destructive part-object which is maintained split off in the lung, from the rest of the self, on purpose to save from destruction the other parts of the psychic and bodily ego. The evolution of the treatment and the prognosis of the illness depend on the intensity of these psychotic mechanisms which underlie the process of somatisation. The author evokes, in conclusion, the consequences of these findings upon evolution of social medicine and of psychosomatic research and theory.

718

Bellak L. **Psychiatric aspects of tuberculosis.** Soc Casework 31:183-189, 1950.

▶ psychotherapy, social casework

Some psychiatric aspects of tuberculosis, as encountered in a social agency, have been discussed. No specific personality type or psychiatric disorder was observed among the 46 patients seen by the author for consultation or psychotherapy, nor in the 250 patients discussed in detail with social workers. The psychological reaction to being informed of the diagnosis of tuberculosis is met by a series of defense mechanisms often in terms of pre-existing fantasies, and sometimes experienced as a catastrophic change in body image. With this change of body image an increase in secondary narcissism, oral needs, passivity, and regression is observed as is to be expected on the basis of psychoanalytic hypotheses. The problems of the return to the family after an absence of months or years have been mentioned, with particular reference to the complication of the family relationships in adolescents. Psychotherapy is aimed at the isolation of the irrational aspects of the responses to an admittedly difficult reality situation—the peculiarly strong transference problems in the patient who is reduced almost to helplessness by his illness. Psychosomatic problems need simple, convincing explanations first, and then further interpretation. In the case of the adolescent, the family usually needs help also and, if this is impossible, his separation from the family needs to be encouraged. Depression and denial of the illness as self-harming behavior need prompt attention.

719

Benjamin JD, Coleman JV, Hornbein R. **A study of personality in pulmonary tuberculosis.** Am J Orthopsychiatry 18:704-707, 1948.

▶ psychotherapy

Extracted summary: Our most interesting single finding, in partial confirmation of an observation by Luehrs, concerns the relationship of hostility to the course of the disease. We have the definite impression from our cases that inhibited conscious hostility exerts an unfavorable influence; on the contrary, the capacity to express conscious hostility has a favorable influence. In several instances we were able to follow this correlation in psychotherapy with surprising consistency, and in no case did we find any contradiction to it. It is clear, however, that an observation of this sort will require many more cases for its confirmation. If confirmed, it will again raise the question of the mechanisms involved. We emphasize the status of the hostility because in two of our subjects, with deeply repressed hostility, the course was an excellent one. Parenthetically, the fact that this status is identical with that described by Alexander in his essential hypertension cases is one more bit of evidence that in psychosomatics as in psychopathology in general we are at best dealing with necessary, but not with sufficient, conditions. In conclusion, it is relatively simple to demonstrate the importance of personality factors in the onset and course of pulmonary tuberculosis, and the resultant necessity for a psychiatric orientation in the treatment and rehabilitation of many patients. What is much more difficult is to generalize from the individual to the group in the attempt to define some specific psychosomatic relationships of varying significance and generality. In part, the results of this investigation are negative in this respect; in part, however, suggestive positive findings have been reported. Future study may confirm and, it is to be hoped, elaborate upon them.

720

Berle BB. **Emotional factors and tuberculosis: a critical review of the literature.** Psychosom Med 10:366-373, 1948.

▶ review: psychoanalysis, doctor-patient relationship, milieu therapy, psychotherapy

Extracted summary: The importance of these several observations and hypotheses in relation to the development and course of tuberculosis remains to be determined. However, no progress can be made in the understanding of the relation of emotional factors and tuberculosis unless the physiologic accompaniments of emotional stress are included in the detailed study of the problem of virulence, since this will be the only way in which the effect of "undue emotional strain," recognized since the third century as

influencing the course of this disease, can be broken down into its component parts.

721

Brown L. **The mental aspect in the etiology and treatment of pulmonary tuberculosis.** Int Clin 3:149-174, 1933.

▶ supportive psychotherapy, suggestion, doctor-patient relationship

Extracted summary: Suggestion and persuasion are powerful allies in the treatment of pulmonary tuberculosis. Many unpleasant symptoms are amenable to suggestion. The various phobias demand immediate psychic treatment. It is better to grant slight liberties to a bed patient than to lose all the benefit of bed rest. A return to a state of psychic turmoil at home means usually a speedy return to the cure. Upon the personality of the tuberculosis expert rests much of the success of treatment.

722

Bumbacescu N, Blumenfeld S. **The psychologist and psychology of the pulmonary tuberculous patient.** Rev Med Chir Soc Med Nat Iasi 74:747-750, 1970. (in Romanian: no English abstract)

▶ psychotherapy

723

Coleman JV, Hurst A, Hornbein R. **Psychiatric contributions to care of tuberculous patients.** JAMA 135:699-703, 1947.

▶ psychotherapy, psychological management

In summary, we have presented a cross section of psychiatric problems relating to every phase of the care and management of the tuberculous patient, from the time of diagnosis to his return to the community as a person with arrested tuberculosis. We have emphasized that psychiatric insight is not an occasional need but that it is of continuous importance in any program of comprehensive care in tuberculosis. The consistent and systematic utilization of psychiatric resources, applied to every phase of medical care and oriented to the understanding of the person who is ill, imposes a greater area of responsibility for the physician but promises enrichment in the concept of the practice of medicine and significant extension of therapeutic services to the patient.

724

Coleman JV, Hurst A, Whedbee JS. **Tuberculosis and dependency.** Psychosom Med 12:189-198, 1950.

▶ psychotherapy, social casework

Extracted summary: [T]he treatment of chronic dependency patterns, considered apart from the challenge of their psychodynamic understanding, is probably a more appropriate field for casework than for psychiatry. The present case makes it clear that an early period of dependency gratification is essential for these patients, and a casework approach which is too eager to confront clients with situational realities will probably not be helpful. This is also true of psychotherapy. The advantage of casework, however, in these situations is that the patient does have a major problem of readjustment to community living, and the understanding by the worker of community resources, in their potentialities and limitations, can provide a very comfortable framework for the patient's readaptive strivings.

725

Crouzatier A. **Psychoanalyses and psychotherapies of patients with recent onset of pulmonary tuberculosis.** Rev Fr Psychanal 33:463-504, 1969.

▶ psychotherapy, psychoanalysis

A great majority of patients with pulmonary tuberculosis, and more significantly those with frequent relapses or chronic evolution, present a personality structure akin to character neurosis of the frigid, narcissistic type, fixated at a very early level of affective development. The fragility of this seemingly stable, relatively symptom-free structure breaks down when external pressures for affective relations cannot be denied any more except by escape into psychosis. A decompensatory process with neurotic symptomatology precedes the pulmonary episode so consistently as to be considered an integral part of the crisis. Absence of father, "smothering" mother, frustration, a sense of basic deficiency are listed as contributing factors to this character structure. The traditional treatment of tuberculosis provides the therapeutic atmosphere for the developing of object relations and emotional maturation. Those who have not received this psychological benefit from the somatic treatment may be helped by psychotherapy, even psychoanalysis, with the possible introduction of parameters.

726

Day G. **Observations on the psychology of the tuberculous.** Lancet 251:703-706, 1946.

▶ psychotherapy, milieu therapy

Extracted summary: Even if we cannot accept [the] thesis fully, I think we must agree to the generalization that every individual reacts to a disease according to his personality; from which it must follow that the psychoneurotic, when given a touch of tuberculosis, will exploit his disease process to suit his pattern of living—or of dying. Moreover, such a patient may develop a secondary reactive personality, of which the disease is a complementary and necessary part, as in the "Dornford Yates syn-

drome" described earlier. Obviously, if such a patient is to recover from his tuberculosis, we must treat more than the local lesions and the toxic manifestations. His concurrent psychological disease must be alleviated, and alleviated in good time, if he is to recover and not become chronic or incurable. Time itself is notoriously a great healer in cases of emotional maladjustment that are not basic. The period of retreat in a sanatorium—that mother figure—brings about changes in both the inner and outer lives of many, probably most patients. They overcome the disease when they are ready. But for quite a few cases it would be as well if psychiatric help and guidance were at hand to expedite their readjustment.

727

Day G. **The psychosomatic approach to pulmonary tuberculosis.** Lancet 1:1025-1028, 1951.

▶ milieu therapy, supportive psychotherapy

Extracted summary: How then does ordinary adult-type phthisis develop? There are two schools of thought. One maintains that generally—owing to "lowered resistance" (that convenient legal fiction)—there is leakage of endogenous bacilli from the primary focus to other tissues (via blood-stream, bronchial tree, or lymphatic channels). The other school says that generally it is due to a superinfection by a massive dose of fresh bacilli from outside, perhaps again helped by temporarily lowered resistance. Such evidence as we have is sufficiently labile to support both schools. I think we are agreed that both mechanisms operate but we cannot agree which is the more usual. And it is a matter of some importance to the psychosomatic approach. Under one scheme an individual needing pulmonary tuberculosis can develop it merely by lowering his resistance and allowing his primary lesions to leak, whereas under the other scheme he must, in addition, go out and find some more bacilli.

728

De Freitas O Jr. **Introduction to the psychobiological study of pulmonary tuberculosis.** Neurobiologia 9:296-304, 1946. (in Spanish: no English abstract)

▶ psychotherapy

729

Douady D, Jeanguyot MT, Lacalmontie J, Rosembaum SB, Thibier R. **Role of psychotherapy in a collective of adolescents with tuberculosis.** Therapeutique 47:623-626, 1971. (in French: no English abstract)

▶ psychotherapy, milieu therapy

730

Dubo S. **Psychiatric study of children with pulmonary tuberculosis.** Am J Orthopsychiatry 20:520-528, 1950.

▶ psychotherapy, group therapy

This study has attempted to offer some additional insight into the psychic content of the child with pulmonary tuberculosis. In these 25 cases there is no indication of a characteristic pre-illness personality pattern. The reaction to the illness, however, is characteristic and is marked by overwhelming anxiety, morbid preoccupations and fears of death. Attempts at denial and projection mechanisms are common. There are severe identification problems with striving to identify with the normal. Regressive tendencies are present but are resisted with a strong drive to maintain independence. The child with tuberculosis feels different and stigmatized and tends to take personal responsibility for the illness, often with hostility toward parents displaced inward. These psychological problems find expression in behavior patterns observed in medical treatment and account for many of the difficulties in management. It is emphasized that tuberculosis presents a special problem in children because of its abstract quality to them. The severity of the illness is not reflected subjectively in symptoms; and the intangible nature of the threat to life, with the drive to action in the face of danger denied expression in the rest treatment, makes psychological adjustment difficult. Tuberculosis constitutes a severe threat to the child's ego, and reaction patterns can be understood as attempts to deal with anxiety, to establish normal identifications, and to preserve the integrity of the ego. It would seem clear in these cases that the problems of anxiety and conflict revealed have a marked influence on the course and response to treatment in childhood tuberculosis and that the need for psychotherapy as part of the treatment program is indicated. Finally, we can hope that insight into the inner life and preoccupations of the tuberculous child may be of help to the physician responsible for his total care.

731

Eyre MB. **The role of emotion in tuberculosis.** Am Rev Tuberc 27:315-329, 1933.

▶ counseling

1. The human organism responds as a unitary whole to its environment, rather than as separated into concepts of "mind" versus body. 2. Because man, being animal plus, has a bigger brain, he can within limits choose the direction of his growth-energy and develop his nervous system by use, short of fatigue. 3. Emotion is a form of energy, discharging in muscle and gland. It is essential to recognize the dynamic quality of emotion in tuberculosis. 4. It is essential also to recognize the principles that emotion and preparation to act are brought about by stimulation of the sympathetic nervous system. 5. That the body, when prepared for violent action by the sympathetic, suffers when action is thwarted or postponed. 6. That tuberculosis is a disease peculiarly fitted through its long duration, disturbance of social relations, financial burden, and segregation, to foster emotional stress. 7. That tuberculosis prevents effective discharge of energy through physical activity, and therefore requires re-routing. 8. That fear, anger, hate are the most disrupting emotions in tuberculosis, and that fear is practically universally present. 9. That spes phthisica is a disguise for fear, and that the same mental state is present in other chronic diseases having like conditions. 10. That a specific toxin is not essential to produce emotional symptoms commonly attributed to tuberculosis. 11. That it should be possible to compare from the dynamic angle emotional symptoms in all chronic illness, regardless of specific toxins. 12. That in reeducation lies relief and that it is necessary to show the patient how to deal with his emotional problems by tracing their sources, substituting new feeling-habits, and by offering outlets for his energy which shall be satisfactory to him on his own intellectual level.

732

Finer BL, Nylen BO. **Cardiac arrest in the treatment of burns, and report on hypnosis as a substitute for anesthesia.** Plast Reconstr Surg 27:49-55, 1961.

▶ hypnosis

Extracted summary: If further surgery is needed in a case of successfully treated cardiac arrest, hypnotic analgesia may be tried. One of our cases reported here underwent five operations consisting of excisions and skin grafts, with hypnosis as the only form of anesthesia.

733

Flarsheim A. **Ego mechanisms in three pulmonary tuberculosis patients: a contribution to the study of the psychosomatic process.** Psychosom Med 20:475-482, 1958.

▶ psychotherapy

The thesis of this paper is that certain changes in ego operations constitute a part of the chain of events whereby the loss of an object relationship is followed by a somatic illness. This is based on the observation of time correlations between integrating and disintegrating emotional forces, and remission and exacerbation of respiratory illness. An hypothesis is advanced regarding the mechanism of connection between the state of ego integration and the physical illness. It is postulated that: A. Susceptibility to respiratory illness in these patients is increased when there is what we consider psychologically to be ego depletion. Resistance to the physical illness is correlated with replenishment of ego energy from the narcissistic reservoir. B. Two mechanisms whereby psychological integrative mechanisms may contribute to this energy depletion and restoration are advanced. These are: 1. In the first two patients the loss of a supportive relationship led to lowered self-esteem, hopelessness, and a distraught state, considered to be evidences of ego depletion, and also to breakdown of behavioral controls. The latter added to the ego depletion, and the process then became circular. 2. In the third patient the loss of a supportive relationship led to lowered self-esteem, hopelessness, feeling of lack of motivation or purpose for working, and lack of energy to work, considered to be evidences of ego depletion. Despite this depleted state, the patient continued the expenditure of great effort and became ill.

734
Hartz J. **Tuberculosis and personality conflicts.** Psychosom Med 6:17-22, 1944.

▶ psychotherapy

A brief review of the divergent views in the literature of the past few decades indicates the need for further documentation of the relationship between personality conflicts and pulmonary tuberculosis. Three cases are described which indicate that an individual may react to life situations with an anxiety state or other personal behavior in such a way as to interfere with healthy living; and these reactions may thereby become a most significant factor in the onset and course of clinical tuberculosis. The individualistic character of these personality reactions does not encourage one to expect valid general formulations for the direct correlation of personality traits with tuberculosis infection. In addition, a special limitation to extensive statistical study of such correlations is clearly seen:—the "official" case history usually misses the more significant personal issues, and these come to light only in personal relationships or in special personal types of psychiatric study.

735
Hurst A, Henkin R, Lustig GJ. **Some psychosomatic aspects of respiratory disease.** Am Pract 1:486-492, 1950.

▶ psychotherapy

1. The respiratory tract, as an organ system through which symptoms of psychogenic origin are expressed, is carefully reviewed. 2. The literature on the subject, as well as case material, has been presented. 3. It is important that considerably more co-ordinated studies be done by psychiatrists and physicians interested in such problems.

736
Jelliffe SE, Evans E. **Psychotherapy and tuberculosis.** Am Rev Tuberc 3:417-432, 1919.

▶ psychoanalysis

Extracted summary: The depressing effect of the inhibited emotions upon physiological activity has been well established, and it should be the duty of the physician to improve metabolic changes through psychical control as through physical. While the chronic toxemia of tuberculosis is irritating to the nerve cell and produces general disharmony in the cellular activity, so also is a depressed emotional condition disturbing to cellular activity. In a psychoanalysis patients are able to see that these emotional disturbances result in a weak attitude toward life, desiring always their own gratification and unable to sacrifice the infantile wish. Psychoanalysis cannot change the physical results which are produced by the tuberculous process, but it can greatly improve the functional activities and the physiological processes by relieving the patient of the great drain on his nerve energy through making known to him the unconscious conflict between the heretofore unknown infantile wishes and the demands of conscious life.

737
Kalachnikoff P, Laugie H, Lengrand J, Leclerc P. **A propos of persistent tuberculous cystitis and its treatment in a sanitorium.** J Urol Nephrol (Paris) 74:283-287, 1971. (in French)

▶ psychotherapy

738
Kishimoto K, Tsuboi H, Fukatsu K. **Psychosomatic medicine of tuberculosis: a trial of psychotherapy based on oriental thought.** Nagoya Med J 13:201-208, 1967.

▶ psychotherapy

Extracted summary: In the psychological dimension, the doctor must analyse complexes due to psychic trauma received in childhood. Sometimes it is necessary for the patient to solve his own realistic conflicts. This results in self-insight.

739
Kobayashi M. **Psychotherapy for tuberculosis patients.** Shinryo Shitsu 6:459-465, 1954. (in Japanese: no English abstract)

▶ psychotherapy

740

Ludwig AO. **Emotional factors in tuberculosis.** Public Health Rep 63:883-888, 1948.

▶ doctor-patient relationship, psychotherapy, social casework

Extracted summary: Whenever indicated, the patient should be given an understanding of how his own personality, personal problems, or conflicts enter into and influence his disease. Consciously or unconsciously he may be using his tuberculosis for a purpose: for escape, for self-punishment, or even for purposes of retaliation toward the family or others. It may serve him as the long sought excuse to sink into helpless dependency. With such problems he needs objective, sympathetic, outside help; and treatment has not been fully efficient if it is not given. The addition of psychiatrists to the staffs of sanatoriums would greatly further the recognition and care of these problems. Finally, I would urge that every doctor and nurse who works with tuberculosis, or indeed with any chronic disease, should receive at least rudimentary training in the emotional aspects of illness and the psychology of rehabilitation. Ideally again, one would welcome the incorporation into the body of medicine of a basic core of knowledge and understanding not only of the psychology and personality of the sick, but also of the normal person. The correlation of the meaning of emotional factors in chronic disease is still a very new field and much detailed psychiatric study is needed of tuberculosis in order to delineate accurately and usefully these inter-relationships. Observations in regard to this aspect of disease can and should be made and recorded by the entire therapeutic team engaged in treating chronic illness if continued progress in improving treatment of the whole patient is to be attained.

741

Marks JB. **Special problems in group work with tuberculosis patients.** Int J Group Psychother 2:150-158, 1952.

▶ group therapy

Extracted summary: From our experience it may be possible to make some generalizations about group work with tuberculous patients. First, it is almost inevitable that patients will see group work as another form of treatment, something that is given to them, and that they can be passive or resistive. In a sense, they both passively invite and actively fear therapeutic intervention in their own lives. The leader can safely deal with the "good" patient and the hostile one not by falling in with their passive or active expectations but rather by setting up an objective body of information and observations which they themselves can use in their own way. This was the essence of the didactic approach. Again, the fact that therapy in a hospital situation is, in a sense, imposed from outside means

that the initial efforts must be directed toward bringing individuals into a therapeutic situation. A process of desensitization must take place both to the discussion of the members' own problems and to the social attitude toward psychotherapy. Since this is essentially a cultural attitude, a group with its partly independent subculture is useful in setting up the interpersonal supports to resist it. Although resistance to psychotherapy was at first a group one, this later became transformed into a group pressure for psychotherapy. When two or three new members were introduced to the group they soon responded to the group climate within a few sessions and participated effectively in the discussions.

742

Minor CL. **The psychological handling of the tuberculous patient.** J Med Soc NJ 14:427-438, 1917.

▶ doctor-patient relationship, milieu therapy

Extracted summary: In no disease is the relation between mind and body, between the psychical and the physical so close and so important, as in pulmonary tuberculosis, and he who would successfully treat this disease must be prepared to pay as much attention to his patient's psychic side, to his mental attitude and to his reaction to his sickness as does the neurologist with his cases.

743

Moorman LJ. **The psychology of the tuberculous patients.** Am Rev Tub 57:528-533, 1948. (editorial)

▶ psychotherapy

744

Muhl AM. **Tuberculosis from the psychiatric approach.** Psychoanal Rev 16:397-403, 1929.

▶ psychotherapy

Extracted summary: [The] children did remarkably well with psychotherapeutic treatment. They reacted so well to suggestions that when the right kind of encouragement was presented they responded in an amazing way. Their suggestibility was invaluable too in helping to clear up the fears and worries and to build up new types of personality. If all children with incipient tuberculosis could be reeducated emotionally at the same time that their physical health was being built up, there would be a greatly diminished adult tuberculosis problem.

745

Muhl AM. **Fundamental personality trends in tuberculous women.** Psychoanal Rev 10:380-430, 1923.

▶ psychotherapy

In view of the fact that there were certain common characteristics in this group of thirty in which such great variety as to age, station, social status, nationality and occupation existed, I feel justified in drawing the following conclusions: 1. That in tuberculous women there are certain fundamental personality trends which are common to all, no matter what the apparent type of reaction may be. 2. That they have a two-fold mixed personality which shows strongly marked introverted qualities suggestive of a precox-like pattern on the one hand and extroverted tendencies with a manic-depressive-like swing of greater or less intensity on the other. 3. That the mixed personality is responsible for an immense misuse of energy-imprisoning and burying on one side, recklessly expanding on the other, thus leaving a very small or no surplus for emergencies, either physical or mental. 4. That the patients may present the most varied picture to the casual observer—gay, sad, suspicious, frank, hypomanic, depressed or shut-in-according to which group of trends is in the ascendancy, introvert or extrovert. 5. That if the patient does develop a psychosis or psychoneurosis she may present apparently quite varied pictures at different times, for the reasons mentioned above. 6. That the most characteristic trends can not always be disclosed by questioning, but that it requires analysis to get at them. 7. That the common features are inertia, fatigability, oscillating mood, perseveration, irritability, converted sex trends in the form of masochism and sadism, suggestibility, hypersensitiveness, regressive and suicidal trends, depression and abnormal respiratory behavior. 8. That other very frequent characteristics are ambition, evidence of dissociative trends, memory impairment and day dreaming. 9. That wherever there is a combination of suggestibility, with both masochism and sadism well marked, there is also found evidence of dissociative trends with strong bisexual features. 10. That the regressive trends are very deeply rooted and are influenced and modified by the patients' suggestibility, feeling of inferiority and sensitiveness. 11. That the so-called optimism of the tuberculous patient is chiefly a myth or at least only a compensatory feature, because depressions and suicidal trends in the unconscious were found in all of these patients. 12. That psychotherapy has a distinct place, in addition to routine treatment, in the treatment of the tuberculous patient; and 13. That not until we are prepared to cope with all three phases of the disease, physical, mental, and biochemical, will we be able to really understand and adequately care for our patients.

746

Munro DGM. **The psycho-pathology of pulmonary tuberculosis, with special reference to treatment.** Lancet 201:556-557, 1921.

▶ psychotherapy, psychoanalysis, autosuggestion

Have we then done all that is possible up to the present for patients suffering from this disease who are placed under our care in sanatoriums or otherwise? I do not think

so. I believe we have in psychotherapy a remedy for the alleviation at least of many of the distressing accompaniments of this disease, and one which can materially assist our efforts for the patient's restoration to a moderate degree of health, with arrest of the progress of the disease. It may fairly be asked what part can be played by psychotherapy in an organic disease of this nature. Although Krafft-Ebing and Forel are stated to have carried out certain experiments intended to show that organic changes can be brought about by suggestion, they have had to admit that the results were not very satisfying; it is, I think, also generally acknowledged by psychotherapists that this form of treatment cannot directly affect morbid organic changes. But even if this fact is admitted, we should not, I think, strain the law of psycho-physical parallelism by assuming the close co-relation in disease of the psychic factor and the bodily functions—in short, by holding that psychotherapy can in fact react favourably upon the purely physical side of such a disease as pulmonary tuberculosis.

747

Pinney EL. **Paul Schilder and group psychotherapy: the development of psychoanalytic group psychotherapy.** Psychiatr Q 50:133-143, 1978.

▶ group psychotherapy, psychoanalysis

Discusses the development of psychoanalytic group psychotherapy, including examples of J. H. Pratt's work with tuberculosis patients and I. Wender's therapeutic groups. Although Wender was aware of transference and resistance phenomena, he did not interpret or demonstrate their meaning to his group patients. P. Schilder is considered to be the first to interpret resistance, transference, and dreams in his group sessions. Schilder's publications are discussed in reference to their effects on current mainstream group psychotherapy.

748

Pinney EL. **The beginning of group psychotherapy: Joseph Henry Pratt, M.D., and the Reverend Dr. Elwood Worcester.** Int J Group Psychother 28:109-114, 1978.

▶ group psychotherapy

Describes early developments in the field of group psychotherapy, including its first use in 1905 when Pratt formed a group for tuberculosis patients. The group sessions, which were called classes, focused on member interaction and were modeled on the Methodist Episcopal church system for religious instruction. Using Pratt's methodology, Worcester formed a group in 1906 for persons suffering from mental disorders. Worcester's method (called a health conference) included member self-revelation, prayer, lectures, and group activities, which were held in conjunction with individual sessions. By 1917, group psychotherapy had achieved international recognition and was being practiced in several hospitals.

749

Scherding JP. **On cooperation between the phthisiologist and psychiatrist in French health care establishments.** Wien Klin Wochenschr 80:620-627, 1968. (in German: no English abstract)

▶ consultation-liaison, psychotherapy

750

Seidenfeld MA. **The psychological reorientation of the tuberculous.** J Psychol 10:397-405, 1940.

▶ counseling

The results of psychological services given the patient are generally a reduction in restlessness and nostalgia, a rise in morale due to the hope engendered by the process of increasing the patient's opportunities for employment, greater confidence in recovery because his physician is giving him tangible assurance that he is getting better.

751

Shultz IT. **The emotions of the tubercular: a review and an analysis.** J Abnorm Soc Psychol 37:260-263, 1942.

▶ review: psychotherapy, counseling, milieu therapy

In summarizing, certain facts are discernible: (1) The sanatorium population is more emotionally maladjusted than the general population. These emotional deviations differ tremendously in kind and degree. (2) Some earlier studies suggest that, as a result of bodily lesions and concomitant toxic effects, the mind is affected in a particular way, giving rise to a condition of exaggerated happiness or euphoria which is specific to the disease. (3) Other investigators see evidence of a relationship between emotional patterns and the disease, either for weal or woe. Correct mental attitudes actually aid the cure, while the opposite facilitates the progress of the disease. (4) More modern authors take the view that tuberculosis merely accentuates what emotional maladjustments were present before the onset of the disease. The personality of the patient is the determining factor. Normal or abnormal adjustment depends upon the previously formed emotional habits, which produce emotional crises. (5) Recently there is a trend toward a broader therapy involving educational and vocational rehabilitation as a factor in emotional readjustment. (6) There is increasing evidence that psychology has a significant place in this program.

752

Studt HH. **Psychological factors in pulmonary tuberculosis (IV): Prodromal and concomitant symptoms, disease course, psychotherapy and summary.** Z Psychosom Med Psychoanal 19:201-219, 1973. (in German: no English abstract)

▶ psychotherapy

753

Thompson BA. **The relationship of tuberculosis to nervous and mental diseases.** Med J Rec 129:690-693, 1929.

▶ psychotherapy, doctor-patient relationship

Persuasion is a part of the therapeutic armamentarium which probably most doctors use. The suggestibility of the tuberculous patient is unquestionable and very important. Not more suggestive, however, than many others who are ill over a long period of months. Here again the physician is of paramount importance, a warm and lively interest, sympathetic understanding and imparting of faith and hope, and above all an abundance of charity.

754

Trojanek S. **Role and work of a psychologist in the diagnosis and rehabilitation of tuberculous patients.** Gruzlica 42:1147-1154, 1974. (in Polish)

▶ group psychotherapy, milieu therapy

The aim, task, and conditions of work of a clinical psychologist employed at tuberculosis sanatoria and hospitals are presented in relation to the type of the institution. A set of psychological tests, useful in the work of a psychologist among tuberculous patients, was worked out. The groups of problems, commonly referred to the psychologist by the patients who expect help in dealing with their problems, are enumerated. The author calls attention to the way of interpreting the result of psychological examinations and discusses the problem of the practical use of psychological diagnosis. The pattern of individual programme of rehabilitation in tuberculosis was worked out. It is proposed to include one of the forms of group psychotherapy, a so called therapeutic society, into the process of rehabilitation. The necessity of psychological examinations in patients with non-specific chronic respiratory diseases is mentioned.

755

Weigel BJ. **Neuropsychiatry in tuberculosis: a survey of two hundred patients.** Med J Rec 121:40-42, 1925.

▶ psychotherapy, milieu therapy

Psychotherapy was employed in forty-eight of the patients. Some of these patients were located outside of the institution and it was very difficult to treat them satisfactorily. A complicating factor so often met in this series was the presence of members of the families accompanying the patients and being in constant attendance upon them. This handicaps one in attempting to treat by isolation, which is, of course, good practice in these cases. Nevertheless, markedly favorable results were obtained in at least twenty-seven of these patients. This is considered wellworth while and leads one to believe that intensive psychotherapy in proper surroundings is a great aid in treating the tuberculous. This paper is a plea for men in tuberculosis sanatoria to familiarize themselves with neuropsychiatry and undertake the study of the psychologic makeup of every patient. The successful men in practice many times possess keen insight into the patient's psychobiological makeup and practice psychotherapy instinctively. This probably constitutes the greatest weapon outside of specific therapy in the physician's armamentarium when he is confronted with organic disease. However, not all are blessed with this gift but training along neuropsychiatric lines will fill this long felt need. Conclusions: 1. Functional nervous disease occurs with great frequency among the tuberculous. 2. The disturbances in bodily function by a neuropsychiatric state can no doubt constitute a predisposing factor in tuberculosis. 3. Psychoneurotics are sometimes wrongly diagnosed as tuberculous and find their way into institutions for the treatment of tuberculosis. 4. It is a question as to just how much of a role these patients play in statistics reported from institutions where neuropsychiatric diseases are not recognized. 5. Neuropsychiatric diagnoses in patients with tuberculosis and proper psychiatric treatment are a definite help in the treatment of their tuberculosis. 6. The psychoneurotic has a definitely worse prognosis for his tuberculosis than the individual with approximately normal personality.

756
Wilbur BM, Salkin D, Birnbaum H. **The response of tuberculous alcoholics to a therapeutic community.** Q J Studies Alcohol 27:620-635, 1966.

▶ group therapy, milieu therapy

382 out of 841 men with tuberculosis, admitted to the Veterans Administration Hospital in San Fernando during 1957-1959, were diagnosed as alcoholics. An experimental group of 120 were assigned to a therapeutic-community ward program as beds became available. In contrast to the conventional ward management received by the 141 in the control group, the experimental ss had daily informal group meetings with the therapists, occupational therapy, and "an atmosphere designed to create free expression of feeling, shared responsibility and deeper understanding. It was concluded that the form of therapeutic community described may be effective in helping high-maturity-nonarrestee alcoholics to complete treatment for tuberculosis, but it can have a detrimental effect on the behavior of arrestee alcoholics. A better understanding of the individual characteristics of patients, treatments and therapists, and the complex interaction among them, can guide the development of more varied and more selective procedures for the treatment of alcoholic tuberculous patients."

757
Wilkes WO. **Psychotherapy in the treatment of tuberculosis.** Tex State J Med 15:331-335, 1919-1920.

▶ psychotherapy, suggestion, doctor-patient relationship

Extracted summary: Psychotherapy, on the other hand, helps the patient to cure his own disease "by improving the functions of his own body cells through orderly psychic influences." It relieves many functional disorders, and affections of the second personality—the subconscious individual—and will aid in the cure of organic diseases in all cases where there is conscious cerebration. The combination of the two methods—material medicine and psychotherapy—is the ideal procedure and will give by far the largest measure of success. Every successful practitioner of medicine makes use of psychotherapy, whether consciously or unconsciously. To be a successful practitioner one must have a measure of personal magnetism and individual impressivness, or psychic force. These qualities act psychotherapeutically, and the successful doctor of the old school used both to the fullest extent, though entirely ignorant of the large work that defines much of his therapeutic endeavors. If pushed for a definition he would probably have called it "hoss sense." And "hoss sense" is the very best equipment a doctor can have for the alleviation of disease. Unfortunately, we are not all born with it in equal ratio, but all of us can cultivate the use of mental suggestion.

Other Infectious Disorders

758
Arone di Bertolino R. **Psychosomatic treatment of recurrent herpes simplex.** Minerva Med 72:1207-1212, 1981. (in Italian)

▶ psychotherapy, hypnosis

Psychological causes are often found to be responsible for the recurrence of herpes in clinical practice. This, and the fact that certain factors concerning recurrence itself are not clear, has led Terni to suggest that psychogenic factors are essential in determining the frequency and extent of such recurrences, and that without prejudice to its undoubtedly viral nature, recurrent herpes simplex may be regarded as a psychosomatic disease. The underlying criteria, practice, clinical progression and positive results obtained with psychotherapy and hypnosis in the treatment of 24 cases of recurrent herpes simplex are described in support of this view. The effectiveness of the method employed indicates that the hypothesis put forward is correct.

759
Blank H, Brody MW. **Recurrent herpes simplex: a psychiatric and laboratory study.** Psychosom Med 12:254-260, 1950.

▶ psychotherapy

Ten patients were studied independently by a dermatologist and by a psychiatrist. With one possible exception, an amazing uniformity was found in the psychologic pattern. The entire group were found to be of a hysterical character structure, very immature, passive, dependent, highly suggestible, and over-reactive to small stimuli. Over-intensified erotic desire at the genital stage of development and inevitable frustration caused regression. The psychologic conflict was expressed predominantly in oral terms. Genital satisfaction became inhibited by shame and guilt feelings. With the loss of genital satisfaction there was an intensification of oral and possibly skin erotism. The patient described in detail (Miss AA) felt no conscious shame for her promiscuous sexual behavior but did react with recurrent herpes. Not only were the erotic feelings worked out in oral terms, but hostility was also recognized as an oral concept. Indicative of the high degree of unresolved infantile sexuality, transference phenomena dominate the picture. Proper management of the transference is capable of giving almost immediate relief of symptoms. Disturbing the positive transference causes increased anxiety, shame, and guilt and precipitates an outbreak of herpetic lesions. In these people the usual mode of defense to ward off danger is by being good, sweet persons. However, their very defenses become erotized and they become "sweet enough to eat." This is manifest in superficial observation of their overt appearance. The specific mechanism for herpetic eruptions seems to be a return of repressed oral impulses in oral receptive people, a projection of oral sadistic tendencies with guilt, and shame for erotic feelings. The physiology of the mechanism whereby the skin reacts to this feeling of guilt and shame is unknown.

760
Geocaris K. **Circumoral herpes and separation experiences in psychotherapy.** Psychosom Med 23:41-47, 1961.

▶ psychoanalysis

The patient presented in this report was a young woman who developed circumoral lesions of herpes simplex during important separation experiences related to her psychotherapy. In the setting of analytically oriented psychotherapy, the therapist had the opportunity of studying these occurrences within the context of the patient's life situation and her fantasies, dreams, and free associations.

761
Gould SS, Tissler DM. **The use of hypnosis in the treatment of herpes simplex II.** Am J Clin Hypn 26:171-174, 1984.

▶ hypnosis, suggestion, imagery

Hypnosis training was used to treat the painful lesions and emotional symptoms associated with herpes simplex II in two females, ages 32 and 26. Three weekly sessions of hypnosis and daily practice sessions were initiated in the first case. During this time, the patient experienced a decline in the subjective level of pain and severity of the lesions, as well as an elevation in mood level. On three-month followup, she reported no pain or skin eruptions and significantly less feelings of stress and anxiety. The second case utilized two sessions of hypnosis and daily practice sessions, and similar results were obtained. A traumatic event caused a relapse in the latter patient, but she was again able to use hypnosis to bring the virus back under control and to experience an elevation in mood level as well. A seven-month followup indicated no eruptions and an improvement in self-esteem.

762
Janicki MP. **Recurrent herpes labialis and recurrent aphthous ulcerations: psychological components.** Psychother Psychosom 19:288-294, 1971.

▶ psychotherapy, counseling

The relevant research literature is reviewed to determine the psychological components in 2 psychophysiological disorders, recurrent herpes labialis and recurrent aphthous ulcerations. Two major variables emerge: that emotional stress is usually associated with outbreaks of both, and appears to be the precipitating agent; and that counseling and psychotherapy appear to have an effect upon the nature of the recurrences and oftentimes upon their cessation. The need for further controlled experimentation is indicated.

763
Saul LJ. **Psychogenic factors in the etiology of the common cold and related symptoms.** Int J Psychoanal 19:451-470, 1938.

▶ psychoanalysis

(1) Evidence is presented which confirms the observation that emotional factors may be of prime importance in certain cases of the "common cold" (including sore throat and laryngitis), i.e., the "cold" may be essentially a neurotic symptom. (2) That psychogenic factors may be of appreciable frequency and importance in the etiology of colds is indicated by a brief statistical survey of the practices of six psycho-analysts: every one of fifteen patients who had repeated colds before analysis, had few or none after analysis (average years of follow up, three). (3) In the nine patients reported, colds occurred regularly in situations of frustration of strong, mostly unconscious, receptive demands with more or less repressed rage. In the opinion of the author, the evidence in these cases shows that the relationship is causal. This observation in no way implies that all emotional states of receptive thwarting result in colds, nor obviously that this etiology is in any sense exclusive. The emotional factor is only one of several (infectious agents, irritants, allergins, temperature changes, etc.), operating separately or in combination, and may be of greater or lesser importance or prominence in any individual case. Nor are the emotions and mechanisms here described necessarily the only ones which can produce the picture of the cold. In the cases reported in which the emotional factors played a prominent role, the symptoms seemed more closely related to allergic than to infectious conditions, although nothing positive can be concluded on this point. (4) The emotional impulses stimulate physiological activities in other regions of the body. These result in the other symptoms which frequently accompany colds: gastro-intestinal disturbances (anorexia, nausea, diarrhea, colitis, constipation), headache, and in women, leucorrhoea. The fatigue, malaise, etc., are often, at least in part, manifestations of mild depression. Fever, apparently truly psychogenic, occurred in two cases. The whole condition is utilized in the services of masochism, passive indulgence, secondary elaboration and various other secondary gains. (5) Some incidental observations are made on psychogenic factors in catarrhal vaginitis and leucorrhoea.

Books and Book Chapters on Infectious Disorders

764
Hartz J. **Psychological aspects of pulmonary tuberculosis.** In: ED Wittkower, RA Cleghorn (eds.), Recent Developments in Psychosomatic Medicine. Philadelphia: Lippincott, 1954.

765
Hendricks CM. **Psychosomatic aspects of tuberculosis and its complications.** In: EW Hayes (ed.), Fundamentals of Pulmonary Tuberculosis and its Complications. Springfield, Illinois: Thomas, 1949.

766
Huebschmann H. **The Mind and Tuberculosis.** Stuttgart: Enke, 1952.

767
Mann T. **The Magic Mountain.** New York: Knopf, 1927.

768
Sparer PJ (ed.). **Personality, Stress and Tuberculosis.** New York: International Universities Press, 1956.

769
Wittkower ED. **A Psychiatrist looks at Tuberculosis.** London: National Association for the Prevention of Tuberculosis, 1949.

Skin
Diseases

Acne

770

Albrecht H, Schonfelder T. **Excoriative acne of young women—from the psychiatric viewpoint.** Arch Klin Exp Dermatol 223:509-526, 1965. (in German: no English abstract)

▶ psychotherapy

771

Brown BW. **Treatment of acne vulgaris by biofeedback-assisted cue-controlled relaxation and guided cognitive imagery.** Diss Abstr Int 42:1163, 1981.

▶ behavior therapy, biofeedback, relaxation, imagery, attention-comparison

A cognitive-behavioral adjunctive intervention involving biofeedback-assisted relaxation and cognitive imagery procedures for the treatment of acne vulgaris was investigated in this study with 30 patients, already receiving traditional dermatological treatment, as participants. A three-group design was used which consisted of a treatment (relaxation-imagery), a rational behavior group therapy attention-comparison, and a medical intervention control (medication and lesion extraction) group. The treatment and attention-comparison group subjects were administered the Sixteen Personality Factor Questionnaire at pre- and posttreatment in order to explore personality changes as a function of the psychological intervention that they received. These subjects also engaged in daily home practice procedures in addition to their laboratory treatment sessions. Both these groups received an identical number of laboratory and home practice sessions, and similar experimenter-induced expectations and demand characteristics during treatment. None of the hypothesized therapeutic components of the treatment group were present in the attention-comparison group. The treatment and attention-comparison group subjects received the same medical intervention as the third group of acne patients who were routinely monitored to control for dermatological treatment effects. As hypothesized, the treatment group showed a significant reduction in acne severity as compared to the attention-comparison and the medical control group. A second hypothesis, which held

that the attention-comparison and control group conditions would not significantly differ from each other was also confirmed. The hypothesis which held that treatment group subjects would exhibit equally low electromyographic biofeedback levels while engaging in either cue-controlled relaxation or guided cognitive imagery was also supported. Significant changes were found across treatment on each of the four second-order personality factors assessed. Data regarding subjects' self-grading of acne severity, expectations for treatment effectiveness, and frequency of home practice was obtained and analyzed for treatment and attention-comparison group subjects. The results of this research provided strong support for the efficacy of biofeedback-assisted relaxation-imagery therapy as an adjunctive treatment for patients with chronic acne vulgaris. Future research was suggested.

772

Ellerbroek WC. **Hypotheses toward a unified field theory of human behavior with clinical application to acne vulgaris.** Perspect Biol Med 16:240-262, 1973.

▶ psychotherapy, suggestion, placebo

There is little doubt in my mind about the number and variety of negative reactions this paper will provoke. However, whether critics speak of faith healing, hypnotism, suggestion, or placebo effect, the results might still arouse some interest. My fullest cooperation is offered to those who wish to make clinical trials, but for a "fair" test, it should be noted that the essentials are an enthusiastic therapist who does not fear intense involvement with his patients and who will go to great lengths to help them, as well as patients who have been thoroughly convinced of the earnestness and capabilities of their physician and of the results that it is possible to achieve. Finally, note that this paper is not about acne vulgaris: it is about how people get "sick" and how they get "well." If this admittedly controversial approach has a major value, it is in the demonstration that Graham's study of "attitudes" came very close to solving the problem of psychosomatic specificity. My own idea is that a "disease" is determined by all the specific psycholinguistic and behavioral events in the life history of the patient, including his total interaction with his field within and without. There are those who will say that such an explanation explains nothing. But it appears to me as the only rational explanation of human behavior, including "disease," and that—since postures, voices, behaviors, words, and thoughts are all modifiable variables—there is therefore no such thing as an untreatable disease. After many years in surgery, and now in psychiatry, I still have the same goal: not the treatment of acne, but the elucidation of mechanisms of disease, both "mental" and "physical." It is my carefully considered opinion, mad as it may sound, that this mechanism—ubiquitous in human beings—is the long-sought-for hidden factor behind major system malignancies, and that the road to cancer control and prevention is open to us now. The message is: Don't be depressed—why get cancer?

773

Hollander MB. **Excoriated acne controlled by post-hypnotic suggestion.** Am J Clin Hypn 1:122-123, 1959.

▶ hypnosis, suggestion

Extracted summary: In general, symptom displacement through hypnosis seems of questionable advisability. The symptom is serving a function which may not be at all obvious, and if that symptom is displaced its function may be taken over by something even more undesirable. There is also the ever-present possibility that the non-psychiatric physician may, in displacing a symptom, precipitate something too hot for him to handle. The specific situation of excoriation of acne does not seem to fall into this general category. It bears little resemblance to ordinary neurotic excoriation. What started the picking originally was the same thing which is bothering the patient now, the appearance of the face. Without regard to the associated difficulties which may have attached themselves to the picking, this appears to be a self-contained situation in which improvement in the appearance of the face allays anxiety about it, so that the need to pick is actually diminished. This is a preliminary report, for two cases are not enough to justify anything more than encouragement to investigate further. The experience in these two cases, though, has been so far superior to the results usually seen in such instances as to warrant continuing along this line of post-hypnotic suggestion.

774

Hughes H, Brown BW, Lawliss GF, Fulton JE. **Treatment of acne vulgaris by biofeedback relaxation and cognitive imagery.** J Psychosom Res 27:185-191, 1983.

▶ biofeedback, relaxation, imagery

A multielement intervention involving biofeedback-assisted relaxation and cognitive imagery treatment of acne vulgaris was investigated in this study with 30 patients (aged 17-41 yrs) receiving medical dermatological treatment. Ss were matched on age, sex, and pretreatment acne severity and randomly assigned to groups. Treatment consisted of 12 sessions over 6 wks and resulted in a significant reduction in acne severity as compared to the attention-comparison and medical control groups. Treatment-group Ss continuing home practice until follow-up maintained their gains, whereas those who discontinued failed to maintain gains.

775

Jelliffe AM, Soutter C, Meara RH. **An investigation into the treatment of acne vulgaris with Grenz x-rays.** Br J Dermatol 81:617-620, 1969.

▶ suggestion

From these results it would appear that Grenz rays in the dosage used have no effect, but that 50 kV x-rays perhaps have some beneficial effect upon acne vulgaris. In an attempt to assess other factors which might influence the response, 33 patients who responded symmetrically on both sides in the Grenz x-ray series, were examined in detail. The patient's sex and the duration of the improvement are indicated in Figure 3. In this group of patients, it must be accepted that the side treated by Grenz rays did no better than the side treated by suggestion alone. The better response of female patients is obvious.

776

Montgomery L. **Psychoanalysis of a case of acne vulgaris.** Psychoanal Rev 23:274-285, 1936.

▶ psychoanalysis

Extracted summary: In [the patient's] case, as the unconscious figure gradually emerged in its complete aliveness and was slowly with much difficulty inserted into her reality, the morbid material was gradually eliminated and her acne cleared completely ... Nineteen months after the analysis, the patient reports no recurrence of acne lesions nor any of the other symptoms. We might postulate that at least certain psychosomatic symptoms may run a chronic course precisely because they satisfy a definite need of the unknown second figure that dwells within. Further study along this line may disclose that the specific form which somatic symptoms take is determined by the specific form of satisfaction the unconscious figure demands, that is, the psychosomatic interrelationship might lie between the two personalities existing within the total personality. The one, the unconscious figure in its relationship to the inner physiological functions; the other, the conscious figure in its relationship to the environment.

777

Sontag LW. **The purpose and fate of a skin disorder.** Psychosom Med 7:306-310, 1945.

▶ psychotherapy

This is a case report of a woman whose life was marred by a severe and disfiguring skin disease, one considered by leading dermatologists to be due to a cutaneous circulatory disturbance. The original appearance of the condition and its recurrence coincided with periods of severe emotional stress associated with sexual problems. Any one of the following interpretations of the significance of this relationship might be made. 1. That the relationship was a coincidence. 2. That the emotional distress was disturbing to all metabolic processes and nutrition, and that the acne rosacea was only one aspect of such a generalized disturbance. 3. That the acne resulted from autonomic-induced cutaneous vasodilation, incident to periods of disturbed emotional state. 4. That the acne was a purposeful action of the unconscious, a punishment and a safeguard, accomplished through autonomic control of the cutaneous vascular bed. The title of this paper suggests that Elaine's acne rosacea may have been a purposeful process. However, while it is my intention to suggest and discuss this possibility, I do not wish to imply that it is necessarily the correct one.

Alopecia Areata

778

Basset F et al. **Some considerations concerning the psychosomatic study of alopecias: preliminary note.** Ann Med Psychol 2:283, 1969. (in French)

▶ psychotherapy

Reviews the significance of hair in linguistic expressions, mythology, and religion, briefly analyzes the psychosomatic literature, and presents 10 cases (3 children) of the diverse alopecias seen at a psychosomatic service created in a Strasbourg dermatology clinic. The majority of the patients were depressed and anxious, with enuresis common among the young ss. The obvious mother attachments, the question of death phantasms in alopecia raised by the frequent "osseous" Rorschach responses, and the problem of castration are also discussed, culminating with a study on the possible function of hair as a "partial object."

779

Cohen IH, Lichtenberg JD. **Alopecia areata.** Arch Gen Psychiatry 17:608-614, 1967.

▶ psychotherapy

2 Ss who had developed alopecia areata were studied and treated by intensive psychotherapy. Both had been treated for other reasons and developed alopecia near the end of psychotherapy. In further therapy it was found that the symptom served an adaptive function signaling the need for more therapy. There was strong motivation, an intense facility for treatment, and a tendency to somatization. Following the onset of the alopecia, memories were brought to consciousness which had not been available before, demonstrating a complex intertwining of separation and castration anxiety. There was a family background of sexual overstimulation, magical properties assigned to body parts, and special significance of hair linked to mother. While the case material suggests that the alopecia in these Ss was a psychologically induced symptom, it is possible that the relative importance of psychological and physical factors may vary from patient to patient.

780

Jokipaltio L. **Rejection of femininity in a 6-year-old girl.** Schweiz Z Psychol Anwendung 25:322-335, 1966. (in German)

▶ psychoanalysis

Presents the case history of a 6-yr-old girl admitted to the psychiatric department of the Basle Children's Hospital because of alopecia areata and phobias. During the 2 1/2 yr. of psychoanalysis, her fears were seen to be castration fear. As a result of the analysis she was able to progress to a normal female development; the alopecia areata receded and the girl was happier; she made contact with other people more easily and her performance improved.

781

Macalpine I. **Is alopecia areata psychosomatic? A psychiatric study.** Br J Dermatol 70:117-131, 1958.

▶ psychotherapy

An investigation of 125 cases of alopecia areata including 25 of alopecia totalis and universalis produced no evidence for the widely held view that psychological factors—mental illness, anxiety or mental shock—play a significant part in causing or precipitating the disorder. These clinical findings are supported by the fact that alopecia occurs in the lowest-grade mental defectives living in the constant milieu of colonies. Although our findings are mainly negative, a survey of our patients' histories for mental stress which did not precipitate an attack of alopecia areata seems to justify the more positive statement that it is unlikely that mental stress plays an important part. Yet much may be done psychotherapeutically to help patients adjust to their condition. Our conclusions may best be expressed in Hutchinson's (1893) words, written forty years after he had started his first intensive study of alopecia areata: "The entire absence of any form of ill-health in the subjects of alopecia areata induces me to put wholly aside any inquiry on that score. We may, I think, entertain absolute incredulity as to what is called the neurotic form of this disease. It attacks young people more frequently than others, and they are usually those in whom neither headache nor any species of neurotic disturbance has been observed. It does not appear to me to be worth while in such a malady to ask an adult patient as to overwork, mental worry, and the like. Such influences may be found, if sought for, in the majority of those who consult us, and I feel very certain that when they chance to be coincident with alopecia they do not stand to it in the relation of cause."

782

Pasqua MC, Beltrani G. **Total alopecia areata: personality study and attempted psychotherapy.** G Ital Dermatol 46:210-212, 1971. (in Italian)

▶ psychotherapy

Personality studies in an 8-year-old subject with total alopecia areata of two years standing are reported. Investigation of the patient's family and school background showed a close relationship between his lack of adaptation and the disease.

783

Stowe JE, Goldenberg E. **Systematic desensitization as a component for treatment of alopecia areata: a case study.** Psychol Rep 46:875-881, 1980.

▶ systematic desensitization, relaxation

Examined the effects of systematic desensitization and relaxation on hair growth in a 20-yr-old male with a 4-yr history of alopecia areata. Six bald scalp patches were photographed over 6 mo; 2 ordered hierarchies involving interpersonal and compulsive themes were presented in 8 treatment sessions. Results indicate nearly complete hair regrowth over the 6 mo, with no new appearances of bald patches. Both rate and duration of growth exceeded that reported in dermatological literature, suggesting that autonomic activity associated with anxiety and nervousness are correlated with physiological changes precipitating hair loss.

Burns

784

Ben-Hur N, Izak M. **Hypnosis in severe burn cases.** Harefuah 89:301-303, 1975. (in Hebrew: no English abstract)

▶ hypnosis

785

Bernstein NR. **Observations on the use of hypnosis with burned children on a pediatric ward.** Int J Clin Exp Hypn 13:1-10, 1965.

▶ hypnosis

Hypnotic suggestions have been employed in the management of children being treated in hospitals for burns. Several cases are described, and observations made about the interplay of forces between the staff, the patient, and the therapist, as well as the expectations of the patients to assess how these factors influenced the use of hypnosis. Hypnosis appears to be a particularly useful means for reaching isolated and depressed children with burns and for improving the morale of the staff team working with these children. The results may be along specific lines in terms of pain tolerance and improved eating, or in general improvement of cooperativeness and mood on the part of the child.

786

Bernstein NR. **Management of burned children with the aid of hypnosis.** J Child Psychol 4:93-98, 1963.

▶ hypnosis

1. Hypnosis is a useful aid in managing children hospitalized for severe burns. 2. General co-operativeness and improved morale in the children result, and more interest from the staff helps diminish loneliness and improve cooperativeness in patient and personnel. 3. Pain tolerance may be increased and appetite improved. 4. Three patients are described in which this approach was used. 5. Some conceptual and clinical aspects of using hypnosis are discussed.

787

Bird EI, Colbourne GR. **Rehabilitation of an electrical burn patient through thermal biofeedback.** Biofeedback Self Regul 5:283-287, 1980.

▶ biofeedback, relaxation

A 22-year-old male subject, with high-voltage electrical burns to one wrist, utilized differential relaxation and visual biofeedback to increase skin temperature in the damaged hand. Through 14 thermal biofeedback and passive relaxation sessions, the subject was able to produce temperature increases in his damaged hand of up to 21° F, which considerably diminished the pain. Healing, feeling, and movement control seemed to progress with extreme rapidity, suggesting that axoplasmic transport was greatly enhanced.

788

Crasilneck HB, Stirman JA, Wilson BJ, McCrane EJ, Fogelman MJ. **Use of hypnosis in the management of patients with burns.** JAMA 158:103-106, 1955.

▶ hypnosis, suggestion

Hypnotic and posthypnotic suggestion were successfully used in burned patients as an anesthetic agent and as an analgesic. Eight patients were included in the present study, six of whom were excellent hypnotic subjects; however, the other two were not amenable to this therapy. Suggestion during hypnosis was used to stimulate tremendous appetites in persons otherwise not inclined to eat. Furthermore, suggestions were made to provide motivation to use and exercise injured parts previously immobilized by pain. Hypnosis was successful as a psychotherapeutic agent in correcting some of the detrimental emotional responses and psychological adaptation mechanisms to thermal injury. The potential value of hypnosis in severely burned or chronically ill persons is to be investigated further.

789

Dahinterova J. **Some experiences with the use of hypnosis in the treatment of burns.** Int J Clin Exp Hypn 15:49-53, 1967.

▶ psychotherapy, hypnosis

Our experience with hypnosis as a means of eliminating pain during surgical procedures for the treatment of severe burns has been favorable in 3 out of 4 cases discussed. These include patients who had relatively chronic, serious, and severe burns. We concluded that hypnosis can be an important and useful adjunct in the psychotherapeutic treatment of burns.

790

Ewin DM. **Emergency room hypnosis for the burned patient.** Am J Clin Hypn 26:5-8, 1983.

▶ hypnosis

Hypnosis can be a most valuable method in the emergency room treatment of the burn patient. This paper addresses certain issues and methods of hypnotic therapy within such a setting.

791

Hammond DC, Keye WR, Grant CW Jr. **Hypnotic analgesia with burns: an initial study.** Am J Clin Hypn 26:56-59, 1983.

▶ hypnosis, suggestion

This study was an initial attempt to experimentally evaluate the effects of hypnotic analgesia and suggestion of coolness on inflammation and healing of burns. Six subjects were equally sunburned on both thighs and then hypnotic suggestions given for analgesia in only one thigh. None of the subjects reported pain in the analgesic burn area. There was a significant ($p < .01$) and consistent trend of lower temperatures in the analgesic thigh, and a significantly ($p < .01$) greater proportion of the redness ratings were lower in the hypnotically anesthetized thigh compared to the control thigh. Thus all three signs of inflammation were diminished. The results should be interpreted cautiously because of the small sample size, but give tentative support to the belief that hypnotic analgesia may reduce burn inflammation and possibly promote healing. Recommendations for future research are given.

792

Jorgensen JA, Brophy JJ. **Psychiatric treatment modalities in burn patients.** Curr Psychiatr Ther 15:85-92, 1975.

▶ operant conditioning, desensitization, counseling, hypnosis, imagery, psychotherapy

Behavioral approaches are most effective in handling many of the problems that arise in the intermediate stage. The particular problem in which behavioral techniques should be considered is resistance to treatment (e.g., refusal to eat or recalcitrance about the Hubbard tank and physical therapy). Too often, the problems create control struggles between the patient and staff. Attention to specific behaviors, a careful plan for a behavioral approach, and, most important, a clear cooperative follow-up of the plan by the staff are necessary for behavioral techniques to succeed. Several useful behavioral techniques are operant conditioning, desensitization, rational guidance, and modeling.

793

Jorgenson JA, Brophy JJ. **Psychiatric treatment of seriously burned adults.** Psychosomatics 14:331-335, 1973.

▶ operant conditioning, desensitization, modeling, confrontation, psychotherapy

There is a wide spectrum of problems during recovery from severe burns. At one end, the acute phase tends to present with psychiatric problems which are related to the multiple medical-surgical difficulties. Often, psychiatric consultation involves a close alliance with the surgical team in diagnosing the type of psychiatric condition, particularly correctible brain syndromes. While they should not substitute for correction of such reversible conditions, phenothiazines and sedative-tranquilizers are effective in alleviation of the brain syndrome and allaying anxiety. They are an adjunct to adequate analgesia and good supportive care. At the other end of the spectrum lies the long recuperative phase just before and after hospital discharge. A patient's optimism at leaving the hospital following his long ordeal is not indicative of a good prognosis. The individual's premorbid adjustment and to a lesser degree disfigurement and dysfunction determine the ability to cope with readjustment problems following hospitalization. Aftercare psychiatric treatment, usually psychotherapy, is often poorly planned and executed. In between both ends of the spectrum, a host of intermediate phase problems occur including: inadequate analgesia, aversive conditioning to painful situations, staff-patient conflicts, and the patient's own depression, grief, hostility, and regression. All three treatment modalities: psychotropic drugs, behavioral approaches and individual psychotherapy are useful during this phase.

794

LaBaw WL. **Adjunctive trance therapy with severely burned children.** Int J Child Psychother 2:80-92, 1973.

▶ hypnosis

Severely burned children are among the most massively traumatized ever treated clinically. Organic and psychic injury are combined in them in a desperately needful package. Trance therapy (medical hypnosis for practical use)

was employed as an adjunct in the comprehensive treatment of twenty-three such children. Anxiety, depression, and regression were the children's emotional hallmarks. They often viewed their injuries punitively. Their self-images were dimmed. The purpose of this pilot study was to determine if the induced regressive state achieved through trance therapy could serve as an effective partial alternative to this naturally occurring regressive state, thereby curtailing the unhealthy concomitants of the latter. This was found to be the case, as the patients' difficulty with clinically offensive symptoms—such as pain, eneuresis, encopresis, and inanition related to poor food and fluid intake—was diminished, lessening their morbidity. Trance therapy is the treatment of choice for the regressive anorexia and involuntary soiling of the gravely injured individual.

795

Margolis CG, De Clement F. **Hypnosis and the treatment of burns.** Burns 6:253-254, 1980.

▶ review: hypnosis, autohypnosis

A scan of the literature on clinical hypnosis points to the usefulness of hypnosis in reducing pain in patients with burn injuries. Two cases involving patients who experienced thermal injury and subsequent complications are reported. Both represented management problems to the staff at the St. Agnes Burn Unit in Philadelphia. In their cases, characteristic of a significant number, hypnosis was successfully used to reduce pain and anxiety.

796

Margolis CG, Domangue BB, Ehleben C, Shrier L. **Hypnosis in the early treatment of burns: a pilot study.** Am J Clin Hypn 26:9-15, 1983.

▶ review: hypnosis, imagery, suggestion

A review of the literature indicates that hypnosis, which has long been successfully used for pain control in burn patients, might also be able to alter the body's physiological response to burn injury. The present study is designed to determine if a single, early, hypnotic induction can alter the physiological response of the patients to their thermal injury. The hypnotic induction used visual imagery with suggestions of coolness and comfort according to a standard protocol. All patients were seen within 12 hours post burn. A total of 17 patients were enrolled in the study, 11 of whom accumulated sufficient data to be included in the analyses. Matched controls were selected on the basis of age and percent body surface area burn. Six of the 11 experimental subjects included in the analyses were judged by clinical observations to be at least mildly hypnotized whereas the remaining five did not. There were no significant differences between length of stay, fluid input or urine output between the total experimental group and their matched controls. However, Day 2 urine output (24-

28 hours post burn) was significantly higher for the 6 hypnotized subjects than for their matched controls. It is hypothesized, since urine output is related to edema and fluid retention, that hypnosis was able to exert a physiological effect on the response of these five patients to their burn injury. Further work needs to be done on the potential for hypnosis in burn care.

797

Merz B. **Hypnosis for burn patients: healing body and spirit.** JAMA 249:321-323, 1983. (News)

▶ hypnosis

798

Moore LE, Kaplan JZ. **Hypnotically accelerated burn wound healing.** Am J Clin Hypn 26:16-19, 1983.

▶ hypnosis

This study was designed to assess the efficacy of hypnotically induced vasodilation in the healing of burn wounds. Patients were selected on the basis of having symmetrical or bilaterally equivalent burns on some portion of their right and left sides. Since one side only of the body was treated by hypnotically induced vasodilation, the patient served as his own experimental control. In this single blind study, the hypnotist and patient knew the side selected for treatment, the evaluating surgeon and nursing staff did not. Four of the five patients demonstrated clearly accelerated healing on the treated side, the fifth patient had rapid healing to both sides. It is concluded that hypnosis facilitated dramatic enhancement of burn wound healing.

799

Pennisi VR. **On behavior modification therapy in the recalcitrant burned child.** Plast Reconstr Surg 58:216, 1976. (letter)

▶ psychotherapy

800

Schafer DW. **Hypnosis use on a burn unit.** Int J Clin Exp Hypn 23:1-14, 1975.

▶ hypnosis

Hypnosis was utilized with 20 severely-burned patients on a modern burn unit. 14 were benefited in the control of pain, especially during dressing changes. Half of these were either somnambulists or were capable of enough depth to control pain posthypnotically. The other half were benefited during the state of hypnosis even though their level was around 3 on a scale of 5. This second half of "successes" found relief via a personalized recording when the author was not present. The 6 failures were, with one exception, under the age of 21. Morale, regression, and ward adjustment were improved by the presence of the author as both a psychiatrist and also a hypnotist.

801
Shorkey CT, Taylor JE. **Management of maladaptive behavior of a severely burned child.** Child Welfare 52:543-547, 1973.

▶ behavior modification, counterconditioning

Consistent use of discrimination and counterconditioning procedures decreased the child's anxiety responses under the social condition and reduced the number of times that the infant became upset during the brief treatment periods every 2 hours. Changes in the child's behavior were not observed until the second day of the regime. At that time, crying lessened during the social period and the child began to watch silently as staff members entered her room. Two days later the child smiled during this period for the first time. By the fourth day the staff began to induce smiling by playing a peek-a-boo game, and by the end of the 2 weeks the child appeared comfortable and smiled during these visits. Behavior during treatment remained unchanged. The infant's ability to differentiate between treatment and feeding procedures allowed resumption of skin grafting. The discrimination procedures were continued for 1 1/2 months until the child was in relatively good physical condition, showed little fear of hospital personnel and ate satisfactorily. The last weeks of hospitalization were relatively painless and the discrimination procedure was dropped 2 weeks before the child was released. The use of the behavior-modification techniques in this case not only produced changes in the behavior of the child that allowed treatment to be resumed, but was a source of reinforcement for the staff.

802
Varni JW, Bessman CA, Russo DC, Cataldo MF. **Behavioral management of chronic pain in children: case study.** Arch Phys Med Rehabil 61:375-379, 1980.

▶ behavior therapy, reinforcement

Although chronic pain in children often has a clear etiology, environmental factors may influence the continuation of pain behaviors. The present study investigated socioenvironmental factors which influenced the pain behavior of a 3-year-old girl subsequent to severe burns. Behavioral treatment strategies consisted of rearranging reinforcement contingencies so as to reduce pain behaviors and increase observed "well" behaviors, including those related to orthopedic and physical therapies. The significance of the findings is discussed in terms of rehabilitating pediatric patients with chronic pain.

803
Wakeman RJ, Kaplan JZ. **An experimental study of hypnosis in painful burns.** Am J Clin Hypn 21:3-12, 1978.

▶ hypnosis, autohypnosis, relaxation

The present study examines the usefulness of hypnosis in the control of acute pain in thermal and electrically burned patients as an adjunctive analgesic during the routine care of burn wounds. It was hypothesized that the use of hypnosis would lead to significant reductions in the amount of drugs needed as compared to patients using medication only. Anxiety and discomfort associated with daily tanking, debridement, and dressing changes were expected to be reduced because of the introduction of hypnotic procedures. The experimental study also examined the variables of age and percent of burns. Two studies were conducted including patients with 0-30% total body burns and 31-60% burns. A variety of hypnotic techniques were used. Both studies revealed significantly lower percentages of medication used ($p < .01$) by the hypnotic groups than control groups. The 7-18 year-old patients used significantly less medication ($p < .05$) than the adult groups. The implications of the findings, and usefulness of hypnosis and ego strengthening techniques for improvement of self-confidence and improved body image were considered.

804
Walker LJS, Healy M. **Psychological treatment of a burned child.** J Pediatr Psychol 5:395-404, 1980.

▶ behavior modification, relaxation training, bibliotherapy, play therapy

An 8-year-old girl who was hospitalized with second- and third-degree burns covering 80% of her body was treated with a combination of behavior modification, relaxation training, bibliotherapy, and play therapy techniques. The appropriate utilization of the various psychotherapeutic approaches in response to the predictable sequence of the emotional needs of a pediatric burn patient and the parents is discussed.

805
Weinstein DJ. **Imagery and relaxation with a burn patient.** Behav Res Ther 14:481, 1976. (case report)

▶ imagery, relaxation

806
Weisz AE. **Psychotherapeutic support of burned patients.** Mod Treat 4:1291-1303, 1967.

▶ psychotherapy, hypnosis, consultation-liaison

Psychotherapeutic support of burned patients is required due to the severity and extent of the adaptive problems caused by the burn injury. The physician in charge of the comprehensive treatment program is best situated to manage psychologic problems as an integral part of overall therapy. Management suggestions are made for the acute post-burn crisis period, the prolonged period of hospital treatment and recovery, and for the stage of discharge planning. Special considerations with children and their families are described. The role of the psychiatrist both as an indirect consultant vis-a-vis the burn treatment team, and as a direct consultant are explored.

807

Wernick RL, Jaremko ME, Taylor PW. **Pain management in severely burned adults: a test of stress inoculation.** J Behav Med 4:103-109, 1981.

▶ stress inoculation

A treatment program of stress inoculation for the pain experienced by 16 severely burned adults was carried out by the nursing staff of a burn and trauma unit. Results showed that treated subjects improved on measures of unauthorized pain requests, physical and emotional self-ratings, "tanking" ratings, compliance with hospital routine, and state and trait anxiety, whereas non-treated subjects showed little improvement.

808

Wisely DW, Masur FT, Morgan SB. **Psychological aspects of severe burn injuries in children.** Health Psychol 2:45-72, 1983.

▶ review: hypnosis, behavior modification, relaxation, bibliotherapy, play therapy

The psychological literature on the severely burned child is reviewed. Four phases of the traumatic process are defined: the preinjury phase which refers to relevant premorbid aspects of the burn victim; the acute phase, which centers on the medical treatment directed toward physiological stabilization; the intermediate phase, in which skin grafts and other extremely painful medical procedures are performed and wherein severe psychological and behavioral problems are likely to emerge; and the rehabilitative phase, characterized by the child's reentry into or withdrawal from the social milieu. For each of these stages, common psychological reactions, potential psychological interventions, and research needs are presented. The role of the health psychologist in each phase is discussed.

809

Zahourek RP. **Hypnosis in nursing practice—emphasis on the "problem patient" who has pain (I).** J Psychosoc Nurs Ment Health Serv 20:13-17, 1982.

▶ hypnosis, autohypnosis, relaxation, imagery

Extracted summary: [The author] worked successfully with severely and moderately burned patients and later expanded the program to "difficult" patients whom [she] and the nursing staff felt might benefit from a program of relaxation and/or hypnosis.

810

Zahourek RP. **Hypnosis in nursing practice—emphasis on the "problem patient" who has pain (II).** J Psychosoc Nur Ment Health Serv 20:21-24, 1982.

▶ hypnosis, autohypnosis, suggestion, relaxation

The program of treating burned patients with hypnosis was expanded to treating multi-problem and chronic pain patients on the same surgical unit at Denver General Hospital. The majority of patients received some benefit. Many gained control over intense pain and many increased their sense of self-esteem and mastery. The behavioral problems diminished and the staff became reinterested and reinvolved with these very needy people. Whether or not nurses elect to practice hypnosis, the principles are familiar and can be added to the repertory of nursing practice. Physical and psychological relaxation relieves distress and potentiates patients' comfort with or without pain medication. Communicate to the patient that what you are doing builds confidence and increases the probability that treatment will be effective. Furthermore, recognizing imaginary capacities as powerful in promoting comfort adds an option for intervention not always considered or used by nurses. Whether or not nurses describe what they do as "hypnosis," the use of these techniques can be useful to their practice and to the patients in whom they attempt to alleviate suffering and promote comfort and growth.

811

Zide B, Pardoe R. **The use of behavior modification therapy in a recalcitrant burned child: case report.** Plast Reconstr Surg 57:378-382, 1976.

▶ behavior modification, operant conditioning, reinforcement

Extracted summary: Behavior therapy is concerned with modifying maladaptive, inappropriate behavior (i.e., this patient's symptoms), rather than trying to identify the underlying subconscious process that many psychotherapists believe "causes" symptoms. The unconscious ego structures, or defense mechanisms, are not dealt with. For this patient, we used "operant conditioning therapy"— that is, environmental procedures were used to control the consequences of the patient's voluntary behavior. Ultimately, the patient was able to control the consequences himself. The target set of behaviors to be modified (i.e., eating, physical therapy, dressing changes, and general attitude) was identified. A set of rewards was then devised to "control" this behavior. He became constructive rather than self-destructive, and he learned to cope with the discomforts because of the satisfying outcomes. The situation was manipulated to influence his behavior; in this way, his in-hospital life was made happier and more enjoyable.

Condylomata Acuminata

812

Ewin DM. **Condyloma acuminatum: successful treatment of four cases by hypnosis.** Am J Clin Hypn 17:73-83, 1974.

▶ hypnosis, psychotherapy, suggestion

Venereal warts (condyloma acuminata) are reported to be increasing in frequency along with other venereal "infections." They can be difficult to treat by methods other than suggestion. They are caused by the same virus that causes wart infections in other parts of the body and are just as amenable to suggestion therapy, except that there is more emotional energy invested in these warts than others. 4 cures are reported: 1 by direct suggestion, 1 by hypnoanalysis, 1 by waking suggestion, and 1 cured following a dream that was readily interpreted by the patient.

813

French AP. **Treatment of warts by hypnosis.** Am J Obstet Gynecol 116:887-888, 1973. (letter)

▶ hypnosis

814

Klapper M. **Condylomata acuminata and hypnosis.** J Am Acad Dermatol 10:836-839, 1984. (letter)

▶ hypnosis

815

Rapini RP. **Treatment of venereal warts using hypnosis.** J Am Acad Dermatol 10:837, 1984. (letter)

▶ hypnosis

816

Straatmeyer AJ, Rhodes NR. **Condylomata acuminata: results of treatment using hypnosis.** J Am Acad Dermatol 9:434-436, 1983.

▶ hypnosis

We report a 48-year-old woman with venereal warts; hypnosis was used to treat her condition. After four weekly treatment sessions, her warts were eliminated.

Eczema (Atopic Dermatitis)

817

Abramson HA. **Psychogenic eczema in a child.** Ann Allergy 14:375-381, 1956.

▶ psychotherapy, family therapy

I am reluctant to label this case as psychogenic eczema, because I believe that all illness is psychosomatic, with both mind and body components. I feel, however, that here the allergic components were negligible compared with the psychogenic forces. If we understand that psychogenic factors can no more act alone than can somatogenic forces, for practical purposes this is a case of essentially psychogenic eczema in childhood.

818

Allendy R. **A case of eczema.** Psychoanal Rev 19:152-163, 1932.

▶ psychoanalysis

Extracted summary: [The patient's] case is interesting since it shows the influence of psychic factors on diseases considered to be organic. It was almost by accident that Mrs. C. came to be analyzed; owing to her psychopathic antecedents, and above all to the perspicacity of her doctor. One wonders to what extent those diseases, considered to be purely organic, may have arisen from psychical disorders. Such cases bring forward a problem, which, if we could get to the bottom of it, has doubtless great surprises in store for us. It is possible that material causes, toxins, microbes, etc., usually invoked, may only be secondary causes, and that the primordial determinant may be hidden further away, in the depths of psychic life. Perhaps it is always essential that such disorders should exist, in order to bring into being the etiological mechanisms which we believe to be the source of organic disease. It would be still more strange if the suppression of the psychic trouble led to the disappearance of the disease. Already certain writers have brought forward numerous cases in favor of this theory, particularly Groddeck, since 1917, and Maeder. We should note, in the report we have just made, the appearance of the eczema at the same time, or shortly after the tardy weaning; its disappearance at puberty; its reappearance after pregnancy coinciding with serious psychic disorders. Perhaps we ought still to wait a considerable time before speaking of definite recovery, although the disease had lasted ten years, had resisted various treatments, and there was no longer any sign of it at the end of the analysis. Even if a longer delay were necessary for absolute confirmation, the therapeutical question may be reserved and this report still not be considered worthless from the point of view of the psychic genesis of organic disease.

819

Barinbaum M. **A brief report on two psychotherapeutically influenced cases of eczema.** Zentralbl Psychother 5:106-111, 1932. (in German: no English abstract)

▶ psychotherapy

820

Boddeker KW, Boddeker M. **Behavior therapeutical techniques in the treatment of atopic dermatitis, especially of obsessional scratching.** Z Psychosom Med Psychoanal 22:85-92, 1976. (in German)

▶ positive reinforcement, aversive conditioning, relaxation

Presents a descriptive model of compulsive scratching in patients with atopic dermatitis. The limited repertoire of social skills of these patients does not provide them with a strategy to master negative emotions. The resulting diffuse tension is temporarily reduced by scratching; this reinforces the tendency to perceive itching. The immediate relief of tension that follows scratching is followed, with some delay, by feelings of dissatisfaction or guilt associated with scratching the afflicted skin; this further increases the tension. Suggested treatment techniques include positive reinforcement for not scratching, aversive conditioning, relaxation, and training in social skills.

821
Bosse K, Hunecke P. **The pruritus of endogenous eczema patients.** MMW 123:1013-1016, 1981. (in German)

▶ psychotherapy

The psychosomatic aspects of the pruritus symptom of endogenous eczema patients are presented. The phenomenon of "scratching" is analysed descriptively from observations of the behavior of the patient and his family. Psychotherapeutic approaches as a supplement to the dermatological therapy of endogenous eczema are described.

822
Brown DG, Bettley FR. **Psychiatric treatment of eczema: a controlled trial.** Br Med J 2:729-733, 1971.

▶ psychotherapy

Seventy-two patients with eczema were randomly allotted to one of two treatment groups: A, those receiving dermatological treatment only, and B, those receiving the same dermatological treatment plus psychiatric treatment, limited where possible to four months. Cases were followed up at six-monthly dermatological assessments, 57 (79%) for 18 months. The findings suggest that in the presence of overt emotional disturbance, of new psychological or psychophysiological symptoms preceding the rash by up to a year, and of high motivation for it, brief psychiatric treatment improves the outcome in eczema (the proportion clear at 18 months was about doubled), whereas in their absence such treatment may worsen it, especially in the short term.

823
Bunneman O. **Successful use of hypnosis in psychogenic eczema.** Med Welt 8:87, 1934. (in German)

▶ hypnosis

824
Dobes RW. **Amelioration of psychosomatic dermatosis by reinforced inhibition of scratching.** J Behav Ther Exp Psychiatry 8:185-187, 1977.

▶ behavior therapy

A behavioral approach was implemented in the treatment of a 28-yr-old female with a 15-yr history of a chronic psychosomatic skin disorder. Treatment consisted of a self-modification program in which the S solicited reinforcement from peers for decreased scratching behavior. This resulted in amelioration of the eczema for over 2 yrs.

825
Dubnikow EI. **Hypnosis of eczema of nervous origin.** Vrach Delo 15:634-636, 1932. (in Russian)

▶ hypnosis

826
Dubnikow EI. **On the question of healing an eczema of a neurotic origin through hypnosis.** Ther Ggw 73:403-406, 1932. (in German: no English abstract)

▶ hypnosis

827
Dunbar A, Rosenbaum M, Crede R. **Atopic dermatitis.** Psychosom Med 11:293-299, 1949.

▶ psychotherapy

This case deals with a single white man who has suffered from atopic dermatitis since infancy. His emotional conflicts are centered about his relationship to a rejecting, dominating, and controlling mother with whom he still lives in a childlike relationship. The psychodynamic forces evident in the patient's relationship to his mother are unsatisfied dependency needs and repressed and suppressed hostility. Marked sexual conflicts are another evidence of the patient's psychopathology. The patient has utilized his chronic dermatitis and scratching to discharge tension associated with his psychologic conflicts. His skin has become "erotized" as an "organ of expression" of hostile, masochistic, and exhibitionistic trends in his personality. Repressed genital sexuality has been displaced to the skin with scratching occasionally representing a masturbatory equivalent. During the interview with the patient it was learned that the longest period his skin had been in remission was when he lived with his grandmother who was more giving and permissive than his mother. There has been a decrease in the patient's anxiety with a concomitant decrease in the skin symptomatology during the course of psychotherapy with the therapist assuming a permissive and giving role. Patient has gradually been able to openly verbalize hostility to his mother whereas initially the hostility was suppressed and repressed. As his sexual anxiety has diminished he has been able to release sexual tension through genital activity. There have also been recent evidences of strivings for independence on the part of the patient.

828
Fritz GK. **Psychological aspects of atopic dermatitis: a viewpoint.** Clin Pediatr (Phila) 18:360-364, 1979.

▶ psychotherapy

An overview of existing research on the psychological aspects of atopic dermatitis is presented. Conclusive evaluation of specificity hypotheses, relating to emotional conflicts or personality types, is lacking, yet these theories continue to exert their influence. A reactive-interactive model is elaborated whereby a number of psychological processes exacerbate and maintain the disorder. Management strategies and psychiatric involvement are discussed.

829

Goodman HP. **Hypnosis in prolonged resistant eczema: a case report.** Am J Clin Hypn 5:144-145, 1962-1963.

▶ hypnosis

Extracted summary: At the present time, some eighteen months after the institution of hypnotherapy, [the patient] is free from skin symptoms and she is neither taking nor using medications. She does, however, still make use of the posthypnotic suggestions of fingertip application whenever she feels a need or notices a possible beginning rash. She also insists upon returning for hypnotherapeutic reinforcement sessions three or four times a year.

830

Gray SG, Lawlis GF. **A case study of pruritic eczema treated by relaxation and imagery.** Psychol Rep 51:627-633, 1982.

▶ biofeedback, relaxation, imagery

Treated a 25-yr-old white, married female for chronic pruritic eczema through the use of frontalis EMG, relaxation, and imagery training. The biofeedback readings, ratings of the pruritus, and ratings of skin smoothness were made over 10 sessions. Although the EMG measures did not decrease significantly, the rash disappeared completely. A 1-yr follow-up confirmed disease control.

831

Greenhill MH, Finesinger JE. **Neurotic symptoms and emotional factors in atopic dermatitis.** Arch Dermatol Syph 46:187-200, 1942.

▶ psychotherapy

Thirty-two patients with atopic dermatitis were studied to evaluate the influence of emotional factors on this disease. The patients were investigated by means of questionnaires which embraced the dermatologic, medical and psychiatric history, the presence of neurotic symptoms and the personality characteristics of each patient. Controls included 16 patients with lupus erythematosus, 20 psychoneurotic patients and 20 normal persons. Patients with atopic dermatitis show psychoneurotic symptoms more frequently than do the patients with lupus erythematosus or the normal controls, although they do not approach the psychoneurotic group in frequency or consist-

ency of symptoms. The greater proportion of the patients with atopic dermatitis who presented neurotic symptoms had compulsive-obsessive symptoms, whereas practically none were found to have symptoms of hysteria. The patients with lupus erythematosus also showed compulsive-obsessive tendencies. The patients with atopic dermatitis were found to have hostile tendencies, feelings of inadequacy and depressive trends. Blushing and exhibitionism occurred no more prominently in the group with atopic dermatitis than in the groups with lupus erythematosus and psychoneurosis. There was a definite correlation between events which evoked feelings of anger and depression and exacerbations of the eruption in the patients with atopic dermatitis.

832

Guy WB, Shoemaker RJ. **A psychophysiological concept of atopic eczema.** Arch Dermatol 77:34-41, 1958.

▶ psychotherapy, doctor-patient relationship, group therapy

1. Atopic eczema (disseminated neurodermatitis) is a psychophysiological skin disorder of complex and incompletely understood etiology. Severe exacerbations of the disease are associated with depression, social withdrawal, masochistic attack upon the skin, and a state of relative immobilization. Remissions are associated with increased aggressiveness, increased physical activity, the assertion of more personal independence, and restitution of more adequate personality defenses. Behavioral transitions between these two polarities are indicative of the trend of the disease and the efficacy of treatment. 2. Supportive psychotherapy has provided a valuable adjunct to the standard medical treatment of atopic eczema in our experience. Therapeutic responsiveness has been an influence of psychotherapy with these patients, and improvement or remission of skin symptoms has been associated with improvement in their over-all personality adjustment. 3. Interdisciplinary collaboration has resulted in more adequate therapy than either specialist can provide when working in isolation. 4. Psychotherapy, which gives definition to the force of the traditional doctor-patient relationship, is adaptable to the treatment regimen of physicians interested in the problem of atopic eczema. These problem patients require special attention and adequate emotional support in addition to routine medical managment. Group therapy is especially useful in selected cases and in those situations where the physician is limited in time and confronted by large numbers of patients.

833

Guy WB, Shoemaker RJ, McLaughlin JT. **Group psychotherapy in adult atopic eczema.** Arch Dermatol Syph 70:767-781, 1954.

▶ group therapy, psychotherapy, consultation-liaison

1. The comprehensive treatment of atopic eczema is best served by a therapeutic regime that includes both der-

matological treatment and supportive psychotherapy. 2. Group psychotherapy, modified to meet the special needs of a relatively homogeneous test group of female atopic eczema patients, has proved to be an effective treatment method. 3. The establishment of a satisfactory working relationship between dermatologist and psychiatrist, in a common setting, has combined to give more adequate service than either discipline has provided when working in isolation. 4. Adequate appraisal of the patient is a requisite to selection of the most appropriate form of psychotherapy. Although group psychotherapy may provide optimal emotional support as well as maximum economy, individual psychotherapy remains more acceptable to certain patients. 5. Therapeutic success appears to bear heavily upon the physician's ability to cope with the excessive demands and the well-known unresponsiveness of these patients. An iatrogenic factor stems from unconscious hostility and some form of rejection of the patient by the physician. 6. Remissions of atopic eczema occur when frictional dependency ties are severed, compensatory emotional support is gained, and infantile wishes find greater satisfaction in aggressive outlets.

834
Haynes SN, Wilson CC, Jaffe PG, Britton BT. **Biofeedback treatment of atopic dermatitis: controlled case studies of eight cases.** Biofeedback Self Regul 4:195-209, 1979.

▶ biofeedback, relaxation

Eight atopic dermatitis patients were exposed to a no-treatment baseline phase, a phase incorporating nonspecific treatment factors, and a phase involving frontal EMG feedback and relaxation instructions. Significant remission of dermatological problems was found across the entire program. Ratings of itching level decreased within but not across treatment sessions, and variable correlations across Ss were found between frontal EMG and itching level. Results suggest that the disorder may be amenable to behaviorally oriented treatment.

835
Heigl-Evers A. **Some psychogenetic and psychodynamic connections in the clinical picture of endogenous eczema.** Z Psychosom Med Psychoanal 12:163-178, 1966. (in German: no English abstract)

▶ psychoanalysis

836
Homburger A. **Lichenoid eczema as a psychogenic dermatosis.** Z Neurol Psychiatr 82:105-116, 1923. (in German: no English abstract)

▶ psychoanalysis

837
Ironside W. **Eczema, darkly mirror of the mind.** Australas J Dermatol 15:5-9, 1974.

▶ psychotherapy

In conclusion, I wish to outline a principle of the psychosomatic approach. It is best stated as a series of conditions as follows: If (1) Multiple aetiological factors including genetic and constitutional predisposition are operative, and if (2) the organ system is directly influenced by emotional factors mediated by the C.N.S. and participates in emotional expression, and if (3) intrapsychic processes such as self-concept, identity, and eroticism involve the organ system, and if (4) the organ system is likely to be the object of conversion and conditioning because of emotional arousal consequent on intrapsychic problems, and if (5) social values and standards are linked with the organ system, then that system is vulnerable to psychosomatic ailments. The skin is uniquely positioned to be an organ system that can become part of a psychosomatic process. It would appear, on the basis of our present knowledge, that eczema can, in some instances, be predominantly psychosomatic. Though, as a mirror of the mind eczema is darkly, I believe that continued psychophysiological studies of it will lead to a deeper understanding of its complex of causes and to a heightened effectiveness in its therapy. As a mirror of the mind it will then reflect more clearly.

838
Israel L, Couadau A. **Considerations on psychosomatic object relations, a propos of a case of eczema.** Rev Med Psychosom 8:377-393, 1966. (in French)

▶ psychotherapy

There may be a specific psychosomatic structure existing alongside other neurotic, psychotic structures whose nature may be elucidated through the study of relationships to objects. A detailed analysis of the information which emerged through the psychotherapy of a case of eczema illustrates the thesis.

839
Kartamischew AJ. **Hypnotherapy for eczema.** Dermatol Wochenschr 102:711-714, 1936. (in German: no English abstract)

▶ hypnosis

840
Kaszuk C. **Jeannette and Christiane.** Rev Med Psychosom 13:411-422, 1971. (in French: no English abstract)

▶ psychotherapy

841

Kelman H, Field H. **Psychosomatic relationships in pruriginous lesions.** J Nerv Ment Dis 88:627-643, 1938.

▶ psychotherapy

The life history of a patient is given from psychiatric viewpoint as well as the details of the development of his skin lesion (generalized eczema, type prurigo Besnier). The results of fifty interviews are summarized in an attempt to show the method of approach to a patient who is neither willing nor sees the need for treatment and who is unable to cope with the problem of marriage as it implies parenthood, responsibility and masculinity because of a strongly developed feeling of inadequacy and a low self-estimate. The psychodynamics of the case are discussed using the symptom of pruritus as a means of understanding psychosomatic relationships. The literature on the psychogenic aspects of skin disease is mentioned as it relates to this case. It is emphasized that a skin disease or in fact any disease cannot be considered apart from the patient who suffers with it.

842

Kepecs JG, Rabin A, Robin M. **Atopic dermatitis: a clinical psychiatric study.** Psychosom Med 13:1-9, 1951.

▶ psychotherapy, hypnosis

1. Twenty cases of atopic dermatitis fell into two main groups, an emotionally labile, tending to hysteria, and a rigid, tending to compulsiveness. Clinically, 14 cases were predominantly labile, 5 were predominantly rigid, 1 was unclassified. The Rorschach examiner independently arrived at the same grouping as the psychiatrist. The patients in the more labile group were afflicted with dermatitis for a much greater portion of their lives than were members of rigid group. 2. The characteristic family constellation included a strongly hostile-dependent relationship to the mother. 3. The characteristic major conflict was in the sphere of heterosexual relations. Strong strivings for sexual relationships were frustrated to various degrees. In the small, more rigid group, sexual problems were less on the surface, major tensions being related to work and responsibility, with conflicting feelings about work situations leading to skin outbreaks. These more rigid patients appeared to have made better sexual adjustments than those in the large hysterical group, in whom exacerbations of the skin disease occurred most characteristically in situations of real or potential heterosexual contacts. 4. Suppressed weeping was a prominent symptom. Weeping expressed a desire to overcome separation from a loved object, basically the mother. 5. Itching and scratching were manifestations of anger at mother figures or heterosexual objects. Because of guilt and fear this anger was handled masochistically, expressing itself in self-destructive scratching, which may be secondarily erotized.

Hostile attitudes were usually conscious, and much anger was expressed in interviews, dreams, and the Rorschach test. Objectively the patients were often timid and shy. They tended to handle their feelings by suppression, beneath which, in the more labile group, was a marked emotional hyperreactivity close to the surface.

843

Klinge JE. **Atopic dermatitis.** J Am Inst Hypn 12:128-131, 1971.

▶ relaxation, psychotherapy, hypnosis

Discusses treatment of atopic dermatitis, variously called infantile eczema, neurodermatitis, or atopic eczema, as if S (a) had underlying dry skin, (b) had a slight allergy to everything which touches him, and (c) needed help. An attempt is made to determine the reason for the problem, then giving the S relaxation, and treating problem areas with analgesic. Tension states between mother and child are reduced by hypnosis and hypnotherapy. 3 brief case histories of children are presented. It is strongly suggested that the mother undergo hypnosis since she worries about the child's condition and often thinks it is worse than it is. With relaxation, the mother loves the child more normally and feels better toward the child; in turn, the child will become increasingly improved by himself. It is felt that food allergy tests do very little in determining the cause of atopic dermatitis and may result in depriving the person of needed nutrition.

844

Koldys KW, Meyer RP. **Biofeedback training in the therapy of dyshidrosis.** Cutis 24:219-221, 1979.

▶ biofeedback

Biofeedback training for hand warming and relaxation was used with five patients with severe dyshidrotic eczema who were poorly responsive to conventional therapy. Improvement was seen in all five patients, especially those who most noted flaring of their disease under stress. Biofeedback is being used in the treatment of diverse stress-related disorders, and may have potential in dermatologic diseases.

845

Kuijpers BR. **Constitutional eczema: clinico-psychological findings.** Ned Tijdschr Geneeskd 112:976-981, 1968. (in Dutch)

▶ psychotherapy

Seventy patients with constitutional eczema, between the ages of 17 and 35 years, were examined by psychological tests; no specific emotional conflict situation was found, nor any particular type of personality. However, distinct neurotic disorders could be observed in the persons examined.

846
Kuypers BRM. **Atopic dermatitis: some observations from a psychological viewpoint.** Dermatologica 136:387-394, 1968.

▶ psychotherapy

The therapist should aim to release in the patient the emotions from their confinement. The patient learns to recognize his own emotions and not to reject them or timidly control them, and to master a more supple and less diffident adjustment. Sometimes a clinical treatment of both somatic and psychotherapeutic type is most indicated. Above all, when the current life situation is a too heavy load a clinical admission gives the patient the opportunity to solve quietly his problems and to begin again with a clean skin. We have achieved hopeful results in this way with the above-mentioned age group of 13-40; already during the admission of the patient an intensive psychotherapeutic treatment should be begun, to be followed up in the polyclinic. We are convinced that there is little sense in trying to view constitutional eczema as something merely somatically or psychically conditioned. It is our experience that mind and emotions play a definite role on the course of atopic dermatitis; the evidence does not necessarily imply that emotion causes the disease, but it becomes readily apparent that the state of mind may have a definite and remarkable effect on the course of the disease.

847
Manuso JS. **The use of biofeedback-assisted hand warming training in the treatment of chronic eczematous dermatitis of the hands: a case study.** J Behav Ther Exp Psychiatry 8:445-446, 1977.

▶ biofeedback, relaxation

A 60-yr-old female with a 6-yr history of chronic eczematous dermatitis of the hands was successfully treated by a relaxation technique and by digital temperature biofeedback training to increase hand temperature, the latter lasting 13 wks. A 6-mo follow-up indicated that the treatment effects were maintained.

848
Mariz J. **Psychogenic eczema (in relation to two cases treated by psychotherapy).** Med Cir Farm (Rio de Janeiro) 141:28, 1948. (in Portuguese: no English abstract)

▶ psychotherapy

849
McLaughlin J, Shoemaker R. **Personality factors in adult atopic eczema.** Arch Dermatol 68:506-516, 1953.

▶ review: supportive psychotherapy, doctor-patient relationship

Extracted summary: 1. The syndrome of atopic eczema represents a psychophysiologic skin disorder occurring in conjunction with primitive polymorphous personality patterns, in which there are evident a minimum of classic psychoneurotic characteristics. 2. The general pattern of personality defect seen in these patients is similar to that described for a variety of psychosomatic disorders, namely, excessive passivity and clinging dependency, coupled with a crippling inhibition of aggressive and erotic drives. 3. The more specific pattern of the eczema-pruritus-scratch complex seems importantly related to the dynamics of depression, even when given specific elaboration in the service of conflictual erotic and aggressive strivings. 4. A close temporal relationship can be demonstrated repeatedly between stressful life situations and the occurrence or exacerbation of atopic eczema in the patients of this series. Characteristically, these life situations are not catastrophic, but, instead, reflect the normal complications of maturation. The common factor to the various situations is that each represents an actual or threatened disruption of the emotional ties between patient and the object of his excessive dependency. 5. In the life patterns of the patients of this series there could be demonstrated a chronic and persisting unhealthy child-parent relationship, characterized by a relative or actual rejection of the patient by the parents, chiefly the mother.

850
Miller RM, Coger RW. **Skin conductance conditioning with dyshidrotic eczema patients.** Br J Dermatol 101:435-440, 1979.

▶ biofeedback

Thirty-three patients with dyshidrotic eczema were trained either to decrease or to increase the electrical conductivity of the skin. Skin conductance has been found to be related to epidermal water content as well as emotional variables, both of which have suggested links to eczema. Subjects trained to decrease skin conductance showed clinical improvement more often than the controls who were trained in the opposite direction. They also showed a significant decrease in measured conductance and anxiety. The controls showed increased anxiety and no significant changes in skin conductance level.

851
Miller RM, Coger RW, Dymond AM. **Biofeedback skin conditioning in dyshidrotic eczema.** Arch Dermatol 109:737-738, 1974. (letter)

▶ biofeedback

852

Mirvish I. **Hypnotherapy for the child with chronic eczema: a case report.** S Afr Med J 54:410-412, 1978.

▶ hypnosis, counseling

Chronic eczema in a child usually produces much discomfort and distress. Associated behaviour problems further complicate the issue. A comprehensive approach to treatment is therefore essential. Hypnotherapy may be a useful adjunct in the overall management. An illustrative case history is presented. Combining hypnotherapy with child guidance and medical treatment led to the relief of symptoms and improved behavioural pattern in a boy aged 10 years.

853

Motoda K. **A case report of the counter conditioning treatment of an eczema patient by hypnosis.** Jpn J Hypn 15:46-49, 1971.

▶ hypnosis, conditioning

A 26-year-old female patient with eczema chronicum had been treated by a dermatologist for two and one-half years. Because of continuous scratching of the diseased area none of the medication prescribed by the dermatologist had been effective. The patient was given counter conditioning treatment by the author using hypnosis to provide an hallucination of pain when the diseased area was scratched. After the counter conditioning treatment the patient stopped scratching the diseased area allowing the prescribed medicine to take effect and the eczema was cured. The eczema has not reappeared in the eight months following the completion of the counter conditioning treatment.

854

Pines D. **Skin communication: early skin disorders and their effect on transference and countertransference.** Int J Psychoanal 61:315-323, 1980.

▶ psychoanalysis

Eczema in the first year of life results in a basic disturbance of the earliest mother-infant relationship, a disturbance that is renewed with every transitional phase of the life-cycle. The pervasive fear of disintegration or loss of the self, and the need to be contained and held, affects subsequent character formation. Infants who experience extended periods of bodily soothing learn to translate psychic pain into visible bodily suffering and so arouse concern and care. This is illustrated by direct observation of women patients suffering from skin diseases and their interaction with women doctors in hospital. In the analysis of patients who have had such an infantile experience, whether they know it or not, a disturbance in concepts of

the self linked with narcissistic difficulties and acute sensitivity to object relationships may be anticipated. The mother's human disappointment in her baby's appearance gives rise to an unsatisfying and unsatisfactory self image which remains unaltered in the true self. Transference and countertransference problems derived from the analysis of a female patient are described in order to illustrate these themes.

855

Podoswa-Martinez G, Beltran G. **A new therapeutic approach to eczema in pediatrics.** Bol Med Hosp Infant Mex 33:213-226, 1976. (in Spanish)

▶ psychotherapy

Considering the disease as a psychophysiologic reaction of the skin, a psychologic therapeutic approach was used in 15 children with epidemiologic problems of atopic eczema.

856

Rosenthal MJ. **A psychosomatic study of infantile eczema (I): The mother-child relationship.** Pediatrics 10:581-591, 1952.

▶ counseling, doctor-patient relationship

Extracted summary: The lack of cuddling and caressing in most of the cases studied was felt to be an important factor in causing the eczema. However, other factors such as constitutional predisposition and allergy were possibly equally important. Certain therapeutic suggestions were made on the basis of the hypothesis.

857

Rostenberg A Jr. **Psychosomatic concepts in atopic dermatitis—a critique.** Arch Dermatol 79:692-699, 1959.

▶ review

What then can one say about the role of emotions in atopic dermatitis? I do not believe that any specific formulations can be made. I believe, and I have stated elsewhere, the emotional factors are only one facet of a dynamic interplay of factors conducing to pruritus in a genetically determined soil. The same inheritance that determines the dry quasi-ichthyotic skin with its vulnerability to pruriginous stimuli also determines that most people with such skins are atopic persons and may also favor a psychogenic maturation that in turn may lead to a commonness of emotional reactions to certain conflictual stimuli. To lift any one of these inherited determinants out of the total constellation of the syndrome atopic dermatitis and to give it undue importance or to assign it pride of place so that it seems to dominate or to exercise a causal influence is to indulge in special pleading and deserves Mencken's derisive comment. "There is a solution for every human problem—neat, plausible, and wrong."

858

Shoemaker RJ. **The meaning of psychotherapy in the management of atopic eczema.** Allerg Asthma (Leipz) 2:241-247, 1956. (in German: no English abstract)

▶ psychotherapy, group therapy

859

Vaugh VC. **Emotional undertones in eczema in children.** J Asthma Res 3:193-197, 1966.

▶ supportive psychotherapy, doctor-patient relationship

Some of the ways in which emotional problems may complicate eczema are discussed. Attention is called to the need for preventing the skin condition from becoming the focal point of conflict between parent and child. Aids to this will be the setting of reasonable goals consistent with the knowledge that eczema is often self-limited in the infant but in the older child sometimes a very chronic condition in which responsibility for skin care and other aspects of the therapeutic regimen will need to be increasingly transferred from parent to child.

860

Waisman M. **Atopic dermatitis: clinical aspects and treatment.** Postgrad Med 52:180-184, 1972.

▶ supportive psychotherapy, doctor-patient relationship

Extracted summary: Office psychotherapy is an indispensable part of treatment. Brief, friendly, casual discussion at each visit often uncovers smoldering emotional problems relating to home, school, job, or love life. The physician's interest, sympathy, support, encouragement and advice can be consequential for initiating clinical improvement. The aim is for the patient to identify and change the direction of his inwardly channeled aggression. An understanding physician helps to strengthen the patient's tolerance of his emotional troubles, enabling him to live more comfortably with his skin.

861

Williams DH. **Management of atopic dermatitis in children: control of the maternal rejection factor.** Arch Dermatol Syph 63:545-560, 1951.

▶ counseling

During recent years the concept of "humanism" in medicine has become increasingly associated with the scientific viewpoint. A growing study of the tangible somatic expressions of emotional interpersonal relationships is a part of this increasing association. There has been an in-

creasing reexamination of unexplained or partially understood dermatoses in which emotional factors have been evident. Atopic dermatitis belongs to this group of dermatoses. The mother is the closest and most prominent personality in the environment of the infant and growing child. Maternal rejection has been shown to be a usual observation in children with clinical forms of atopy. Repressed hostility to the mother or a mother figure is present in most adults with atopic dermatitis. In this study of a group of children with atopic dermatitis the common observation of maternal rejection was confirmed. It is suggested that this rejection by the mother elicits in the child anxiety and hostility, which have two components of expression—one, the somatic component, exhibiting itself as the characteristic pruritus of atopic dermatitis, and the other, the psychic component, exhibiting itself as wilful (aggressive) behavior. A program of therapy, directed mainly toward the correction of the mother's behavior to the child, is outlined. It consists of instructing the mother concerning (a) the basic emotional needs of a child, (b) the effect on the child of these needs' not being provided and (c) the means of providing them. A comparison is made between a group of children treated by indirection in this manner and a control group of children not treated thus. The results of this study suggest that the management of the maternal rejection factor in children with atopic dermatitis is an important adjuvant to existing therapeutic procedures.

862

Wittkower E, Edgell PG. **Eczema: a psychosomatic study.** Arch Dermatol Syph 63:207-219, 1961.

▶ psychotherapy

The psychosomatic histories of 90 patients with disorders of the "eczema family" were compared with those of 50 controls. Specific situations were seen to precipitate the onset or relapse of eczema: threats to life and existence, threats of loss of an outside source of support or disturbance to inner established patterns, such as blows to self esteem or conflicts over sex and aggressiveness. A hereditary predisposition to the development of eczema and respiratory disorders existed in the group studied, particularly well marked among those who had childhood eczema. Persons with childhood eczemas showed a high incidence of "difficult" family positions. Eczema patients as a whole tended to have either "unwanted" or "spoiled" children and to have been more strongly attached to one parent than to the other. A correlation was demonstrated between the childhood environment and the transparency of the adult personality. The "spoiled" children tended to be of the "undisguised" eczema type. The "unwanted" children were more likely to adopt "disguises." The basic character was that of the insecure clinging child always in need of reassurance and affection. The "disguises" adopted included "limelight seeking," "self driving" and, most commonly, "resentment." The patient's behavior under examination and in social, occupational, sexual and marital spheres is considered in detail. The emotional consequences of a disfiguring rash are discussed. Attention is drawn to the unintentional psychological value of routine dermatological treatments. Brief psychotherapy was found to be practicable on an outpatient basis and was felt to have benefited 2/3 of a small group of patients. The universality of the eczema conflicts and personality types is noted and some speculation attempted to account for the nature of this illness.

863
Wittkower ED, Hunt BR. **Psychological aspects of atopic dermatitis in children.** Can Med Assoc J 79:810-816, 1958.

▶ review: psychotherapy

Extracted summary: Patients suffering from atopic dermatitis have no doubt, as far as their local lesion is concerned, been successfully treated by dermatologists or allergists in innumerable instances. Yet removal of the skin lesion, however effective, does not do away with the emotional factors which propagate it. Hence, one might venture to state that the rate of recovery could be improved if due regard were given in the treatment of the patient to the emotional factors involved. In this way the scope of the treatment by dermatologists and allergists could be profitably enlarged. Yet there remains a group of patients in whom, on account of the severity of their emotional disorder, intervention by a psychiatrist becomes an obvious necessity. We feel that any patient proving resistant to the efforts of a psychosomatically oriented allergist or dermatologist over a period of time should be further evaluated by a psychiatrist. It is preferable to commence psychiatric treatment before family relationships have deteriorated and before more than two to three years have passed.

Neurodermatitis

864

Ackerman NW. **Personality factors in neurodermatitis—a case study.** Psychosom Med 1:366-375, 1939.

▶ psychotherapy

Extracted summary: The patient showed slight betterment of her skin condition with medical treatment. Later, with intensive psychotherapy she showed simultaneous improvement of considerable degree in both her behavior and her skin.

865

Butov IuS. **Dynamics of immunological indices in patients with neurodermatitis during electronarcosis, hypnosis and corticosteroid therapy.** Vestn Dermatol Venerol 42:48-52, 1968. (in Russian: no English abstract)

▶ hypnosis

866

Dunkel ML. **Casework help for neurodermatitis patients.** J Soc Casework 30:97-103, 1949.

▶ social casework, consultation-liaison

Although the etiology of neurodermatitis is obscure and the role of emotional factors controversial, certain typical personality problems occur with some consistency in a group of forty-five patients with rather severe attacks of neurodermatitis. These gross examples illuminate the meaning of subtler manifestations in less ill patients. Conflict over dependency and a painful suppression of resentment are outstanding characteristics which the caseworker is particularly fitted to affect favorably as his part in collaborating with the dermatologist in understanding and treating the total patient.

867

Hobler WR. **Management of emotional factors in localized neurodermatitis.** Arch Dermatol Syph 59:293-300, 1949.

▶ supportive psychotherapy, consultation-liaison

Localized neurodermatitis is an external expression of emotional tension. As the eruption becomes established, a tenacious habit pattern of itching, scratching and more itching develops, in addition to the emotional tension. Most patients with localized neurodermatitis have a superficial type of emotional problem causing their pruritus. This can usually be elicited in a few minutes by simple questioning if the physician appears completely unhurried. Examples of some of the commoner types of cases are given. Treatment must be directed toward the breaking of the habit pattern of itching and scratching by local means and the patient guided to better emotional adjustment in order to reduce the number of recurrences. Elimination from the diet of coffee and other stimulants is important. Patients with deep emotional problems should be referred to a psychiatrist immediately, so that maximum benefit can be obtained through combined psychiatric and dermatologic care.

868

Horan JS. **Management of neurodermatitis by hypnotic suggestion: report of two cases.** Br J Med Hypn 2:43-46, 1951.

▶ hypnosis, psychotherapy

The literature on neurodermatitis is discussed briefly with reference to psychotherapeutic treatment. Two cases are reported, in which lesions subsided under hypnotic suggestion.

869

Joseph ED, Peck SM, Kaufman MR. **A psychological study of neurodermatitis with a case report.** J Mt Sinai Hosp 15:360-366, 1949.

▶ psychotherapy, hypnosis, suggestion

A woman with neurodermatitis of two and one-half years' duration is presented. Guilt over her child's illness apparently precipitated the skin disorder. Other psychologic factors in the illness are presented and discussed. During the course of psychotherapy she developed an acute psychotic episode. The implications of this for the therapy of psychosomatic disease are discussed.

870

Kline MV. **Delimited hypnotherapy: the acceptance of resistance in the treatment of a long standing neurodermatitis with a sensory-imagery technique.** Int J Clin Exp Hypn 1:18-22, 1953.

▶ hypnosis, psychotherapy, imagery

A case of experimental hypnotherapy of a chronic neurodermatitis has been presented within which the resistance of the patient was accepted as reasonable. Therapy was structured by the patient's limitations and the results, at least in this one case, justified the procedure. It is suggested that a more global perception of resistance be recognized apart from its unconscious meaning and that cognitive aspects of resistance be evaluated and utilized in treatment planning. The problem of an artifact neurotic reaction in resistance oriented therapy is discussed.

871

Lehman RE. **Brief hypnotherapy of neurodermatitis: a case with four-year followup.** Am J Clin Hypn 21:48-51, 1978.

▶ psychotherapy, hypnosis

A 20-yr-old single woman was treated for persistent and severe neurodermatitis. M. H. Erickson's (1954) pseudo-orientation in time technique was used to consolidate and extend partial therapeutic gains resulting in complete system remission, which was maintained at a 4-yr follow-up. While reoriented, the client also successfully predicted the time at which the dermatitis would disappear.

872

Milberg IL. **Group psychotherapy in the treatment of some neurodermatoses.** Int J Group Psychother 6:53-59, 1956.

▶ group psychotherapy

With the small number of patients, and a short period of treatment, it is far too early and too hazardous to evaluate the meaning of the results obtained. However, I feel that the method described yielded sufficient positive results to warrant further studies so as to gain better understanding of both the etiological and therapeutic mechanisms in these conditions. At this time several therapeutic factors are worth noting. Of prime importance is that this therapy was carried out in a group setting where a common therapeutic goal was achieved. This achievement, I feel, was enhanced by the fact that the patients were above average intelligence, perception and sensitivity, and all had a drive to get well. Furthermore, the transference reaction toward the therapist, which was not at all times on a positive level, was not divided among several physicians.

873

Miller ML. **Psychodynamic mechanisms in a case of neurodermatitis.** Psychosom Med 10:309-316, 1948.

▶ psychoanalysis

The detailed psychoanalytic study of this case of neurodermatitis corroborates many of the findings in the literature. The specific way in which the repressed aggression toward father figures was handled was by [the patient's] attacking himself through the skin and exhibiting an unconscious passive feminine attitude. The regressive fantasies connected with the feminine attitude were an expression of early infantile sadistic attitudes toward female figures and identification with them, as an attempt to deal with the problem of aggression toward male members of the family.

874

Nickel WR. **Neurodermatitis—a concept.** Cutis 21:677-680, 1978.

▶ supportive psychotherapy

The skin is an obvious "shock organ" for emotional stresses, as well as the other organ systems. Lividity, blushing, blanching, "goose flesh" are common observations. Personal emotional stress is carried in the mind of the patient, but often, after a period of time, this stress becomes manifest as skin disease. This delay interval is usually two to four weeks, if the histories are accurate. The patient can often be benefited by accepting the relationship of emotional stress and skin disease, along with appropriate treatment.

875

Obermayer ME. **Psychotherapy of functional dermatoses: its value and limitations as applied to neurodermatitis.** Calif Med 1:28-30, 1949.

▶ psychotherapy

Etiologically, neurodermatitis is interpreted as an often manifestly hereditary diathesis which is frequently complicated and exacerbated by disturbances of the patient's emotional and psychic structure. The following traits are commonly exhibited, singly or in combination: a tendency toward excitability and an exaggerated capacity for response to stimuli, polyvalent dermal hypersensitivity, a propensity to vascular disturbances, a personality somewhat obsessional in structure and evidence of deep-seated emotional conflict. Shallow psychotherapy, an indispensable adjunct to the treatment of neurodermatitis, can be successfully applied by any dermatologic physician adequately endowed with patience, sympathy and tact. This method does not achieve a cure, but, properly applied, it can immeasurably improve the patient's lot.

876

Purchard PR. **Neurodermatitis with a case study.** Psychiatr Q 38:518-527, 1964.

▶ review: psychotherapy, consultation-liaison

A review of the literature and a case study of neurodermatitis was presented. Neither revealed a clearly discernible dynamic formulation specifically responsible for neurodermatitis. Rather, four major characteristics were seen in varying quantities: 1. The skin most definitely can become highly eroticized and can be used as a site of expression of emotional conflict. 2. Such conflicts usually involve a dependent hostile relationship with a dominant controlling and rejecting parent, often the mother or mother surrogate. 3. Guilt, masochism, and displaced sexual conflicts, especially masturbatory, are frequently emphasized in these patients. 4. Exhibitionism seems to be served in almost every case, even if only symbolically. The case presented was of a 26-year-old male with a 75 per cent neurodermatitis. He first had an allergic rash in infancy, eczema in his early childhood, asthma at seven and neurodermatitis at 21. Asthma attacks and rash exacerbations correlated amazingly with environmental stresses to the extent of having rash flare-ups with a skin-conscious mother and asthma attacks with an asthma-conscious mother surrogate. Combined dermatologic and psychiatric treatment brought successful results. Psychiatric consultation is recommended in cases of generalized neurodermatitis.

877

Ratliff RG, Stein NH. **Treatment of neurodermatitis by behavior therapy: a case study.** Behav Res Ther 6:397-399, 1968.

▶ aversive conditioning, reciprocal inhibition, relaxation

Extracted summary: The results suggest that the application of progressive relaxation, as employed in the present context, provides an effective means for eliminating compulsive scratching in a case of neurodermatitis. Thus, the progressive reduction in the occurrence of a behavioral component which affected the physical aspects of the disorder permitted the prescribed medication to gradually promote improvement in the patient's skin condition.

878

Robertson G. **Emotional aspects of skin disease.** Lancet 2:124-127, 1947.

▶ psychotherapy

Patients with intractable dermatitis may sometimes be found to labour under a deep sense of grievance. Inquiry into the emotional difficulties associated with the onset of the dermatitis may cause an acute exacerbation. On the other hand, when these difficulties are resolved or even when the patient is given insight into them, the dermatitis may rapidly clear. Often industrial dermatitis cannot be satisfactorily explained by the action of the irritant substances to which the skin is exposed. The underlying cause may be an emotional disturbance.

879

Rosenbaum MS, Ayllon T. **The behavioral treatment of neurodermatitis through habit-reversal.** Behav Res Ther 19:313-318, 1981.

▶ behavior therapy, habit-reversal

Azrin and Nunn's habit-reversal technique was used to treat four clients with neurodermatitis. Following a single treatment session, scratching associated with this skin condition was markedly reduced for three clients, whereas this reduction occurred for the fourth client 4 days following treatment. Results at 6-month follow-ups showed that scratching was eliminated for the client with the mildest case, whereas this behavior remained at low levels for the other three clients.

880

Sacerdote P. **Hypnotherapy in neurodermatitis: a case report.** Am J Clin Hypn 7:249-253, 1965.

▶ hypnosis

A young woman with neurodermatitis of the face and back of seven years' duration was successfully treated with three sessions of hypnotherapy after other measures had failed. The techniques are described; the improbability of any psychiatric or somatic complications with competent use of hypnosis is discussed; and the values of hypnosis in medical practice are stressed.

881

Scarborough LF. **Neurodermatitis from a psychosomatic viewpoint.** Dis Nerv Syst 9:90-93, 1948.

▶ psychotherapy

Reports on psychosomatic medicine stress the fact that other psychoneurotic symptoms are present in these cases which is also the fact in the three cases reported. Hostile tendencies were the most marked feature present in all of these cases and there seems to be a definite correlation between events which evoked the feelings of anger and the exacerbation of the eruption on the patient. There were also symptoms of depression and in at least one case evidence of obsessive and compulsive symptoms. The exacerbation of the depressive feelings usually followed the anger and the eruption. In these patients there was a prominence of sexual maladjustment, strong feelings of hatred, fear and guilt, conflict over masturbation and in all instances some secondary gain brought about by the illness.

882
Schechter MD. **Psychoanalysis of a latency boy with neurodermatitis.** Psychoanal Study Child 27:529-564, 1972.

▶ review: psychoanalysis

Recounts in detail the successful treatment of an 8-yr-old boy with severe itching and scratching symptoms which had long resisted medical measures. Diagnostically, the dermatitis was viewed as a reaction to castration anxieties and a failure to settle his Oedipal conflict. He seemed to have reached the phallic-Oedipal phase of ego development before the onset of acute symptoms, making it a case of infantile neurosis rather than a "psychosomatic" disorder. During treatment, cooperation with psychoanalytic procedures came from all concerned in the case. Both the dermatologist and the parents willingly accepted direction from the analyst. Prior treatment failures facilitated transference, and identification enabled the child to exercise his own capacity for self-analysis. Analytic help continued to be available after cessation of the disease and termination of treatment, but was needed on only 3 occasions. Reasons for the short- and long-term effectiveness of this analysis are discussed. There is a brief review of relevant psychoanalytic literature on dermatitis.

883
Schoenberg B, Carr AC. **An investigation of criteria for brief psychotherapy of neurodermatitis.** Psychosom Med 25:253-263, 1963.

▶ psychotherapy

Neurodermatitis patients were treated in brief psychotherapy, following a specific method of treatment designed to encourage and reinforce the expression of hostility toward contemporary life conflicts. Significant differences were found between those who were successfully treated and those who were not. Of those investigated factors related to outcome, two (intensity of overt hostility as inferred from initial interviews and hostile-content responses on the Rorschach test) showed significant differences, although not in the direction predicted. Such factors are inferred motivation for treatment, likelihood of dangerous acting out, verbal resources, and the likelihood of a psychotic decompensation did not appear to be related to outcome. There was no evidence of significant symptom substitution or of dangerous acting out in the course of treatment. Results support the hypotheses that patients with neurodermatitis can be treated in brief psychotherapy with successful remission of their symptom and that patients who do not improve or who discontinue the pre-

scribed form of treatment differ significantly from those who complete it successfully.

884
Sivak VP. **Psychotherapy and balneotherapy in the treatment of children with neurodermatitis in a specialized health resort pioneer camp.** Vopr Kurortol Fizioter Lech Fiz Kult 2:63-64, 1984. (in Russian: no English abstract)

▶ milieu therapy, psychotherapy

885
Skripkin IuK. **The effect of combined treatment with electric sleep and hypnosis on the results of electroencephalography in patients with neurodermatitis.** Vestn Dermatol Venerol 39:3-10, 1965. (in Russian)

▶ hypnosis

Studies of electroencephalography influenced by combined treatment with electric sleep and hypnosis were carried out in 60 patients with neurodermatitis. Before treatment signs of the inhibition process prevailed in 21 patients, and the prevalence, sometimes significant, of the irritation process was observed in 25 patients, whereas wakening of both processes was observed in 11 patients. In three patients with restricted neurodermatitis the EEG values were normal. Under the effect of the above-mentioned therapy a considerable portion of patients showed, in addition to the favourable therapeutic effect, a significant improvement or normalization of the EEG. These positive changes in the EEG occurred later than the improvement in the dermatic process. Some patients (23 persons) had some signs of distortion and the electroencephalographic curve which required repeated courses of hypnotherapy and electric sleep in combination with low, gradually decreasing doses of corticosteroid hormones.

886
Thoma H. **The lack of specificity in psychosomatic disorders exemplified by a case of neurodermatitis with a twenty year follow up.** Psyche (Stuttg) 34:589-624, 1980. (in German)

▶ psychoanalysis

The author proposes a nonspecific psychosomatogenesis in opposition to Franz Alexander's specificity hypothesis. As illustration he presents the history of a man whose neurodermatitis was at first treated unsuccessfully with conventional means. Following a psychoanalytic intervention he has remained asymptomatic for twenty years.

887

Walsh MN, Kierland RR. **Correlation of the dermatologic and psychiatric approaches to the treatment of neurodermatitis.** Med Clin N Am 34:1009-1017, 1950.

▶ psychotherapy

The correlation of psychiatric and dermatologic management of patients with neurodermatitis has been discussed. Emphasis has been placed on our concept of neurodermatitis and on the role of the dermatologist himself in the evaluation and treatment of the minor psychiatric aspects of the disorder. For the most part the dermatologist should be capable of caring for both the dermatologic and psychiatric aspects of this condition, but he should recognize the value of psychiatric help in the management of those patients who require major psychotherapy. The general principles of management of patients with neurodermatitis have been reviewed.

888

Walsh MN, Kierland RR. **Psychotherapy in the treatment of neurodermatitis.** Proc Staff Meet Mayo Clin 22:578-584, 1947.

▶ psychotherapy

Fifteen patients with generalized neurodermatitis which had failed to respond satisfactorily to dermatologic therapy were treated with the addition of psychotherapy. Psychopathology which appeared to have causative meaning in relation to the dermatologic reaction was demonstrable in all . . .

889

Watson DL, Tharp RG, Krisberg J. **Case study in self-modification suppression of inflammatory scratching while awake and asleep.** J Behav Ther Exp Psychiatry 3:213-215, 1972.

▶ behavior modification

Self-directed modification programs are of increasing interest, and can be of use even in rather serious conditions. The subject of the case reported here maximized the self-direction, since she designed, maintained and terminated her own treatment, using only brief non-professional consultation. The young woman suffered from a neurodermatitis of 17 yr duration. Scratching her limbs while awake and asleep inflamed and infected her skin. A 20-day contingency program reduced scratching to zero, and eliminated itching. Eighteen-month follow-up revealed two brief recurrences, quickly suppressed by re-institution of the self-modification program. She is currently asymptomatic.

890

Woolhandler HW. **Neurodermatoses: their concept and management.** Penn Med J 51:1108-1113, 1948.

▶ supportive psychotherapy

Extracted summary: The minor problems referred to are rarely of such magnitude as to require the services of a trained psychiatrist. Their simplicity may actually cause them to be overlooked, unless the examiner constantly bears in mind that this type of patient exaggerates all stimuli, and what may appear to be of little consequence is to him a matter of serious import. With a little effort the dermatologist can not only learn to recognize these problems but he can attain appreciable success in aiding the patient to arrive at a solution.

Pruritus

891

Allen KE, Harris FR. **Elimination of a child's excessive scratching by training the mother in reinforcement procedures.** Behav Res Ther 4:79-84, 1966.

▶ reinforcement

It was hypothesized that one means of making professional service available to a greater number of individuals was through training the parents to use operant guidance techniques for dealing with the problem behavior of their children. A five-year-old girl whose face and neck as well as other parts of her body were covered with open sores and scabs from almost one year of scratching herself was treated by the mother, who was trained to withhold all reinforcement contingent upon the child's scratching herself but to reinforce other, desirable behavior. As the scratching decreased, the mother was instructed in appropriate techniques for thinning out the reinforcement schedule. At the end of 6 weeks the child's face and body were clear of all scabs and sores. Four months later the scratching behavior had not recurred.

892

Arndt JL, Polano MK. **The psychotherapeutic treatment of a case of pruritus vulvae.** Ned Tijdschr Geneeskd 3:2675-2678, 1950. (in Dutch)

▶ psychotherapy

Description of a woman patient who for 22 years had been suffering from pruritus vulvae, for which she had been operated upon twice, and who recovered after a few psychotherapeutic sessions. Some remarks on the importance of psychological factors in itching and itching dermatoses.

893

Bien E. **The clinical psychogenic aspects of pruritus vulvae.** Psychoanal Rev 20:186-196, 1933.

▶ psychotherapy

In short, the essential, psychogenic nonsymptomatic pruritus vulvae has an aspect of depression which is to be placed above the pruritus in the cases observed, and therefore the pruritus has to be considered as the incentive or cause of a psychosis of involution in the sense of a "melancholia expruritus" or a periodic depression. Sack, in discussing the therapy of psychogenic dermatoses, raised the question of the therapeutic competence, and justly considered the psychogenic dermatoses as the psychotherapeutic sphere of action of the dermatologist. Also Werther was of the opinion that one sometimes succeeded in healing a patient with the small amount of therapy of the practicing dermatologist; however, it would be more to the point to treat the pruritus vulvae described above from the psychopathic angle, always keeping in mind Walthard's warning to refrain from any local pseudo-treatment of the pruritus vulvae, as this might do more harm than good.

894

Calnan CD, O'Neill D. **Itching in tension states.** Br J Dermatol 64:274-280, 1952.

▶ psychotherapy

The results of investigation and treatment of 30 patients with itching of the skin are described. Six of those had excoriations of the skin, 10 had simple pruritus without skin lesions, and 14 had itching with lichenification. Emotional tension was the principal determinant of the illness in all the patients. In 23 patients the onset of the skin disorder occurred at a time of special stress. Relapses and exacerbations, in all 30, were related to situations arousing prolonged emotional tension. After treatment 19 were much improved, 5 improved, and 6 unchanged. The patients who benefited least from treatment were those with simple pruritus.

895

Cantor AJ. **Psychosomatic aspects of pruritus ani.** Rev Gastroenterol 16:778-782, 1949.

▶ psychotherapy

Pruritus ani is a symptom and not a disease. The etiology is often complicated by emotional factors. A new classification is introduced, including chronic psychopathology, recent psychogenic problems, neurogenic cases, path of least resistance cases, and projection cases. These are fully discussed. The therapy of each of these problems is detailed. Close cooperation between the proctologist and the psychiatrist is often indicated. In all cases, however, the patient must be given immediate relief. This is best obtained by the operation of tattoo-neurotomy.

896
Czubalski K. **Psychosomatic aspects of pruritus.** Psychiatr Pol 8:551-556, 1974. (in Polish)

▶ review: psychotherapy

897
Dengrove E. **Psychosomatic aspects of dermographia pruritus.** Psychosom Med 9:58-61, 1947.

▶ psychotherapy

1. Two case histories are presented which throw light upon the etiology of dermographia and pruritus. 2. It is suggested that these symptoms may arise in passive and dependent persons with allergic family history consequent upon a separation reaction involving loss of support and gratification.

898
Dugois P, Amblard P, Boucharlat J. **Pruritus en culotte of purely psychogenic origin.** Bull Soc Fr Dermatol Syphiligr 74:372-373, 1967. (in French: no English abstract)

▶ psychotherapy

899
Espin Montanez J, Iranzo Prieto V. **A case of anal pruritus of psychic origin.** Actas Luso Esp Neurol Psiquiatr 28:184-191, 1969. (in Spanish)

▶ psychotherapy

900
Estrin J. **Hypnosis as a supportive symptomatic treatment in skin diseases.** Urol Cutan Rev 45:337-338, 1941.

▶ hypnosis

Extracted summary: Hypnosis was used...in five cases of skin disease in order to attempt to allay the distressing symptoms of pruritus and pain which accompanied the lesions. Due to uncontrollable circumstances, except for the first case, hypnosis could be used only once during the illness. The results, though temporary, were . . . definite and dramatic . . .

901
Lamontagne Y. **Treatment of prurigo nodularis by relaxation and EMG feedback training.** Behav Anal Mod 2:246-249, 1978.

▶ relaxation, biofeedback

A 61-year-old female, suffering from prurigo nodularis for 25 years and treated with various drugs without improvement, received 10 sessions of frontal EMG feedback and learnt to carry out home relaxation excercises. This procedure led to an improvement in the patient's disease which was maintained at the 6-month follow-up. It is suggested that research should be undertaken to explore the potential of biofeedback in the treatment of patients with dermatologic disorders.

902
Lantz JE. **Extreme itching treated by a family systems approach.** Int J Fam Ther 1:244-253, 1979.

▶ family therapy

Presents the case of a 16-yr-old female who developed extreme itching and scratching behavior triggered by the occurrence of manifested parental conflict. S's scratching also served the family function of helping the parents avoid marital conflict. Family treatment consisted of helping the parents negotiate and resolve marital conflict issues in front of S so that she could experience the benefits of dealing with a family conflict in a functional way. The approach helped S decrease her anxiety about conflict situations and resulted in a significant decrease in itching and scratching behavior. In addition, the parents reported an improved marital relationship since S's itching no longer interrupted the parents' attempts to negotiate marital conflict issues.

903
Moller P. **Psychotherapy for pruritus.** Acta Derm Venereol (Stockh) 31:268-271, 1951.

▶ psychotherapy, hypnosis, autogenic training

Extracted summary: The 2 methods [hypnosis and autogenic training] supplement each other in an excellent manner. The hypnosis will comparatively quickly render the patient symptom-free, but requires the doctor's constant co-operation, while the autogenous training, indeed, has a weaker hypnotic effect, but, on the other hand, requires no aid from the doctor when first thoroughly practiced. If one has succeeded in convincing the patient that his disease is psychogenic, he will feel more rationally treated than by the use of ointments and liniments. The feeling that, after instructions, he may unaided control his disease will give him a self-confidence, which more than anything else will contribute to his recovery from the neurosis. The proof of the success of this treatment must be partly that it induces quiet and undisturbed sleep, and partly that it is able to make the patient permanently symptom-free, or at least to reduce the itching to an inconsiderable trouble compared with that causing the neurosis.

904
Musaph H. **Psychodynamics in itching states.** Int J Psychoanal 49:336-339, 1968.

▶ psychoanalysis

Extracted summary: During the last fifteen years I have had the privilege of co-operating regularly with dermatologists, psychoanalysts and psychologists from the University of Amsterdam and this co-operation stimulated thinking about problems of psychosomatic medicine in general and of skin disease in particular. We have examined hundreds of patients suffering from severe itching states, the origin of which was not clear to the dermatologists. In trying to find out the nature, dynamics and therapeutics we found the combination of ethological and psychoanalytical discoveries of value.

905
Musaph H. **Psychogenic pruritus.** Dermatologica 135:126-130, 1967.

▶ psychotherapy

Pruritus psychogenicus is a disease characterized by fits of severe pruritus with no skin or internal disorder except lesions caused by scratching. Patients present a typical character structure which is described. Many specific emotional conflict situations cannot be solved adequately because of their character structure. Treatment is a two-way process. The dermatologist has to help to remove the skin lesions; the psychiatrist has to try to help the patient solve his problems more satisfactorily.

906
Obermayer ME. **Treatment of pruritis.** Med Clin North Am 26:113-122, 1942.

▶ psychotherapy, doctor-patient relationship

In the management of pruritus and of pruritic dermatoses the following admonitions should be borne in mind: First, determine the cause; and if that should prove impossible in the beginning, at least rule out the presence of any internal disorder which might be responsible. Second, give the patient symptomatic relief by prescribing sedatives and by using local applications which will soothe but under no circumstances irritate. Third, study any patient who has chronic recurrent pruritus from the functional point of view. A common sense evaluation of complicating or underlying emotional difficulties will often aid in restoring the functional stability of the nervous system. The emotional catharsis which a patient may experience through his relationship to an understanding and sympathetic physician can be an important factor in his recovery from a chronic recurrent pruritus of "obscure origin."

907
Rosenbaum M. **Psychosomatic factors in pruritus.** Psychosom Med 7:52-55, 1945.

▶ psychoanalysis

The case histories of two patients suffering from pruritus vulvae have been presented in which the psychogenesis of the disorder was that of an hysterical conversion symptom.

908
Salerno EV. **A case of pruritus vulvae treated by psychotherapy.** Prensa Med Argent 37:150-158, 1950. (in Spanish)

▶ psychotherapy

909
Schneider E, Kesten B. **Polymorphic prurigo: a psychosomatic study of three cases.** J Invest Dermatol 10:205-214, 1948.

▶ psychotherapy

Ten patients with a chronic, generalized, polymorphic, itching dermatitis are reported in whom the disease corresponds to that previously described under such varied nomenclature as generalized erythroderma; distinctive exudative discoid and lichenoid chronic dermatosis; and allergic dermatitis simulating lymphoblastoma. After some months residence in the Southwest away from unsatisfactory emotional environment, seven patients became free from this eruption. Of this group, five have remained in the Southwestern states and are ostensibly cured. The other two patients returned to the East, one to her old surroundings, where she has had a recurrence of the eruption, the other to an emotionally satisfactory environment where he has remained well. The remaining three patients underwent a psychosomatic study. After therapy two of the three have remained well while living in their habitual environment. This study indicates that emotional conflict is of singular importance in the evolution of polymorphic prurigo and that psychotherapy is a major factor in its successful treatment.

910

Seitz PFD. **Psychocutaneous aspects of persistent pruritus and excessive excoriation.** Arch Dermatol Syph 64:136-141, 1951.

▶ psychotherapy

Extracted summary: Successful psychotherapeutic management of patients with persistent pruritus and excessive excoriation involves a permissive therapeutic relationship with the patient in which corrective emotional experiences may occur. By the physician's consistent acceptance of him in the face of his expressed inferiority and rage, the patient learns to accept himself and to find constructive rather than personally destructive methods for expressing aggressiveness. If as a result of the permissive therapeutic atmosphere the patient begins to act out his resentments in social settings, an eventuality consistently associated with improvement of the psychocutaneous disorder, limits must be set in order to prevent the development of antisocial behavior. From the psychotherapeutic standpoint, it is especially important that the physician understand that insight alone is not tantamount to cure. Benefit from psychotherapeutic management in such cases derives principally from the corrective emotional experiences associated with the skillfully controlled relationship between the patient and his physician.

911

Sonneck HJ. **Psychotherapy for psychogenic pruritus.** Dermatol Wochenschr 124:693, 1951. (in German)

▶ psychotherapy

912

Stern E. **Pruritus: a psychosomatic study.** Acta Psychother 3:107-116, 1955.

▶ psychotherapy

Psychosomatic study of 42 cases of pruritus. Such cases only were included in the investigation as did not show any signs of another dermatosis (eczema, lichen, etc.). The author stresses the importance of psychological factors in the etiology of pruritus, whereby however the presence of somatic factors is by no means excluded (e.g., small skin lesions or dermatological anomalies). He studies in the first place the personality of the patients, their life history; he shows the importance of past experience for the development of the "terrain" as well as the importance of precipitating factors, which are almost always present. The principal part is played by disturbances in the sexual field and the aggressivity. In many cases the pruritus and the scratching may be looked upon as a substitute for the sexual act or masturbation, the scratching itself as the expression of aggressivity directed against the individual himself, as a source of simultaneous pleasure and displeasure; it expresses at the same time a feeling of guilt and of a tendency towards self-inflicted punishment.

913

Winkler F. **Universal cutaneous pruritus.** Monatschr Prakt Dermatol 52:223-234, 1911. (in German)

▶ psychoanalysis

The Freudian school has given exact proof that once exercised and later given up autoerotic satisfaction can recur in an attack of hysteria. The restriction of localized pruritus to those zones used in early childhood for autoerotic satisfaction is related to the occurence of sexual desire during itching attacks and should be addressed from this point of view. Therefore, the cutaneous pruritus is a partial manifestation of a larger neurosis. The patient must be handled like a neurotic (Freud) and the neurosis cured to get at the localized disease.

Psoriasis

914

Benoit LJ, Harrell EH. **Biofeedback and control of skin cell proliferation in psoriasis.** Psychol Rep 46:831-839, 1980.

▶ biofeedback

Examined the effect of skin-temperature-biofeedback training on cellular proliferation in 3 psoriasis patients: a 60-yr-old male and 2 females aged 21 and 28 yrs. It was hypothesized that (a) Ss would be able consciously to decrease skin temperature of psoriatic tissue and (b) there would be a positive correlation between rate of cellular proliferation and temperature change. Results show that biofeedback training was effective in decreasing the surface temperature of psoriatic tissue. Temperature-training effects generalized from the location of the thermistor to the contralateral limb. Rate of cellular proliferation decreased from pre- to post-training biopsies. Improvement in psoriatic plaques was observed up to 4 mo post-training.

915

Dengrove E. **Emotional aspects of psoriasis.** J Am Soc Psychosom Dent Med. 23:126-132, 1976.

▶ hypnosis, psychotherapy

Describes 2 case histories in which hypnotherapeutic techniques, together with attempted resolution of associated emotional conflict, produced at least temporary recovery from psoriasis.

916

Epstein KN. **The use of skin temperature biofeedback in the treatment of psoriasis.** Diss Abstr Int 40:3470-3471, 1980.

▶ biofeedback, relaxation

Psoriasis is a prevalent inflammatory dermatosis of unknown etiology. Many recognized medical treatments for psoriasis exist. However, none are effective with all patients, none prevent recurrences, and many entail the risk of serious side-effects. Several studies have found that many patients and physicians have noticed that psychological factors seem to influence the course of psoriasis. However, Baughman and Sobel (1971), in the most recent attempt to study the relationship between stress and psoriasis, failed to demonstrate more than a modest relationship between these two variables. The current investigation consisted of two parts. In Experiment 1, the effects of using skin temperature biofeedback training plus relaxation techniques as an adjunct to standard medical treatment were assessed. It was found that during the one month training period, the mean Psoriasis Severity Scale score decreased 41% compared with only 7% for the control group, $t(18) = 1.12$, $p < .02$. Further, during the treatment period, skin temperature and reactive hyperemia threshold times were monitored in order to investigate the role that dilatation and constriction in the peripheral vasculature might play in mediating the course of the disease. It was found that the group instructed in relaxation and skin temperature biofeedback techniques increased skin temperature, $t(18) = 1.08$, $p < .02$, and decreased reactive hyperemia threshold times, $t(17) = -1.79$, $p < .001$, relative to the control group. Also, those patients in whom psoriasis improved, whether or not they received biofeedback, experienced a greater increase in mean skin temperature, $t(18) = .85$, $p < .05$, than the group in which psoriasis did not improve. These results support the conclusion that routine medical treatments for psoriasis can be made significantly more effective by using them in conjunction with relaxation and skin temperature biofeedback training. Furthermore, since the correlations between changes in the peripheral vasculature and both psoriasis severity and exposure to these psychological treatments were found to be significant, it then appears that changes in cortical functioning, fluctuations in the degree of dilatation of the peripheral vasculature, and the course of the disease are all intimately related. In Experiment 2, the reproducibility and validity of the Baughman and Sobel (1971) study, cited above was tested. Again, only a modest degree of correlation between annual stress and severity of psoriasis scores was obtained. However, in the current investigation it was found that patient estimations of change in psoriasis severity over a one month period are highly unreliable, $r = .20$, $p < .20$, relative to a trained and experienced dermatologist. The computed degree of correlation between annual stress and severity of psoriasis scores is dependent partially upon the accuracy of the patient's estimation of change in psoriasis from year to year. Furthermore, an additional source of error was probably introduced into the original study due to the use of retrospective estimations by the patients of their stress and psoriasis levels during each of the preceding five years. Therefore, the results of the Baughman and Sobel study may not be accurate due to methodological difficulties with that study.

917
Frankel FH, Misch RC. **Hypnosis in a case of long-standing psoriasis in a person with character problems.** Int J Clin Exp Hypn 21:121-130, 1973.

▶ psychotherapy, hypnosis, autohypnosis, imagery

Describes the use of hypnosis in treating a 37-yr-old male schoolteacher, socially withdrawn and pathologically sensitive to public opinion, with stubborn and widespread psoriasis. Sensory imagery was used to replicate the feelings in his skin that he experienced while sunbathing—an activity which had proved somewhat beneficial in the past. The patient was taught to induce the hypnotic state by himself and did so 5-6 times/day. The psoriatic lesions improved markedly as did his progress in psychotherapy.

918
Hughes HH, England R, Goldsmith DA. **Biofeedback and psychotherapeutic treatment of psoriasis: a brief report.** Psychol Rep 48:99-102, 1981.

▶ biofeedback, supportive psychotherapy

The client was a 31-year-old white male evidencing multiple psoriatic plaques. The condition was considered severe and had been resistant to previous dermatological treatments. Following a baseline period of 3 wk., 30 treatment sessions were conducted over a 7-mo. period. Each treatment session consisted of 20 min. of skin temperature training at the target plaque site and 15 min. of supportive psychotherapy focused on personal adjustment problems. Photographs of the plaque area and skin temperature recordings were taken during each session. Ratings of the photographs indicated marked improvements of dermatological signs. Despite efforts to reduce skin temperature, small but consistent increases were obtained. It was not possible to assess the relative contribution of biofeedback training, psychotherapy, cognitive variables, or uncontrolled life events. It is hypothesized that a general stress-reduction model might be more useful in the development of an effective treatment of psoriasis. Follow-up checks are needed.

919
Jelliffe SE, Evans E. **Psoriasis as an hysterical conversion symbolization: a preliminary report.** NY Med J 14:1077-1084, 1916.

▶ psychoanalysis

We begin to see, here, the regression of the libido from [the patient's] work and environment, and later the lost libido strives to effect a transference to the young, unmarried brother. He, however, does not prove a sufficient outlet, perhaps from his own efforts to free himself from the family. He loses his health and has a severe illness in a hospital; she has no one to depend upon and reverts to the past, where the father was the ideal, and finally constructs a sexual exhibitionistic substitute—a resymbolization in the form of red spots on the skin—psoriasis.

920
Kartamischew AJ. **Hypnotherapy in psoriasis.** Dermatol Wochenschr 102:260-262, 1936. (in German: no English abstract)

▶ hypnosis

921
Kline MV. **Psoriasis and hypnotherapy: a case report.** J Clin Exp Hypn 2:318-322, 1954.

▶ hypnosis, psychotherapy

A chronic case of psoriasis in a forty-five-year-old woman has been reported upon wherein there has been demonstrated a definitive relationship between emotional factors and the onset of the psoriasis. Despite resolution of the precipitating distress, the psoriasis remained unabated for more than twenty years until successfully treated with hypnotherapy. Some of the theoretical issues related to both the origin and therapeutic rationale have been discussed.

922
Kohli DR. **Psoriasis, a physiopathologic adaptive reaction: six year cure by retraining.** Northwest Med 66:33-39, 1967.

▶ behavior therapy, hypnosis, relaxation, autosuggestion

Psoriasis has not yet been proven to be due to viral, bacterial, mycotic, or parasitic invasion, or to chemical, thermal, meteorological, or unusual physical trauma. It does not appear to be an allergic reaction and its victims do not appear to be socially, economically, or emotionally much different from the rest of us. It does have the characteristics of an adaptive reaction and retraining offers help to those willing to accept carefully directed instruction. Four cases illustrate the possibility. One, a totally incapacitated, middle aged male, has been totally relieved for six years. The others were less spectacular because less ravaged by the disease but all responded favorably while following the regimen that employed retraining only and used no medication.

923
Laugier P. **The treatment of psoriasis.** Ann Dermatol Syphiligr (Paris) 103:547-566, 1976.

▶ review: psychotherapy

924
Leuteritz G, Shimshoni R. **Psychotherapy in psoriasis—results at the Dead Sea.** Z Hautkr 57:1612-1615, 1982. (in German)

▶ psychotherapy, group therapy, relaxation, imagery

In 75% of patients with psoriasis beginning at the head, the psoriatic lesions were preceded by a substantial change in the way of life of these patients, throughout a critical period of life experiences, whereas in 46% of patients with psoriasis starting on the body the lesions were proceeded by continued stress situations arising from fear of failure. 33% of these patients had gone through a critical life event. 39 out of 75 patients interviewed, revealed a psoriasis proceeding from the head. A relaxation and visualisation program as a part of group therapy is described.

925
Munjal GC. **Psoriasis: a preliminary report on its treatment with psychotherapy and certain drugs.** Trans All-India Inst Ment Health 7:16-24, 1967.

▶ psychotherapy

10 patients suffering with psoriasis, when treated with a combination of psychotherapy and psychotropic drugs (trifluoroperazine, chlordiazepoxide, and trimeprazine) showed remarkable improvement.

926
Novotny F. **General aspects of treatment of psoriasis.** Cesk Dermatol 51:56-61, 1976. (in Czech)

▶ milieu therapy, psychotherapy

The author explains the advantages of combined external and internal treatment of psoriasis including physical therapy and psychotherapy with regard to the site of action of the drugs in the pathophysiological process. He recommends an individual approach to therapy, depending on the stage, form and severity of the disease, on the assessed trigger agents, age and occupation of patients and drug tolerance. He mentions criteria for the use of cytostatic preparations and cortisonoids. He evaluates the advantages of in-patient treatment and recommends the establishment of a special sanatorium for psoriasis. He

draws attention to the necessity of preventive therapeutic procedures to prevent relapses and in this connection emphasizes the necessity to dispensarize psoriatic patients.

927
Poussaint A. **Emotional factors in psoriasis: report of a case.** Psychosomatics 4:199-202, 1963.

▶ psychotherapy

Extracted summary: [A] patient is presented who had a five-year history of chronic, non-remitting psoriasis which cleared almost entirely after she was admitted to the hospital for five weeks and treated successfully for a reactive depression.

928
Schulte MB, Cormane RH, Van Dijk E, Wuite J. **Group therapy of psoriasis: duo formula group treatment (DFGT) as an example (I).** J Am Acad Dermatol 12:61-66, 1985.

▶ group therapy

Between 1978 and 1982 an experiment on group treatment for and by psoriasis sufferers was conducted, based on a pyramid of previous investigations since 1968. Each group was facilitated by a duo consisting of a fellow sufferer and a physician, both having trained together. The subjects practiced the procedure described, directed toward self-care and mutual aid facilitated and supported by the duo, in a series of ten 2-hour weekly sessions. A pretest/posttest control group design was used. Comparing the results of the quantitative analysis of the experimental groups with those of the control groups, the experimental groups showed significant change. The results of the qualitative analysis showed that decrease of anxiety correlated with mastering of the skills involved. The key element affecting outcome was the balance in cooperation within the duo, the expertise of the patient lying in his personal experience of the condition, and the expertise of the physician in his knowledge and skills. One of the method's main characteristics was the intrinsic complementarity of the duo partners.

929
Shafii M, Shafii SL. **Exploratory psychotherapy in the treatment of psoriasis—twelve hundred years ago.** Arch Gen Psychiatry 36:1242-1245, 1979.

▶ psychotherapy

Presents a translated case history from an original Persian text written in 1155 A.D. (M. Qazwini, 1969) demonstrating the relationship between the outbreak of psoriasis and the existence of interpersonal conflicts. The techniques of developing therapeutic alliance and confrontation, clarification, dynamic interpretation, and exploration of intrapsychic and interpersonal conflicts are in accord with present concepts of exploratory and dynamic psychotherapy.

930

Sobrado EA, Benedetti S, Geronazzo G, Rolando D. **Psychological study of psoriasis.** Med Cutan Iber Lat Am 9:111-116, 1981. (in Spanish)

▶ psychotherapy

Due to the need to epistemologically delimitate the theoretical instrument, in order to understand the phenomena from a psycho-analytical reading, 65 complete psychological studies and 12 psychotherapeutic developments in a group of patients with psoriasis symptoms are analysed. The psychodiagnostic constants at the intellectual area, in the perceptivo-motor integration and the structure and the dynamics of the personality are proved, where there appears the constitution of a symbiotic link and the formation of a psychic apparatus with a feeble ego, and very old defense mechanisms which form an ambiguous personality with identity problems. The authors try to understand theoretically the material accounting for the skin function and its relationship with the body ego and the frustrated processes of the propioceptive sensibilization which fall upon the frustrating phase of the development that later, by a compulsory repetition, would be reproduced in the psoriasis symptoms. The behaviours which give character to the psoriasic management, both from the patient point of view and the physician's are analysed, in order to consider the psychotherapy in psoriasic patients.

931

Vogel PG. **Psychodynamic aspects of psoriasis vulgaris.** Z Psychosom Med Psychoanal 22:177-189, 1976. (in German)

▶ psychoanalysis

A psychodynamic model for psoriasis vulgaris is developed, based on a case report of psychoanalytic treatment of a patient with a first manifestation of the disease. The probable significance of schizoid aggressive impulses is discussed.

932

Waxman D. **Behaviour therapy of psoriasis.** Postgrad Med J 49:591-595, 1973.

▶ hypnosis, psychotherapy, desensitization

In the case described, an account is given of psoriasis in a female aged 38 who presented with a history of a rash of increasing severity for 20 years, originating during a period of severe emotional stress in a susceptible personality type. During the whole of this period, there was never a time when she had been clear, and exacerbations had been most severe during her two pregnancies. She was treated under hypnosis by a six-point schedule. This involved analysis and discussion, with interpretive (insight) psychotherapy and desensitization by reciprocal inhibition as described by Wolpe. As well as the disappearance of the rash, overall improvement in personality was a notable impression gained from the self-rating Personality Schedule score at the end of treatment.

933

Wisch JM. **Hypnosis for psoriasis.** Dermatol Wochenschr 100:234-236, 1935. (in German)

▶ hypnosis

The question of the nature and treatment of psoriasis is not definitely resolved. Four cases of trauma-induced psoriasis successfully treated by hypnosis are discussed.

934

Wittkower E. **Psoriasis.** Lancet 1:566-569, 1946.

▶ psychotherapy

It is fascinating to speculate why patients with psoriasis fall ill in the way they do—i.e., to understand the psychological meaning of their complaint. But there is no uniformity of emotional conflict. In the light of our present knowledge one can only state that individuals in whom the hereditary element is very powerful may develop psoriasis in any case, whereas others need a catalyst to mobilise a dormant predisposition to psoriasis. More often than is generally known, emotional crises of a nature specific to the individual affected seem to assume this function. In other words, if an individual is emotionally maladjusted for reasons unrelated to the psoriasis, the emotional maladjustment may, but need not, take charge of the psoriasis and determine its onset and further relapses. The parallel to other conditions, such as allergic manifestations and diabetes mellitus, is obvious.

935

Zuili N, Nachin C. **Work of the so-called phantom in the unconscious and psychosomatics: a propos of psoriasis.** Ann Med Psychol (Paris) 141:1022-1028, 1983. (in French)

▶ psychoanalysis

The theory of "ghost" in the heart of the unconscious relates the precocious psychic legacy of mental misfunctioning through the unconscious to unconscious relationship with a relative inhabited by a mourning that has not been worked through. These misfunctionings can express themselves thanks to various psychopathological demonstrations, but through psychosomatical illnesses as well. As shown by the authors in some cases of psoriasis: determinism that could associate—a genetical predisposition of the future patient,—a notion of family or personal history having to do with events such as burns, fire.

Warts

936
Allington HV. **Review of the psychotherapy of warts.** Arch Dermatol Syph 66:316-326, 1952.

▶ review: psychotherapy

Extracted summary: In order properly to evaluate any therapy for warts, further knowledge is needed regarding the epidemiology and natural history of untreated warts. Facts are needed regarding immunology in order to help explain wart behavior with particular reference to spontaneous cure. Results of treatment must be accurately recorded and properly controlled. In experimental studies, methods of psychotherapy must be chosen carefully in order to avoid introducing questionable nonpsychic influences. Conversely, controlled series will be difficult to obtain without subjecting the patients to some psychic stimuli. The close cooperation of persons fully trained in psychiatry should be sought. It would be desirable to know whether wart patients in general show any significant psychological deviations from the normal. A psychiatrist should be able to help in choosing methods and techniques of psychotherapy which may be more suitable and effective than those described to date and of setting up adequate controls. The question of possible harm to the patient from improper psychotherapeutic procedure, as raised by Obermayer, should be carefully considered. Until a specific remedy for warts is discovered and made available for general use, their treatment will continue, at times, to be a difficult and distressing problem. The evidence that psychotherapy is an effective method of treatment for warts is inconclusive. More study is needed before the suitability and limitations of this procedure can be established.

937
Bleiberg J. **Witchcraft, warts and wisdom.** J Med Soc NJ 54:123-126, 1957.

▶ suggestion, folk medicine

Extracted summary: Viruses enter a cell and can alter the chemistry of that cell according to their needs. This alteration in chemistry may take place immediately after the penetration of the cell; or the host cell may go on functioning normally, undergoing numerous normal mitoses, until a trigger mechanism activates the dormant virus, causing it to multiply at the expense of the host cell. The first premise, then, is that the wart virus is present in the epidermal cells of many individuals, as a dormant parasite. It must then be postulated that the trigger is a chemical molecule. Such molecules could be elaborated as a result of emotional stress, with or without local injury, causing the warts to appear. If therapy is properly applied, be it salicylic acid plaster or a grasshopper bite, so as to inspire hope and confidence, the causative emotional tension is neutralized. The favorable climate for the virus' growth is eliminated. The warts disappear. It is not impossible that some substances may locally diminish the ability of the virus to grow. Certainly, podophyllin may function that way, at least in the non-cornified genital warts. The virus then may be destroyed, or it may return to a dormant state within the cell, lurking there, ready for re-activation with the proper stimulus. Only by assuming that the chemical effects of emotional stress play a part in the etiology of warts, is it reasonable to explain the effectiveness of suggestion in their treatment. Linus Pauling has pointed out that we are on the threshold of molecular medicine. We must begin to think in terms of the chemistry of suggestion.

938
Bloch B. **Curing warts through suggestion.** Klin Wochenschr 6:2271-2275, 1927. (in German: no English abstract)

▶ suggestion

939
Bonjour J. **Warts: their etiology demonstrated by cure through suggestion.** Schweiz Med Wochenschr 54:748-751, 1924. (in French: no English abstract)

▶ suggestion

940
Bonjour J. **The cure of warts by suggestion.** Schweiz Med Wochenschr 57:980-981, 1927. (in French: no English abstract).

▶ suggestion

941

Breitbart EW. **Modern treatment of warts.** Z Hautkr 57:27-37, 1982. (in German)

▶ suggestion, hypnosis

A short historical review of the treatment of wart virus is given including suggestive and also x-ray-therapy.

942

Chandrasena R. **Hypnosis in the treatment of viral warts.** Psychiatr J Univ Ottawa 7:135-137, 1982.

▶ hypnosis, psychotherapy

16 males and 16 females (8-25 yrs old) with common, palmar, or plantar warts of 18 mo average duration were treated with daily hypnosis either individually or in groups. 56% responded satisfactorily to treatment over an average of 9.5 sessions. Depth of hypnosis was related to outcome, and previous dermatological applications offered no adjuvant effect to subsequent hypnotherapy. Palmar and plantar warts responded poorly to hypnotherapy, while common warts on the other areas of the body were more responsive.

943

Ciecierski L. **Treatment of common warts.** Wiad Lek 25:63-65, 1972. (in Polish)

▶ psychotherapy

944

Clarke GHV. **The charming of warts.** J Invest Dermatol 45:15-21, 1965.

▶ suggestion

Experiments designed to test whether warts can be charmed away are considered. The results of such an experiment indicate that suggestion or charming does not succeed. After further consideration of previously published work, a possible explanation of the success of the treatment of warts by suggestion is that because warts have a limited life, treatment initiated near the end of this life results in cure. This cure is often and erroneously attributed to the immediately preceding therapy.

945

Cohen SB. **Warts.** Am J Clin Hypn 20:157-159, 1978. (editorial)

▶ hypnosis, suggestion

946

Dreaper R. **Recalcitrant warts on the hand cured by hypnosis.** Practitioner 220:305-310, 1978.

▶ hypnosis

Extracted summary: In any case, whatever the pros and cons of antibody and cell mediated immunity, it would seem difficult to accept that either of the above mechanisms could cause the geographically selective destruction of warts as happened in the case of Mrs. M. Is it conceivable that the cure under hypnosis (or indeed with wart charming) may lie in some neurogenic mechanism? This would seem to offer the only explanation of selectivity. Take, for instance, the one wart left on Mrs. M.'s ring finger. What nervous mechanism could be involved. The sympathetic nervous system which would therefore implicate the sweat glands? Under hypnosis patients can be made to produce anatomically localized sympathetic effects such as vasodilation and sweating in one hand or one side of the face. It is noticeable how many people with warts have hot sweaty hands and feet. A leading article (British Medical Journal, 1961) commented that there has been no satisfactory trial on the effect of internal medication on warts and suggested that attention to the sweating of soles and palms might be worth-while. However, a trial of the sweat diminishing agent propantheline, which blocks the cholinergic sympathetic nervous supply to the sweat glands, was found to be disappointing, a fact that I have confirmed on 25 of my own patients. However, one fact of importance merits further research. A localized tumour that is virus induced can be caused by hypnosis to regress completely while a nearby similar tumour remains. If the precise reason for this regression could be determined the findings might have significance in the wider field of cancer research, as well as affording a clue to the more efficient cure of warts.

947

Dudek SZ. **Suggestion and play therapy in the cure of warts in children: a pilot study.** J Nerv Ment Dis 145:37-42, 1967.

▶ play therapy, placebo, suggestion

Treatment of warts using a combination of play therapy, placebo medication, and suggestion was attempted with 24 children brought to a skin clinic for the surgical removal of warts. 20 were seen to completion of therapy. Treatment was administered under 2 techniques: (1) suggestive therapy combined with threat of surgery on 2nd visit (provided no warts had shown curative changes), and (2) suggestion without threat of surgery. A total of 10 cases completely lost their warts, 4 lost only some prior to discharge, and 6 cases were unchanged within the set time limit. The average cure rate was 7 wks. Adequacy of emotional rapport may be a relevant factor in effecting cure.

While it seems valid to infer that psychological factors were instrumental in effecting somatic change, it is not at all clear what parts placebo medication and emotional variables played. Further research in this area is recommended.

948
Goldman L. **Area diagrams as a technique of psychotherapy in the treatment of warts of the hands in children.** Urol Cutan Rev 5:90-91, 1950.

▶ suggestion

Extracted summary: With a pencil the outlines of the hands and wrist (even other areas of the extremities) are traced carefully. The child is told to mark off on the drawing the exact location and approximate size of each wart. He is told that when this is finished he is to send the diagrams to the doctor. A bland or colorful topical medication may or may not be ordered for use at home after the drawings are made. The patient is told the doctor will examine his drawings carefully. When the drawings are received the doctor writes back in formal style, directly to the child that the drawings were examined, the warts counted. If the physician desires, he may add also that the paper was thrown in the fire and all burned up and that three to four weeks later the warts should disappear.

949
Goss EO. **Wart charming.** Radiography 22:75-77, 1956.

▶ folk medicine

Extracted summary: In the West country wart charming is accepted by a large majority of the rural population as a routine therapeutic measure. Application for more orthodox forms of treatment under the National Health Scheme is not necessarily a reflection on charming, although it may indicate that no convenient charmer lives in the neighbourhood. These notes, which cover charming and other unorthodox remedies, refer to the common wart or verruca vulgaris, which generally occurs on the back of the hands, but may occur on the face or elsewhere, varying in size from a pinhead to a filbert. They are usually discrete but may group to form large swellings. They are inoculable from one spot to another and from one individual to another. Treatment can be divided into the following classifications: X-rays, cautery, surgery, CO_2 snow, acids or lotions, surgical diathermy. I will not enlarge upon these well-tried methods but consider the more unorthodox forms of therapy which can be classified under the following headings: local applications, white magic, symbolism.

950
Grumach L. **Treatment of warts by suggestion.** Munch Med Wochenschr 74:1093-1094, 1927. (in German: no English abstract)

▶ suggestion

951
Hellier FF. **The treatment of warts with x-rays: is their action physical or psychological?** Br J Dermatol 63:193-194, 1951.

▶ suggestion

1. Attention is drawn to the present epidemic of warts.
2. Any beneficial effect of fractional doses of x-rays on warts is the result of suggestion in the majority of cases.

952
Johnson RF, Barber TX. **Hypnosis, suggestions, and warts: an experimental investigation implicating the importance of "believed-in efficacy."** Am J Clin Hypn 20:165-174, 1978.

▶ hypnosis, suggestion, meditation

Suggested to 22 volunteer Ss (mean age 22.5 yrs) that their warts would disappear if they imagined them tingling for a few minutes each day. Half the Ss received the suggestion after they had been exposed to a formal hypnotic induction procedure and the remaining half (controls) received the same suggestion after they were told simply that they were to be treated by a method called "focused contemplation." Three of the 11 hypnotic Ss and none of the 11 "focused contemplation" Ss lost their warts during the experimental period. It is suggested that the relatively greater effectiveness of the hypnotic treatment may have been due to its "believed-in efficacy"; that is, Ss who lost their warts strongly believed that warts could be cured by hypnosis whereas the focused-contemplation Ss did not believe that their treatment was especially effective in curing warts.

953
Konig KJ. **The treatment of the common wart.** Z Haut Geschlechtskr 44:247-254, 1969. (in German: no English abstract)

▶ suggestion

954
Leidman IuM. **Hypnospsychotherapy as a means of treating warts in children under ambulatory conditions.** Vopr Okhr Materin Det 18:57-59, 1973. (in Russian: no English abstract)

▶ hypnosis, psychotherapy

955
Leidman IuM. **Experience in the treatment of warts in children by suggestion.** Vestn Dermatol Venerol 42:86-89, 1978. (in Russian)

▶ hypnosis, suggestion

Thirty-four children with warts were treated by hypnosuggestion. Suggestion in the state of hypnosis was combined with conditional reflex therapy. Seances of hypnosis were group and individual. One to three seances in treatment of flat warts was successful in 100% cases. Less effective was treatment of periungual and sole warts. In 23 children with vulgar and flat warts complete cure was achieved. In 11 children hypnosuggestive treatment produced poor or no effect. Warts disappeared within 1 week to 2-3 months. There were no scars or spots at sites of disappearing warts. No correlation was found between the success of treatment and the depth of hypnotic sleep.

956
McDowell M. **Juvenile warts removed with the use of hypnotic suggestion.** Bull Menninger Clin 13:124-126, 1949. (also Br J Med Hypn 2:23-25, 1951)

▶ hypnosis, suggestion

Extracted summary: There is sufficient evidence to warrant a suspicion that the skin condition was playing a psychodynamically active symptomatic role in [the patient]. If this suspicion could be substantiated, it would certainly make the disappearance of [warts] in response to suggestive or other magic-like procedures much more understandable.

957
Memmesheimer AM, Eisenlohr E. **An inquiry into the suggestive treatment of warts.** Dermatol Z 62:63-68, 1931. (in German: no English abstract)

▶ suggestion

958
Obermayer ME. **Verruca plana of the face treated by posthypnotic suggestion.** Arch Dermatol Syph 60:1222-1224, 1949.

▶ hypnosis, suggestion

Extracted summary: Since a preliminary interview revealed no psychoneurotic features, the psychiatrist expressed the belief that while the treatment could produce no ill effects, its chance of success was small. At the end of the first interview, the patient was told to imagine for a few minutes before bedtime each night that her face was covered by cold compresses and was beginning to itch and tingle. At her second visit, she gave the encouraging report that she had had the sensation of itching. An attempt at hypnosis was followed only by a state of deep relaxation without sleep, during which it was suggested that her face would feel cold, her skin would itch and the warts would begin to fall off. The patient began the third and last consultation by stating that the warts had commenced to become scaly. Once more hypnosis was attempted, and a state of light sleep was produced. It was then suggested that her face would feel cold and turn pale

and that the lesions would itch and fall off within two weeks. The patient was awakened and told that no further interviews were contemplated because her warts would shortly disappear. Two weeks later her skin was clear of all lesions.

959
Obermayer ME, Greenson RR. **Treatment by suggestion of verrucae planae of the face.** Psychosom Med 11:163-164, 1949.

▶ hypnosis, suggestion

Extracted summary: We do not wish to suggest that the findings we report are new nor to propose the routine use of suggestion in the treatment of verrucae. However, in view of the well-known shortcomings and unreliability of all "approved" methods of treating warts, we do believe that suggestive therapy should be retained among available measures and continue to be applied and studied in carefully selected cases.

960
Rowe WS. **Hypnotherapy and plantar warts.** Aust NZ J Psychiatry 16:304, 1982. (letter)

▶ hypnosis

961
Samek J. **Suggestive healing of warts.** Dermatol Wochenschr 93:1853-1857, 1932. (in German)

▶ hypnosis

This normally occurring, spontaneous healing of warts can be speeded up with accompaniment (according to Delbanco, Hallerstaedter and Galewsky) of a clearly inflammatory reaction. Inflammatory stimulation of a very low degree, it is assumed, can contribute to the healing of warts. "The important thing about the suggestive treatment of warts is the fact that through a psychic influencing, a purposeful inflammation occurs."

962
Schmidt LM. **Warts: their diagnosis and treatment.** Pediatr Ann 5:782-790, 1976.

▶ psychotherapy

Warts are common skin lesions caused by a papova virus. Their clinical appearance is variable. There is no definitive therapy. Therapy must be individually modified to get the best result with the least discomfort to the patient. Most warts will spontaneously resolve after an average of two years, so any therapy that has serious side effects or results in scarring should not be used. New modes of therapy, particularly immunotherapy, look promising but are still in the experimental stage.

963
Sheehan DV. **Influence of psychosocial factors on wart remission.** Am J Clin Hypn 20:160-164, 1978.

▶ suggestion, conditioning

The effects of psychosocial events on the natural history of warts and the physiological mechanisms that mediate them are observed in 2 case studies. Psychosocial factors not only accelerate the remission of warts but may also reinforce their presence and proliferation as in case 1. In that case, a 14-yr-old girl believed that a beloved grandfather had given her warts as a secret life-bond between them. When the grandfather died, the warts underwent natural extinction. Vasomotor changes during and following nonspecific hypnotic suggestions in case 2 involving a 25-yr-old man lend confirmation to earlier speculations and hypotheses on the nature of one mediating physiological mechanism in wart remission. The merits of an operant conditioning paradigm of so-called "hypnotic" behaviors are discussed.

964
Sinclair-Gieben AHC, Chalmers D. **Evaluation of treatment of warts by hypnosis.** Lancet 2:480-482, 1959.

▶ hypnosis, suggestion

14 cases of warts were treated by hypnosis. It was suggested to the patient that the warts on one side of the body (the worst affected) would disappear. The other side served as a perfectly matched control. In 9 of the 10 patients in whom deep or moderate hypnosis was achieved, the warts on the "treated" side disappeared while those on the control side remained unchanged. This treatment was effective in all cases where the patient was hypnotised deeply enough to perform, on awakening, some action that had been suggested to him.

965
Staukler L. **A critical assessment of the cure of warts by suggestion.** Practitioner 198:690-694, 1967.

▶ suggestion

An attempt has been made to induce unilateral disappearance of common warts by using two forms of suggestion under controlled conditions. Twenty-four of the original 91 patients defaulted without trace after three months; 22 of the remaining 67 lost their warts, but all did so on both sides. No case of unilateral disappearance was seen. It is suggested that these results show that this attempt to charm warts failed and that the "cures" depended upon spontaneous resolution. With the possible exception of Sinclair-Gieben and Chalmers (1959) who used hypnosis (not simple charming) I know of no convincing evidence that charming works.

966
Sulzberger MB, Wolf J. **The treatment of warts by suggestion.** Med Rec 140:552-556, 1932.

▶ suggestion

Extracted summary: The fact that suggestion, without recourse to any other therapy, cures an appreciable percentage of warts stands established. This fact is not a supernatural but a natural one which can be explained in several ways. This is, in our opinion, the most important advance embodied in these studies. For, as soon as one recognizes that these cures are not the results of witchcraft or magic, one has gained material for objective study. And such studies may lead to the discovery of fundamental biological phenomena.

967
Surman OS, Gottlieb SK, Hackett TP. **Hypnotic treatment of a child with warts.** Am J Clin Hypn 15:12-14, 1972.

▶ review: hypnosis

The present case report describes a nine year old girl with multiple common warts. The lesions were refractory to routine dermatologic treatment but appeared to respond dramatically to hypnotherapy. The patient's schoolwork concomitantly improved. The authors present a brief discussion of the literature and indicate some problems for future study.

968
Surman OS, Gottlieb SK, Hackett TP, Silverberg EL. **Hypnosis in the treatment of warts.** Arch Gen Psychiatry 28:439-441, 1973. (also Advances 1:19-26, 1983)

▶ hypnosis

This study was designed to test the hypothesis that warts are treatable by hypnotherapy. Seventeen experimental patients with bilateral common or flat warts were hypnotized weekly for five sessions and were told that the warts would disappear on one side only. They were reexamined three months from the time of the first hypnotic session. Seven patients who were untreated were also reexamined at the end of three months. Fifty-three percent of the experimental group improved. No improvement was observed among untreated controls. These findings support the hypothesis that warts respond to hypnotherapy. Whereas specific lesions could not be influenced selectively, the findings suggest that hypnosis has a general effect on host response to the causative virus.

969

Tasini MF, Hackett TP. **Hypnosis in the treatment of warts in immunodeficient children.** Am J Clin Hypn 19:152-154, 1977.

▶ hypnosis

Three patients (12- and 14-yr-old females and a 12-yr-old male) with an immunologic deficit developed multiple warts which proved refractory to all therapy. The warts disappeared in response to hypnosis in all 3 cases, and there was no recurrence after 8 mo of follow-up.

970

Tenzel JH, Taylor RL. **An evaluation of hypnosis and suggestion as treatment for warts.** Psychosomatics 10:252-257, 1969.

▶ hypnosis, suggestion

Used suggestion under hypnosis on 1 side and suggestion without hypnosis on the opposite side in 28 patients with bilateral warts, to test the predication of unilateral regression on the side treated with hypnosis. Results are consistent with the natural life cycle of warts. There was no increase in regressive rate following either suggestion alone or under hypnosis. It is concluded that neither hypnotic suggestion nor suggestion alone are efficacious therapies for the removal of warts.

971

Ullman M. **On the psyche and warts.** Psychosom Med 21:437-488, 1959.

▶ review: hypnosis, suggestion, doctor-patient relationship

The literature on the suggestion therapy of warts has been reviewed and the areas of general agreement among the various investigators have been noted. With due consideration to the rate of spontaneous recoveries (as near as this can be determined by studying large groups of patients with warts), the cure of warts can be brought about by psychological means generally associated with the term "suggestion." Some authors go so far as to imply that this is the most important factor underlying the successful treatment of warts by x-ray, drugs, and even surgery. All agree that in one way or another an affective response must be set up in the patient. An attempt was made to reconsider the work of earlier investigators from the viewpoint of the nature and goal of the personal relationships established. For the most part, they represented a heightening of the authoritarian relationship between doctor and patient in an effort to reproduce clinically some of the psychological factors which obtain in lay healing, e.g., the combination of submission and helplessness on the part of the subject and the aura of omnipotence and infallibility

on the part of the healer or healer-symbol. The ritual involved in the various lay approaches and the procedures employed in the medical techniques to effect a cure by suggestion both result in the temporary suspension of the discriminative, critical, and evaluative faculties of the patient in favor of certain emotional reactions engendered by the situation. These reactions are as yet not very clearly defined. The considerations here presented warrant the further exploratory use of hypnosis as a procedure incorporating many of the elements that appear to be involved in the various accounts of the cure of warts by suggestion.

972

Ullman M, Dudek S. **On the psyche and warts (II): Hypnotic suggestion and warts.** Psychosom Med 22:68-76, 1960.

▶ hypnosis, suggestion

Hypnosis was attempted in 62 patients with warts. Deep hypnosis was established in 15. Within a four-week period after the therapeutic suggestion was given, 8 of these 15 patients showed complete remission of their warts, in contrast to the occurrence of 2 cures in the 47 patients who could not be deeply hypnotized. The findings suggest that the hypnotic relationship may play a significant role in facilitating the curative process in certain patients with warts. The inability to cure some patients under the same or similar conditions, the occurrence of cures under other conditions, and the phenomena of so-called spontaneous cure indicate that factors other than those involved in the specific hypnotic procedure undoubtedly played a role. These factors urgently require further experimental clarification.

973

Vollmer H. **Suggestive treatment of warts in childhood.** Kinderarztl Prax 4:64-68, 1933. (in German: no English abstract)

▶ suggestion

974

Vollmer H. **Treatment of warts by suggestion.** Psychosom Med 8:138-142, 1946.

▶ suggestion

Warts in children can be cured by suggestion. The results seem to be better in children than in adults. Verrucae planae juveniles respond to treatment by suggestion in a higher percentage of cases and within a shorter time than verrucae vulgares. Children below three years of age and feebleminded individuals are not suited for this treatment. Warts have a tendency to heal spontaneously. However, the average duration of untreated warts is more than ten times longer than that of warts treated by suggestion.

The great number of other methods which have been recommended in the literature for the treatment of warts are probably unspecific, and, with the exception of radiotherapy and surgery, act mainly as disguised suggestion. It is assumed that cure by suggestion and spontaneous healing are similar processes, and that successful suggestion merely accelerates the spontaneous healing of warts by causing hyperemia in the surrounding tissues. This opinion is supported by histological findings of Samek.

975
Wilkening K. **Therapy of juvenile warts.** Dtsch Med Wochenschr 103:317, 1978. (in German: letter)

▶ suggestion

976
Yalom ID. **Plantar warts: a case study.** J Nerv Ment Dis 138:163-171, 1964.

▶ psychotherapy

This paper describes the psychodynamics and course of therapy of a patient painfully incapacitated with plantar warts. Data are presented which suggest the psychogenicity of the patient's disorder and which elucidate some of the probable factors operative in choice of the symptom. As is often the case with recalcitrant symptoms and psy-chophysiologic complexes, the central theme is one of loss and depression, the symptom operating as a depressive equivalent. A practical problem arose out of the patient's dysfunctional communicative methods: intravenous pentothal and Ritalin administered prior to each interview facilitated a successful therapeutic outcome.

977
Zwick KG. **Hygiogenesis of warts disappearing without topical medication.** Arch Dermatol 25:508-521, 1932.

▶ suggestion

1. As the methods of magic treatment for warts are identical in principle with the methods of treatment by suggestion, their results are also identical. 2. Magic treatment fortifies and supplements "suggestion" by employing mechanical manipulations causing trauma, which alone may cause the disappearance of warts. 3. Autohemotherapy is useful in the treatment for warts, even though it is not uniformly successful 4. The disappearance of warts following the treatment by magic, by suggestion, by injection of the patient's blood or of foreign protein derived from other sources, as well as the so-called spontaneous disappearance of warts, are causatively linked with a change in the host of the warts. 5. Unless the host overcomes all the invaders, the warts return sooner or later.

Combined Skin Disorders

978
Abramowitz EW. **The use of placebos in the local therapy of skin diseases.** NY State J Med 48:1927-1930, 1948.

▶ placebo, psychotherapy

Placebo is defined as material which works by the mechanism of suggestion and is a temporary chemical psychotherapeutic device. There are "pure" and "impure" placebos. Both types of placebos have their place in the local therapy of skin diseases. If the eruption is of psychologic etiology, more skillful psychotherapy is required, either by the dermatologist or the psychiatrist. Certain patients cannot receive placebo therapy because of negative attitude toward the physician. Many prescriptions with active ingredients contain placebo elements.

979
Allison SD. **Psychosomatic dermatology circa 1850.** Arch Dermatol Syph 68:499-502, 1953.

▶ review

There has been presented a review of some of the remarks of Erasmus Wilson, a famous mid-19th century physician and philanthropist, on the emotional origin and alleviation of dermatologic distress. One hundred years ago the emotional origin of urticaria and eczema was recognized, as well as the psychic cure for warts.

980
Arone di Bertolino R. **Hypnosis in dermatology.** Minerva Med 74:2969-2973, 1983. (in Italian)

▶ hypnosis

Almost all skin diseases are caused by a variety of factors with psychogenic factors having a great influence on progression and the development of chronic conditions. After remarks on this aspect, the techniques employed in hypnosis therapy are described and psychosomatic skin diseases are outlined. Personal experience in the treatment of viral skin diseases is then described in detail and some aspects of the treatment of bacterial, reactive and psychosomatic diseases are presented. Behavioural disturbances related to dermatological problems and essential pruritus are also mentioned.

981
Bar LHJ, Kuypers BRM. **Behaviour therapy in dermatological practice.** Br J Dermatol 88:591-598, 1973.

▶ conditioning, assertiveness training, desensitization

Behaviour therapy provides important psychotherapeutic possibilities for the treatment of dermatological disorders. Compulsive scratching and trichotillomania can be treated by aversive conditioning, or by the token economy technique. The treatment of blushing is described: assertive training is useful for patients with symptomatic erythema and erythrophobia. Hyperhidrosis can be treated by assertive training and systematic desensitization.

982
Barber TX. **Hypnosis, suggestions, and psychosomatic phenomena: a new look from the standpoint of recent experimental studies.** Am J Clin Hypn 21:13-27, 1978.

▶ hypnosis, suggestion

Reviews a series of investigations indicating that suggestion (a) can block the skin reaction (dermatitis) that is produced by poison ivy-like plants, (b) can give rise to a localized skin inflammation that has the specific pattern of a previously experienced burn, (c) can be effective in the cure of warts, (d) can ameliorate congenital ichthyosiform erythrodermia ("fish skin disease"), and (e) can stimulate the enlargement of the mammary glands in adult women. Experiments are also summarized supporting the hypothesis that the aforementioned suggested phenomena may be due, in part, to localized alterations in blood flow to the skin and other organs that can occur when certain types of suggestions are accepted.

983
Barber TX. **Changing "unchangeable" bodily processes by (hypnotic) suggestions: a new look at hypnosis, cognitions, imagining, and the mind-body problem.** Advances 1:7-40, 1984.

▶ hypnosis, suggestion, imagery, biofeedback, placebo

The author reports that hypnotic suggestions can influence diseases of the skin (allergic dermatitis, ichthyosiform erythrodermia, pachyonychia congenita, warts) and outlines an explanation of how blood flow to specific areas of the skin can be controlled through suggestion.

984
Barinbaum M. **A preliminary report on the significance of Freudian psychoanalysis in dermatology.** Dermatol Wochenschr 95:1066-1067, 1932. (in German)

▶ psychoanalysis

The advantage of the methods of Freudian psychoanalysis is that they show the energy source of an illness. One patient sticks to his skin disease to get a pension, another to be rid of an unpleasant job, a third so that he need not support his separated wife. Freudian psychoanalysis is good for dermatology for two reasons: its well-worked-out methods of investigation and the essential relationship between the skin disease and the endocrinovegetative apparatus.

985
Belliboni N. **Possibilities of hypnosis in dermatology.** Rev Psicol Norm Patol 4:147-164, 1958. (in Portuguese)

▶ hypnosis

986
Bernstein ET. **The emotional factor in skin diseases.** J Nerv Ment Dis 89:1-13, 1938.

▶ psychotherapy, doctor-patient relationship, suggestion

Extracted summary: Successful therapy in psychogenic and related dermatoses often depends on the harmonious relation between patient and physician. The medicinal armamentarium is wide and varied, including the use of numerous sedatives, local anesthetics, drugs affecting the vagosympathetic balance, such as ephedrin, ergotamine tartrate, etc., and organotherapy when endocrine disturbances are associated. Concerning the indications and contraindications for these drugs, discussion would be superfluous as the audience is fully familiar with them. Instead, it is proposed to discuss certain methods of psychotherapy which I use in my practice.

987
Bethune HC, Kidd CB. **Psychophysiological mechanisms in skin disease.** Lancet 2:1419-1422, 1961.

▶ hypnosis, autohypnosis, suggestion

A mechanism is discussed whereby psychological stresses can produce skin lesions in areas of somatic weakness. In states of emotional "high drive," suggestion produces "ideovisceral" and "ideovascular" effects in these susceptible areas. Experimental evidence for this has led to a method of treatment by inducing perceptual distortion. Cases are described which illustrate the modes of action.

988
Bonjour J. **Influence of the mind on the skin.** Br J Dermatol Syph 41:324-326, 1929.

▶ suggestion

Extracted summary: In conclusion we may say that patients suffering from the above-mentioned skin diseases are persons whose nervous systems are affected either through an emotion or through some other cause of excitement. My experiments have conclusively demonstrated that the skin expresses in its vascular response and its tissues the suggestions given and also that it is influenced by fear or ancestral belief, so that it really is the mirror of the soul.

989
Bunch JR. **Brief psychotherapy in dermatology.** Rocky Mt Med J 64:78-81, 1967.

▶ psychotherapy, doctor-patient relationship, consultation-liaison

Extracted summary: This is not the treatment of choice for a decompensated person whose basic defenses have cracked. The patient must be able to mobilize his assets and cope with his trials. He may be insomniac and anxious, but if he is still functioning this modality is worthy of a trial. Do not use this method in severe neurotic states of long standing, phobias, hysterical paralysis or poorly matured persons who have to be thawed out. Do not use this method for a patient who has a psychosis of any kind, nor for the severely depressed person, the schizoid, or even the passive dependent person. Use every means at your command to get these patients to a competent psychiatrist. Brief therapy is also contraindicated in the deeply ingrained neurotic, the suicidal, the patient with organic brain disease, or any psychopathologic state such as addiction or perversion. A severe psychosomatic illness is not to be treated by this means (ulcerative colitis). However, brief therapy may be used as a preparation for deeper therapy. The brief therapist should attack the problem just as if he were going to do the deeper treatment and may thereby make psychotherapy in more experienced hands more acceptable to the patient. The initial interview may not reveal the depth of the patient's disturbance but if at any time the physician becomes aware of it, or meets too much resistance from the patient, he should withdraw and accept the fact that brief psychotherapy is a definitely limited method of treatment.

990

Bunneman O. **Psychogenic dermatoses: a biological study and a treatise on the symptomatology of hysteria.** Z Gesamte Neurol Psychiatr 78:115-152, 1922. (in German: no English abstract)

▶ hypnosis

991

Bunneman O, Jadassohn J, Jolowicz E, Memmesheimer AM, Sack WT, Werther J. **Successes and limits of psychotherapy in skin diseases.** Dermatol Wochenschr 94:20-26, 1932. (in German)

▶ psychotherapy

The question if and how far organic sicknesses, skin diseases included, can be psychotherapeutically influenced rests on the body-soul problem, and can only be solved in a cognitive-theoretical manner. A psychotherapy based on this approach must proceed from the idea that somatogenic and psychogenic suffering do not exist side by side, but that every manifestation in life is both of these at once. Success in psychotherapy is often dependent on the severity of a given complex. It is not possible, therefore, to predict the success of psychotherapy of a skin disorder and to demarcate its boundaries.

992

Cheek DB. **Possible uses of hypnosis in dermatology.** Med Times 89:76-82, 1961.

▶ hypnosis, suggestion, autosuggestion

In essence, the use of hypnosis in the therapy of skin diseases can be outlined as a building up of self-respect and a pyramiding of hope. The methods described here are applicable to the entire scope of human illness as much as they are to dermatology. The reason for this appears to be that the normal status of animal life is its optimum balance with its environmental stresses. Hypnosis is one of the means by which that balance can be regained in illness by a constructive use of imagination and by releasing the enormous potential of the deepseated animal drive to survive. There are critical times when hypnosis can save a life.

993

Christensen BE. **The psyche and the skin.** J Am Med Wom Assoc 10:117-122, 1955.

▶ psychotherapy, doctor-patient relationship

No one would question the close physiologic relationship between the psyche and the skin. However, we are rather hesitant in accepting the fact that there may also be a pathologic relationship between the two: that prolonged emotional stimuli with their concomitant physiologic changes may actually produce structural changes in the skin. Detailed case studies seem to confirm the importance of such psychogenic factors in some of the dermatoses. It has therefore been postulated that therapy cannot be totally effective unless some form of psychotherapy is used in conjunction with more conventional forms of treatment. The psychotherapy needed for these patients is not beyond the scope of the general practitioner, and he should use minor psychotherapy as readily as he uses minor surgery.

994

Cipollaro AC. **The place of health resort therapy in dermatologic disorders.** JAMA 134:249-253, 1947.

▶ milieu therapy

Extracted summary: In general it may be said that the cases in which the patient will benefit most from a sojourn at a health resort are those in which change of locale, removal from physical or psychic irritants and the establishment of a scientifically regulated regimen, supplemented by treatment with therapeutic waters, can be expected to improve primarily the patient's general health and sense of well-being and secondarily his dermatosis. I shall therefore describe briefly a group of cutaneous diseases that should respond better to treatment under ideal resort conditions than to ordinary office treatment.

995

Cleveland DEH. **The psychosomatic aspect of dermatologic therapy.** Can Med Assoc J 62:122-127, 1950.

▶ doctor-patient relationship, psychotherapy, consultation-liaison

It is impossible to outline dogmatically any line of procedure to be followed in all cases. Simple reassurance, as has been remarked, is seldom adequate; dealing with the true psychoneurotic by the employment of so-called "common sense" is as vague as the term itself and does no good. One must recognize the limitations of superficial or minor psychotherapy such as may be learned and practised by the dermatologist, and know that the true psychoneurotic urgently demands the skill and experience and special techniques of the psychiatric specialist. In the simpler cases of emotional and personality disorders which do not yield to minor psychotherapy and the dermatologic disorder continues or becomes persistently relapsing, yielding to no ordinary dermatologic therapeutic measures, the psychiatrist will be a valuable consultant. He will assist the dermatologist in selecting and developing the lines of approach which he may learn to use successfully.

996
Coles RB. **Group treatment in the skin department.** Trans St Johns Hosp Dermatol Soc 53:82-85, 1967.

▶ review: group therapy

Groups of psoriasis and acne patients are described. The psoriasis patients attended regularly, and much hard group work developed. They benefited from the supporting community of the group. In the case of acne, the attendance was transient. The young people found the two hours' discussion helpful as a learning process, but they never "condensed" themselves into an ongoing group.

997
Cormia FE. **Basic concepts in the production and management of the psychosomatic dermatoses.** Br J Dermatol 63:83-92, 129-151, 1951.

▶ psychotherapy

1. Observations have been made on 137 patients with various types of psychosomatic dermatoses; 100 of these have been completely studied. 2. The most common complaints were ano-genital pruritus (40); lichen Vidal (18) and neurotic excoriations (15). 3. The presenting dermatosis was the sole cutaneous psychosomatic manifestation in 71.8% of the cases. 4. Other psychosomatic manifestations, severe psychoneuroses or psychoses were present in 43% of the various syndromes and in 45.2% of 104 patients. 5. Severe family maladjustments were present in 57% of the patients, maladjustments in early life in 62% and long-standing adult maladjustments in 80%. 6. Major conflicts occurred in early life in 44% of the group, in adult sexual life in 52%, in domestic life in 37%, in the work sphere in 30%, and in the social life in 11%. 7. Recent psychic trauma of a major degree occurred in 12% of the patients. 8. Major precipitating factors in the psychic realm were noted in 20% of the group, and were far outweighed by major conflicts in early life (44%) and by severe long-standing maladjustments in adult life (61%). 9. A positive correlation between the personality type and individual dermatoses were present in only a few syndromes. 10. Eighty-five patients were followed for periods varying from 1 month up to 3 years, with an average of 6 months. 11. In the followed group, no response to treatment was noted in 26%, symptomatic improvement or cure was obtained in 27%, symptomatic improvement or cure followed by relapse or development of other psycho-

somatic symptoms in 17.6% and basic improvement or cure in 29.4%. 12. No patient with generalized or scattered pruritus, lichen Vidal, phobic manifestations, or dermatitis factitia was either fundamentally improved or cured. 13. The importance of early preventive therapy is stressed. 14. Specific needs for future research in the field are outlined.

998
Cormia FE. **Psychosomatic factors in dermatoses: a critical analysis of diagnostic methods of approach.** Arch Dermatol Syph 55:601-620, 1947.

▶ psychotherapy

Extracted summary: In conclusion, it will be seen that the psychosomatic approach has many advantages over other methods of investigation. It requires only a moderate amount of experience and a liberal dash of common sense and can be obtained in from one to three hours. Moreover, it lends itself well to the management of all but the more long-standing, recalcitrant conditions, for which prolonged psychoanalysis is indicated. Lastly, a patient is under the guidance of a single physician. As such, continued doses of psychotherapy can be administered and environmental adjustments made while roentgenologic and other symptomatic methods of treatment are being given.

999
Cormia FE. **The role of psychosomatic factors in dermatoses.** Conn Med J 14:1051-1061, 1950.

▶ psychotherapy, doctor-patient relationship

A survey of the basic mechanisms of importance in the production of psychosomatic dermatoses has revealed that these syndromes are in every way comparable to psychosomatic disease in general. By and large, successful management depends more on an understanding of the "whole" patient and attempts to affect a basic reorientation towards his individual problems, than to special dermatologic "know how." Such procedures as x-ray therapy, the use of antihistamine preparations, injection techniques and other dermatologic tools are distinctly of secondary importance as compared with the more fundamental type of therapy as above described.

1000
Diakonov MF. **4-year experience with the treatment of some dermatoses with sleep therapy in association with hypnotic suggestion.** Vestn Dermatol Venerol 39:47-50, 1965. (in Russian)

▶ hypnosis, suggestion

During 4 years the author used electric sleep in combination with hypnosuggestive therapy for the treatment of

134 patients with dermatic diseases, including 96 patients with different forms of eczema, 21 with neurodermatitis, 12 with extensive forms of lichen ruber planus, 2 with urticaria and 3 with skin pruritis. Clinical cure was achieved in 73 patients, considerable improvement in 46, improvement in 12, no effect in 3 patients.

1001

Duller P, Gentry WD. **Use of biofeedback in treating chronic hyperhidrosis: a preliminary report.** Br J Dermatol 103:143-146, 1980.

▶ biofeedback, relaxation

Preliminary findings attesting to the successful therapeutic use of biofeedback training in reducing symptoms of chronic hyperhidrosis are reported. Eleven of the fourteen adult patients trained with biofeedback were able to demonstrate clinical improvement in their excessive sweating 6 weeks after termination of treatment. Relaxation was suggested as the active ingredient in the biofeedback treatment effect. These findings support a recent report of the successful use of biofeedback in treating patients with dyshidrotic eczema.

1002

Eletsky VY. **Effect of hemosorption on the time-course of neuropsychic disturbances in patients with psoriasis and neurodermatitis.** Zh Nevropatol Psikhiatr 83:1687-1691, 1983. (in Russian)

▶ psychotherapy

Found that 102 of 150 patients with either psoriasis or neurodermatitis had neurotic reactions, neurotic developments, psychopathic reactions, or psycho-organic syndromes. A relationship was found between premorbid features of the personality, the severity and duration of the skin disease, and the type of neuropsychic disturbances experienced by ss. The time course of the disturbances in the process of treatment is discussed. Best results for a regressive time course in the neuropsychic disorders and improvement in skin disease were obtained by psychocorrective treatments and hemosorption therapies.

1003

Eller JJ, Silver S. **Psychosomatic diseases of the skin.** Behav Neuropsychiatry 1:25-36, 1970.

▶ consultation-liaison

This paper deals with the inter-relationships between psychologic factors and skin disease. Psychosomatic diseases of the skin may be divided into four categories, depending upon the fundamental type of psychologic influence. The first category consists of exaggerations of the normal involuntary transient cutaneous manifestations of emotional states, blushing and sweating. Presumably, the abnormality lies both in the physiologic, as well as the psychologic domain. The second category consists of those cutaneous manifestations of more prolonged and abnormal emotional states, such as neuroses, psychoses, and nervous habits. Basically, the skin itself is normal, but is injured by the patient himself. The third category includes those skin diseases which may be to some extent mysteriously activated or aggravated by emotional states. A number of skin diseases are particularly prone to psychologic influences. Lastly, there are those skin disorders which, through the disfigurement they produce, or the intensity or chronicity of their symptoms, have profound psychologic effects. The psychiatrist and the dermatologist working together in many such cases will serve the best interest of the patient.

1004

Engels WD. **Psychosomatic illness review (II): Dermatologic disorders.** Psychosomatics 23:1209-1219, 1982.

▶ psychotherapy

The contribution of emotional factors to many dermatologic disorders has long been recognized, although the specific relationships and mechanisms remain to be clarified. Sensitive dermatologists have incorporated psychotherapeutic approaches into their management of a variety of skin disorders, and in some cases psychiatric consultation or treatment may be called for. Various dermatologic conditions, such as pruritus, hyperhidrosis, atopic dermatitis, urticaria, rosacea, alopecia areata, psoriasis, and associated conditions, including "dermatologic nondisease" are reviewed with a focus on the psychic substrate present in many of them. The appropriate integration of psychotherapy into the treatment is discussed for each condition.

1005

English OS. **Role of emotion in disorders of the skin.** Arch Dermatol Syph 60:1063-1076, 1949.

▶ psychotherapy

Extracted summary: As the role of emotions in cutaneous conditions becomes more widely accepted, we shall have more psychotherapeutic efforts and hence more reports of results of treatment. This will be good for the morale of both dermatologists and patients alike. As things stand, the patient still has too little faith in what can be done for his condition by a psychotherapeutic approach. It is really hard for him to look at his emotions, since he is too busy looking at his skin and sees little reason why he should shift his attention to his emotions, which he considers as secondary to the state of his skin. But as word gets around that one's disposition can be expressing itself in the skin, the physician can obtain more cooperation in the psychotherapeutic treatment. The emotional factor is a variable one, and no one is trying to assert that skin diseases are due to emotions alone. But when emotion is a factor, it is one that must be dealt with; if well dealt with, it may be the factor which will give the most practical results in comfort and hence in satisfaction to both patient and physician. Dermatologists and psychiatrists must stimulate and help each other to carry on more therapy of the emotional forces which are using the skin for their expression. Psychotherapy is not a simple, easily mastered tool, and the patient is not always a willing subject for therapy. But, if we try to ascertain what the role of emotions can be in conditions of the skin, we will cure the condition in occasional subjects, improve it in some, make it easier to live with in others and find the specialty of dermatology altogether more interesting through the pleasure which comes from taking a greater interest in human emotions in our daily work as physicians.

1006

Escande JP. **Institutional organization of a hospital dermatology service with a responsibility for psychosomatic care.** Sem Hop Paris 60:916-919, 1984. (in French)

▶ psychotherapy

Clinicians trained in dermatology and having submitted themselves to psychoanalysis have developed an original psychosomatic approach to skin disease at the Tarnier Hospital (Cochin-Port Royal University Hospital Center). Its mainspring is detection and management of the patient's distress. The author analyzes the conditions under which it was possible to carry out this experiment and the implications of this approach which is directed at achieving a change in the way the department is run rather than adding one more specialized appendage to the outpatient care activity.

1007

Fernandez GR. **Hypnotism in the treatment of the stress factor in dermatological conditions.** Br J Med Hypn 7:21-24, 1956.

▶ hypnosis, suggestion

The skin plays an important role in the psychosomatic disorders. More research is necessary before the stress factor can be demonstrated in the numerous other dermatoses of unknown aetiology. It is encouraging to note that the skin is particularly responsive to suggestion; some investigators have been able to raise blisters on it by means of hypnosis, and feelings of burning and intense irritation can also be induced or suppressed by this means. This opens up a new vista of hope in the treatment of the bullous dermatoses of unknown aetiology, like pemphigus, which

is so often fatal, and the distressing conditions of dermatitis herpetiformis, herpes zoster and simplex. To what extent warts are due to stress remains to be seen, but their removal by suggestion is a well demonstrated fact. Certain types of naevi appear at various stages of childhood and adolescence, and are described as congenital lesions of the skin. It was encouraging to note a few years ago the removal of a large and disfiguring naevi in a young boy, by means of hypnosis, when all other measures proved futile.

1008

Fernandez GR. **Hypnotherapy in dermatology.** Br J Med Hypn 9:38-40, 1958.

▶ hypnosis

Extracted summary: In the treatment of pruritic dermatoses, ranging from simple localized itching, to generalized feelings of intense burning and irritation, from lichen simplex chronicus, to the more severe forms of urticaria, allergic disorders and acute generalized eczemas, hypnotherapy is invaluable, both alone but, better still, with supportive therapy in the form of local applications, and internal medication.

1009

Frumess GM. **The role of emotion in dermatoses.** JAMA 152:1417-1420, 1953.

▶ psychotherapy

Commonly encountered emotions such as insecurity, anxiety, hostility, and guilt may cause stimulation of the autonomic nervous system, leading to flushing, sweating, itching, and excoriating. Physical agents through which emotions mediate these effects are acetylcholine released at parasympathetic nerve fiber endings; sympathin produced by sympathetic stimulation; synergism between acetylcholine and histamine; and the mechanical and allergic effects of sweat retained under pressure. Several skin disorders believed to be of emotional origin exhibit fairly characteristic personality patterns. An effort has been made to relate the clinical entity to the emotional pattern in herpes simplex, rosacea, urticaria, childhood eczema, adult neurodermatitis, and localized neurodermatitis. In most such cases it is desirable that one physician supervise both the somatic and psychic aspects of therapy. Functional dermatoses such as delusions of parasitosis, syphilophobia, dermatitis factitia and neurotic excoriations result from deep-seated neuroses or psychoses and should be referred to the psychiatrist for treatment.

1010

Gay Prieto J. **Psychosomatic dermatology.** Medicamenta (Madr) 10:231-234, 1952. (in Spanish)

▶ psychotherapy, suggestion

1011
Gordon H. **Hypnosis in dermatology.** Br Med J 1:1214, 1955.

▶ hypnosis, suggestion, psychotherapy

Extracted summary: Hypnosis was started in the form of simple suggestion. Varying degrees of hypnotic trance were obtained, and during the hypnotic state the suggestion was given that the skin condition would resolve and return to normal and that irritation, if present, would go. In most of the conditions treated pruritus was a marked feature, and it was certainly found that the anti-pruritic effect of simple hypnosis was often very striking. It soon became apparent that under hypnosis the doctor-patient rapport was considerably enhanced. Patients became much more willing, so to speak, to "let their hair down." Consequently psychotherapy was added to hypnosis.

1012
Gottesman AH, Menninger K. **The dermatologist and the psychiatrist.** Arch Dermatol Syph 59:367-371, 1949.

▶ psychotherapy

The awareness that there is an essential relation between emotions and cutaneous conditions would seem to be a first consideration for adequate therapy. Once this is recognized, various possibilities of treatment present themselves. These possibilities include (1) symptomatic treatment of the cutaneous lesion alone, regardless of possible emotional maladjustment, (2) combined treatment of the medical and psychologic components by the dermatologist, (3) concurrent treatment of the patient by both dermatologist and psychiatrist and (4) treatment by the psychiatrist alone. Of these four possibilities of treatment, the combined medical and psychologic therapy by the dermatologist is probably the one most frequently indicated. But competence in the proper handling of the emotional factors by the dermatologist can come only from an understanding of fundamental psychiatric principles.

1013
Gould WM, Gragg TM. **A dermatology-psychiatry liaison clinic.** J Am Acad Dermatol 9:73-77, 1983.

▶ psychotherapy, consultation-liaison

A dermatology-psychiatry liaison clinic at Stanford University is described. The clinic provides an opportunity for dermatology residents to learn about the psychological aspects of the specialty and to witness at first hand technics of interviewing, strategic questioning, and listening.

1014
Hachez E. **Psychotherapy and the dermatologist.** Zentralbl Haut Geschlechtskr 9:166-171, 1950. (in German)

▶ psychotherapy

1015
Hellier FF. **The relation of dermatology to psychiatry.** Br Med J 2:583-585, 1944.

▶ psychotherapy, consultation-liaison

Extracted summary: The recognition of the type of patient is easy, but how can one help him? The application of ointments and x rays will literally only touch the surface of the condition; if we are to obtain permanent benefit we must tackle the patient as a whole and consider his personality and environment. The problem may be divided into two parts: the discovery of the immediate factor which caused the present attack, and the wider aspect of the adjustment of the patient's attitude to life and his skin condition. The former is often surprisingly simple; the patient is only too willing to pour fourth his troubles to a sympathetic listener, and, helped by a few judicious questions, soon reveals marital or financial worries, a period of strain, or some emotional shock which seems to bear a direct relation to the current attack and which the patient is ready to accept as such. The solution to these problems is often possible, using common sense and a little persuasion. More difficult is the problem of altering the patient's outlook and mode of existence so that he may be protected from stresses and strains which his hypersensitive make-up cannot support. One aims at giving the patient insight into his condition, reassuring him that it can be controlled if he goes about it the right way, and modifying his environment. In many cases this common-sense psychology will succeed; but in others one is faced with a severe anxiety state, and it is sensed that there are hidden stresses in the patient's mind that one has failed to expose. One is often reduced to giving these patients bromide—a confession of failure—and it is in such cases that one turns for help to the trained psychiatrist.

1016
Hornstein OP. **What can dermatology expect from psychotherapy?—A plea.** Z Hautkr 55:913-927, 1980. (in German)

▶ psychotherapy, doctor-patient relationship

The philosophy of rationalism, increasingly dominating also in medicine since the 19th century, has led to a dualistic way of thinking about the organic and psychical phenomena of maladies, so hampering a more profound comprehension by physicians of the psycho-somatic sources of many diseases in human beings. Due to their bioscientific education most physicians are trained to study the diseases of their patients by means of physico-chemical and other "objectifying" methods. Scientists are often inclined to identify the totality of different diagnostic results with the virtual actuality of an individual morbid state, so failing to notice that whatever they find also depends on the methodology of solving a question. Psychic implications, if any, of dermatological disorders are usually interpreted as either secondary responses to organic disorders or neurophysiological transformations of mental stress and other emotional disturbances on bodily behaviour including some patterns of cutaneous reactivity. It ranks with the most important recognitions of the psychosomatic medicine that both the physician's and patient's subjective personality are intrinsically involved in the very complex condition of an individual health recovery. A patient's non-compliance with medical advice or drug prescription may often be based on a hardly realized emotional irritation of the doctor-patient-interaction. This pathology of unconscious personal interaction may defeat the success of therapeutic management, though "objectively" being adequate, in many cutaneous diseases. So-called Balint seminars held by physicians under tutorial advice of a psychotherapeutic expert prove useful for better understanding the pathogenous interdependency of visible symptoms and emotional condition in patients suffering from dermal or other physical disturbances. By aid of such medical training programs with mainly patient—and not disease-centered—case consultations the participants will better be able not only to recognize the psychical problems of their patients but also to reflect on their own behaviour that may trouble the efficiency of medical care.

1017
Ikemi Y, Nagakawa S, Higuchi K. **Psychosomatic study of so-called allergic dermatoses.** Rev Med Psychosom 7:45-51, 1965. (in French)

▶ psychotherapy

I have experimentally re-evaluated the significance of the suggestive mechanism in the development of psychosomatic conditions in some skin disorders, mainly so-called allergic conditions. The results of these experiments are as follows: (1) The pattern of the interaction of constitutional and psychological, especially suggestive factors could be statistically demonstrated in contact dermatitis. It was histologically proven that suggestion or psychological conditioning can induce definite organic skin pathology which closely resembles those induced by actual touch to noxious trees. (2) Similar significance of suggestive mechanisms was found in a few other allergic conditions. The considerable effectiveness of suggestive therapy for certain varieties of alopecia was statistically re-confirmed. (3) A systematically planned psychotherapeutic approach to control psychological factors in these conditions was found to be practically useful depending upon the degree of predominance of psychological factors and constitutional components. (4) The replacement of symptoms was frequently observed during the course of psychosomatic disorders, especially allergic conditions, and therapeutic approach to them. This phenomenon itself often may have beneficial effect not only on the patients but also on the physicians as well.

1018
Kartamischew AJ. **Treatment of some skin diseases by suggestion under hypnosis.** Vestn Dermatol Venerol 5:7-12, 1952. (in Russian)

▶ hypnosis, suggestion

1019
Kelley WE. **Psychosomatic medicine: skin and its appendages.** Nebr Med J:182-183, 1950.

▶ psychotherapy

Extracted summary: The abnormalities mentioned are skin manifestations of a psychic problem, and can best be met with complete cooperation between the psychiatrist, the dermatologist and the patient. Once the condition is recognized, it is up to the psychiatrist to find out why this condition exists.

1020
Klauder JV. **Psychogenic aspects of skin diseases.** J Nerv Ment Dis 85:249-273, 1936.

▶ psychotherapy

In a discussion of the psychogenic aspects of skin diseases the following phases will be considered: the influence of the skin on the psyche, the influence of the psyche on the skin, clinical aspects of the relation of psychologic phenomena to skin diseases.

1021
Klauder JV. **Psychoneurotic manifestations in dermatology with particular reference to treatment with suggestive and educative measures.** Arch Neurol Psychiatry 12:99-102, 1924.

▶ psychotherapy, suggestion, relaxation, patient education

Psychotherapy may be of considerable value in the treatment of certain skin diseases, objectively as well as subjectively manifested. A psychic cause of such common skin diseases as pruritus and urticaria should be included among the many causes of these diseases. Not only is psychotherapy of value in the treatment of the psychogenic types of the aforementioned diseases, but also in other conditions encountered by the dermatologist. Such conditions as neurotic excoriations should be considered, as for example, trichotillomania, trichokryptomania, and dermatothlasia.

1022

Klauder JV. **The cutaneous neuroses with particular reference to psychotherapy.** JAMA 85:1683-1690, 1925.

▶ psychotherapy, counseling, suggestion

Extracted summary: The history of these patients should be taken with the aforementioned possibilities in mind; attention should particularly be directed at the circumstances associated with the onset of the pruritus or urticaria, the circumstances associated with its continuation, and its specificity referable to the time and place of its occurrence. Indeed, these remarks pertain not only to pruritus or urticaria, but also to other cutaneous phenomena, as will later be shown. If a psychic origin of the complaint is suspected the patient may well benefit by the application, on the part of the physician, of the principles of Janet and of Dejerine. Psychotherapy is of considerable value in reconditioning the psychologic reaction, in producing a transformation of the mental attitude, in dispelling fear or dread, or in distracting the psychic fixation. This is accompanied by suggestion or more especially by reeducation. A full comprehension of the psychogenesis of the complaint is urged on the patient.

1023

Kline HS. **Psychogenic factors in dermatitis and their treatment by group therapy.** Br J Med Psychol 22:32-52, 1949.

▶ group therapy, psychotherapy

The psychological factors present in seventeen cases of dermatitis have been studied in detail. Although these cases were referred for different reasons, they all showed evidence of psychiatric illness, the symptomatic nature of which varied widely. It is considered that, apart from those cases definitely due to physical or chemical agents, dermatitis is only one symptom of a psychosomatic disorder occurring in a certain type of personality. Individuals suffering from dermatitis are usually over-conscientious, worrying, obsessional, and though overtly passive and anxious to please have a good deal of latent hostility and ambivalence. They show gross disturbance of their sexual life, have difficulty in dealing with their aggressive impulses and give evidence of inner conflicts around exhibitionism. Intensive individual psychotherapy, aided by group therapy, is believed essential for radical treatment. Immediate results are encouraging, but the ultimate prognosis in terms of total personality adjustment is doubtful.

1024

Klinge JE. **The sexual aspects in the practice of dermatology.** J Am Inst Hypn 13:11-15, 1972.

▶ psychotherapy, hypnosis, suggestion

Discusses the close relationship between the subconscious mind and the skin. 3 cases are described in which the skin diseases (lichen planus and psoriasis) were related to fears of pregnancy, rape by a step-father, and homosexuality. It is suggested that the skin lesions served the functions of protection, prevention, and/or punishment. Additional cases are presented to illustrate this theory. It is concluded that many skin conditions may be caused or aggravated by emotional problems and that hypnoanalysis and suggestion may be beneficially used in their treatment.

1025

Koblenzer CS. **Psychosomatic concepts in dermatology: a dermatologist-psychoanalyst's viewpoint.** Arch Dermatol 119:501-512, 1983. (also Advances 1:77-78, 1984)

▶ review: psychotherapy, consultation-liaison

Few experienced clinicians remain unimpressed both by the influence of psychological and social factors on the physical state and by our relative inability to deal adequately with this aspect of the practice of dermatology. This article reviews the historical development of psychosomatic concepts, describes some theories concerning the process whereby somatization takes place and why a particular disease is "chosen," reviews some of the relevant basic science findings, offers a working classification of psychocutaneous disease, and, finally, makes some suggestions as to how we may become more effective in handling this important part of our clinical practice.

1026

Krafchik H. **Psychosomatic factors in dermatology.** S Afr Med J 24:533-535, 1951.

▶ doctor-patient relationship, psychotherapy, relaxation

Extracted summary: Every patient who consults his doctor is in a state of fear. He is thereby rendered more susceptible to suggestion and the correct attitude of the doctor can profoundly affect his autonomic nervous system through his emotions, and thereby almost every chemical reaction throughout his body may be modified. A frequent and intimate discussion with the patient, and reassurance, will often produce an unbelievable feeling of well-being and strength in a patient and contribute much to the resolution of skin eruptions produced by emotional upsets. In a recent discussion on the subject "The Dermatologist and the Psychiatrist" by Grottesman and Menninger, the general consensus of opinion arrived at was that the importance of psychiatrical methods of treatment in dermatology cannot be overrated, and that the dermatologist was the proper person to handle his own cases.

1027

Kuypersen BR, Bar LH. **The psychologist in the dermatological clinic: methods and possibilities of treatment.** Ned Tijdschr Geneeskd 116:1268-1271, 1972. (in Dutch)

▶ psychotherapy, consultation-liaison, behavior therapy

Psycho-social factors sometimes play an important part in skin diseases. It appears that this fact is not yet generally recognized, to the detriment of the patients. A number of criteria are listed which may help the physician discover possible emotional problems. This may lead to useful cooperation between the dermatologist and the psychologist in the examination and treatment of such patients. Psychological methods are described, and special reference is made to a number of methods of treatment belonging to the recently developed behaviour therapy methods, which prove to be of considerable value in the treatment of certain dermatological patients.

1028

Leonenko PM. **Hypnosuggestive therapy in treatment of skin diseases.** Akad Beloruss (Minsk) 6:281-291, 1959. (in Russian)

▶ hypnosis, suggestion

1029

Lewis GM, Cormia FE. **Office management of the neurodermatoses.** NY State J Med 47:1889-1894, 1947.

▶ psychotherapy

An office technic for the management of the neurodermatoses is outlined. This embraces a preliminary appraisal of the patient to exclude primarily physical diseases or to evaluate their relative importance in the causation of the presenting disease. A special investigation is then documented and the details are exemplified by illustrative case reports. It should be emphasized that these procedures, while not as time-consuming as psychoanalysis and related technics, cannot be effective with brief consultations. With the combined psychosomatic and symptomatic methods of therapy, the results of treatment were decidedly good, 50 per cent of the group being cured or markedly improved while 22 per cent were slightly or not improved. The remaining 28 per cent lapsed from observation; of these, 14 per cent may be considered as complete failures, while the other 14 per cent were seen only in consultation or have moved from the neighborhood. While the management of the neurodermatoses is still difficult and the results uncertain in many instances, it is hoped that the methods of interpretation and therapy advocated in this paper will be of practical value to the dermatologist.

1030

Lo Presti G, Campione A. **Personal clinical experiences with some cases of psychosomatic dermatoses.** Minerva Dermatol 42:167-172, 1967. (in Italian: no English abstract)

▶ psychotherapy

1031

MacKenna RMB. **Psychiatry and the skin.** Proc R Soc Med 43:797-799, 1950.

▶ psychotherapy, consultation-liaison

Extracted summary: Psychiatrists tend to forget, for example, that an eczema may be psychogenic in origin but the symptoms and signs may be perpetuated by mechanisms of infection, auto-sensitization and superimposed contact dermatoses which the patient's mind cannot control. If these secondary effects are not dealt with at the same time as the primary psychological cause, the patient—although he cooperates fully with the psychiatrist—may continue to suffer severely from eczematous eruptions. So I suggest that in dermatology—as in many other branches of medicine—the role of both parties, psychiatrists and dermatologists, should be the role of players in a team, and in that team we would do well to include the biochemists.

1032

MacKenna RMB, Macalpine I. **Application of psychology to dermatology.** Lancet 1:65-68, 1951.

▶ psychotherapy

Extracted summary: Ideally, this psychological and dermatological approach to skin disease should be a double approach made by a single clinician. For reasons of training this is hardly ever possible. Hence it is necessary to establish fruitful cooperation between the dermatologist and the clinical psychologist. This may seem a banal statement, but in reality there might easily enter into such common work a sense of rivalry concerning the scientific priority and validity of the two disciplines. Since some of the differences between the two approaches are fundamental, they will be discussed first. Secondly, the actual task of the clinical psychologist to a skin department will be dealt with. Thirdly, some scientific methods suitable for such work will be examined.

1033

Macalpine I. **Psychiatric observations on facial dermatosis.** Br J Dermatol Syph 65:177-182, 1953.

▶ psychotherapy

(1) Psychiatric experiences in the course of investigation by psychotherapy of 35 patients with facial dermatoses of

various kinds are described. (2) The importance of unconscious factors and the similarity between the formation of psychosomatic and psychotic symptoms is stressed. (3) Anger was the common underlying emotion. (4) In all patients there was a direct relation to depression. Injudicious management may remove symptoms but precipitate a true depression. (5) The symptom may be assessed as a masked depression. (6) Paranoid attitudes about the facial lesion are regarded as pathognomonic of psychosomatic as opposed to organic lesions. (7) Specific personality types could not be found.

1034
Manferto G. **Hypnosis in dermatology.** Minerva Med 66:3864-3865, 1970. (in Italian)

▶ hypnosis

The cases treated with hypnosis in the Dermatological Division of the Vercelli General Hospital are reviewed. The results obtained in 6 cases of Lichen Ruber Planus, 4 cases of alopecia areata and 2 cases of circumscribed neurodermitis are reported.

1035
Mason AA. **Hypnosis and allergy.** Br Med J 1:1675-1676, 1963. (letter)

▶ hypnosis

1036
Menninger K. **Observations of a psychiatrist in a dermatology clinic.** Bull Menninger Clin 11:141-147, 1947.

▶ psychotherapy

Extracted summary: It would seem clear that dermatologists and psychiatrists should pool their skills in a cooperative effort. The great dependence of the dermatologist upon the discriminating observation which he has brought to such a high degree of perfection, has to a certain extent proved his undoing. No one is more aware of this than the thoughtful dermatologists themselves, because while it is true that correct diagnosis frequently leads with automatic celerity to proper treatment, it does not do so in the great burdensome eczematoid group ... On the other hand, the psychiatrist who acts as a consultant or visitor in the dermatological clinic quickly learns that the techniques of his own routine practice are not capable of direct transfer to the dermatological problem. The patient with the skin lesion has oriented all of his thinking about that lesion, and it is exceedingly difficult for him to depart from this preoccupation. Furthermore, one is constantly aware of difficulty in limiting the biographical study for the psychiatric interview. By taking a detailed, circumstantial history of the present illness, one indeed learns that many things have happened in the patient's life which might be considered unusual emotional stresses. The question always is what role these stresses actually played with reference to current or previous skin eruptions.

1037
Michael JC. **Emotional stress and allergic cutaneous manifestations.** South Med J 22:282-283, 1929.

▶ psychotherapy

Extracted summary: More and more in my practice, difficult cases of chronic urticaria, eczema and cutaneous pruritus are being elucidated by study of the psychic state of the patient. The principal factors concerned in the pathogenesis of allergy are well known. Attention is directed here to that modicum of cases in which grief, sex conflict, disappointment, worry and other emotional stress are the presumably predisposing factors upon which the allergic state develops. In this necessarily brief presentation it is impossible to go further into the many aspects of the subject, some of them debatable, and therefore I will proceed to illustrate my experience by several cases chosen for the purpose.

1038
Milberg IL. **Group therapy in the treatment of some dermatoses.** Skin Oct:307-310, 1963.

▶ group therapy

A method has been presented using a combined dermatological and psychotherapeutic approach in the treatment of some chronic disabling cutaneous conditions. These skin ailments consist of somatic reaction which is closely allied with emotional malfunctioning in a sometimes indivisible two-way relationship. There was no common denominator apparent in the relationship of the psychodynamic factors present and the cutaneous symptoms. This concept of body-mind unity, which has led to such positive results, is so important that it deserves special emphasis which we have attempted to realize in this combined treatment program.

1039
Mirakhmedov UM, Belova LV. **Psychotherapeutic problems in dermatology.** Vestn Dermatol Venerol November:62-66, 1982. (in Russian)

▶ psychotherapy

The authors describe different methods of psychotherapy in dermatological practice, propose their wider use and search for an individual creative approach to each patient.

1040

Mittelman B. **Psychoanalytic observations on skin disorders.** Bull Menninger Clin 2:169-176, 1947.

▶ psychoanalysis

1) The conflicting trends that were found correlated with the skin disorders here presented were the longing for affection and care, the fear of abandonment and attack, feelings of helplessness, hostility, aggression, hurt self-esteem, guilt, self-depreciation and self-debasement with anal coloring, and erotization of the skin. The fantasy content was that of obtaining love and care through warmth and cutaneous contact. 2) The skin reactions changed their character with changes in the external traumatic situation and the internal conflict pattern. 3) Once a skin pathology was established, the same pathological reaction could occur with shift in the dominant conflict pattern. 4) Broad, emotional needs and drives, such as need for love and care, hostility, erotic strivings, anxiety and guilt, were vital in the dynamics of the skin pathology, and the same broad needs led to anxiety attacks, depressive reactions, and characterological manifestations.

1041

Moller P. **Psychosomatic dermatology.** Ugeskr Laeg 112:892-895, 1950. (in Danish)

▶ psychotherapy, autogenic training, hypnosis

Although an increasing number of papers has been published concerning the relationship of psyche to skin disease, no paper has hitherto been published suggesting the use of psychotherapy for some of these diseases. In some cases of protracted intense itching, in which physical changes by no means correspond to the subjective complaints and where careful physical examination gives no hint with regard to the aetiology, the ordinary dermatological treatment shows no results at all. In such cases psychotherapy is recommended and the author mentions some case histories in which such treatment has been successful. The object is to teach the patients a kind of sleeping ritual, so that they do not scratch themselves in the night, and to create a new conditioned reflex replacing the scratching reflex in the daytime. For this purpose exercises of relaxation (Schultz's autogenous training) and hypnosis are used. The system yields satisfactory results in some cases of neurosis caused by itching.

1042

Musaph H. **Behavior therapy in psychodermatology.** Ned Tijdschr Geneeskd 116:1769-1771, 1972. (in Dutch: no English abstract)

▶ behavior therapy

1043

Musaph H. **Psychodermatology.** Psychother Psychosom 24:79-85, 1974.

▶ review: psychotherapy

A description of the history of psychodermatology and of the three phases of research conceptualization—the anecdotal phase, the methodological phase, and the present integrative phase—are given. A typical example of a psychodermatological approach towards itching and scratching is given, an example which shows that a simple, specific, recurring causal relationship between precipitating factors and reaction patterns does not exist.

1044

Myers WK. **The psychosomatic aspect of skin disorders.** Med J Aust 38:476-480, 1951.

▶ psychotherapy, consultation-liaison

Extracted summary: Sometimes the dermatologist, if he has the time, can, by a few brief questions, find a cause for the persistence of the patient's dermatosis; but in a number of cases this requires expert psychiatric examination. From a practical viewpoint two drawbacks become evident; these are the patient's unwillingness, on the grounds of expense, to consult more than one doctor, and a certain resentfulness at the explanation that his complaint is influenced by the "nerves." (Incidentally, there are a number of patients who revel in this suggestion and like very much to hear it.) The resentful patient fails to see why his complaint should, as it were, be blamed upon himself, and consults another dermatologist ... In conclusion I wish to state that I believe that the object of these papers and any subsequent discussion is to appeal for a compromise between the rationalism of Virchow and the idealism of Coue, and to make a practical attempt to evolve a combined approach by both dermatologist and psychiatrist.

1045

Neumann J, Weiker A. **Psychotherapy and skin diseases.** Dermatol Wochenschr 122:951, 1950. (in German)

▶ psychotherapy

1046

Obermayer ME. **Functional factors in common dermatoses.** JAMA 122:862-864, 1943.

▶ psychotherapy, counseling

Extracted summary: In approaching the problem of functional disease, the physician must call on his store of patience, sympathy and tact. Once the suspicion is aroused that the patient's disorder may have a functional basis, every effort should be expended to gain his confidence so that the extent of the nervous disturbance may be determined. Treatment of a full blown neurosis or psychosis is distinctly the province of the psychiatrist, who alone has had the specific training and experience necessary to enable him to assume full responsibility for the patient with severe mental disease. Consequently common sense and discrimination must be exercised in deciding which patients must be referred directly to the psychiatrist and which ones will be suitable subjects for the relatively shallow psychotherapy which the practicing physician can administer along with his treatment of the cutaneous disorder. Fortunately the majority of patients with functional dermatoses have only mild emotional disturbances, which can be alleviated by the understanding and interested physician. Therapy of such disorders is not difficult, but not all physicians have the attributes which are essential for carrying it out successfully. Intelligent sympathy and understanding are the two prime requirements without which no physician can hope to carry out successful psychotherapy. A functional disease is a true disease; its symptoms are very real to the patient, and adopting the attitude that he is "not really sick" will vitiate any attempts to get at the underlying emotional problems. A sympathetic understanding implies not a "hand holding" point of view but a realization that the patient needs assistance in solving his difficulties.

1047

Preston K. **Depression and skin disease.** Med J Aust 1:326-329, 1969.

▶ psychotherapy

1. A series of 500 patients with psychosomatic skin disorders has been reviewed. 2. Over 40% of all patients show obvious features of depression, and a further 25% show masked depression. 3. The depression seen in these skin disorders is mild in type and often responds dramatically to treatment. Associated with this improvement is a more rapid resolution of the skin eruption. 4. If depression is looked for carefully in all cases of psychosomatic skin disorders, its true incidence will be realized. 5. As has been shown with other functional illnesses, depression may manifest under the guise of a skin disorder.

1048

Renshaw DC. **Sex and the dermatologist.** Int J Dermatol 19:469-471, 1980.

▶ counseling

Extracted summary: The dermatologist has a large "territory" to cover as a "body doctor." Adding the dimension of comfortable, appropriate sex education and discussion in the office may assist a patient, spouse and family to

benefit from the helpful studies of this decade in the frontiers of sexual medicine.

1049

Rogerson CH. **Psychological factors in skin diseases.** Practitioner 142:17-35, 1939.

▶ psychotherapy

The few examples which have been quoted may serve to illustrate some of the relationships which may exist in this field. As was stated at the beginning, skin lesions may be wholly determined by psychological difficulties or the psychological factors may play a contributory part in their origin. In other cases the lesion may arise from physical causes, and may then be used secondarily to serve a psychological end. With so many varieties of lesion and such varying relationships it must be clear that the sharp definition between organically-determined lesions and psychogenically-determined lesions cannot be upheld, nor is it reasonable to suppose that one set of constitutional factors can be at work in those patients with psychogenically-determined skin diseases. It is far more fruitful to study each individual case in order to learn what organic factors and what psychological factors are present and how important a part each is playing. When this has been done it becomes possible to compare groups of cases in which similar factors or similar lesions have been shown to occur.

1050

Russell BF. **Emotional factors in skin disease.** Br J Psychiatry 9:447-452, 1975.

▶ review: psychotherapy

Inherent personality difficulties and unsatisfactory interpersonal relationships are the basis on which psychogenic dermatoses develop. The majority fall within the designation "frictional dermatoses," being manually produced or aggravated. Such individuals tend to vent their aggression on themselves. In others emotional influences are shown as vasolability, sweating or horripilation. In skin diseases of the reactional type emotional influences represent only one of several influences which may activate or aggravate the skin condition. With an holistic approach, psychogenic factors need their due share of attention, side by side with genetic, infective, biochemical, toxic, allergic and other influences.

1051

Russell JD. **Psychosomatic aspects of dermatology.** Med J Aust 38:478-480, 1951.

▶ psychotherapy

Extracted summary: [T]he psychiatrist, with his awesome jargon and his air of mystery, has tended to deter the average medical practitioner from attempting to understand simple elucidations of personality and environmental stresses. However, the elements of the psychiatric approach can be learnt readily if one has sufficient interest and a real desire to understand, and is prepared to spend time listening to the patient. Under such circumstances it should rarely be necessary to refer your patients to a psychiatrist.

1052
Sack WT. **The method of research on psychogenic dermatoses.** Arch Dermatol Syph 154:410-420, 1928. (in German)

▶ psychotherapy, hypnosis, suggestion

The modern doctor must investigate the "hysterical nature" of a symptom along the difficult and thankless path which leads to the clearing up of the psychogenic mechanism of the symptom.

1053
Sack WT. **Psychotherapy and skin disease.** Dermatol Wochenschr 84:16-22, 1927. (in German: no English abstract).

▶ psychotherapy

1054
Sadger J. **Skin-, mucous membrane- and muscle eroticism.** Jahrb Psychoanal Psychopathol 3:525-556, 1912.

▶ psychotherapy

Case report of a young woman treated by analysing salient aspects of her childhood and, in particular, her relationship with her domineering mother.

1055
Schilder P. **Remarks on the psychology of the skin.** Psychoanal Rev 23:274-285, 1936.

▶ psychoanalysis

Extracted summary: Psychogenic manifestations on the skin have always a meaning. This meaning may be conscious, it may lie in a symbolic and instinctive sphere. There is no fundamental difference between a change imagined on the skin, between a merely so-called psychogenic manifestation, and a so-called organ neurosis. They are all centrifugal but reach the periphery, the organ as such. There are no emotions and imaginations which are merely psychic. The psyche is an organic agent. But there is no change in the body which does not reflect in the psychic attitudes. There exists only one organism and this is a psychophysical one.

1056
Schneider E. **Psychodynamics of chronic allergic eczema and chronic urticaria.** J Nerv Ment Dis 120:17-21, 1954.

▶ psychotherapy

That psychologic factors are of importance in the genesis and course of chronic allergic eczema and chronic urticaria is pretty much accepted by most investigators of these dermatoses. However, when it comes to the specific psychic factor or factors involved, there is hardly any agreement at all. As one reviews the literature there is scarcely a conflict experienced by man that has not in some way been implicated. Sadomasochism, exhibitionism, masturbatory guilt, sexual anxiety, repressed resentment, and many others have been delineated as a specific determinant. One reason for this is probably the fact that the more intensively a patient is studied the more one finds. The question to be answered is whether there is any specific dynamic factor or factors common to the disease process. Thus far there is no information on this point comparable to what we know, for example, about peptic ulcer or hypertension. My aim in this paper was to present some clinical material which indicates that there is a specific force involved, namely, anxiety and guilt connected with hostile aggressive impulses. Continued investigation will determine whether still more basic components are involved. Thus far it is interesting to note how an acute explosive psychic force is so intimately related to an acute explosive reaction in the skin.

1057
Scott MJ. **Hypnosis in dermatologic therapy.** Northwest Med 56:701-706, 1959.

▶ hypnosis

[P]hysicians will find hypnosis to be not a panacea, but a valuable adjunct to conventional dermatologic therapy in judiciously selected cases. Certain aspects of hypnosis still remain controversial and unexplained, a situation not unique in the field of medicine. Orientation in psychodynamics is a basic prerequisite for successful hypnotherapy and hypnosis can be abused if it is not individualized.

1058
Secter II, Barthelemy CG. **Angular cheilosis and psoriasis as psychosomatic manifestations.** Am J Clin Hypn 7:79-81, 1964.

▶ hypnosis, autohypnosis, suggestion

Extracted summary: When other bases for dermatological lesions do not seem to apply, the possibility of psychogenic origin may be considered. This case report also exemplifies the fact that many capable hypnotic subjects resent the idea of being hypnotized. This patient's personality needs obviously required that the situation remain in her control at all times.

1059
Seitz PFD. **An experimental approach to psychocutaneous problems.** J Invest Dermatol 13:199-205, 1949.

▶ psychotherapy, hypnosis, suggestion

An experimental method has been outlined for enlarging our knowledge and understanding of psychocutaneous reactions. Existing experimental approaches have been briefly and critically reviewed, and the present method is proposed as a further step toward objectifying and broadening psychosomatic dermatologic research. Perhaps needless to say, an experimental procedure of this type should be undertaken only by those physicians who are specially qualified in the psychiatric technics involved. The method consists of (1) psychiatric study of patients with non-dermatologic, psychosomatic disorders, during which the nature of the emotional conflict, as well as the psychodynamic meaning and purpose of the symptoms, are ascertained; (2) hypnotic substitution of various cutaneous phenomena for the original non-dermatologic symptom; and (3) correlation of information gained from (1) and (2). It has been possible to replace psychogenic chorea with circumscribed dermatitis and with blushing in this way, and to arrive at psychodynamic explanations for the success of these replacements.

1060
Seitz PFD, Gosman JS. **Can the dermatologist do psychotherapy?** Arch Dermatol Syph 66:180-190, 1952.

▶ supportive psychotherapy

We answer the question, "Can the dermatologist do psychotherapy?" with a qualified "Yes." The important qualifications which we attach to our affirmative answer are specified and illustrated. The qualifications for the dermatologist are that he must enjoy helping people, be able to sit quietly and listen comfortably, not become excessively anxious in doing this kind of work, be gratified and rewarded by his own life situation, and be relatively free from serious psychological problems in himself; he must have obtained training and supervision in dynamic psychiatry and psychotherapy. The qualifications for the patient are that his illness is not too long-standing; the past history is one of relatively good social, occupational, marital, and sexual adjustment, and his emotional conflicts are primarily current. The patient to be treated by the dermatologist must not have psychoses, severe neuroses, or psychopathic disorders; he must not have delusions of parasitosis, acrophobia, longstanding atopic dermatitis, anal and genital pruritus syndromes, or dermatitis herpetiformis. The qualifications for the psychotherapy are that it

consist in supportive methods which reinforce mature aspects of behavior, promote organization and harmony, and strengthen the forces of repression. It may provide mild ventilation and catharsis in connection with current conflicts; it must avoid penetrating, excavating, extensively cathartic, and uncovering methods. The physician should not strive primarily for insight.

1061
Sharlit H. **The impact of psychiatry on therapy in dermatology.** NY State J Med 50:1926-1928, 1950.

▶ psychotherapy, consultation-liaison

Extracted summary: Sufficiently convincing reports are already available in the literature to justify the conclusion that research clinics in dermatology must include a psychiatrist among their personnel. Psychosomatic studies are trying and time-consuming, and crucial to an ultimate appraisal of these psychosomatic studies on dermatologic cases will be the ingenuity used in the selection of cases for study and a proper interpretation of the clinical results. The laws of psychodynamics, say the psychiatrists, as implied earlier in this report, find clinical application, not alone to the obvious cases involving self-mutilation, admitted or denied, or cases of unknown etiology characterized by chronicity, but supposedly to such cases that involve known etiology but present persistence or repeated recurrences in spite of apparently adequate somatic therapy.

1062
Shorvon HJ, Rook AJ, Wilkinson DS. **Psychological treatment in skin disorders with special reference to abreactive techniques.** Br Med J 2:1300-1304, 1950.

▶ psychotherapy

The literature on the psychological aspects of skin conditions contains few references to treatment. The application of the abreactive technique in treatment of certain skin disorders is described, and an attempt has been made to define the criteria for its employment. Five illustrative cases are reported. The value and limitations of psychological methods of treatment are discussed, and it is suggested that the abreactive technique offers a practical and useful method of treatment.

1063
Silverman AJ. **Psychiatric factors in dermatologic disorders.** Am J Med Sci 226:104-110, 1953.

▶ review: hypnosis, suggestion, psychotherapy, consultation-liaison

Extracted summary: Thus, it is seen that many methods have been found to be efficacious. The dermatologist may find simple, reassuring supportive therapy to be quite valuable. More distressed patients will be referred to the psychiatrist to be evaluated for psychotherapy. A few startling cures by hypnosis are found. However, all are agreed that both disciplines should and must collaborate. Neither psyche nor soma should be ignored; the patient is regarded as a psychosomatic unit. Psychiatrist and dermatologist, working together in a well designed clinical and basic investigation, will do much to accelerate our acquisition of knowledge regarding the skin in sickness and health.

1064
Skalicanova M, Nagyova H, Kordova E. **Suggestive and group psychotherapy in some children's somatic diseases.** Cesk Psychiatr 73:174-177, 1977. (in Slovak)

▶ group therapy, suggestion, psychotherapy

Used suggestion and relaxing medication in group therapy in the treatment of 28 children (ages 8-14) with warts on hands and faces and 8 adolescents (ages 15-18) suffering from excessive hand sweating. Contrary to failure to achieve complete cure and frequent recidivism when treated by dermatology, the children with warts showed early and permanent remission of symptoms. Results of psychotherapy of excessive hand sweating were less favorable.

1065
Skryleva TN, Sharonov BG, Shevarova VN, Suvorova KN. **Late results of sanatorium-resort treatment of patients with eczematous diseases and psoriasis in Sochi.** Vestn Dermatol Venerol 11:60-62, 1982. (in Russian)

▶ milieu therapy

The immediate and late results of treatment of 44 patients with eczematous disease at the Sochi resort were studied. The effectiveness of the resort therapy was found to be much higher in those patients who had received active drug therapy immediately before going to the resort. The resort treatment exerts a favourable influence on the course of dermatoses prolonging the remission, decreasing the number and duration of exacerbations, and cases of temporary incapacity.

1066
Slany E. **Pediatric psychotherapy within the scope of dermatology.** Hautarzt 26:419-422, 1975. (in German)

▶ psychotherapy

The possibilities of psychotherapy of children with psychosomatic skin diseases on an outpatient basis are reported. Twenty children in their pre-school and school years were treated over a period of one to two years using

conversational therapy and the Sceno test (from G. v. Staabs). The results underline the necessity of identification and working up of conflicts in order to prevent recurrences or shifting of the disease.

1067
Slorach J. **Emotional aspects of skin disease.** Lancet 2:296, 1948. (letter)

▶ psychotherapy

1068
Smirnov LD, Golod ER. **Effectiveness of peloidotherapy in patients with some chronic dermatoses at the Saki resort.** Vestn Dermatol Venerol 45:71-74, 1971. (in Russian)

▶ milieu therapy

1069
Smith H. **The psychosomatic factor in dermatology.** Union Med Can 80:1399-1402, 1951. (in French: no English abstract)

▶ psychotherapy

1070
Sneddon IB. **The mind and the skin.** Br Med J 1:472-475, 1949.

▶ psychotherapy, reassurance

Extracted summary: The most important feature is to realize that the handling of the psychodermatoses differs in no way from that of other psychosomatic disease. These patients are constitutionally less able to face life's problems than the average run of humanity, and are not persons with only an inflamed patch of skin. A firm but kindly sympathetic approach is necessary, and it takes time to extract the life story and the salient problems which have led up to the onset of the dermatosis. It is impossible to gain the patients' confidence with other people—particularly relatives—present, and it may not be until the second or third interview that they will unburden themselves.

1071
Sokolianskii MN. **Results of suggestion therapy in treatment of certain dermatoses in a district hospital.** Vestn Dermatol Venerol January:83-84, 1974. (in Russian)

▶ hypnosis, suggestion

Hypno-suggestive therapy was given to 22 patients (13 with eczema, 4 with urticaria, 2 with psoriasis, 2 with herpes zoster, 1 with abundant loss of hair), aged from

20 to 47 years. In the majority of the patients favourable therapeutic effect was achieved.

1072
Steinhardt MJ. **The skin as an organ of expression of feelings: case presentation.** Ann Allergy 20:248-251, 1962.

▶ supportive psychotherapy

This case history is presented as an example of the psychophysiologic manifestation of certain types of dermatitis and urticaria. It also illustrates the multiplicity of factors such as foods, inhalants, drugs, infection, and emotional stress that are encountered in the etiologic study of urticaria. It also shows clearly the characteristic personality pattern and manner in which feelings seek expression through the skin. The patient's immature and infantile need to be loved and admired is shown by her excessive demands and narcissism. Her exhibitionism is evident from her flair for dramatics, her wish to entertain in grand style, and her striving for display (also the skin). There is another element present in her skin sensitivity and that is the erotic and sensuous pleasure derived from touching her skin. This is apparent from her predilection for the soft, luxurious, and refined, and her aversion for the coarse. There is also the feeling that she was wrongly treated in not possessing the wealth of her friends. She feels herself trapped and doomed to a life of penny-pinching by her husband's illness and lack of drive and ambition. She considers her husband's repeated attacks of coronary thrombosis as an attack against herself and against her rightful place in her social scheme. The hostility of the patient against her husband, family, and friends was evident during the interviews. Undoubtedly, the imposed social restraints and her resulting repressions made her direct her hostile feelings against herself by inflicting punishment upon her skin.

1073
Stokes JH. **Functional neuroses as complications of organic disease: an "office" technique of approach with special reference to the neurodermatoses.** JAMA 105:1007-1013, 1935.

▶ supportive psychotherapy, doctor-patient relationship, relaxation

Extracted summary: For the past fifteen years, a special interest in the functional neuroses and in behavior problems has led me to develop, from a variety of sources, a technic of "office" analysis and treatment of this now recognized element among the many causes of cutaneous disease. A sufficient number of patients have considered this feature of the management of their cases at my hands as an important element in their permanent recovery or satisfactory adjustment to encourage me to present the mode of approach for trial in cases in which circumstances do not permit or justify the calling of a neuropsychiatric consultation and special or sanatorium treatment. With apologies, under the pressure of condensation, a highly didactic form is used, without citation of case illustrations or discussion of percentage results.

1074
Stokes JH. **The personality factor in psychoneurogenous reactions of the skin.** Arch Dermatol Syph 42:780-801, 1940.

▶ psychotherapy, counseling, relaxation

It is hardly to be expected that the busy specialist will wish to apply even the simpler methods of office analysis by leads and catharsis described in my previous paper. It is possible, however, to draw up a species of general prescription for the psychoneurogenous phase of the eczema-asthma-hay fever person's difficulties and a similar set for those of the tension personality, and this I do in full awareness of the risk I run in offering ready-made solutions for such complex problems.

1075
Stokes JH. **The effect on the skin of emotional and nervous states (II): Masochism and other sex complexes in the background of neurogenous dermatoses.** Arch Dermatol Syph 22:803-810, 1930.

▶ psychotherapy

1. Three examples representing stages in complexity and in clarity of demonstration of a sexual psychosis as an element in the maintenance if not the actual origin of itching are offered. 2. In one of the cases, a masochistic-sadistic complex appeared to be superposed on a generalized dermatitis of apparently diathetic and focal infectious background (late eczematid of Rost). 3. In a second and more completely studied case, a substitution of scratch pleasure for sexual orgasm, possibly under a combination of hereditary predisposition with a mother-fixation inhibiting normal relief in marriage, was observed to constitute what Sack has described as a true onanistic equivalent—"cutaneous masturbation." No other explanation of the cutaneous picture, except a possible minor food allergy, could be identified despite the most searching and repeated investigation.

1076
Stokes JH. **Nervous and mental components in cutaneous diseases.** Penn Med J 35:229-233, 1932.

▶ supportive psychotherapy

Extracted summary: Inasmuch, then, as linkage between mental and nervous function and the actual cutaneous tissue lesion is still so largely intangible, and the action of emotional and nervous states so unweighable and untestable, it is essential that extraordinary caution be used in accepting a nervous cause for a cutaneous phenomenon. Just as "hunch" and intuitive dermatologic diagnosis, not based on reasoned analysis after painstaking observation of the physical lesion, is the weakest there is, so "hunch" tactics in the recognition and evaluation of a neurogenous component are the weakest there are. Refuse, therefore, to yield to the intrinsic lure of the mental side of a case. In the etiologic analysis, place the neurogenous inquiry among the last, covering all other possibilities first, but never omit it.

1077
Stokes JH, Pillsbury DM. **The effect on the skin of emotional and nervous states (III): Theoretical and practical consideration of a gastro-intestinal mechanism.** Arch Dermatol Syph 22:962-993, 1930.

▶ psychotherapy

Extracted summary: The larger our experience and the more careful our search, the more we are inclined to believe that in the urticarias and urticarial dermatitides of middle life, in the diathetic eczemas and rosacea, and even in dermatoses which, like epidermatophytosis, seem far removed from psychologic considerations, the tension make-up, the personality defect, the conflict and anxiety, the repression and the complex have their place as causal influences, to be sought out and rectified side by side with, and sometimes even before, the correction of the more apparent physical dysfunctions.

1078
Teichmann AT, Bosse K. **Skin disease and communication.** Hautarzt 25:427-429, 1974. (in German: no English abstract)

▶ psychotherapy

1079
Thoma H. **Psychotherapy in dermatology.** Arztl Fortbild 16:97-101, 1968. (in German: no English abstract)

▶ psychotherapy

1080
Tobia L. **Hypnosis in dermatology.** Minerva Med 73:531-537, 1982. (in Italian)

▶ hypnosis

Skin diseases rarely present serious clinical diagnostic problems for the specialist. All too frequently, however, they are impossible to diagnose aetiologically, since so many are of psychosomatic origin. In the light of the close relationship between skin and nervous system, the neurophysiological and neuropsychological mechanisms forming the basis of the most commonly encountered dermatological somatizations are described.

1081
Van Moffaert M. **Psychosomatics for the practising dermatologist.** Dermatologica 165:73-87, 1982.

▶ review: psychotherapy, doctor-patient relationship, consultation-liaison

Extracted summary: [The] practical view on psychodermatology, as explained in this paper, is based on 10 years of close collaboration with the dermatologists of the University Dermatology Department. It aims at establishing a feasible psychosomatic approach for the practising dermatologist who has neither the facilities for easily accessible consultation-liaison psychiatry, nor the desire to turn his/her practice into a psychotherapeutic setting.

1082
Van Moffaert M. **The importance of permanent psychiatric consulting in the dermatologist clinic.** Arch Belg Dermatol 30:215-220, 1974.

▶ consultation-liaison, psychotherapy, behavior therapy

The need for a permanent psychiatric consultant in the department of dermatology is put forward on the basis of the undeniable influence of mental stress in general on the cause and the treatment of certain dermatological diseases. With artefacts, psychogenic itching, alopecia and certain psychosomatic diseases a complementary therapy has been realised by a combined dermatological and psychiatric approach.

1083
Van Moffaert M. **Psychiatric consultation in the dermatology clinic.** Tijdschr Geneeskd 31:587-595, 1975. (in Dutch)

▶ psychotherapy, consultation-liaison

One hundred patients under treatment in the department of dermatology were referred to the psychiatric clinic for a variety of reasons. The indications were mainly the simultaneous existence of a skin disease and a psychiatric clinical picture, skin complaints without any organic disorder, artefacts, and skin diseases that no longer reacted to any classical therapy. We have tried to classify these heterogeneous cases which presented a great variety of dermatological affections and psychiatric problems. The tentative conclusions from our study are that psychic stress can have a strong impact on the development and the relapse of skin diseases. It appears that the cooperation between dermatologist and psychiatrist is particularly indicated for the treatment of psychogenic itching, alopecia and automutilation.

1084
Vogel PG, Beckmann H. **Psychotherapy and psychopharmacotherapy in dermatology: psychotherapeutic aspects and indications.** Hautarzt 27:519-524, 1976. (in German)

▶ psychotherapy

Different dermatoses, known as psychodermatoses, are classified into psychodynamic and psychopathological aspects. The symptoms are differentiated in: psychosomatic-, psychotic-, hiding a psychoneurosis, psychovegetative- and secondary symptom. The only and important instrument for diagnosis is the interview. An example of a patient with chronic urticaria is given. The differentiation is important to indicate the therapy: psychotherapy or psychopharmacological therapy.

1085
Volkmann H, Eissing KW. **Contributions to psychotherapy of skin diseases.** Dtsch Militararzt 7:314-318, 1942. (in German)

▶ psychotherapy

1086
Walsh MN, Kierland RR. **Minor psychotherapy in dermatology.** Mod Med 123:123-125, 1950.

▶ psychotherapy, counseling, suggestion

Extracted summary: Every practitioner must be prepared to administer minor psychotherapy, and he should familiarize himself with the fundamentals of psychodynamics and the technics of minor psychotherapy. The methods of minor psychotherapy are calculated to relieve the patient from the emotional load of his unresolved conflicts. Everything the physician says or does within sight or hearing of the patient, or that he does to or for the patient, constitutes psychotherapy, which may be good or bad to the extent that it relieves the patient's anxiety or adds to it. Reassurance is one of the most widely employed psychotherapeutic methods, while suggestion therapy and technics of removal of external strain, the provision of guidance and advice, the giving of information, the fostering of socialized living, persuasion, and reeducation all have influence. For some patients, confession and ventilation may be employed cautiously, so that the patient may put his problems into words and thus crystallize his attitudes. This procedure when done too early or too rapidly may result in an exacerbation of the cutaneous disorder. When done cautiously, repeated confession and ventilation may desensitize the patient to sensitive stresses and conflicts.

1087
Weissberg G. **Practical aspects of psychosomatic dermatology.** NY St J Med 61:2420-2427, 1961.

▶ doctor-patient relationship, counseling

In summary, I should like to say that in spite of the various difficulties encountered, a psychosomatic orientation is helpful in the diagnosis and management of patients. This approach requires time, a certain amount of intuition, and curiosity in what is going on beneath the skin of the patient. It also requires caution, the ability to listen rather than to talk, and the foresight to think twice before asking or answering questions. There will be disappointments, but they will be outweighed by added gratifications.

1088
Whitlock FA. **Skin disorders and the mind.** Australas J Dermatol 14:5-10, 1973.

▶ psychotherapy

Extracted summary: One word of caution needs to be said before concluding. Too often it is assumed that manifestations of emotional disturbance in the course of a skin condition require that the patient should be treated by psychological techniques. Nothing in fact could be further from the truth. My definition implies that the aetiology of psychosomatic disorders is multiple and that excessive concentration on one aetiological variable to the exclusion of others does the patient no great benefit. The judicious combination of dermatological and psychological treatment seems to be ideal and to be aimed at and it would be a great mistake to assume that the matter can be left in the hands of the psychiatrist while the patient's external or internal treatment by applications or drugs can be left in abeyance. To put the matter more succinctly, in the words of an anonymous writer, "Have faith in the Lord but use sulphur for the itch."

1089
Wittkower E. **Psychiatry and the skin.** Proc R Soc Med 43:799-801, 1950.

▶ psychotherapy

In all, 74 patients, suffering from the four skin diseases discussed, were treated by psychotherapy. The treatment was carried out along analytical lines similar to the principles laid down in Felix Deutsch's "Applied Psycho-Analysis." The psychotherapist concentrated on those aspects of the personality which were regarded as essential for the symptom formation. 60 out of the 74 patients taken on for treatment have benefited by it. 52 of the 60 sucessfully treated patients could be followed up, at least three months after termination of treatment. Of these 35 had maintained their improvement or had continued to improve. Of the four skin diseases discussed, rosacea responded best and pruritus ani worst, to brief psychotherapy.

1090

Wittkower ED. **Psychological aspects of skin disease: I, Seborrhoeic Dermatitis: II, Psoriasis: III, Pompholyx.** Bull Menninger Clin 11:148-176, 1947.

▶ psychotherapy

Extracted summary: Pompholyx was considered as a neurosis by Tilbury Fox who first described it in 1873. Since then it has been the subject of much study. More recently the original idea that pompholyx is a psychosomatic disorder has gained ground.

1091

Wittkower ED. **Skin and psyche.** Urol Cut Rev 56:94-98, 1952.

▶ psychotherapy

In all, 74 patients suffering from the four skin diseases discussed were treated by psychotherapy. Many others had to be rejected for a variety of reasons: because the patients were either too old or too young, of too low intelligence, or unable to attend regularly because their illness was of very long standing or because no clear psychosomatic connection could be established. In some cases it was felt that in view of the compromise function of the skin symptom the patients were psychologically better off with their skin malady than without it. Owing to the set-up of the unit, only brief treatment could be offered to our patients. The treatment was carried out along analytical lines similar to the principles laid down in Felix Deutsch's "Applied Psychoanalysis." The psychotherapist concentrated on those aspects of the personality which were regarded as essential for the symptom formation. The patients attended the outpatient department once or twice a week and were asked to lie down on a couch and to associate freely; but no attempt was made to go into the intricacies of their personality deviations. In a few patients group therapy was used: in only two ECT was regarded as indicated. The results obtained were fairly satisfactory. Sixty patients out of the 74 patients taken on for treatment were benefited by it. It was possible to recall 52 of the 60 successfully treated patients for a follow-up by a dermatologist, at least three months after termination of treatment. Of these 35 had maintained their improvement or had continued to improve, while 17 had relapsed. Of the four skin diseases discussed, rosacea responded best and pruritus ani worst—for obvious reasons—to brief psychotherapy.

1092

Wright CS. **Therapy of psychosomatic dermatoses.** Arch Dermatol Syph 60:303-306, 1949.

▶ psychotherapy

Extracted summary: When psychotherapy is introduced in the treatment of cutaneous conditions, efforts to treat the skin itself are being relaxed and a new element is introduced for the discovery of precipitating factors; this procedure doubtless often makes a contribution toward correction of the underlying exhaustion. One does not then rely so much on drugs and other treatments applied to the skin, but thoughts of physician and patient are turned toward the mental irritations which may be finding their way to the skin either through the phenomenon of conversion involving symbolization or through well known pathways of the autonomic nervous system to pervert circulation, glandular activity or both, or to cause trophic changes. If the physician looks sympathetically and helpfully for nervousness as an etiologic factor, the patient will generally help and with each visit will bring added information or clues as to the relation of emotional distress and symptoms. The psychiatrist has found that time to allow for reorientation in thinking is important and that a speedy solution to emotional problems is infrequent. Hence, there is no reason to be discouraged with psychotherapy because it does not remove the patient's symptoms immediately. Dermatology and psychiatry may seem to be widely separated specialties, but they have in common a few acute manifestations of symptoms and many chronic ones which yield slowly to therapy.

1093

Wright CS. **Psychosomatic factors in dermatology.** South Med J 42:951-958, 1949.

▶ psychotherapy, consultation-liaison

The theory of "psychosomatic medicine" is being increasingly accepted by the dermatologist. A chart is presented indicating those dermatoses that may be considered as pure psychoses, those in which the psychic and somatic factor vary in predominance and those in which a psychic factor may be present but is questionable. The type of therapy chosen depends upon the degree of mental affection. Some cases require only the psychiatrist once the diagnosis is made; some require collaboration between the dermatologist and psychiatrist; and some the dermatologist is capable of handling alone. I make a plea for greater collaboration between the specialties of dermatology and psychiatry in the management of the dermatoses recognized to have both a psychic and somatic factor.

1094

Wright CS. **Psychosomatic aspects of dermatoses.** Clinics 3:711-727, 1944.

▶ psychotherapy, relaxation, consultation-liaison

Numerous dermatoses have their origin in a psychic disturbance. Others are due to a combination of psychic and somatic causes and the dermatologist who fails to take both into consideration may fail to benefit the patient. An attitude of sympathy and understanding toward the patient who has a psychic disturbance whether it be the cause or result of a dermatosis is most important. The present textbook classification of dermatologic neurosis is unsatisfactory and requires further study and review. Closer cooperation between the dermatologist and the psychiatrist such as exists between the dermatologist and the allergist should be helpful in solving many dermatologic neuroses, and perhaps lead to a more workable classification.

1095

Zaidens SH. **Dermatologic hypochondriasis: a form of schizophrenia.** Psychosom Med 12:243-253, 1950.

▶ supportive psychotherapy

Dermatologic hypochondriasis is an acute recurrent anxiety state occurring in some latent schizophrenic patients. It may be precipitated by acne vulgaris, hypertrichosis, seborrhea of the scalp, or other cutaneous changes. Investigation of the 11 patients included in this report elicited a history of latent schizophrenia prior to the dermatologic disturbance plus hereditary and constitutional factors frequently associated with schizophrenic syndrome. The acute anxiety state resulted from two related sources: loss of status through threatened or marred attractiveness; and inability to compete along any other level of adaptation. Treatment consists of dermatologic correction in addition to protection and supportive type of psychotherapy.

Other Skin Disorders

1096

Albrecht K. **Hysterical skin gangrenes.** Arch Psychiatr Nervenkr 64:544-569, 1921-1922. (in German)

▶ psychotherapy

Skin gangrenes often appear in hysterical patients; some consider them to be spontaneous, others to be artificial. The clinical picture of the disease is the same for both the artificial and the spontaneous skin gangrene. The symptoms and affectations may take place over a period of many years—hence it is difficult for the physician to form a complete picture.

1097

Arone di Bertolino R. **Hypnotherapy in a girl, 22 months old, with molluscum contagiosum.** Minerva Med 72:1213-1215, 1981. (in Italian)

▶ hypnosis

The practice and informing theories of hypnositherapy, successfully adopted in a case of molluscum contagiosum in a girl of 22 months, are reported.

1098

Arone di Bertolino R. **Psychotherapy of molluscum contagiosum in children.** Minerva Med 73:1849-1851, 1982. (in Italian)

▶ psychotherapy

The psychotherapeutic technique successfully used in the treatment of 8 cases of molluscum contagiosum is described. A special technique for implanting ideas in the minds of children under four, which may be extended to the treatment of other conditions, is described with comments.

1099

Baron C. **The skin as an organ of expression.** Ky Med J 47:192, 1949. (case report)

▶ psychotherapy

1100

Barragan M. **Towards effective treatment in child psychiatry.** Neurol Neurocir Psiquiatr 17:69-82, 1976. (in Spanish)

▶ psychoanalysis

The author suggests that psychoanalytic theory, developmental theories and family dynamics theories are insufficient to allow for a comprehensive treatment of children. Adding elements of systems theory, he proposes that in every case, individual, familial and ecological factors be devised to solve problems in each area. He illustrates the approach with the clinical report of a successfully treated case of vitiligo.

1101

Bettley FR. **Ichthyosis and hypnosis.** Br Med J 2:615, 1952. (letter)

▶ hypnosis

1102

Carr EG, McDowell JJ. **Social control of self-injurious behavior of organic etiology.** Behav Ther 11:402-409, 1980.

▶ reinforcement, time-out

Treated the self-injurious scratching behavior of a normal 10-yr-old boy using a combination of time-out for scratching and tangible reinforcement for reductions in the number of body sores. The efficacy of this treatment was demonstrated using a reversal design. At 9-mo follow-up the number of body sores was negligible. Although the scratching was initially elicited by organic factors (contact dermatitis), analysis suggested that the behavior was influenced by social reinforcement. These data support the general principle that many problems that have an organic etiology may acquire operant characteristics and become amenable to behavioral intervention.

1103

Cataldo MF, Varni JW, Russo DC, Estes SA. **Behavior therapy techniques in treatment of exfoliative dermatitis.** Arch Dermatol 116:919-922, 1980.

▶ behavior therapy

We report here a case study in which behavior therapy techniques were used to treat the persistent and severe scratching of a patient with long-standing exfoliative dermatitis. A multiple-baseline clinical design across different body areas was used to evaluate the behavioral treatment program. This program consisted of (1) training the patient to monitor his scratching behavior and to use an incompatible response and distraction procedure contingent on the occurrence of scratching, and (2) differential attention by the therapist, so that the therapist's attention was contingent on intervals of nonscratching, and the therapist ignored the patient when he did scratch. The results indicated that the program was effective in almost completely eliminating scratching when a variety of therapists were and were not present. This suggests that the procedures used might easily be taught to the nursing staff.

1104

Cormia FE, Slight D. **Psychogenic factors in dermatoses.** Can Med Assoc J 33:527-530, 1935.

▶ psychotherapy

1. An ill-defined eruption of long standing proved to be the result of emotional conflict. 2. The diagnosis was confirmed by the rapid involution of lesions when the limbs were protected from excoriation. 3. The patient was of a masochistic type and obtained relief of sexual tension through excoriation, thus producing lesions which resisted all forms of local treatment, and on which various diagnoses had been made, including that of "tuberculosis of the skin." 4. The case illustrates the fact that sexual tension may be relieved through an extragenital mechanism.

1105

Fleischer D. **Psychotherapy of disorder of the skin, probably lupus erythematosus.** Ned Tijdschr Geneeskd 85:566-567, 1941. (in Dutch)

▶ psychotherapy

In a case of skin affection of the nose, probably lupus erythematodes, a connection with an unconscious inferior sexual desire could be proved. With the aid of psychoanalysis the desire could be overcome, after which the skin affection disappeared in 8 days.

1106

Freeman J. **Ichthyosis and hypnosis.** Br Med J 2:615, 1952. (letter)

▶ hypnosis

1107

Gajwani AK, Sehgal VN. **Hypnosis: a new therapeutic approach in vitiligo.** Cutis 14:572-573, 1974.

▶ hypnosis

The present case brings our attention to psychosomatic factors which may be operating in such cases of vitiligo areata. Such factors have often been incriminated in this disease though no particular personality patterns are described. The fact that psychotherapeutic procedure has resulted in successful repigmentation of vitiliginous spots, further reaffirms that the psyche plays a decisive role in precipitation of vitiligo. Furthermore, as it is a well documented fact that all vitiligo patients do not respond to photosensitizers, we feel the need of an alternative procedure and psychological intervention in such cases is recommended for further trials.

1108

Gibbs DN. **Reciprocal inhibition therapy of a case of symptomatic erythema.** Behav Res Ther 2:261-266, 1965.

▶ reciprocal inhibition

Treatment by reciprocal inhibition of the infrequently reported condition of symptomatic erythema is described. Diagnosis and interpretation of the social learning of the symptoms, and the rationale and procedures, are given. An evaluation of the therapy is made.

1109

Gotz H. **Suggestive management of onychomycoses?.** Dtsch Med Wochenschr 94:1136, 1969. (in German: no English abstract)

▶ suggestion

1110

Hornstein OP. **Development of the psychosomatic concept of perioral dermatitis.** Z Psychosom Med Psychoanal 22:93-98, 1976. (in German)

▶ psychoanalysis, psychotherapy

In recent years, "perioral dermatitis" though practically unknown in the past, has been observed rather frequently in female patients. It has proven remarkably refractory against external dermatotherapy, and numerous attempts to analyse the causality have failed. However, we very often noted certain characteristics of personality structure and social attitude in the patients afflicted with the disease. Both clinical findings and various signs of vegetative dystonia suggested psychoneurotic rather than purely somatic causes. We therefore set about to elucidate the psychic and other clinical symptoms of our patients in cooperation with a psychoanalyst and a clinical psychologist. Throughout a period of several years, this interdisciplinary teamwork helped us develop biographically and psychoanalytically oriented case studies in so-called Balint seminars. We thereby gained a better understanding of the psychodynamics in each of our cases, which enabled us to treat the disease successfully. We consider "perioral dermatitis" a primarily psychosomatic disorder which, in most cases, responds well to short-term psychotherapy. Other findings reported in dermatological literature are controversial as to their causal interpretation, even when assuming an origin by infecting microbes. We regard bacterial and other findings as sequelae which may give rise to clinical exacerbation, yet not as genuine causes of the disease. Our conception is strongly supported by the success of psychotherapy, through which the symptomatic tetracyclin and/or corticosteroid treatment has been rendered superflous.

1111
Ikemi Y, Nakagawa S. **A psychosomatic study of contagious dermatitis.** J Med Sci 13:335-352, 1962.

▶ suggestion

We have experimentally proven the definite effect of psychological factors, especially the influence of auto-suggestion, upon the development of contagious dermatitis. From the results of our experiment, it seems to be possible to resolve some problems of this condition which were not explainable from the purely physiological standpoint.

1112
Jabush M. **A case of chronic recurring multiple boils treated with hypnotherapy.** Psychiatr Q 43:448-455, 1969.

▶ hypnosis, autohypnosis, psychotherapy, imagery

Extracted summary: Would not similar improvement have occurred in this case without hypnotherapy? One can only speculate. However, it appears that the interpolative techniques involving sensory imagery, coupled with intensification of previous ego-exhilarative affect catalyzed by a heightened positive transference generated by the hypnotic relationship, contributed to a "desensitization" process wherein the rigid and chronic behavioral response of the psyche-skin interaction was altered.

1113
Kartamischew AJ. **A case of arsphenamine dermatitis healed by hypnosis.** Arch Dermatol Syph 174:36-37, 1936. (in German)

▶ hypnosis, suggestion

Before injections of salvarsan [for syphilis] the patient was subjected to a hypnotic "seance" and given the suggestion that the injection would proceed without complications, and the patient would smell no bad odor (patient complained earlier of a bad smell during the injection); the same treatment was continued with positive results.

1114
Kartamischew AJ. **Treatment of lichen ruber planus by means of hypnosis.** Dermatol Wochenschr 96:788-791, 1933. (in German: no English abstract)

▶ hypnosis

1115
Kidd C. **Congenital ichthyosiform erythroderma treated by hypnosis.** Br J Dermatol 78:101-105, 1966.

▶ hypnosis, suggestion

Since Bernheim (1889), workers using techniques of suggestion with or without hypnosis have reported remissions in certain skin diseases. The actual mechanisms underlying this process are ill-understood, though it is presumed that the effect of suggestion on the patient activates the nervous system and allows complex physiological adjustments to take place. It is easy to understand that psychological methods may be successful in the treatment of skin diseases initiated or maintained by a combination of psychological and organic factors. It is less easy to understand how a congenital and hereditary organic condition such as ichthyosiform erythroderma can be so spectacularly affected by a psychological process. The experience of the two patients here described provides some considerations in this respect.

1116
Krantz W. **Are mollusca contagiosa susceptible to suggestive treatment?** Dermatol Wochenschr 120:311, 1949. (in German)

▶ suggestion

1117
Latimer PR. **The behavioral treatment of self-excoriation in a twelve-year-old girl.** J Behav Ther Exp Psychiatry 10:349-352, 1979.

▶ behavior modification, behavioral analysis

Presents a case study of a 12-yr-old girl in whom self-excoriation began 6 yrs prior to treatment in association with a superficial dermatitis secondary to a dog bite. The maladaptive scratching and picking were maintained primarily by the attention and concern of the parents who were otherwise shy and undemonstrative. Behavioral treatment, centering on reinforcing desirable behavior and noncritical communication, was successful. The importance of a complete behavior analysis in selecting and directing several discrete interventions is emphasized.

1118
Lerer B, Jacobowitz J. **Treatment of essential hyperhidrosis by psychotherapy.** Psychosomatics 22:536-538, 1981.

▶ psychotherapy

This report illustrates the potential amenability of certain cases of essential hyperhidrosis to psychotherapeutic intervention. It also demonstrates the wealth of dynamic understanding concerning the nature of the disorder and the conflicts underlying it that can be derived from such an approach. We recommend such intervention for hyperhidrotic patients who meet the criteria for psychotherapy in terms of motivation and capacity for insight.

1119
Lorand S. **The psychogenic factors in a case of angioneurotic edema.** J Mt Sinai Hosp 2:231-236, 1936.

▶ psychotherapy

Extracted summary: One can only speculate as to why in this case the symptom of angioneurotic edema was chosen to express psychological conflicts, aggressions, and resentments. One may also speculate about the erotization of the skin, which in this case may not be much of a mystery as [the patient] was very much concerned about her complexion and highly attentive to her face and other parts of her body, being easily alarmed by the slightest appearance of pimples ... It should be emphasized that the structure of the several psychological mechanisms which were found responsible for the symptoms in this case is not presented here as typifying all cases of angioneurotic edema, not even a group of cases. It is found to be true in the case presented here. Its discovery made possible a therapeutic approach rewarded by apparently good results.

1120
Malament IB, Dunn ME, Davis R. **Pressure sores: an operant conditioning approach to prevention.** Arch Phys Med Rehabil 56:161-165, 1975.

▶ operant conditioning

A training system for the prevention of pressure sores has been designed to teach the paralytic person to relieve pressure intermittently from his ischium while sitting in a wheelchair. The system automates the training of wheelchair pushups, and conditions the person into exercising, based upon modified avoidance learning procedures. Results indicate that the paralytic person can be trained to pushup intermittently and efficiently using this system,

thus reducing the incidence of pressure sore formation. Further long-term study is needed to assess the effectiveness of the training system as a preventative program for pressure sores.

1121
Mason AA. **A case of congenital ichthyosiform erythroderma of Brocq treated by hypnosis.** Br Med J 2:422-423, 1952.

▶ hypnosis

From this response to hypnosis one of two inferences may be drawn. Either there is a hitherto unsuspected psychic factor in the aetiology of the disease or this is a case of a congenital organic condition being affected by a psychological process. A combination of both these factors is of course a third possibility. Whichever is true, the improvement in this case seems to be totally unprecedented, and was effected after the failure of all recognized methods of treatment.

1122
Mason AA. **Ichthyosis and hypnosis.** Br Med J 2:57-58, 1955. (letter)

▶ hypnosis

1123
Mullins JF, Murray N, Shapiro EM. **Pachyonychia congenita: a review and new approach to treatment.** Arch Dermatol 71:265-268, 1955.

▶ review: hypnosis, suggestion, psychotherapy

The treatment of pachyonychia congenita as reported in the English language is reviewed, and a case of pachyonychia congenita in a 13-year-old boy is reported. The case was treated by suggestive therapy with improvement after failure with the more conservative methods of therapy.

1124
Musaph H, Molhuysen-van der Walle SMC, Barendregt JT. **Bullosis psychogenica and epidermolysis bullosa.** Psychosom Med 19:30-37, 1957.

▶ psychotherapy

Extracted summary: [In the case described] it is obvious that psychotherapy has not cured the anxiety hysterical neurosis, nevertheless the freeing of symptoms has been accomplished by stimulating the ego to become strengthened and the super-ego to become more tolerant. For the patient this means a socialization which increases the possibility of further growth of personality.

1125

Pearson GHJ. **Some psychological aspects of inflammatory skin lesions.** Psychosom Med 2:22-33, 1940.

▶ psychotherapy

Two cases are reported in which the patients irritated and injured inflammatory lesions of the skin. Their behavior to their skin lesions was a form of childish autoerotism to which they turned because they found it impossible to have adequate emotional reactions and social relationships in their real life. Their inability to react adequately emotionally was due to fear; in one case largely a real fear of the consequences of any reaction because of an over-restricted environment, in the other, because of a fear of the superego. One case is presented in which the patient solved her emotional difficulties by converting the emotional problem into an itching painful skin lesion. She had conflict between her desire to leave home and accomplish her desires, and her fear of her superego which was based on fear of social disapproval and a childish fear of her mother. The solution of the emotional problems enabled the two first patients to cease their irrational behavior toward their skin lesions and cured the skin lesions of the third patient.

1126

Robertson IM, Jordan JM, Whitlock FA. **Emotions and skin (II): The conditioning of scratch responses in cases of lichen simplex.** Br J Dermatol 92:407-412, 1975.

▶ conditioning, extinction

Lichen simplex is generally regarded as a condition initiated and perpetuated by scratching and emotional tension. It was felt that the scratching might partly be a conditional response to itching and other signals, and that feelings of guilt, anxiety and hostility would be prominent features in these patients. Conditioning experiments designed to establish scratch responses to an itch stimulus (ICS) and a tone (CS) showed that lichen simplex patients conditioned more readily and extinguished more slowly than controls. These findings were more marked when the itch stimulus was applied to affected as compared with normal skin. It was not possible to distinguish differences in the psychological tests between patients and controls. The possible significance of these findings is discussed.

1127

Ryzhkova EI, Liagushkina MP. **Comprehensive therapy of rosacea (a clinical and morphological study).** Vestn Dermatol Venerol June:16-22, 1978. (in Russian)

▶ psychotherapy

1128

Schneck JM. **Ichthyosis treated with hypnosis.** Dis Nerv Syst 15:211-214, 1954.

▶ hypnosis

Extracted summary: A thirty-three year old patient with life-long ichthyosis showing consistent, repetitive, seasonal variations, was treated with hypnotic techniques. He demonstrated a comparative over-all improvement of forty to forty-five per cent counterbalancing maximum seasonal scaling. There were specific points of interest in connection with his improvement and many questions to be answered in relation to the significance of the results for this case and others, and for possible future clinical and experimental investigations.

1129

Schur M. **Chronic, exudative, discoid and lichenoid dermatitis (Sulzberger-Garbe's syndrome): case analysis.** Int J Psychoanal 31:73-77, 1950.

▶ psychoanalysis

Extracted summary: 1) [T]he method applied by me of relying mainly on analysis of representative cases of an entity, proved to be fruitful. It is being applied to other—and should be to all—dermatological entities, and beyond that, to any so-called psychosomatic syndrome. It will teach us more than statistics based on generalization can do. 2) For what I believe to be the first time a big incurable dermatological entity of unknown origin could be explained as the dermatological manifestation of a neurosis and treated successfully by psycho-analysis. 3) The concept of the defence mechanism of magic sacrifice seems to be of particular importance in certain psychosomatic disorders.

1130

Stokes JH, Beerman H. **Effect on the skin of emotional and nervous states (IV): The rosacea complex.** Arch Dermatol Syph 26:478-494, 1932.

▶ psychotherapy

Extracted summary: The therapy of rosacea would seem to follow rational lines when it includes (1) adjustment of neurogenous background; (2) correction of the gastro-intestinal phase thus, and by the free administration of hydrochloric acid and calcium and the sharp and lasting restriction of carbohydrates plus the encouragement of acidophilic intestinal flora; (3) elimination of caffeine, hot and spiced foods, alcohol and the gobbling of food; (4) roentgen and topical applications for the seborrheic phase, with special attention to the often neglected scalp, on which the x-rays may be rather freely used, and (5) attention to allergic susceptibilities including especially local contacts (cosmetics, etc.). Relapse most frequently follows, in our experience, (1) failure or inability to correct the neurogenous substrate; (2) indulgence in carbohydrate, and (3) neglect of the acid-calcium regimen.

1131
Thurn A. **Psychogenic aspects of perioral dermatitis.** Z Psychosom Med Psychoanal 22:99-109, 1976. (in German)

▶ psychotherapy, group therapy

A report has been given how patterns of diagnosis contributed by a Balint group led to a better understanding of patients afflicted with perioral dermatitis. The interaction between internalized and unconscious conflicts and specific, actual conflict situations has been elucidated. Various factors of individual biography and contemporary history were seen to play concurrent roles. In agreement with the results of psychological testing, certain personality attributes were observed, which manifested themselves in two types, i.e., a rather passive and a more active one. This is important for the prognosis, because of the correlations existing between personality attributes, the gravity of the disease and success in therapy.

1132
Twerski AJ, Naar R. **Hypnotherapy in a case of refractory dermatitis.** Am J Clin Hypn 16:202-205, 1974.

▶ hypnosis, autohypnosis, psychotherapy

Extracted summary: An important component of the conflict involving anger toward a parent is the fear of rejection by the parent as a result of the hostile feelings. It is therefore possible that an intense unconscious identification with the parent might serve as a defense against separation anxiety. It is further possible that to the unconscious, which is timeless, the immersion in sea water is equivalent to envelopment in amniotic fluid and consequently represents a total inclusion of the individual within the mother. The latter "experience," although never coming to awareness, could be most effective in combatting the separation anxieties resulting from the existence of hostile feelings toward the mother. In his fanciful work "Thalassa," Ferenczi (1938) cites psychoanalytic evidence for the unconscious equation of the amniotic environment with the sea. The patient's interesting reference to a dominating maternal figure as "she gets under my skin," may indicate that her initial mechanism of dealing with the separation anxiety was via a different type of identification, i.e., one wherein mother was incorporated within the patient. The scratching would be a symbolic aggressive act toward the incorporated mother. The ocean bathing would then be seen as accomplishing the goal of identifying and becoming inseparable from mother by an exact reversal of the process, i.e., the patient becoming incorporated within the mother. The latter process eliminated the irritant from within the

patient, removed the aggressive target, and accorded the patient the security against separation, which then allowed her to deal more realistically with her hostile feelings. The explanation for the dramatic recovery must remain hypothetical. About all we can safely conclude is that the direct contact of the ocean water with her skin, as a chemical therapy, was obviously not operative. This case stimulates speculation into the salutory effects of mineral baths and other types of hydrotherapies which have shown beneficial results, as well as the various immersion rituals prevalent in many cultures since time immemorial.

1133
Volmat R, Laugier P, Allers G, Ellena V, Vittouris N, Barale T. **Palmar dyshidrosis, resistant to dermatologic therapy, disappearing after 2 nondirective psychotherapeutic consultations.** Bull Soc Fr Dermatol Syphiligr 75:667-670, 1968. (in French: no English abstract)

▶ psychotherapy

1134
Wilsch L, Hornstein OP. **Statistical investigations and therapy results in perioral dermatitis.** Z Psychosom Med Psychoanal 22:115-125, 1976. (in German)

▶ psychotherapy

Presents data on 279 patients treated for perioral dermatitis at a university hospital. With the exception of 2 men and a 5-yr-old girl, all were adult females, most of them 25-39 yrs old. Prior to admission for treatment, the disease had been apparent for longer than 1 yr in 45% of the Ss. Prior unsuccessful treatment with corticosteroids was reported by 72% of the Ss; 22% had suffered steroid damage. Sleep disorders, headaches, constipation, excessive perspiration, and other vegetative nervous system symptoms were reported in 90% of the cases. Compared to other groups of patients in the same hospital, Ss tended to have more education and higher professional or occupational positions. Treatment by local dermatica (free of corticosteroids) and psychotherapy resulted in a complete recovery from the target skin disorder in 90%. The recovery occurred later in those without than in those with other vegetative symptoms, possibly because the latter group could more easily somatize their still partly unresolved internal conflicts in the other symptoms.

1135
Wink CAS. **Congenital ichthyosiform erythroderma treated by hypnosis.** Br Med J 2:741-743, 1961.

▶ hypnosis

Extracted summary: In the two cases described ... it seemed unlikely that there was a psychological factor in the aetiology, and both showed some definite conformity to the suggestions, though this conformity was not exact, for the response included improvement extending outside the designated areas, and a relative failure in other areas which were intended to respond. Finally, though there was a mild improvement in undesignated areas, it was quite overshadowed by the changes in those intended to benefit.

1136
Wink CAS. **A case of Darier's disease treated by hypnotic age regression.** Am J Clin Hypn 9:146-150, 1966.

▶ hypnosis, suggestion

Darier's disease is very briefly described and the possible role of Vitamin A in its treatment is mentioned. A single case and its response to five different therapeutic approaches are the subject of this paper. A surprising result is reported when hypnotic age regression is used. The limitations of this study are pointed out and no conclusions are offered.

1137
Wittkower E, MacKenna RMB. **The psychological aspects of seborrhoeic dermatitis.** Br J Dermatol Syph 59:281-293, 1947.

▶ psychotherapy

Extracted summary: It looks as if the seborrhoeic patient does not only feel ostracized because of his skin affection, but that he is prone to develop his skin affection because he feels—and has always felt—ostracized. The malady disturbs the social relationships of the patient still further, and relegates him in many cases to the position of a pariah. Though outwardly protesting against this state of affairs and actually suffering through it, the seborrhoeic may inwardly accept the infliction as being well deserved.

1138
Woodburne AR, Philpott OS. **Cheilitis glandularis: a manifestation of emotional disturbance.** Arch Dermatol Syph 62:820-828, 1950.

▶ psychotherapy

A report of three cases of cheilitis glandularis pointing to the uselessness of an organic approach to this disease and illustrating the remarkable effect of the release of severe emotional tensions in the rapid and permanent cure of this condition is presented.

Books and Book Chapters on Skin Disorders

1139
Achterberg-Lawlis J, Kenner C. **Burn patients.** In: DM Doleys, RL Meredith, AR Ciminero (eds.), Behavioral Medicine: Assessment and Treatment Strategies. New York: Plenum, 1982.

1140
Alexander F. **Emotional factors in skin diseases.** In: F Alexander, Psychosomatic Medicine: Its Principles and Applications. New York: Norton, 1950.

1141
Ambrose G, Newbold G. **Hypnosis in dermatology.** In: G Ambrose, G Newbold, A Handbook of Medical Hypnosis: An Introduction for Practitioners and Students. 3rd ed. Baltimore: Williams & Wilkins, 1958.

1142
Barber TX. **Changing "unchangeable bodily" processes by (hypnotic) suggestions.** In: Sheikh A (ed.), Imagination and Healing. Farmingdale, New York: Baywood, 1984.

1143
Bunney MH. **Treatment of warts by psychological means.** In: MH Bunney, Viral Warts: Their Biology and Treatment. Oxford: Oxford University Press, 1982.

1144
Couper L, Davies JHT. **Psychiatric treatment in dermatology.** In: Proceedings of the Tenth International Congress of Dermatology. London: British Medical Association, 1953.

1145
Crasilneck HB, Hall JA. **The use of hypnosis in dermatologic problems.** In: HB Crasilneck, JA Hall, Clinical Hypnosis: Principles and Applications. Orlando, Florida: Grune & Stratton, 1975.

1146
Deutsch F, Murphy WF. **Atopic dermatitis.** In: F Deutsch, WF Murphy, The Clinical Interview. Vol. 1. Diagnosis. New York: International Universities Press, 1955.

1147
Ewin DM. **Clinical use of hypnosis for attenuation of burn depth.** In: FH Frankel, HS Zamansky (eds.), Hypnosis at its Bicentennial. New York: Plenum, 1978.

1148
Fischer-Williams M, Nigl AJ, Sovine DL. **Disorders of the integumental system.** In: M Fischer-Williams, AJ Nigl, DL Sovine, A Textbook of Biological Feedback. New York: Human Sciences Press, 1981.

1149
Grossbalt TA, Sherman C. **More than Skin Deep: A Mind/Body Approach for Healthy Skin.** New York: Morrow. (in press)

1150
Hecht M. **Psychiatric aspects of dermatology.** In: L Bellack (ed.), Psychology of Physical Illness. Orlando, Florida: Grune & Stratton, 1952.

1151
Hughes H, Gray S, Rafael Toledo J, Olen E. **Psychological Treatment of Skin Disorders.** Washington, DC: American Psychological Association, 1981. (36-page review)

1152
Hurley HJ. **Management of neurodermatitis.** In: JH Nodine, JH Moyer (eds.), Psychosomatic Medicine: The First Hahnemann Symposium. Philadelphia: Lea & Febiger, 1962.

1153
Kartamischew AJ. **Hypnosis and Suggestion in the Therapy of Dermatoses.** Moscow: Medgiz, 1953.

1154
Kroger WS. **Hypnosis in dermatology.** In: WS Kroger, Clinical and Experimental Hypnosis in Medicine, Dentistry, and Psychology. 2nd ed. Philadelphia: Lippincott, 1977.

1155

Kroger WS, Fezler WD. **Dermatological disorders.** In: WS Kroger, WD Fezler, Hypnosis and Behavior Modification: Imagery Conditioning. Philadelphia: Lippincott, 1976.

1156

Kroger WS, Freed SC. **Pruritus vulvae.** In: WS Kroeger, SC Freed, Psychosomatic Gynecology. Philadelphia: Saunders, 1951.

1157

Lachman SJ. **Psychosomatic skin disorders.** In: SJ Lachman, Psychosomatic Disorders: A Behavioristic Interpretation. New York: Wiley, 1972.

1158

Luthe W, Schultz JH. **Skin disorders.** In: W Luthe, JH Schultz, Autogenic Therapy: Medical Applications. Vol. 2. Orlando, Florida: Grune & Stratton, 1969.

1159

Mannon JM. **Caring for the Burned: Life and Death in a Hospital Burn Center.** Springfield, Illinois: Thomas, 1985.

1160

Musaph H. **Itching and Scratching: Psychodynamics in Dermatology.** New York: Karger, 1964.

1161

Musaph H. **Psychodermatology.** In: OW Hill (ed.), Modern Trends in Psychosomatic Medicine. Vol. 3. London: Butterworth, 1976.

1162

Musaph H. **Itching and other dermatoses.** In: ED Wittkower, H Warnes, Psychosomatic Medicine: Its Clinical Applications. Hagerstown, Maryland: Harper & Row, 1977.

1163

Norton A, Hall-Smith P. **A psychiatric view of skin disorder.** In: D O'Neill (ed.), Modern Trends in Psychosomatic Medicine. London: Butterworth, 1955.

1164

Obermayer ME. **Psychocutaneous Medicine.** Springfield, Illinois: Thomas, 1955.

1165

Risch C, Ferguson J. **Behavioral treatment of skin disorders.** In: JM Ferguson, CB Taylor (eds.), The Comprehensive Handbook of Behavioral Medicine. Vol. 2. New York: SP Medical and Scientific Books, 1981.

1166

Rook A, Wilkinson DS. **Psychocutaneous disorders.** In: A Rook, DS Wilkinson, FJG Ebling (eds.), Textbook of Dermatology. Philadelphia: Davis, 1968.

1167

Sack WT. **Psychotherapy and Skin Disease.** Halle: Marhold, 1927.

1168

Schaefer CE, Millman HL, Levine GF. **Skin disorders.** In: CE Schaefer, HL Millman, GF Levine (eds.), Therapies for Psychosomatic Disorders in Children. San Francisco: Jossey-Bass, 1979.

1169

Scott MJ. **Hypnosis in dermatology.** In: LM LeCron (ed.), Techniques of Hypnotherapy. New York: Julian Press, 1961.

1170

Scott MJ. **Hypnosis in dermatology.** In: JM Schneck (ed.), Hypnosis in Modern Medicine. Springfield, Illinois: Thomas, 1953.

1171

Seitz PFD. **Psychological aspects of skin diseases.** In: ED Wittkower, RA Cleghorn (eds.), Recent Developments in Psychosomatic Medicine. Philadelphia: Lippincott, 1954.

1172

Walton D. **The application of learning theory to the treatment of a case of neurodermatitis.** In: HJ Eysenck (ed.), Behavior Therapy and the Neuroses. New York: Pergamon, 1960.

1173

Weiss E, English OS. **Special senses—ear, eye, skin.** In: E Weiss, OS English, Psychosomatic Medicine: The Clinical Application of Psychopathology to General Medical Problems. Philadelphia: Saunders, 1950.

1174

Whitlock FA. **Hypnosis and skin.** In: FA Whitlock, Psychophysiological Aspects of Skin Disease. Philadelphia: Saunders, 1976.

1175

Whitlock FA. **Some implications for treatment.** In: FA Whitlock, Psychophysiological Aspects of Skin Disease. Philadelphia: Saunders, 1976.

1176

Wittkower ED, Russell B. **Emotional Factors in Skin Disease.** London: Paul B Hoeber, 1953.

1177
Wolpe J. **A case of neurodermatitis.** In: J Wolpe, Theme and Variations: A Behavior Therapy Casebook. New York: Pergamon, 1976.

1178
Zheltakov MM. **The use of hypnosis and conditioned-reflex therapy in dermatology.** In: RB Winn (ed.), Psychotherapy in the Soviet Union. New York: Philosophical Library, 1961.

1179
Zhukov IA. **Hypnotherapy of dermatoses in resort treatment.** In: RB Winn (ed.), Psychotherapy in the Soviet Union. New York: Philosophical Library, 1961.

Combined
Immunologic
Disorders

1180

Angell M. **Disease as a reflection of the psyche.** N Engl J Med 312:1570-1572, 1985. (editorial)

▶ relaxation, imagery

1181

Bowers KS, Kelly P. **Stress, disease, psychotherapy, and hypnosis.** J Abnorm Psychol 88:490-505, 1979.

▶ psychotherapy, hypnosis, suggestion, relaxation, imagery

There has been a growing appreciation of how psychologically produced stress reactions can enhance vulnerability to disease, especially via imbalances engendered in immune responsiveness. The importance of psychological factors as potential antecedents of disease has in turn implied the possibility that psychological modes of treatment may benefit people suffering from a variety of physical illnesses [asthma, cancer, and others]. Although many types of psychological interventions hold some promise in this regard, the present article presents considerable evidence for the importance of suggestion and hypnotic ability in the healing or amelioration of various somatic disorders. It is argued that even in some treatment interventions that are not explicitly hypnotic, suggestion and hypnotic ability may be hidden factors that help to promote successful healing. Consequently, hypnotic ability may be an individual difference variable that influences treatment outcome in a manner not heretofore recognized by many investigators and clinicians involved in helping the psychologically and physically ill.

1182

Clawson TA, Swade R. **The hypnotic control of blood flow and pain: the cure of warts and the potential for the use of hypnosis in the treatment of cancer.** Am J Clin Hypn 17:160-169, 1975.

▶ hypnosis

Cites case histories to show that hypnosis can control massive bleeding and pain and can remove warts, probably by stopping blood flow to them. It is suggested that blood flow to cancerous tumors could likewise be controlled, destroying them outright, or that such control could be a useful adjunct to chemo- or radiotherapy.

1183

Covino NA, Dirks JF, Fisch RI, Seidel JV. **Characteristics of depression of chronically ill medical patients: an elaboration of personality styles.** Psychother Psychosom 39:10-22, 1983.

▶ consultation-liaison, psychotherapy

In an earlier study, 13 distinct patterns of depression were found among 132 asthma, tuberculosis, and pain patients. The subscales of Scale 2 of the Minnesota Multiphasic Personality Inventory (MMPI) which were developed at the Massachusetts Mental Health Center were the basis for the classification via 0-type cluster analysis. The present work projected these patterns to the standard three validity and ten clinical scales of the MMPI. In addition, Dirk's panic-fear and Kleiger's alexithymia scales were scored. It was demonstrated that these 13 patterns of depression had important personality correlates associated with them. A useful point of view to take in medical care of the chronically ill is also offered.

1184

Covino NA, Dirks JF, Kinsman RA, Seidel JV. **Patterns of depression in chronic illness.** Psychother Psychosom 37:144-153, 1982.

▶ doctor-patient relationship

An understanding of the existence of depression is essential to the medical management of patients with chronic illness. This study found thirteen unique patterns of depression in depressed persons being treated for chronic medical conditions [asthma, tuberculosis, pain]. Of the 132 persons sampled, 96.2% fell clearly into one of these groups. The fact that these people manifested their clinical depression in such a variety of ways argues against a unilateral approach to the treatment of affective distress among those with a chronic medical illness. While patients manifest their affective distress in a variety of ways, self-esteem issues are significantly involved in almost half of the identified patterns.

1185
De Piano FA, Salzberg HC. **Clinical applications of hypnosis to three psychosomatic disorders.** Psychol Bull 86:1223-1235, 1979.

▶ hypnosis

Reviews outcomes and methodological soundness of studies of hypnosis in the treatment of skin disorders, headaches, and asthma. Some studies focused on changing physiological functions, others on increasing insight in their patients, and others on altering patients' perceptions of their symptoms. Methodological weaknesses included lack of control groups, nonrandom assignment of patients to treatment conditions, and confounding of treatment effects or lack of control for placebo effects. Additional weaknesses centered around the use of single outcome measures and the failure to assess the specific roles of mediating variables. Most studies showed positive treatment effects. However, there was equivocal evidence that hypnosis can directly influence autonomic functioning. Hypnosis may be valuable in facilitating one's capacity to gain insight into how one's symptoms developed and are maintained. In addition, hypnotic procedures have resulted in some success when used to indirectly alleviate symptoms by altering how individuals perceive their disorders and how these disorders affect their lives.

1186
Edwards H. **Alternative medicine: the science of spiritual healing.** Nurs Times 71:2008-2010, 1975.

▶ spiritual healing, doctor-patient relationship

Extracted summary: The healing gift is born of the feelings of inner compassion and sympathy for the sick. This is expressed through a deep inner yearning to help take away pain, suffering and sickness; the spiritual motive which urges so many good men and women to enter the medical and nursing professions and train to become healers. It follows that many nurses and doctors possess the healing potential, even though they may not be aware of it. There is a reason for everything and there is a reason why patients seem to get better more easily under one nurse than another. Some patients gather strength more quickly and so avoid postoperative shock when there is an affinity between the patient, a doctor and a particular nurse.

1187
Fry L, Mason AA, Pearson RSB. **Effect of hypnosis on allergic skin responses in asthma and hay fever.** Br Med J 1:1145-1148, 1964.

▶ hypnosis, suggestion

Forty-seven subjects with known skin sensitivity to pollen and/or house-dust were divided into five groups and tested with four strengths of allergen. The prick-test method was employed. In the first part of the investigation a group of unhypnotized subjects were compared with a group who had suggestions made under hypnosis that their skin reactions to the allergen would not occur when tested a second time. A significant diminution in the size of the weal was obtained in the hypnosis group at the lower two strengths of allergen. In the second part of the investigation the subjects were divided into three groups. All were hypnotized, no suggestions regarding skin reactions were given to one group, the second group were given suggestions that only on one arm would the skin reactions be less or not recur, and in the third group the suggestion was made about the reactions on both arms. There was found to be a similar decrease in the response to prick-tests after hypnosis in all three groups.

1188
Hall HR. **Hypnosis and the immune system: a review with implications for cancer and the psychology of healing.** Am J Clin Hypn 25:92-103, 1982.

▶ review: hypnosis, imagery

Reviews literature on the use of hypnosis to modify immune responses with respect to allergic responses, dermatological conditions, and inhibition of the Mantoux reaction. The relationship between stress, the production of adrenal corticoid hormones, the suppression of the immune system and the progression of cancer suggests that methods of reducing stress and corticoid production could play an important role in cancer treatment. The author reports on research that investigated the use of hypnosis on increasing immunity function in 20 healthy 22-85 yr olds. Findings indicate that hypnosis and visualization may result in an increase in immune function for certain individuals. Methodological issues raised in this area of research are discussed, along with the principles in the psychology of healing.

1189
Iles JD. **"If a man have a strong faith." Can Med Assoc J 105:343, 1971.** (letter)

▶ faith healing, suggestion, hypnosis

1190
Marchal J. **Efficacy of mental imagery, used as therapeutic method in psychosomatic medicine.** Riv Sper Freniatr 94:1292-1309, 1970. (in French)

▶ imagery, psychotherapy

1191

Mason AA. **Hypnosis and suggestion in the treatment of allergic phenomena.** Acta Allergol Suppl 7:332-338, 1960.

▶ hypnosis, suggestion

Extracted summary: When the action of hypnotism is analysed, it becomes apparent that its results are largely due to suggestion in a powerful form. The whole nature of the hypnotic trance with its inherent regression of the patient on the one hand and the idealization of the hypnotist on the other militates towards a degree of hyper-suggestibility rarely seen in other therapies, except perhaps occasionally in faith-healing. In fact, it has a greater effect than faith-healing which also depends largely on suggestion for its results, for today people are more impressed with science than with spiritual belief when it comes to taking medicine.

1192

McLean AF. **Hypnosis in "psychosomatic" illness.** Br J Med Psychol 38:211-230, 1965.

▶ hypnosis, suggestion, doctor-patient relationship

In a series of young patients suffering from asthma of early onset and mainly intermittent type—but in some, bronchitis or emphysema was present in addition—direct suggestion under hypnosis was followed by an immediate and marked improvement. Its continued use, for many years in some cases, has been followed to date by only one gross relapse, which was probably avoidable. There is evidence that the mere anticipation of hypnotic treatment initiated the improvement, but experience in the treatment of various skin diseases suggests that what tends to prevent relapse in the hypnotic treatment of psychosomatic disease is a factor connected with the doctor-patient relationship and the emotional needs of the patient, not necessarily specifically hypnotic, though the use of even light hypnosis increases rapport. Such, it is suggested, may be the decisive factor—unlikely to be identified without the use of detailed case-studies—in those rare cases of congenital skin disease which respond (as none of the three included in the present series did) to direct hypnotic suggestion. The lasting improvement which followed this treatment in several cases of other skin diseases, and the temporary remission in one of two cases of ulcerative colitis, might justify the initiation of large-scale controlled studies, particularly as in one case the skin improved area by area as suggested under hypnosis. In that case hypnotic abreaction was later introduced while in another ventilation of the patient's feelings was encouraged under hypnosis and intravenous methylamphetamine; in both, evidence that the improvement and its persistence (for 10 years to date) are related to the treatment is more definite than in the other skin cases, in some of which such ex-

ploratory methods might also have been used with benefit. These, however, would have little place in the treatment of the asthmatic group, as most were children, even if hypnosis in most had not been light.

1193

Miller ML. **A psychological study of a case of eczema and a case of neurodermatitis.** Psychosom Med 4:82-93, 1942.

▶ psychoanalysis

The psychoanalysis of patients with certain skin diseases offers a good opportunity for study, since the outbreaks are readily observable when they occur on the exposed parts and may be correlated with the patient's emotional states. This report deals with the study of the dynamic psychological factors connected with a case of eczema and a case of neurodermatitis.

1194

Ollendick TH, Gruen GE. **Treatment of a bodily injury phobia with implosive therapy.** J Consult Clin Psychol 38:389-393, 1972.

▶ implosive therapy

Employed implosive therapy in the treatment of an 8-yr-old male having a severe bodily injury phobia of 3-yr duration. This phobia was expressed in the behavioral symptoms of sleepless nights, hives, and asthmatic bronchitis. Following 2 sessions of implosive therapy, the number of sleepless nights diminished from 5-7/wk to 2/wk. In addition, there was no recurrence of hives or asthmatic bronchitis during treatment nor after a 6-mo follow up. Further follow-up data reveal a complete remission of the sleepless-night behavior and substantial improvement in peer relationships and self-concept.

1195

Rogerson CH. **Role of psychotherapy in the treatment of asthma-eczema-prurigo complex in children.** Br J Dermatol 4:368-378, 1934.

▶ review: psychotherapy

Extracted summary: One may therefore justly conclude that the paroxysms of this disease may be, and often are, brought on by psychological stimuli, and further that a state of anxiety so alters the threshold of the unstable nervous sytem that what under other circumstances might be sub-minimal stimuli of other kinds, become capable of producing the attack. Appropriate psychotherapy directed to the environment as much as to the child itself is in many cases capable of preventing the attacks, and in nearly all cases will render more effective the orthodox physical remedies.

1196
Sack WT. **On the psychic and nervous components of the so-called allergic skin diseases and their treatment.** Br J Dermatol Syph 40:441-445, 1928. (address)

▶ review: psychotherapy

1197
Saul LJ. **Some observations of the relations of emotions and allergy.** Psychosom Med 3:66-71, 1941.

▶ psychoanalysis

On the basis of studies now available on the role of emotions in allergic symptoms, the working hypothesis is presented that states of repressed, intense frustrated longing are of central importance. This was found in studies of certain cases of common cold, asthma, hay fever, and urticaria. The choice of sites for the symptoms seems to be determined by more specific factors. But whatever the factors in the choice of site for the symptom, the repressed longing, basically for the mother, frustrated or threatened with frustration, plays a central role. The longing is only one factor in the production of the symptoms. It operates in some cases independently of, and other cases together with specific allergic sensitivities. It is related to allergic sensitivity perhaps through increasing this sensitivity in the individual. It also operates apart from allergens by producing similar symptoms. It is a biological factor which apparently influences and complements allergic sensitivity at least in certain cases.

1198
Stewart H. **Some uses of hypnosis in general practice.** Br Med J 1:1320-1322, 1957.

▶ hypnosis, suggestion, psychotherapy, relaxation

Extracted summary: In this series the psychosomatic cases—that is, asthmas and eczemas—have responded well to suggestion and hypnotic psychotherapy. The teaching of autorelaxation to the asthmatics was very valuable to some of them. Among the psychiatric cases those with a history of a specific emotional trauma did particularly well after abreaction, and cures were rapidly obtained. In the pure anxiety states it was not so successful, as the deeper technique of hypno-analysis was undoubtedly required and the time factor here became of greater importance. But in the relief of anxiety-tension complicating an organic disease, hypnosis was very useful and appears to have a wide application here, since in many organic disorders the anxiety grossly aggravates the organically determined symptoms.

1199
Studt HH. **A comparison of the conflict situations initiating bronchial asthma and pulmonary tuberculosis.** Psychother Psychosom 19:321-341, 1971. (in German: no English abstract)

▶ psychotherapy

1200
Tuft HS. **The asthma, eczema, urticaria, rhinitis syndrome.** Penn Med J 62:177-180, 1959.

▶ psychotherapy, doctor-patient relationship, supportive psychotherapy, milieu therapy, psychoanalysis

Extracted summary: [Conditions in which psychologic factors are predominant (chronic urticaria, intractable asthma, adult atopic dermatitis)] can be managed only by competent psychotherapeutic approach in the following manner: 1. Establishment of rapport with the parents of a child or with the adult patient himself on a level which permits a full discussion of emotional problems as related to factors aggravating or inducing symptoms. 2. Separation of the patient from the environment temporarily to gain control. The hospital, vacation period, summer camp, boarding school, relatives' home, etc., are facilities which can be used depending upon the age and background of the patient. 3. Psychotherapy during which the patient must be helped to understand feelings and the relationship of feelings to both behavior and symptoms. This goal is accomplished largely by reflecting feelings and commenting upon those responsible for certain behavior patterns during play therapy for young children, or counseling for older patients. 4. Psychoanalysis for the few who will not respond to lesser measures.

1201
Woodhead B. **The psychological aspect of allergic skin reactions in childhood.** Arch Dis Child 21:98-104, 1946.

▶ psychotherapy, family therapy

Extracted summary: The following study is based on the investigation of cases of allergic skin disorder in children and young adults which have been referred to me from the Dermatological Department of Guy's Hospital. All were cases which had received physical treatment for some time and were not improved. During my observations the physical treatment was not altered unless it was stopped altogether. Twenty-six cases were investigated; they included cases of infantile eczema, Besnier's prurigo, and two cases of papular urticaria. The word allergic is used as an expression of convenience to denote those symptoms such as eczema, asthma, prurigo, or papular urticaria, which may be produced in sensitive persons by foreign substances, but which, it appears, may also be produced by abnormal psychological states.

Books and Book Chapters on Combined Immunologic Disorders

1202
Abramson HA. **Psychotherapy in allergy.** In: Allergology. Proceedings IVth International Congress on Allergology. New York: Pergamon, 1962.

1203
Black S. **Mind and Body.** London: William Kimber, 1969.

1204
Frazier CA. **Sail away, little ships.** In: CA Frazier, Psychosomatic Aspects of Allergy. New York: Van Nostrand Reinhold, 1977.

1205
Kellerman J, Varni JW. **Pediatric hematology/oncology.** In: DC Russo, JW Varni (eds.), Behavioral Pediatrics. Research and Practice. New York: Plenum, 1982.

1206
Locke SE, Hornig-Rohan M (eds.), **Mind and Immunity: Behavioral Immunology: An Annotated Bibliography 1976-1982.** New York: Institute for the Advancement of Health, 1983.

1207
Luthe W, Schultz JH. **Disorders of the respiratory tract.** In: W Luthe, JH Schultz, Autogenic Therapy: Medical Applications. Vol. 2. Orlando, Florida: Grune & Stratton, 1969.

1208
Mittelman B. **Failures in psychosomatic case treatments.** In: PH Hoch (ed.), Failures in Psychiatric Treatment. Orlando, Florida: Grune & Stratton, 1948.

1209
Papentin F. **Self-purification of the organism and transcendental meditation: a pilot study.** In: DW Orme-Johnson, L Domash, J Farrow (eds.), Scientific Research on Transcendental Meditation: Collected Papers. Vol. 1. Los Angeles: MIU Press, 1974.

1210
Pelletier KR. **Mind as Healer, Mind as Slayer.** New York: Dell, 1977.

1211
Scott MJ. **Hypnosis in Skin and Allergic Diseases.** Springfield, Illinois: Thomas, 1960.

1212
Varni JW. **Hematology/oncology: childhood cancer, hemophilia.** In: JW Varni, Clinical Behavioral Pediatrics: An Interdisciplinary Biobehavioral Approach. New York: Pergamon, 1983.

1213
Varni JW, Katz ER, Dash J. **Behavioral and neurochemical aspects of pediatric pain.** In: DC Russo, JW Varni (eds.), Behavioral Pediatrics: Research and Practice. New York: Plenum, 1982.

1214
Weiss E, English OS. **Skin disorders and allergies.** In: E Weiss, OS English, Psychosomatic Medicine: A Clinical Study of Psychophysiologic Reactions. 3rd ed. Philadelphia: Saunders, 1957.

1215
Wittkower ED, Engels D. **Psyche and allergy.** In: ML Hirt, Psychological and Allergic Aspects of Asthma. Springfield, Illinois: Thomas, 1965.

Cancer

Treatment of Disease

1216
Anonymous. **Unproven methods of cancer management: OC Simonton.** CA 32:58-61, 1982. (editorial)

▶ imagery, relaxation,

1217
Anonymous. **Mind and cancer.** Lancet 1:706-707, 1979. (editorial)

▶ meditation, imagery

1218
August RV. **Hypnotic induction of hypothermia: an additional approach to postoperative control of cancer recurrence.** Am J Clin Hypn 18:52-55, 1975.

▶ hypnosis

A patient with breast cancer was treated with hypnosis to lower skin temperature of an area of skin. The lowering effect was continued for several months.

1219
Baltrusch HJ. **Problems, tasks and limits of psychosomatic cancer research.** Z Psychosom Med 9:285-294, 1963. (in German)

▶ psychotherapy

The problem and tasks confronting psychosomatic cancer research are seen to fall into four major categories including psychological and psychophysiological investigations, psychosomatic animal research, and psychotherapy research in cancer. The effects of personality patterns on the development of cancer and its progress; definition of a "cancer prone personality"; affinity of certain types of malignancy to different personality types; evaluation of psychological states, such as despair and depression, as contributing factors; incidence of cancer in persons with abnormal or psychotic behavior patterns; group investigations on a transcultural basis in different countries, civilizations and societies; investigation of the everyday habits of cancer patients with regard to eating, smoking, and drinking, etc.; and comparision of different age groups characterized by high cancer incidence, such as childhood and old age. As a second area of study on research studies on neurohormonal and immunologic functions, the role of chronic inflammations and trauma, and the previous history of the cancer patient with respect to psychosomatic background data are listed. As to the third area, psychosomatic animal experiments, it is advocated that such experiments be conducted in species "sociologically close" to man. In the fourth category, psychotherapy, it is speculated that if psychosocial factors are able to influence malignancy growth and its course, there are possibly also psychosocial factors which may strengthen the host defense of the organism. The role of psychotherapy in the overall treatment of cancer patients is discussed with regard to the reduction of anxiety and tension, the reinforcement of the patient's will to survive and to cope with life-threatening disease, as well as with regard to secondary prevention and rehabilitation.

1220
Baltrusch HJF. **Some psychosomatic aspects of neoplastic disease with special reference to psychotherapy.** Z Psychosom Med Psychoanal 15:31-36, 1969. (in German: no English abstract)

▶ psychotherapy

1221
Baltrusch HJF. **Psychosocial stress, cancer and coping.** Mitt Ges Bek Krebskr Nordrhein-Westfalen 12:7-12, 1984. (in German)

▶ review: psychotherapy, behavior therapy, consultation-liaison

Extracted summary: In the aftercare of cancer patients two areas are of importance: (1) the rehabilitation of the patient which is not only concerned with physical recovery, but also aims at making the patient able again to take part actively in daily life: (2) secondary prevention with the aim of the evocation of cognitive processes which lead to a change in life styles, detrimental habits and coping behavior. Both aims have to be achieved not only in the medical, but also in the psychological and social spheres in order to effectuate a comprehensive change not only in the patient but also in his family. During the past years psychotherapy in its different forms was appliied to cancer patients within the frame of over-all treatment, aftercare and rehabilitation. However, there seem to be two different forms of application: (a) The promotion of the patient's adjustment to his disease. Help is given predominantly to those patients who show psychic disturbances during the course of their disease, whereas little intervention is done with patients who are overtly adjusted to their illness. In this connection, one may ask whether such a supportive intervention leads to the reinforcement of an emotional state which is more stressing than complaints openly expressed by the patient. (b) Psychotherapeutic intervention aiming at extended survival with better life quality or at recovery. There are hints that under favorable psychologic intervention and with the reduction of tension and anxiety there is an increase of catecholamines and a decrease in corticosteroids, and that the activity of NK cells can be increased, whereas defense patterns, such as denial and emotional withdrawal, are correlated with increased corticosteroid levels and decrease of NK activity. Thus, a favorable psychologic intervention does not only contribute towards an increased well-being of the cancer patient, but possibly also to positive biochemical and immunological changes within the organism. Psychotherapy with cancer patients has always to be focused on the disease and should be applied even in the diagnostic phase. The function of the psychooncologist is only practicable when he is an integrated part of the treatment team.

1222

Baltrusch HJF, Stangel W. **Psychosomatic aspects of polycythaemia vera.** Psychiatr Fenn (Helsinki) Suppl: 133-142, 1981.

▶ psychotherapy, counseling

Extracted summary: As in other malignant conditions psychosocial stress triggers off the clinical onset of polycythaemia vera (PV). The main area of conflict seems to be a deep-lying disturbance of interhuman relationships. PV patients share with persons with other neoplastic sites several common traits, such as abnormal release of anger and hostility, denial of unacceptable affects and a strong commitment to prevailing social norms. There is clinical evidence that also the clinical course of the illness is influenced by psychosocial stress factors. As a consequence, a psychosocial program will be set in train with regard to psychotherapeutic guidance and counselling of PV patients. The relief of tension and anxiety may be beneficial not only for the life quality of the patients, but also for the clinical outcomes of their disease.

1223

Baltrusch HJF, Waltz M. **Cancer from a biobehavioral and social epidemiological perspective.** Soc Sci Med 20:789-794, 1985.

▶ behavior modification

Malignant neoplasms should not be viewed as a "psychogenic" nor as "primarily organic" disease but as an interaction of various forces, in which psychosocial factors may play an important role. To understand the increase in neoplastic disease which has taken place in this century requires a theoretical framework including social, psychosocial and behavioral dimensions, as well as the endocrine and immunologic mechanisms acting as pathogenic pathways. Recent theoretical developments in health psychology and allied disciplines on coping behavior and social support should be integrated into biomedical models of the etiology, pathogenesis, and clinical course of malignant neoplasia. Environmental stressors, as well as mediating variables at the cognitive, affective, behavioral and physiological levels of adaptation, are suggested as major components of a model of multidimensional pathology. A growing body of research on the role of psychosocial factors in adjustment to cancer and its treatment has contributed new insights into possible variables and causal mechanisms which may be relevant in the etiology of the disease. Closeness to parents in childhood and the ability to form close interpersonal relationships in later adult life very possibly influence the ability of the individual to cope effectively with environmental stressors prior to neoplastic disease and with the considerable stresses of being a cancer patient subsequent to diagnosis and treatment. Pathogenic pathways for future investigation include mental health variables, such as self-esteem and sense of control at the psychological level and immunity surveillance at the biological. An integration and cross-fertilization of current work in the etiology of and adjustment to cancer is suggested linking psychosomatic and somatopsychic models.

1224

Bolen JS. **Meditation and psychotherapy in the treatment of cancer.** Psychic 4:19-22, 1973.

▶ meditation, relaxation, imagery

Describes the work of an Air Force doctor who combines meditation and cobalt radiation therapy in the treatment of cancer. It is believed that there is a direct correlation between the patient's attitude and his response to cancer therapy. Results of 152 patients treated for cancer show that, for 150 patients, improved or unimproved conditions correlated with their degree of participation and attitudes toward the treatment. 2 patients improved despite negative attitudes. The meditation program, which involves relaxation exercises and visualizations of peaceful scenes, is outlined. The need for experimental validation is discussed.

1225
Borysenko JZ. **Behavioral-physiological factors in the development and management of cancer.** Gen Hosp Psychiatry 4:69-74, 1982.

▶ review: relaxation response

Recent clinical and animal model studies have demonstrated an effect of behavioral variables on the course of cancer. Unrelieved anxiety, helplessness, depression, and the inability to modulate the expression of anger have been implicated as specific predictors of poor prognosis. The endocrinological sequelae of these emotional states may affect certain parameters of cell-mediated immunity involved in host resistance to neoplasia. Both corticosteroids and catecholamines are likely mediators of behavioral effects on immunological function. Hormonal variations may also affect growth of tumors directly, or through nonimmunological tissue specific mechanisms. Behavioral interventions based on elicitation of the relaxation response provide a means of influencing affective and physiological states that may have particular relevance to cancer. Practice of such interventions reduces anxiety and provides a substrate for coping that enhances the patient's sense of control. Such "immunization" against helplessness can forestall depression. Physiological effects of such behavioral interventions occur both on a direct and an indirect level. Elicitation of the relaxation response per se produces physiological alterations consistent with decreased arousal of the sympathetic nervous system. Furthermore, by reducing fear and helplessness, physiological changes related to such dysphoric states may be minimized.

1226
Bowers KS. **Hypnosis: an informational approach.** Ann NY Acad Sci 296:222-237, 1977.

▶ hypnosis

Extracted summary: The informational view of hypnosis suggests certain treatment possibilities that might otherwise seem implausible. If it is true that semantically received information can be somatically encoded, especially under conditions of deep hypnosis, the possibility exists that some forms of cancer might be helped by hypnotic techniques. Because the previous sentence will undoubtedly cause some eyebrows to rise, let me juxtapose it with the following assertion: To my knowledge, there is not a scintilla of direct scientific evidence that hypnosis can reverse the course of cancer. Moreover, although there are many reports in the literature in which hypnosis successfully alleviated the pain of cancer, there are virtually no claims that the malignancy itself remitted. In fact, death is the almost universal outcome of even extraordinarily successful use of hypnosis as an analgesic for cancer patients. A search of the literature, by no means exhaustive, unearthed only one case in which an apparently permanent remission of cancer at least temporarily coincided with the use of hypnosis. Given this rather bleak evidential state of affairs, why even articulate the controversial proposition that hypnosis might be helpful in at least some forms of cancer. Basically, the reason for doing so derives from several considerations that indirectly suggest the possibility. In the first place, there is a plethora of literature that strongly implies a psychosomatic aspect to cancer. For example, the probability of developing cancer increases considerably after a significant interpersonal loss, a stressful time when there is a lowered resistance to disease generally. The possibility of mobilizing and strengthening the cancer patient's internal resources via hypnotic techniques should therefore not be discounted. For example, one of Collisons' strategies in the treatment of asthmatics by hypnosis was to utilize ego-strengthening procedures and suggestions originally employed by Hartland. Another line of indirect evidence derives from the well-known fact that spontaneous remissions of cancer do take place, although such occurrences are rare. Everson and Cole presented 182 documented cases of such remissions that they were able to glean from the medical literature published since 1900. The existence of such remissions was, until recently, the best available evidence that immunological considerations played an important role in cancer. In effect, it was argued that belated immune reactions to the cancer caused its remission. This explanation of spontaneous remission is consistent with the fact that road-accident victims evidently have a much higher incidence of (previously undetected) cancer than exists in the population at large. The implication of this finding is that the immune system effectively prevents the vast majority of new malignancies from becoming clinically established. The details of the immunological surveillance system that blocks or even reverses the growth of cancer is beyond the scope of this paper. What is interesting is that immunological factors causing certain allergic responses are "amenable to controls." So the principal of psychological control over immunological responses seems established. There are of course, important differences in inhibiting an allergic reaction produced by one antibody, and enhancing the effectiveness of yet another antibody to destroy malignant cells. The apparent effectiveness of hypnosis in the treatment of warts does suggest, however, that immunological efficiency vis-a-vis benign, virally induced tumors can be psychologically enhanced.

1227
Bowers MK, Weinstock C. **A case of healing in malignancy.** J Am Acad Psychoanal 6:393-402, 1978.

▶ psychoanalysis

Presents the case of a young man who, during the course of psychotherapy, developed cancer and subsequently recovered from it. The psychodynamics of the case are discussed in the context of experimental and clinical studies demonstrating a relationship between affect and the body's immunological system. A 19-yr follow-up is presented.

1228
Cassileth BR, Lusk EJ, Strouse TB, Bodenheimer BJ. **Contemporary unorthodox treatments in cancer medicine: a study of patients, treatments, and practitioners.** Ann Intern Med 10:105-112, 1984.

▶ imagery, spiritual healing, doctor-patient relationship

Public education, legislative action, and medical advances have failed to deter patients from seeking unorthodox treatments for cancer and other diseases. To study this phenomenon, we interviewed 304 cancer center inpatients and 356 patients under the care of unorthodox practitioners. A concomitant survey of unorthodox practitioners documented their backgrounds and practices. Eight percent of all patients studied never received any conventional therapy, and 54% of patients on conventional therapy also used unorthodox treatments. Forty percent of patients abandoned conventional care entirely after adopting alternative methods. Patients interviewed did not conform to the stereotype of poorly educated, end-stage patients who had exhausted conventional treatment. Practitioners also deviated from the traditional portrait: of 138 unorthodox practitioners studied, 60% were physicians (MDs). Patients are attracted to therapeutic alternatives that reflect social emphasis on personal responsibility, pollution and nutrition, and that move away from perceived deficiencies in conventional medical care.

1229
Cautela JR. **Toward a Pavlovian theory of cancer.** Scand J Behav Ther 6:117-142, 1977.

▶ positive reinforcement

Reviews anecdotal and research data indicating that stress and lack of reinforcement (depression, loss) are related to the incidence and growth of cancer. Current theories of the etiology of malignant neoplasma involve cellular abnormalities. Pavlovian theorizing concerning the properties of the nervous system is also focused on cellular functioning. Observations from the Pavlovian laboratories indicate that stress (overstrain of excitatory processes and difficulty in nervous system mobility) and excessive and/or protracted inhibition (lack of reinforcement) produce both behavioral and organic abnormalities. A current view on the etiology of cancer that is being considered seriously is the immunocompetence theory which is consistent with Pavlovian theory on conditioning of the immune system. Preliminary research supports this postulation. Treatment of cancer should involve removal of stress and an increase in the level of reinforcement by behavioral means. The general postulation is that stress and/or lack of reinforcement can provide an environment in which abnormal stimulation can increase the susceptibility to and growth rate of cancer.

1230
Cunningham AJ. **Psychotherapy for cancer.** Advances 1(4):8-14, 1984.

▶ review: psychotherapy

Can psychological treatments ameliorate cancer? Alastair J. Cunningham, who recognizes the methodological deficiencies of the clinical studies but who is concerned that their claims may nonetheless be "both true and very important," maintains that another standard should be used to weigh the findings—a standard that might be called the principal of cross-study consistency. Cunningham argues that the results of the clinical studies are consistent with each other and also with the results of prospective studies correlating personality factors with cancer and animal studies investigating the effects of stress on tumor growth. This broad consistency, he suggests, points to a possible core of validity. It indicates, at the very least, that the clinical claims should not be dismissed on methodological grounds and that the time has come to subject the claims to "properly controlled clinical trials."

1231
Davis HK. **Psychiatry, immunology, and cancer.** Tex Med 81:49-52, 1985.

▶ review: behavior modification, relaxation, hypnosis, suggestion, imagery, group therapy, biofeedback, doctor-patient relationship, consultation-liaison

Studies have shown that stress impairs immune system responsiveness and may influence malignant disease. Animal studies, for example, have demonstrated a relationship between stress and accelerated tumor growth, and other studies have suggested a relationship between stress and T and B cell responsiveness. Because of such relationships, physicians treating cancer patients should utilize all available therapies to reduce stress, convey hope, and assure the patient that he or she has allies throughout the illness.

1232
Dowling SJ. **Lourdes cures and their medical assessment.** J R Soc Med 77:634-638, 1984.

▶ spiritual healing

Extracted summary: The latest cure to be passed by the CMIL [International Medical Committee of Lourdes] as medically inexplicable is that of Delizia Cirolli, in September 1982—a child from a village on the slopes of Mount

Etna in Sicily. In 1976 when she was 12 years old she presented with a painful swollen right knee. The CMIL studied the case in 1980 and 1981 and at their meeting in 1982 they decided the Ewing's tumour was the correct diagnosis and concluded that the cure was scientifically inexplicable.

1233
Feder SL. **Psychological considerations in the care of patients with cancer.** Ann NY Acad Sci 125:1020-1027, 1966.

▶ doctor-patient relationship

As physicians, we are concerned with the ultimate outcome of the disease. For the patients, the greatest threat seemed to be not so much that of death, but rather of pain, helplessness, rejection and progressive isolation. Studies of chronically ill people (especially cancer patients who think in terms of disintegration) have shown how intense the fear of abandonment is. It is feared more than death itself. It is usual that we are frightened of things about which we may have some experience or memory. Death is beyond our conscious and unconscious experience (at least subjectively) and cannot be conceptualized; for this reason death is most often equated with abandonment. In the chronically ill person this fear of being unloved and isolated is everywhere. This is what the physician must counteract in every way he can. If our patients are to trust us in this, sympathy and words of reassurance are not enough. If our attitudes and behavior are determined by our knowledge of the patient's fears and his ways of reacting to them, then we impart a feeling of reassurance he cannot obtain in any other way. Facing the truths with the patient, facing the threat of deterioration, reinforces the trust and the feeling of being wanted. Patients must share their experiences; they are too often not sure they are going to find someone with whom to do it. These have been the immediate humanitarian considerations. There is another issue, perhaps more speculative, but of potential great importance. It is the issue to which this monograph has been directed. This is the hypothesis that psychological factors might play a role not only in the onset of malignant disease, but also in its course. Denial mechanisms are always important in cancer patients. But denial is a poor avenue for emotional discharge. Often it is none at all. The same can be said of the situation where a patient's personal and emotional isolation is increased by the observer's inability to accept the emergent emotions. In avoiding an open relationship and in not offering opportunities for emotional discharge we may be encouraging mechanisms unfavorable to the patient's resistance to the disease. It has been suggested that those patients who have adequate avenues for discharge of tension may have a more favorable later course with cancer than those without such adaptive opportunities. Thus, a greater understanding of the reactions to, and methods of coping with, cancer, some of which have been suggested here, may serve to increase this psycho-physiologic adaptability.

1234
Fiore N. **Fighting cancer—one patient's perspective.** N Engl J Med 300:284-289, 1979.

▶ psychotherapy, stress management, relaxation, autogenic training, biofeedback, assertiveness training, suggestion, imagery

Describes the author's experience as a cancer patient (embryonal carcinoma) from diagnosis through the end of chemotherapy. It is emphasized that effective cancer therapy must treat the healthy portions of the patient's body and psyche as well as the diseased cells. Suggestions for using individual psychotherapy sessions at different points in cancer therapy are presented.

1235
Gardner GG, Lubman A. **Hypnotherapy for children with cancer: some current issues.** Am J Clin Hypn 25:135-142, 1982.

▶ hypnosis, autohypnosis, psychotherapy, imagery

Reviews some of the problems that now face clinicians and researchers working in the field of hypnotherapy for pediatric cancer patients. These include (1) understanding and dealing with resistance and refusal, (2) developing preventive hypnotherapeutic strategies for children who will survive cancer, and (3) carrying out research that clarifies the value of hypnotherapy with childhood cancer patients and elucidates when and how specific approaches can best be utilized.

1236
Greer S. **Cancer and the mind.** Br J Psychiatry 143:535-543, 1983. (address)

▶ review

1237
Grossarth-Maticek R. **Social psychotherapy and course of the disease: first experiences with cancer patients.** Psychother Psychosom 33:129-138, 1980.

▶ psychotherapy, suggestion

Introduces a therapeutic approach in the treatment of cancer patients and reports conclusions drawn from the study of 24 Ss treated according to this method. It is suggested that the development of cancer depends to a great extent on the interrelation between environment and patient. A disturbed attitude on the part of the patient toward the environment and himself/herself can adversely influence the development of cancer. The aim of social psychotherapy is to modify such attitudes by psychological means: social support, insight and emotion training, and cooperative suggestion training.

1238

Hall MD. **Using relaxation imagery with children with malignancies: a developmental perspective.** Am J Clin Hypn 25:143-149, 1982.

▶ relaxation, imagery

Describes a relaxation program with a developmental theoretical foundation called "imagery therapy." Its goal is to increase the efficacy of immune mechanisms, thus increasing the survival rate of children with malignancies and/or improving the comfort and quality of their lives. Three constructs—the impact of social stress, the positive development of attachment and the negative effects of separation and loss, and the stages of concept formation relating to the functioning of the human body and the processes of disease and death—underlie this approach to a comprehensive care plan.

1239

Hedge AR. **Hypnosis in cancer.** Br J Med Hypn 12:2-5, 1960.

▶ hypnosis

Extracted summary: All cases showed a marked improvement and in some there was actual tumour regression. Two of them who had been bedridden were able to return to work for several months. Others were able to be up and about and to perform light chores or housework. One woman with breast cancer had multiple tumour nodules over the surface of her chest, yet she later showed a complete disappearance of these metastatic growths (without any hormone therapy, X-ray or adrenalectomy!). In the general discussion with these patients it was pointed out that many people appear to have a natural immunity to cancer, and they often may live for several years without apparent progression. For this reason it was assumed that the apparent immunity was something that could be developed, and even under hypnosis it was suggested that their antibody reaction would become greatly increased and that the biochemistry of the cellular growth would be altered so as to revert to a more mature phase. The picture of the physiological and chemical changes expected was verbally painted for them, and amazingly enough, that appeared to be exactly what was taking place in their tissues! The experiment is still in progress, although three of the patients have already succumbed. Those remaining may or may not continue with us for a lengthy time, but they have already long passed the period when one would have normally expected their demise. It would be foolish to report that this means of therapy is a cure for this dread disease, but it certainly is an incredible aid to the overall care. It is sincerely hoped that others will be encouraged to delve more deeply into this problem and to extend their range of effectiveness in cancer control.

1240

Holland JC. **Why cancer patients seek unproven cancer remedies: a psychological perspective.** CA 32:10-14, 1982.

▶ faith healing, meditation, yoga, doctor-patient relationship

Psychologically, the patient with cancer is apt to feel the worst when it becomes clear that medical treatment can no longer control his disease. As soon as traditional medicine is perceived as being unable to offer either control or cure, both patient and family are likely to begin considering unorthodox and unproven methods for curing cancer. When this happens and the issue of "alternative" therapies is raised, the physician frequently finds that treatment of the disease can become much more complicated. Psychological management of patient and family at this time is of critical importance, since the recommended clinical regimen may be foregone in favor of some "cure." This paper examines social and psychological factors that contribute to this situation.

1241

Howard RJ, Miller NJ. **Unproven methods of cancer management (II): Current trends and implications for patient care.** Oncol Nurs Forum 11:67-73, 1984.

▶ imagery, relaxation, stress management training, group therapy

The second part of this series addresses the currently popular forms of unproven methods in cancer care, highlighted with selected implications for patient care. The Simonton method, macrobiotics, immunoaugmentative therapy, laetrile, and DMSO are explored and evaluated. Implications for nursing practice include assessing the reasons a patient would pursue unproven methods and establishing guidelines for patient education and nursing intervention.

1242

Ishikawa H. **The psychotherapy of advanced cancer.** Rinsho Hoshasen 24:1115-1119, 1979. (in Japanese)

▶ psychotherapy

The psychotherapy of advanced cancer has two faces. One is the psychological influence to the growth of cancer cells and second is the psychotherapy to the dying patient. From these standpoints, the psychosomatic approach must be included in the treatment of the advanced cancer.

1243
Klopfer B. **Psychological variables in human cancer.**
J Proj Tech 21:231-42, 1957. (address)

▶ suggestion

1244
Lansky P. **Possibility of hypnosis as an aid in cancer therapy.** Perspect Biol Med 25:496-509, 1982.

▶ hypnosis, psychotherapy

Examines research that supports the role of hypnosis in the medical treatment of cancer by first discussing how life history patterns and personality traits may play a role in the etiology of disease and may therefore provide a focus for psychotherapeutic intervention. A new strategy is proposed that is based on the "paradoxical intention" technique, whereby patients evoke the psychic equivalent of homeopathy and "love" their tumor to effect self-healing.

1245
LeShan LL, Gassmann ML. **Some observations on psychotherapy with patients suffering from neoplastic disease.** Am J Psychother 12:723-734, 1958.

▶ psychotherapy

Ten patients with malignant neoplasms were studied in over 1400 hours of intensive depth psychotherapy. This led to the recognition of a number of special problems arising during the psychotherapeutic treatment of cancer patients. Some tentative methods of handling these problems are presented and it is hoped that they will prove useful to others working in the same field. The special problems were divided into four areas: (1) The anxieties of the cancer patient. These are predominantly realistic in nature and have to be accepted as such. More support is needed in this form of treatment than is generally given during psychotherapy. (2) The anxieties of the therapist. The therapist must be clear about the goals and values of working with patients who are likely to die in the course of the process. A control therapist is necessary in order that the stress, when one patient dies, does not affect the therapist's relationships with the other cancer patients. (3) The personality of cancer patients. Certain personality factors which have implications for therapy appear with a good deal of consistency in individuals with cancer. These include an unusual amount of deeply repressed hostility, marked feelings of psychological isolation, and despair about having been unable to achieve real satisfactions in life. (4) Special psychosomatic aspects. There is some reason to believe that psychotherapy may under certain circumstances affect the growth rate and development of neoplasms. Therefore a good deal of caution is recommended in deciding how much guilt and hostility may be mobilized during the therapeutic process.

1246
Lerner M. **A report on complementary cancer therapies.** Advances 2:31-43, 1985.

▶ psychotherapy, spiritual healing, imagery, relaxation, yoga, meditation

In his journalistic investigation of complementary cancer therapies, Michael Lerner surveys the types of therapies that are available, broadly estimates their degree of success, and describes the people who use them. His aim is "to provide a balanced account of a controversial medical field." Regarding the people who use complementary therapies, Lerner reports that they characteristically are "intelligent and resourceful patients" and that they are "integrating established and complementary therapies." Regarding the success of the therapies, he reports that "some patients are hurt when complementary therapies are negligently or unscrupulously applied, that a larger number of patients experience transient or lasting 'subjective' benefits, and that a small number experience lasting improvements in health, including partial or complete remission." In his conclusion, he suggests that the careful examination of complementary therapies can have broad humanistic implications. "As we raise the level of discourse regarding complementary cancer therapies, we must inevitably raise the level of discourse about medicine in our time."

1247
Levy SM. **Emotions and the progression of cancer: a review.** Advances 1:10-15, 1984.

▶ review: doctor-patient relationship, relaxation, imagery

Extracted summary: If the argument to this point is correct—that lower survival rates from cancer are associated with depression or helplessness and higher rates are associated with a sense of coping—then the question must be asked: can helplessness and the lack of coping among cancer patients be altered? And if they can, will the change affect the outcome of the disease? The answer to the first question is undoubtedly yes. The strategies for change are numerous. In some, the patient's outlook is the target. The literature indicates that various cognitive interventions—for example, role rehearsal, self-rewards, and thought stoppage—alter depressive or helpless behavior. A recent article by Peterson suggests that medical practitioners adapt for use with patients the type of strategies that dispel helplessness in animals. Peterson suggests that a physician could enlist patients as collaborators in their own treatment, explaining to them that their progress depended on this assistance. Patients thus would be led to feel a greater sense of control over the management of their illness if not over its outcome. Other strategies could more immediately affect the biological substrate. For example, Hoffman et al. showed that in laboratory situations of physical stress, individuals who employed the relaxation response reduced the amount of peripheral nor-epinephrine utilization, thereby minimizing the effects of the stress. Of course patients who used the relaxation response would likely see it as a way of exerting control over their illness and in this sense it could also be a useful method for improving their sense of control. But the technique also directly affects relevant hormonal changes.

1248
Levy SM, Morrow GR. **Biobehavioral interventions in behavioral medicine.** Cancer 50:1936-1938, 1982.

▶ relaxation, hypnosis, biofeedback, conditioning, desensitization, imagery

The committee focused its discussion on biobehavioral factors and/or interventions as important aspects of cancer research in the three general areas of: (1) treatment and disease effects; (2) progression/survival of disease; and (3) development of disease. A consensus of our deliberations in each of these areas is presented in greater detail following a short outline of what we viewed as strengths and weaknesses of the behavioral approach.

1249
Lichstein PR. **Can a physician heal a "hex"?** Hosp Pract 17:125-132, 1982.

▶ supportive psychotherapy, folk medicine

This case illustrates the complexities and dilemmas encountered in the care of a patient with a life-threatening medical disease [hemangiopericytoma], a psychiatric disorder, and a belief that the illness is caused by a hex. Through meetings with this patient, her family, and the staff, the consultant was able to facilitate communication and understanding among those involved in her care. With an increased awareness of her psychiatric problems as well as her folk medical beliefs, the staff was able to attend to the patient's needs in a supportive manner. Once her beliefs were understood and appreciated, effective [medical] therapy could be planned and implemented.

1250
Lustig-Juon E. **Cancer conference in St. Gallen and International Healer Day in Basel.** Krankenpflege (Bern) February:22-24, 1983. (in German)

▶ folk medicine

1251
Magarey C. **Holistic cancer therapy.** J Psychosom Res 27:181-184, 1983.

▶ spiritual healing, doctor-patient relationship

A review of unorthodox holistic cancer therapies suggests that the personality of the therapist is crucial to their apparent success. The spiritually convinced, charismatic healer has all the qualities of a meditator, and physiological measurement has demonstrated that such a healer can induce a state of meditation in his/her patients. Meditation is associated not only with physiological rest and stability, but also with the reduction of psychological stress and the development of a more positive attitude toward life with an inner sense of calmness, strength, and fulfilment.

1252
Margolis CG. **Society for Clinical and Experimental Hypnosis 36th Annual Workshops and Scientific Meetings.** Advances 2:63-66, 1985.

▶ hypnosis, imagery, relaxation, meditation, psychotherapy

Report on workshops at San Antonio, Texas, October 22-27, 1984. Includes presentation by Jeanne Achterberg-Lawlis and Bernard Newton.

1253
Meares A. **Vivid visualization and dim visual awareness in the regression of cancer in meditation.** J Am Soc Psychosom Dent Med 25:85-88, 1978.

▶ meditation

The use of intensive meditation by a patient with advanced cancer was followed by remission of the disease. A relapse occurred when she accompanied the meditation with vivid visualization of healthy cells eating the cancer cells. The alertness caused by the visualization interfered with the state of regression needed for the therapeutic effect (activation of the immune system) of the meditation to occur.

1254
Meares A. **Regression of cancer after intensive meditation.** Med J Aust 2:184, 1976. (letter)

▶ meditation

1255
Meares A. **The quality of meditation effective in the regression of cancer.** J Am Soc Psychosom Dent Med 25:129-132, 1978.

▶ meditation

Extracted summary: The work of Simonton at Fort Worth, U.S.A. and my own work here in Melbourne, Australia, show that cancer growth can be influenced by meditation. The purpose of this article is to describe that particular type of meditation which in my experience is most successful in its effect on cancer growth. Although my work has shown that cancer can be influenced by intensive meditation so that there has been clear evidence of regression of the growth and patients have lived far beyond the life expectancy estimated by experienced oncologists, it must be emphasized that it has not yet been fully established that it can be influenced to the point of cure.

1256
Meares A. **Regression of osteogenic sarcoma metastases associated with intensive meditation.** Med J Aust 2:433, 1978.

▶ meditation

Extracted summary: [I]t would seem that the patient has let the effects of the intense and prolonged meditation enter into his whole experience of life. His extraordinarily low level of anxiety is obvious to the most casual observer. It is suggested that this has enhanced the activity of his immune system by reducing his level of cortisone.

1257
Meares A. **Meditation: a psychological approach to cancer treatment.** Practitioner 222:119-122, 1979.

▶ meditation

In the evolution of something new there must first come a stage of formulating ideas and communicating our incomplete results to our fellows so that we may exchange views with others who may be interested in the same area. Statistical analysis and objective proof must wait. However, the experience with these patients seems to show quite clearly that the growth of cancer can be influenced by this form of intensive meditation—but whether or not it can be influenced to the point of cure has not yet been established.

1258
Meares A. **Regression of cancer of the rectum after intensive meditation.** Med J Aust 2:539-540, 1979.

▶ meditation

Extracted summary: Strangely enough, at present there is no clear indication that one type of neoplasm is more susceptible to this approach than another. This probably means that host resistance and the effect of a profound and sustained reduction of anxiety on the immune system are more important in this work than is the nature of the tumour itself. It may well be that the extreme reduction of anxiety in these patients triggers off the same mechanism as that which becomes active in the rare sponta-

neous remissions. This would be consistent with the observation that spontaneous remissions are often associated with some kind of religious experience or profound psychological reaction. Before the commencement of treatment, it is explained to all cancer patients, and if possible to a relative, that this approach is at present purely experimental. If the patient says that he has been advised to have chemotherapy, and asks for my opinion, he is always told that this is the orthodox treatment. My data have not yet reached a stage at which they can be effectively subjected to statistical analysis, and my own advancing years make any prolonged trial impracticable. In these circumstances, the publication of case reports may bring others to consider this approach as a possible alternative treatment of cancer.

1259
Meares A. **Remission of massive metastasis from undifferentiated carcinoma of the lung associated with intensive meditation.** J Am Soc Psychosom Dent Med 27:40-41, 1980.

▶ meditation

Extracted summary: The therapeutic process in the present case is confused by the patient's subsequent physical treatment, but the case is reported in order to record the initial seven months remission from this highly malignant condition in the absence of any treatment at all except the intensive meditation.

1260
Meares A. **Regression of recurrence of carcinoma of the breast at mastectomy site associated with intensive meditation.** Aust Fam Physician 10:218-219, 1981.

▶ meditation

Extracted summary: The patient attended each weekday for a month for intensive meditation. By this time there was clear evidence of healing. It was arranged that the patient should return to her home in another State, and come back for further treatment in a month's time. However, by then the ulcer had nearly healed, the patient said she was well and felt it was unnecessary to return for further treatment. Figure 2 shows the ulcer completely healed, and the hard raised nodules have disappeared. She has however, recently developed a bony metastasis for which she has had cobalt radiation.

1261
Meares A. **Cancer, psychosomatic illness, and hysteria.** Lancet 2:1037-1038, 1981.

▶ meditation

The onset of cancer is sometimes preceded by psychological reactions similar to those seen in psychosomatic illness and conversion hysteria. Some cancers have regressed after treatment similar to, but more intense than, that used in psychosomatic illness and conversion hysteria. It is suggested that psychological mechanisms resembling those of psychosomatic illness and conversion hysteria may cause some cases of cancer when acting in conjunction with the known chemical, viral, and radiational causes of the disease.

1262
Meares A. **Stress, meditation and the regression of cancer.** Practitioner 226:1607-1609, 1982.

▶ meditation

Extracted summary: It seems likely that a number of different psychophysiological responses are called into play by intensive meditation. The general reduction in the habitual level of anxiety reduces cortisone with consequent freeing of the immune system to act more effectively against cancer. It is the anxiety element of this sequence with which I am at present directly concerned.

1263
Meares A. **A form of intensive meditation associated with the regression of cancer.** Am J Clin Hypn 25:114-121, 1982.

▶ meditation

Elaborates on several cases reported by the present author (1976-1981) regarding the regression of cancer following intensive meditation. This type of meditation is characterized by extreme simplicity and stillness of the mind; it differs from other forms using a mantra, awareness of breathing, or visualization of the healing process. Any logical verbal communication by the therapist stimulates intellectual activity in the patient. Communication is conducted through unverbalized phonation, reassuring words and phrases, and touch. There follows a profound reduction in the patient's level of anxiety that flows into his/her daily life. The nonverbal nature of the meditative experience initiates a nonverbal philosophical understanding of other areas of life.

1264
Meares A. **Psychological mechanisms in the regression of cancer.** Med J Aust 1:583-584, 1983.

▶ meditation

Extracted summary: Psychological regression is an essential feature of deep hypnosis, and also of intensive meditation. The important factor from the point of view of the present discussion is that psychological regression initiates physiological regression. This is well exemplified in the loss of colour vision in intensive meditation. So, in intensive meditation, there is a mechanism which can initiate the physiological regression necessary to re-establish the healing process. Age regression is another well established factor of deep hypnosis. Patients with cancer whose treatment is intensive meditation have reported a similar phenomenon. This is an ontological regression. It seems possible that, at a functional level, the ontological regression may initiate something akin to phylogenetic regression. Besides functioning at a regressed age level, the organism may, in fact, come to function in such a way that the physiological activity of the tissues is carried out at a simpler, more primitive, biological level. Such a concept is relevant to the healing process in general, as the greater propensity for healing in lower forms of life (such as reptiles, crabs, starfish) is a matter of common observation. Some cancers have regressed after intensive meditation in the absence of any orthodox treatment. I have discussed a number of psychological processes, any one of which might possibly be the effective mechanism in bringing about these regressions. We have now grown beyond the idea of seeking single causes of disease, and have generally come to believe that disease results from the interaction of a number of factors, both organic and psychological. If this applies to the cause of cancer, may it not also apply to the cure of cancer? In view of the remarkable propensity of the body for self-healing, perhaps we should return to an earlier medical orientation, and re-examine the healing process as an entity. From such an orientation, we may come to have a better understanding of the healing effect of intensive meditation.

1265
Meares A. **Regression of cancer after intensive meditation followed by death.** Med J Aust 2:374-375, 1977. (letter)

▶ meditation

1266
Meares A. **Atavistic regression as a factor in the remission of cancer.** Med J Aust 2:132-133, 1977.

▶ meditation, spiritual healing

It is suggested that the atavistic regression of the mind in intensive meditation is accompanied by a similar physiological regression, and that this may involve the immune system and so influence the patient's defences against cancer.

1267
Meares A. **Mind and cancer.** Lancet 1:978, 1979. (letter)

▶ meditation

1268
Meares A. **The psychological treatment of cancer: the patient's confusion of the time for living with the time for dying.** Aust Fam Physician 8:801-805, 1979.

▶ meditation

It has been shown that it is possible to influence cancer growth by a form of intensive meditation, although it is not yet established whether it can be influenced to the point of cure. In working with these patients it has been observed that the course of the illness has often been influenced by the patient's confusion of the biologically appropriate time for living and the time for dying. Without recourse to any formal psychotherapy, the family physician aware of this reaction may be able to enhance the immune defences and increase the quality of life of such patients.

1269
Meares A. **What can the cancer patient expect from intensive meditation?** Aust Fam Physician 9:322-325, 1980.

▶ meditation

The results of treatment of 73 patients with advanced cancer who have been able to attend at least 20 sessions of intensive meditation, indicates that nearly all such patients should expect significant reduction of anxiety and depression, together with much less discomfort and pain. There is reason to expect a ten per cent chance of quite remarkable slowing of the rate of growth of the tumour, and a ten per cent chance of less marked but still significant slowing. The results indicate that patients with advanced cancer have a ten per cent chance of regression of the growth. There is a fifty per cent chance of greatly improved quality of life and for those who die, a ninety per cent chance of death with dignity.

1270
Morgenstern H, Gellert GA, Walter SD, Ostfeld AM, Siegel BS. **The impact of a psychosocial support program on survival with breast cancer: the importance of selection bias in program evaluation.** J Chronic Dis 37:273-282, 1984. (Also Advances 1(4):65-66, 1984).

▶ group therapy

A retrospective follow-up study was conducted to assess the impact of a psychosocial support program on survival with breast cancer. One hundred and two nonparticipants were individually matched to 34 participants on several prognostic factors, and both groups were followed from date of cancer diagnosis (1971-1980) until December, 1981. Preliminary findings suggest a strong beneficial effect of the program on survival, which is statistically sig-

nificant. However, this observed effect is due largely to a selection bias caused by the failure to match on the duration of the lag period between cancer diagnosis and program entry. Correcting for this bias in the analysis results in a small, nonsignificant program effect. We are not able to rule out a possible effect, however, because of the relative lack of statistical power and because of a modest, though nonsignificant benefit observed for women who entered the program shortly after diagnosis. Furthermore, the program might have other beneficial effects on the quality of life.

1271
Newton-Bernauer W. **The use of hypnosis in the treatment of cancer patients.** Am J Clin Hypn 25:104-113, 1982.

▶ hypnosis, psychotherapy

Describes how for nearly 8 yrs, cancer patients have been treated at the Newton Center for Clinical Hypnosis in Los Angeles, California, using hypnosis and psychotherapy. Basic concepts, assumptions, and procedures are presented and the issues and problems encountered are discussed. It is concluded that hypnotherapeutic interventions can greatly improve the quality of life for nearly any cancer patient whose physical and psychological condition allows him/her to take advantage of this treatment. Patients can benefit from even brief treatment periods. This treatment can not only lengthen life, but it can also arrest or reverse the disease process.

1272
Peter B, Gerl W. **Hypnotherapy in the psychologic treatment of cancer.** Hypn Kognition 1:56-68, 1984. (in German)

▶ psychotherapy, hypnosis

A report of the author's psychotherapeutic and hypnotherapeutic work with cancer patients. Among the topics discussed are hypnotherapy for the control of pain and other side effects of the disease and its treatment, hypnotherapeutic activation of the body's immune system and unconscious coping mechanism, hypnotherapeutic stimulation of the will to live, and hypnotherapy as a means to support the patient in coping with the illness.

1273
Renneker RE. **Countertransference reactions to cancer.** Psychosom Med 19:409-418, 1957.

▶ psychoanalysis

This paper has described various countertransference manifestations observed within a group of seven analysts engaged in a research project based in the psychoanalysis or psychoanalytical psychotherapy of women with cancer of the breast. Countertransference problems were discussed with regard to psychosomatic research in general, and cancer research in particular. The major countertransference manifestations stem from the peculiar interaction of the particular unconscious research motivation of the analyst in combination with characteristic unconscious meanings attributed to the cancer process. Typical examples are given of this interaction with particular emphasis upon the adaptive and nonadaptive solutions of the countertransference cycle. Insight gained in this area has been applied in a brief discussion of surgeons' problems with cancer patients and countertransference phenomena in general analytic practice.

1274
Renneker RE, Cutler R, Hora J, Bacon C, Bradley G, Kearney J, Cutler M. **Psychoanalytical explorations of emotional correlates of cancer of the breast.** Psychosom Med 25:106-123, 1963.

▶ psychotherapy

Extracted summary: It is our belief that psychotherapy is indicated in all major or life-threatening organic conditions which grow out of the soil of a depression. Treatment should be vigorous, active, and directed primarily against the dynamics of the depression. Psychotherapy is also indicated in a patient with cancer of the breast when psychiatric evaluation discloses a neurotic system decompensating in the areas and ways described in this report. Treatment aims at the replacement of object-fixated, frustrated drives with sublimatory outlets or new relatively conflict-free objects. If psychotherapy contributed to the longevity of any patient, then it possibly accomplished this by raising host resistance through achievement of these aims.

1275
Sacerdote P. **Hypnosis in cancer patients.** Am J Clin Hypn 9:100-108, 1966.

▶ hypnosis, psychotherapy

Suggests dividing patients at the time of their original hospitalization into 3 main groups receiving, respectively, orthodox treatment, orthodox treatment plus psychotherapy, and orthodox treatment plus psychotherapy and hypnotherapy, with final comparison of the results on morbidity, mortality, use of medications, etc., at various time intervals.

1276
Scarf M. **Images that heal.** Psychol Today Sept:33-46, 1980.

▶ imagery, relaxation, psychotherapy

Malignancy, according to the theories of Dr. O. Carl Simonton, is a response to despair, experienced biologically at the level of the cell. Critics of Simonton's method of treating cancer—which calls on patients to visualize the destruction of their offending cells in regular exercises—denounce it as a cruel hoax. Whatever the final verdict, the method raises broader questions about the growing faith in the mind's powers to heal.

1277
Searle C. **The power of the folk healer.** Nurs Mirror 151:30-34, 1980.

▶ folk medicine

1278
Secheny S. **Regression of cancer of the rectum after intensive meditation.** Med J Aust 1:136-137, 1980. (letter)

▶ meditation

1279
Selvey HA. **Psychotherapy in the clinical management of cancer.** J Med Assoc Ga 67:812-816, 1978.

▶ review: psychotherapy, meditation, relaxation response, imagery

Much literature attests to the link of the mind and body in the course of cancer. This suggests the possibility that experiential methods of treatment be added to the growing medical armamentarium dealing with the disease. A method of psychotherapy has been developed to create changes in the psychophysiologic milieu of an individual across a broad front suggested from numerous sources. It is expected that this [will cause] increased host resistance, longer life span and hopefully some "spontaneous regressions." However, while face validity of the treatment appears sound, more statistical evidence is called for.

1280
Shapiro A. **Psychotherapy as adjunct treatment for cancer patients.** Am J Clin Hypn 25:150-155, 1982.

▶ psychotherapy, hypnosis, imagery

Describes the progress of 2 cancer patients in psychotherapy who used the ability to minimize pain and discomfort, maintain a high white cell count despite ongoing chemotherapy, and augment the ability of the body's immune system to fight the disease. All were accomplished through the use of visual imagery in the trance state. Visual imagery was also used to reach feelings that Ss were often unable to verbalize. The gradual shift from despair to hope and even confidence, as well as the development of more assertive behavior, is discussed.

1281
Simonton OC, Matthews-Simonton S, Sparks TF. **Psychological intervention in the treatment of cancer.** Psychosomatics 21:226-233, 1980.

▶ psychotherapy

In a preliminary study of the effects of psychological intervention in the treatment of advanced cancer, it was found that patients so treated survived up to twice as long as would have been expected based on national averages. Better patient motivation, greater confidence in the treatment, and overall positive expectancy are thought to have contributed to the results. An educational model has been developed employing the psychological processes used in the study, and further investigations are under way to assess the effect of the patient's mental health on the course of cancer.

1282
Simonton OC, Simonton SS. **Belief systems and management of the emotional aspects of cancer.** J Transpersonal Psychol 7:29-47, 1975. (address)

▶ imagery, relaxation, psychotherapy, group therapy, family therapy, doctor-patient relationship

1283
Stenlin JS Jr, Brach KH. **Psychological aspects of cancer therapy: a surgeon's viewpoint.** JAMA 197:100-104, 1966.

▶ doctor-patient relationship

With regard to his attitude toward cancer, the patient (and the physician as well) consciously or unconsciously equates the word "cancer" with death—death in its worst form, perhaps next month, next week, or even tomorrow. Frequently, his attitude is based upon erroneous information concerning a friend who had cancer, or upon a distressing recollection of a relative who died of the disease. Open discussion of this problem can go far toward reassuring the patient and allaying his fears. Since most malignant processes apparently develop slowly, the patient should be given to understand that his cancer did not begin yesterday; rather, he has probably been living with it for months or years, and still more important, he will not be dead tomorrow. He should also be made to understand that all cancers are not alike and that many patients with certain forms of the disease, although incurable, have lived productive lives for long periods of time, just as they have lived with chronic nonmalignant processes. Here, the surgeon can suggest that the patient's natural body resistance may be effective in controlling the disease. It is well established that an occasional patient with cancer has a resistance to its spread. Is it not possible that this particular patient may be one of these fortunate ones? The physical

aspects of the patient's cancer and the therapeutic measures available obviously influence the quality of hope he may be offered. At this stage, the surgeon's approach must be directed toward hope for control of the cancer, rather than hope for the cure. First, the surgeon is well justified in pointing out the possibility of control of the cancer by the clinical measures available for this purpose. Aggressive surgical procedures, well-planned radiotherapy, hormones, steroids, and other forms of chemotherapy have proved valuable adjuncts to the supportive care of these patients. The senior author makes no apology for administering chemotherapeutic drugs in moderate doses and under well-controlled circumstances, even to patients with cancers that are known to respond poorly. Their usage in this manner is justified, if for no other reason than to show the patient that a positive attempt is being made to retard the progress of his disease. The physician who refuses to adopt an attitude of hopelessness and despair toward patients with advanced cancer may succeed in adding worthwhile years to the lives of some of those otherwise doomed to early and miserable death, and on rare occasions may bring about cure.

1284
Stierlin H, Wirsching M, Haas B, Hoffmann F, Schmidt G, Weber G, Wirsching B. **Family medicine with cancer patients.** Familiendynamik 8:48-68, 1983. (in German)

▶ family therapy

Since the first report on the family therapy of cancer patients approximately two years ago in this journal (Familiendynamik 6:1-23, 1981) the Heidelberg team has gained new experiences and insights. A predictive study carried out on 63 women admitted for exploratory surgery because of a knot in their breast yielded highly significant results with regard to the occurrence of benign or malignant tumors. The predictions were made on the basis of an interview of 30 to 50 minutes duration carried out before biopsy. Futher, a study of 55 families with chronically psychosomatically ill youngsters permitted comparision with families in which one or more members were suffering from cancer. Similarities as well as differences were noticed. Finally, a project offering family therapy to 50 patients with lung cancer made it possible to experiment with systemic therapeutic procedures in this highly stressed patient group. So far, the results have been encouraging.

1285
Strosberg IM. **Notes on treatment of cancer by hypnosis.** J Am Soc Psychosom Dent Med 29:74-76, 1982.

▶ autohypnosis, psychotherapy

Briefly presents suggestions on how autohypnosis can aid or cause remission of cancer. This method emphasizes the patient's belief in his/her own ability to control the cancer cells. The 5 stages of prospective death are also reviewed: disbelief, anger, self-pity, bargaining, and acceptance.

1286
Warga C. **The role of love and laughter in the healing process.** Advances 1:38-39, 1984.

▶ laughter, counseling

Report of a workshop held at the Sheraton-Boston Hotel, Boston, November 4-6, 1983. Includes presentation by O. Carl Simonton, M.D. on "The role of play in health and healing."

1287
Weinstock C. **Recent progress in cancer psychobiology and psychiatry.** J Am Soc Psychosom Dent Med 24:4-14, 1977.

▶ psychotherapy

A specific pattern preceding the onset of cancer has been identified in many patients: extensive trauma experienced in the 1st 7 yrs of life, impaired trust in parents, and fostered repression of anger. These patients were generally unable to form strong attachments, and one satisfying object relationship occurring in young adulthood was later lost, resulting in hopeless depression. Cancer followed within 6 mo to 8 yrs. Location of the tumor may follow symbolic principles; e.g., in the brain in unfulfilled intellectuals, and in the sex organs in homosexuals. Amelioration of the depression—whether through improved family relations, etc., or psychotherapy—precedes many cases of so-called spontaneous regression of the cancer. Psychotherapy should focus upon mobilization of grief and the search for a new object in life.

1288
Weinstock C. **Psychosocial rehabilitation of cancer patients: a pilot study.** Int Ment Health Res Newsletter 16:10-14, 1974.

▶ psychotherapy

Presents a research outline for psychotherapeutic treatment of cancer patients based on a review of research indicating (a) a link between vital loss, inadequate grieving, and cancer outbreak, and (b) a relationship between remissions of cancer and improvements in patients' existential situations. The proposed study, through careful psychodiagnostic evaluation and psychotherapy, is intended (a) to add to the literature on the perceptual and other tendencies predominant in cancer victims long before any cancer breaks out, and (b) to aid patients with cancer and those suspected to be high-cancer-potential individuals.

1289
Weitz RD. **Psychological factors in the prevention and treatment of cancer.** Psychother Private Pract 1:69-76, 1983.

▶ hypnosis, imagery

Discusses mind and body interaction relative to the development of disease process, particularly cancer. The role of stress as a significant factor in the breakdown of the body's immune system is analyzed. The author's experience with the use of hypnosis and imagery as ancillary therapeutic interventions is described and evaluated. It is noted that personality variables are observed in previous research with cancer patients: many cancer patients have experienced a significant emotional trauma 6-18 mo before cancer is evidenced. It is concluded that individuals have potential in exerting control over their lives and producing a lifestyle that is relatively free of the forces leading to illness. The psychologist has a significant role to play in this emphasis on health maintenance. A national communication network is recommended to consolidate the observations of psychological clinicians working with cancer.

1290
Wirsching M, Stierlin H, Haas B, Weber G, Wirsching B. **Family therapy with cancer patients.** Familiendynamik 6:1-23, 1981. (in German)

▶ psychotherapy, paradoxical intervention

Experience gained in recent years with the treatment of cancer patients and their families are reported. After having been guided initially by the "curing through encounter" model the authors gradually changed to a more strategic approach (partly combined with paradoxical interventions). Clinical aspects illustrate and explain this change. Typical interaction rules, family myths and relational patterns of such families are disclosed. The therapeutic measures attempted are based on the hypothesis that with some of the cancer patients, similiar to other psychosomatic diseases, the course of the illness is affected by psychological factors and particularly by the family situation. This hypothesis has not yet been proved. The present report is meant to provide new stimulation and a possibility of comparison for all those who are working in a similar direction.

1291
Woolley-Hart A. **Meditation and cancer: slowing down the inevitable.** Nurs Mirror 149:36-39, 1979.

▶ meditation, relaxation

Treatment of Side Effects of Disease or Therapy:
Nausea and Vomiting, Insomnia, Fatigue, Eating Problems, Pruritus

1292

Ament P, Milgrom H. **Effects of suggestion on pruritus with cutaneous lesions in chronic myelogenous leukemia.** NY State J Med 67:833-835, 1967.

▶ suggestion

A case study showing the positive effects of suggestion on this condition. Suggestion "therapy was (found to be) at least as helpful as the optimal effects of steroid therapy could have been expected to be without the concomitant adverse reactions of disturbing the endocrinologic balance."

1293

Burish TG, Carey MP, Redd WH, Krozely MG. **Behavioral relaxation techniques in reducing the distress of cancer chemotherapy patients.** Oncol Nurs Forum 10:32-35, 1983.

▶ hypnosis, relaxation, biofeedback, desensitization

Some adverse side effects of cancer chemotherapy are attributed to the pharmacologic properties of the antineoplastic drugs, while others appear to be conditioned or learned. A growing number of clinicians are using behavioral relaxation techniques, including hypnosis, progressive muscle relaxation training, electromyogram (EMG) biofeedback, and systematic desensitization, to reduce the conditioned side effects of cancer chemotherapy. The literature suggests that behavioral relaxation techniques can significantly alleviate some conditioned side effects of chemotherapy including nausea, vomiting, and negative emotions such as anxiety and depression. These behavioral procedures are generally inexpensive, easily learned, and have few if any negative side effects. Several hypotheses for the effectiveness of behavioral relaxation strategies are described and evaluated.

1294

Burish TG, Lyles JN. **Effectiveness of relaxation training in reducing the aversiveness of chemotherapy in the treatment of cancer.** J Behav Ther Exp Psychiatry 10:357-361, 1979.

▶ relaxation

Used progressive muscle relaxation training to reduce the conditioned negative responses developed by a 30-yr-old female cancer patient undergoing chemotherapy. Results indicate that during the therapist-directed relaxation phases and one or both of the s-directed phases, the s showed reductions in negative affect, frequency of vomiting, and postsession physiological arousal. It is concluded that progressive muscle relaxation training may be an effective procedure for reducing the adverse side effects of cancer chemotherapy.

1295

Burish TG, Lyles JN. **Effectiveness of relaxation training in reducing adverse reactions to cancer chemotherapy.** J Behav Med 4:65-78, 1981.

▶ relaxation, imagery

Cancer patients who had developed negative conditioned responses to their chemotherapy either did (relaxation training) or did not (no relaxation training) receive progressive muscle relaxation training and guided relaxation imagery instructions immediately before and during their chemotherapy treatments. Physiological (blood pressure and pulse rate) measures of arousal, frequency of vomiting, and patient-reported and nurse-reported indices of negative affect and nausea were collected during pretraining, training and posttraining chemotherapy sessions. Results indicated that during both the training and the posttraining sessions, patients in the relaxation training condition reported feeling less emotionally distressed and nauseated, and showed less physiological arousal following the chemotherapy infusion, than patients in the no relaxation training condition. The attending nurses' observations confirmed the patients' self-reports. No differences were found in frequency of vomiting between conditions.

These data clearly suggest that the use of relaxation procedures may be an effective means of reducing several of the adverse side effects of cancer chemotherapy.

1296
Burish TG, Redd WH. **Behavioral approaches to reducing conditioned responses to chemotherapy in adult cancer patients.** Behav Med Update 5:12-16, 1983.

▶ review: relaxation, hypnosis, systematic desensitization

Discusses the development of symptoms (such as nausea and vomiting) that may result from chemotherapy and addresses the effectiveness of behavioral interventions. These symptoms appear to result from the pharmacological properties of the drugs as well as from classical conditioning. In the conditioning process, a learned association develops between stimuli related to chemotherapy and the side effects of the anticancer drugs such that the stimuli alone become capable of eliciting the distressing side effects. The development of nausea occurs in about one-third of chemotherapy patients. Recently, behavioral techniques such as progressive muscle relaxation training, hypnosis, and systematic desensitization have been used to treat these side effects. Results of 5 controlled studies support the usefulness of these techniques.

1297
Burish TG, Shartner CD, Lyles JN. **Effectiveness of multiple muscle-site EMG biofeedback and relaxation training in reducing the aversiveness of cancer chemotherapy.** Biofeedback Self Regul 6:523-535, 1981.

▶ biofeedback, relaxation

A 44-year-old female cancer patient was given progressive muscle relaxation training and multiple muscle-site EMG biofeedback to reduce the conditioned negative responses she had apparently developed to her chemotherapy treatments. Following three baseline chemotherapy sessions, the patient was given relaxation training and biofeedback during four consecutive chemotherapy treatments and was asked to practice her relaxation skills daily in the hospital or at home. After the patient felt able to relax on her own, relaxation training and biofeedback were terminated and three follow-up sessions were held. Results indicated that during the chemotherapy sessions in which the patient received relaxation training and biofeedback, she showed reductions in physiological arousal (EMG, pulse rate, systolic blood pressure, and diastolic blood pressure) and reported feeling less anxious and nauseated. Moreover, these changes were maintained during the follow-up sessions. These results suggest that relaxation training plus multiple muscle-site biofeedback may be an effective adjunctive procedure for reducing some of the adverse side effects of cancer chemotherapy.

1298
Cairns GF, Altman K. **Behavioral treatment of cancer-related anorexia.** J Behav Ther Exper Psychiatry 10:353-356, 1979.

▶ behavior therapy

Describes the treatment of an 11-yr-old female anorexic oncology patient using positive social reinforcement, access to play activities, and a token system to reverse weight loss.

1299
Campbell DF, Dixon JK, Sanderford LD, Denicola MA. **Relaxation: its effect on the nutritional status and performance status of clients with cancer.** J Am Diet Assoc 84:201-204, 1984.

▶ relaxation, autosuggestion, imagery

Relaxation was used to promote normal food consumption patterns among persons with cancer. As part of a larger study, 22 persons with cancer were randomly assigned to receive instruction and reinforcement in a relaxation technique to be used preprandially. The relaxation procedure included four components: (a) deep abdominal breathing, (b) tensing and relaxing of various body parts, (c) relaxation by autosuggestion, and (d) voluntary image control. Twelve clients complied with relaxation instructions in part, and 10 did not. Among compliers, 75% experienced desirable weight change over a six-week period. Performance status, measured by the Karnofsky scale, improved for 33% and worsened for 17% over eight weeks. Research has shown relaxation to be an effective measure in relation to pain, hypertension, and other conditions. These preliminary results now suggest that relaxation may also be effective in treating the eating problems of the person with cancer, leading to improvement in weight and performance status.

1300
Cannici J, Malcolm R, Peek LA. **Treatment of insomnia in cancer patients using muscle relaxation training.** J Behav Ther Exp Psychiatry 14:251-256, 1983.

▶ review: relaxation

Mean sleep onset latency was reduced from 124 to 29 min in 15 patients suffering from insomnia secondary to cancer; 15 subjects receiving routine care had means of 116 and 104 min in comparison. Muscle relaxation training was administered in individual sessions on three consecutive days. With 26 subjects available for follow-up 3 months later, the mean differences in sleep latency continued. The relatively greater success in this study than previously reported for a behavioral treatment of insomnia is discussed in light of possible differences between primary insomniacs and those subjects with insomnia secondary to a medical disease.

1301
Chang JC. **Nausea and vomiting in cancer patients: an expression of psychological mechanisms?** Psychosomatics 22:707-709, 1981.

▶ placebo, psychotherapy

Extracted summary: Despite the limited effectiveness of cancer therapy, we are now beginning to learn that a patient can be helped a great deal by a careful psychological approach as part of management of the disease. Aside from nausea and vomiting, there are multitudinous complications. Increased attention to psychological aspects may provide us with keener insights into how to help the gravely ill patient cope with the illness. With broader knowledge, we may be able to better manage not only nausea and vomiting, but also the patient's struggle against cancer.

1302
Cobb SC. **Teaching relaxation techniques to cancer patients.** Cancer Nurs 7:157-161, 1984.

▶ relaxation

Various stress reduction techniques have been advocated to assist patients in dealing with the stress of the cancer experience. One of the most popular stress reduction techniques is relaxation, a technique which may help cancer patients cope with pain and decrease the anxiety and side effects associated with various treatments. Due to increased patient interest and a need for further research in this area, nurses need to be knowledgeable about relaxation techniques. Current relaxation literature is reviewed and a plan for teaching relaxation techniques to patients is proposed.

1303
Cotanch PH. **Relaxation training for control of nausea and vomiting in patients receiving chemotherapy.** Cancer Nurs 6:277-283, 1983.

▶ relaxation

The study reports the use of progressive muscle relaxation (PMR) in reducing nausea and vomiting and anxiety in a group of cancer patients. The patients were identified by their oncologists as experiencing refractory drug-induced nausea and vomiting in spite of the administration of antiemetic therapy. Baseline data was collected during one cycle of chemotherapy as the patients, by virtue of their history, served as their own controls. Data collection measured pre- and post-training physiological arousal and state-trait anxiety levels, food-fluid intake, degree and fre-

quency of nausea and vomiting, and type and quantity of antiemetic therapy 48 hours following drug infusion; change in total body weight, and upper arm skin fold were measured throughout the entire chemotherapy course. The results show that nine of the 12 patients showed some decrease in nausea and vomiting after PMR training. Caloric intake was greater 48 hours post-treatment in all patients. These data are suggestive that PMR may be an effective intervention for nausea and vomiting associated with chemotherapy.

1304
Dempster CR, Balson P, Whalen BT. **Supportive hypnotherapy during the radical treatment of malignancies.** Int J Clin Exp Hypn 24:1-9, 1976.

▶ psychotherapy, hypnosis

Notes that modern medicine has made great strides in developing chemotherapeutic and radiologic measures to arrest or retard the malignant disease process. The patient, however, is often rendered acutely uncomfortable by the side-effects of the treatment. Hypnotherapy is pointed to as a means of supporting the patient in a radical regime by alleviating discomfort, as well as by offering a unique interpersonal environment within which to deal with the issues posed by terminal or potentially terminal illness. A case report is presented and discussed.

1305
Dixon J. **Effect of nursing interventions on nutritional and performance status in cancer patients.** Nurs Res 33:330-335, 1984.

▶ relaxation

Cancer patients, assessed as nutritionally at risk, were randomly assigned to a control group or to one of four intervention groups receiving (a) nutritional supplementation, (b) relaxation training, (c) both nutritional supplementation and relaxation training or (d) neither nutritional supplementation nor relaxation training. Fifty-five subjects completed a four-month intervention period during which they were visited biweekly by a nurse (except control subjects). In repeated measures analyses of variance, significant group-by-time interactions were obtained for weight and arm muscle circumference (a measure of protein stores), indicating that for these measures the groups changed differentially during the intervention period. The group-by-time interaction approached significance on the Karnofsky Performance Status Scale. For all three variables, gain was greatest for the relaxation group; the most severe loss occurred in the control group. These findings suggest that the cachexia of cancer may be slowed or reversed through noninvasive nursing interventions.

1306

Dolan J. **Relaxation techniques in the reduction of pain, nausea and sleep disturbances for oncology patients: a primer for rehabilitation counselors.** J Appl Rehabil Counseling 13:35-39, 1982.

▶ relaxation, autosuggestion, behavior therapy

Describes the use of deep muscle relaxation (DMR) and cue-controlled relaxation (CCR) techniques. These methods may be helpful in reducing anxiety-based problems and some of pain, nausea, and sleep disturbances associated with cancer treatment. The premise of DMR is that muscle tension is in some manner related to anxiety and that a reduction in muscle tension will result in a reduction of experienced tension. CCR, which should be taught after the client has mastered DMR, uses calming self-instructions when the client is faced with an anxiety-provoking situation. These methods offer the advantages that they are easily learned, require no special equipment, and do not interfere with the patient's daily routine or the physician's therapeutic regimen.

1307

Ellenberg L, Kellerman J, Dash J, Higgins G, Zeltzer L. **Use of hypnosis for multiple symptoms in an adolescent girl with leukemia.** J Adolesc Health Care 1:132-136, 1980.

▶ hypnosis

An adolescent girl with chronic myelogenous leukemia was treated with hypnosis for several disease- and treatment-related problems during the last 4 months of her life. Data were collected before and after hypnosis on the nature and intensity of the patient's acute pain and anxiety during bone marrow aspirations, chronic headache and backache, nausea and vomiting during chemotherapy, anorexia, and the discomfort associated with spiking temperatures. Comparisons of baseline and posthypnosis reports suggest that hypnosis was successfully used for acute and chronic pain, anxiety, unpleasant body sensations and, possibly, nausea and vomiting. The hypnotic techniques used, the limitations of hypnosis and clinical issues in this case are presented and discussed.

1308

Feinstein A. **Psychological interventions in the treatment of cancer.** Clin Psychol Rev 3:1-14, 1983.

▶ review: psychotherapy

Eight variables are identified as being implicated in cancer cases where improvement in disease status has been associated with psychological interventions. Research reports bearing on each of these areas are surveyed, and it is suggested that the variables provide a basis for for-

mulating testable propositions. Clinical research programs could measure changes in medical status following interventions that (1) alter stress conditions and their management, (2) work through unresolved grief, (3) stimulate the will to live, (4) promote realistic positive expectations, (5) mobilize mental capacities for psychophysiological control, (6) constructively handle denial, (7) increase appropriate emotional expression, and (8) strengthen specified personal traits. Considerations related to conducting such research are discussed. Although the nature of any relationship between psychological factors and malignant disease remains unclear, palliative psychological interventions that might also have a beneficial effect on medical status are currently available.

1309

Foerster K. **Psychotherapeutic care of leukosis patients treated under conditions of isolation.** Psychother Psychosom Med Psychol 32:35-38, 1982. (in German)

▶ psychotherapy, autogenic training

The author reports on psychotherapeutical observations and experience with 18 leukemic patients who had been treated temporally in germ-free environment (life island). Fourteen patients were under psychotherapeutic treatment during which a supporting psychotherapy with additional learning of autogenous training was carried out. The results are discussed. The problems of the therapeutical team of a hematologic intensive-care unit were pointed out.

1310

Foerster K. **Supportive psychotherapy combined with autogenous training in acute leukemic patients under isolation therapy.** Psychother Psychosom 41:100-105, 1984.

▶ psychotherapy, autogenic training

The author reports on psychotherapeutic observations and experience with 18 leukemic patients who had been treated temporally in a germ-free environment ("life island"). 14 patients were under psychotherapeutic treatment during which a supporting psychotherapy with additional learning of autogenous training was carried out. The results are discussed and the problems of the therapeutic team of a hematologic intensive-care unit are pointed out.

1311

Forester B, Kornfeld DS, Fleiss JL. **Psychotherapy during radiotherapy: effects on emotional and physical distress.** Am J Psychiatry 142:22-27, 1985.

▶ psychotherapy

The authors determined the effects of ongoing weekly individual psychotherapy on the symptoms of patients undergoing a 6-week course of radiotherapy for cancer. Forty-eight patients were given weekly psychotherapy sessions for 10 weeks; another 52 patients served as control subjects. A statistically significant reduction was found in both emotional and "physical" manifestations of distress in the patients receiving psychotherapy compared with the control group. This was true regardless of gender, ward or private patient status, or knowledge of diagnosis. Patient gender and knowledge of diagnosis did affect the pattern and magnitude of the response to psychotherapy.

1312

Friedman MM. **Hypnotherapy in advanced cancer.** Rocky Mt Med J 57:33-37, 1960.

▶ hypnosis, suggestion

The anxieties and intractable pain frequently associated with cancer in its terminal stages can be alleviated by hypnotherapy. The results are roughly proportional to the depth of trance. The method is time consuming and not all patients can be deeply hypnotized. On the other hand, drug requirements are reduced, pain is relieved and the serious emotional problems associated with the disease minimized. Life is prolonged and death is approached tranquilly and without fear.

1313

Gordon AM. **Psychological aspects of isolator therapy in acute leukaemia.** Br J Psychiatry 127:588-590, 1975.

▶ supportive psychotherapy

Treatment under conditions of gnotobiotic isolation can augment the stress of adaptation to a diagnosis of leukaemia. Identification of the psychological problems experienced in isolator treatment can contribute to the effective maintenance of therapy. Individual patterns of adjustment to treatment relate to the psychological defence mechanisms employed to contend with the dependent position enforced by isolation. Psychiatric assessment can assist both patients and nursing staff with the management of their separate difficulties in this unfamiliar treatment situation. Psychological features of isolator treatment in ten patients with acute leukaemia are described and suggestions proposed for psychological management of patients under isolator conditions.

1314

Gordon AM. **Psychological adaptation to isolator therapy in acute leukaemia.** Psychother Psychosom 26:132-139, 1975.

▶ psychotherapy, consultation-liaison

Exteacted summary: A psychiatrist can contribute to an isolator unit in several ways. Psychiatric assessment may be initially requested to help identify patients who might fail to tolerate isolator treatment, especially patients with a previous psychiatric illness. In general, previous psychological disturbance would not appear to contraindicate isolator therapy but the practical difficulties of managing psychotic illness within an isolator could disrupt treatment. The vulnerability of the psychotic patient would require careful assessment. The attitudes of the patient with a manic defence to illness has an understandable appeal to many physicians. Although medical factors are the primary consideration in selection for isolator treatment, it is not surprising to find this group of patients highly represented in this series. A psychiatrist can alert staff to the problems of managing the manic-defended patient and indicate that the apathetic withdrawal of the regressed patient may prove less problematical under isolator conditions. Psychiatric assessment can help predict patient reaction to isolation and joint discussion with medical and nursing staff can increase awareness of adaptive behavior, help staff to understand confusing inconsistencies in patient reaction and assist them in contending with fluctuations in rapport with patients.

1315

Grof S, Goodman LE, Richards WA, Kurland AA. **LSD-assisted psychotherapy in patients with terminal cancer.** Int Pharmacopsychiatry 8:129-144, 1973.

▶ psychotherapy

The paper describes the results of a clinical study exploring the potential of a complex psychotherapeutic program utilizing psychedelic compounds to alleviate the emotional and physical suffering of cancer patients. A total of 60 cancer patients participated in this experimental study. In 44 of these patients, LSD (200-500 micrograms per os) was administered as an adjunct to psychotherapy; in 19 patients, a new psychedelic compound, dipropyltryptamine (DPT) was administered (60-105 mg i.m.). Three of these patients received both LSD and DPT administered on different sessions. The therapeutic results were assessed by means of a rating scale reflecting the degree of the patients' depression, psychological isolation, anxiety, difficulty in management, fear of death, and pain. The ratings were done by attending physicians, nurses, family members, LSD therapists and cotherapists, and independent raters. In addition, the amount of narcotics required in the management of the patient was measured before and after the psychedelic sessions. Systematic rating was carried out in a group of 31 cancer patients treated by LSD. The comparison of the means of individual ratings from pre- to posttreatment showed significant improvement in all the measured parameters for most of the raters. There was a definite reduction of the narcotic medication; it did not, however, reach the level of statistical significance. The pre- to post-treatment comparison of the global indexes used as gross indicators of the degree of emotional and physical distress, indicated that approximately 29% of the patients showed dramatic improvement, and another 41.9% moderate improvement, with 22.6% essentially unchanged. In 6.4% of the patients, global indexes showed a decrement in the posttherapy ratings.

1316
Gybels J, Adriaensen H, Cosyns P. **Treatment of pain in patients with advanced cancer.** Eur J Cancer 12:341-351, 1976.

▶ psychotherapy, relaxation, biofeedback, hypnosis, behavior therapy, consultation-liaison

All of the methods described for the treatment of pain have their shortcomings. The best results are seen when a combination of them is used in the frame of a multidisciplinary pain clinic. The universal approach with analgesic drugs, as used (and misused) by every doctor, can often be corrected and improved by specialists with a larger pharmacological experience. At the same time, the screening for more specialistic intervention is easily realised by the multidisciplinary team, in which the oncologist and family physician are included. In Fig. 5 an attempt is made to summarize the possible modalities of treatment. Nevertheless this is an abstraction of the clinical situation, and it cannot be overemphasized that the treatment of pain has to be individual for each patient.

1317
Hailey BJ, White JG. **Systematic desensitization for anticipatory nausea associated with chemotherapy.** Psychosomatics 24:287-291, 1983.

▶ desensitization

Systematic desensitization (SD) used on a 28-yr-old male with diffuse histiocytic lymphoma enabled him to cope effectively with the anticipatory nausea and vomiting associated with cancer chemotherapy. SD is preferable to drug treatment because it gives the patient a sense of internalized control over his/her body and enables him/her to avoid possible drug effects such as drowsiness.

1318
Hamberger LK. **Reduction of generalized aversive responding in a post-treatment cancer patient: relaxation as an active coping skill.** J Behav Ther Exp Psychiatry 13:229-233, 1982.

▶ relaxation

A male ostomy patient was successfully taught relaxation as an active coping skill to control generalized aversive gastric upset responses which had originally developed in the context of radiation therapy. Because the patient had completed his medical regimen, intervention focused on applied relaxation outside the medical center setting. Treatment involved minimal therapist contact. The results are discussed in terms of assessing aversive side effects which generalize beyond the course of medical treatment, and the contingent aspects of such treatments. The efficiency of relaxation programs, as well as the importance of active patient involvement, are also discussed.

1319
Hoffman ML. **Hypnotic desensitization for the management of anticipatory emesis in chemotherapy.** Am J Clin Hypn 25:173-176, 1982.

▶ hypnosis, desensitization

A hypnotic treatment employing systematic desensitization was used to alleviate anticipatory nausea and vomiting in a middle-aged man undergoing chemotherapy for Hodgkin's disease. After 4 treatment sessions, all nausea associated with chemotherapy was eliminated. Results of this treatment are compared with those of another hypnotic treatment recently reported by W. H. Redd et al. and reasons for differences are discussed.

1320
Holland JC, Rowland J, Plumb M. **Psychological aspects of anorexia in cancer patients.** Cancer Res 37:2425-2428, 1977.

▶ autohypnosis

Transient anorexia occurs in cancer patients secondary to psychological distress. Discomfort, pain, and lack of a sense of well-being contribute to a general dysphoric affective state, although the clinical signs of significant depression consonant with anorexia on the basis of depression are rarely seen in cancer and were not found in a controlled study. The anorexia-cachexia syndrome of advanced cancer derives from causes other than psychological, compounded at times by the side effects of surgery, chemotherapy, and radiation therapy. Management of nutrition in cancer can be improved by judicious use of psychopharmacological drugs to diminish the nausea, vomiting, and anorexia of radiation or chemotherapy. Some drugs appear to have a specific appetite-stimulating effect and should be further investigated (cyproheptadine and 9-tetrahydrocanabinol). Behavioral techniques used in cases of anorexia nervosa seem to have little relevance in adults with cancer, although self-hypnosis appears useful in children. Creation of as pleasant an ambiance as possible around meals, with encouragement to eat, concern for the patient's food preferences, and attention to the most pleasant social setting for the serving of meals is desirable. The value of eating with a family member, friend, or fellow patient and, if desired, of serving wine, which may stimulate both appetite and social interaction, should not be overlooked.

1321

Kaempfer SH. **Relaxation training reconsidered.** Oncol Nurs Forum 9:15-18, 1982.

▶ relaxation, imagery, autohypnosis, biofeedback

Stress management techniques, such as relaxation training, have received attention as possible symptom management strategies in cancer therapy. A review of the reported uses of these techniques with cancer patients yields only a small number of studies, few of which involve systematic research. This finding, as well as anecdotal observations made by the author, suggests that unqualified recommendations for implementation of relaxation training with cancer patients may be premature.

1322

Katz ER. **Conditioned aversion to chemotherapy.** Psychosomatics 23:650-651, 1982. (letter)

▶ classical conditioning, avoidance learning

1323

Kaye JM. **Hypnotherapy and family therapy for the cancer patient: a case study.** Am J Clin Hypn 27:38-41, 1984.

▶ hypnosis, family therapy

Cancer patients often experience uncomfortable side effects of chemotherapy. Using a combination of hypnotherapy and family therapy, the therapist can help the patient deal with the issues of terminal illness. The potential value of a combination of these two approaches used in conjunction with normal medical management is demonstrated in the case presented.

1324

Kellerman J. **Single case study: behavioral treatment of night terrors in a child with acute leukemia.** J Nerv Ment Dis 167:182-185, 1979.

▶ behavior therapy, reinforcement

Describes treatment of a 3-yr-old girl with acute lymphocytic leukemia and a 1-mo history of recurrent nightmares. Symptoms of the disturbance conformed to a clinical picture of slow wave arousal night terrors, or pavor nocturnus. Behavioral treatment aimed at reducing anxiety related to maternal separation and medical procedures, and at reinforcing appropriate sleep patterns, was effective in reducing and eventually eliminating the symptoms. Follow-up revealed no return of nightmares or existence of new problems. A brief review of descriptive,

etiological, and treatment aspects of night terrors is presented, and the hypothesis is put forth that such episodes represent a psychological reaction to trauma. The importance of being aware of age variables in the expression of children's anxiety is noted as is the value of careful tabulation of outcome data.

1325

Kellerman J, Rigler D, Siegel SE, McCue K, Pospisil J, Uno R. **Psychological evaluation and management of pediatric oncology patients in protected environments.** Med Ped Oncol 2:353-360, 1976.

▶ play therapy

Specific aspects of psychological investigation and management of pediatric patients with widely disseminated solid tumors treated in semiportable, laminar airflow patient isolators are discussed. Information was obtained prospectively from a psychosocial study coordinated with a medical investigation of the use of protected environments (PE) employing barrier isolation as an adjunct to intensive anticancer therapy. Included are descriptions of the development of psychological criteria for patient eligibility, psychometric evaluation, longitudinal behavioral observation, pre-entry and predischarge orientation techniques, as well as approaches to the ongoing management of patients and families. No debilitating psychological disturbance has been observed in these patients, and no patients have had to be removed for psychological reasons. Specific transitory psychological changes are noted as are the problems encountered by staff members functioning in such a setting. The adoption of a well-coordinated psychosocial program of investigation and clinical intervention has proved useful in maximizing patient adjustment to prolonged treatment in protected environments.

1326

Klosinski G. **Psychotherapeutic team-consultation including the parents of leukosis children treated under conditions of isolation: an empiric report.** Prax Kinderpsychol Kinderpsychiatr 32:245-251, 1983. (in German)

▶ psychotherapy, consultation-liaison, family therapy

A report on the psychotherapeutic care of 2 leukemic children and on the experiences of a child psychiatric consultant in a hematologic intensive care unit. Frequent psychological problems occur in children who are forced to exist in germ-free isolation therapy. Treatment of these psychological problems in both the children and in their parents is discussed.

1327

Kohle K, Simons C, Weidlich S, Dietrich M, Durner A. **Psychological aspects in the treatment of leukemia patients in the isolated-bed system "life island."** Psychother Psychosom 19:85-91, 1971.

▶ psychotherapy

Report of psychological assessment and supportive psychotherapy in the treatment (intensive chemotherapy under gnotobiotic conditions) of nine patients suffering from acute leukemia. Isolation, extreme dependency on medical and nursing staff, inhibition of motor activity and medical complications aggravate the reaction to the confrontation with the diagnosis. The impact of the specific treatment situation does not only concern the patients but medical and nursing staff as well. Arising problems and means of dealing with them are discussed.

1328

Kutz I, Borysenko JZ, Come SE, Benson H. **Paradoxical emetic response to antiemetic treatment in cancer patients.** N Engl J Med 303:148, 1980. (letter)

▶ classical conditioning

1329

LaBaw WL. **Terminal hypnosis in lieu of terminal hospitalization; an effective alternative in fortunate cases.** Gerontol Clin (Basel) 11:312-320, 1969.

▶ hypnosis, autohypnosis

Presented are two clinical case reports illustrating the initial statement that suggestive therapy for the dying can exceed the value of terminal inpatient care for the patient, attending physician, and observing family. Amplificative discussion follows. Medical hypnosis is described as a useful adjunct in the care and tutelage of a patient anticipating death; its more frequent utilization by physicians is urged.

1330

LaBaw WL, Holton C, Tewell K, Eccles D. **The use of self-hypnosis by children with cancer.** Am J Clin Hypn 17:233-238, 1975.

▶ hypnosis, group therapy

Presents a clinical report relating the experience gained in 24 mo of studying 27 children using contemporary medical hypnosis to combat some aspects of malignancies. The afflicted children were trained in group trance sessions to induce trance in themselves. The trance state resulted in more rest, easier and longer sleep, more adequate food and fluid intake and retention, and greater tolerance for and manageability during diagnostic and therapeutic procedures. Fear, anxiety, depression, overdetermined re-

sponse to discomfort, and anticipatory vomiting prior to treatment were diminished.

1331

LeBaron S, Zeltzer L. **Behavioral intervention for reducing chemotherapy-related nausea and vomiting in adolescents with cancer.** J Adolesc Health Care 5:178-182, 1984.

▶ behavior therapy

Eight adolescents (10-17 years, mean 12.1) with cancer received behavioral intervention for chemotherapy-related nausea and vomiting. Within 3-5 days after the administration of each course of chemotherapy, patients rated (1-10 scale; 1 = none, 10 = maximum) their nausea and vomiting and the extent to which chemotherapy bothered them and disrupted their daily routine. After a baseline (preintervention) assessment of 2-3 courses of chemotherapy, patients received intervention during another 2-3 courses. While no significant reduction of symptoms was found prior to intervention, with intervention there were reductions in nausea ($Z = 2.37$, p less than 0.02), vomiting ($Z = 2.52$, p less than 0.01), bother ($Z = 2.24$, p less than 0.02), and disruption of activities ($Z = 2.38$, p less than 0.02). This preliminary study suggests that chemotherapy side effects in adolescents can be reduced with behavioral intervention.

1332

Leibenluft E. **An atypical eating disorder following cancer chemotherapy.** Psychosomatics 26:147-148, 1985.

▶ behavior modification, relaxation, psychotherapy

Extracted summary: This case demonstrates the complementary nature of various models in explaining the etiology and course of the eating disorder. Such complementary models can be used to design an optimal treatment plan. Here the plan included medication, behavior modification, and psychotherapy, and it yielded a successful outcome. The possibility of spontaneous remission must be considered, but is unlikely, given the patient's consistently worsening psychiatric condition before the combined treatment was instituted. It is also possible that one modality alone effected remission, but this too is unlikely given the fact that each new modality was added after the previous ones alone had been unsuccessful.

1333

Levy SM. **Biobehavioral interventions in behavioral medicine: an overview.** CA 50:1939-1943, 1982.

▶ behavior therapy, hypnosis, systematic desensitization

Extracted summary: An underlying theme throughout this report is the need to understand the biological links between behavior and neoplasia. That is, across all the research areas covered in this paper, the aim should be to understand host differences in cancer susceptibility and course as a function of lifestyle, emotional and behavioral response, and milieu characteristics across population subgroups. These potentially modifiable host differences, ranging from altered immune response as a function of stress to decreased patient stamina as a function of nutritional deficit, present the greatest challenge to behavioral scientists committed to the control of disease.

1334
Liss A. **A psycho-oncological approach using hypnosis and suggestive saturation in the treatment of cancer.** Diss Abstr Int 43:552, 1982.

▶ hypnosis, suggestion, psychotherapy, family therapy

Although there is a growing body of literature supporting a relationship between emotional factors and the cancer process, research studying psychological interventions in treatment of cancer is severely lacking. This study, exploratory in nature, involved the conceptualization, application and evaluation of a psycho-oncological treatment program. This team approach model integrates psychosocial interventions with medical therapies to consider the biological, psychological and social needs of the cancer patient. The patient, a participating team member, along with his/her family, is encouraged to assume an active role in the treatment process. The specific objectives of this study were: (1) to delineate the theoretical, research-based framework and background assumptions of the present intervention model; (2) to describe the treatment program; (3) to demonstrate the application of the psychotherapeutic treatment strategies on a single human subject with lung cancer; (4) to help the patient gain a sense of control over the illness, and consequently, over her life; (5) to the greatest extent possible infer the potential effects of specific interventions. A 59-year-old woman with bronchogenic carcinoma and undergoing medical treatment was the subject of the study. The single case design was employed due to the exploratory nature of this research, aiming primarily at discovering and generating hypotheses. Limitations of this methodology include (1) non-generalizability, (2) lack of controls, (3) subjective method, (4) small sample size. Procedures involved three major components: (1) hypnosis and suggestive saturation, (2) psychotherapy, and (3) family intervention. Data was gathered from the observations of the therapist, patient, family, and attending oncologist. The data was analyzed according to a pre-during-post treatment time frame with respect to the objectives of the study. Within this time frame, favorable trends were observed in four general areas: (1) attitudinal/behavioral change, (2) tolerance of medical treatment, (3) management of side-effects of chemotherapy, (4) effects on certain disease symptoms. Psychological interventions were possibly related to ef-

fecting these trends, and then, to what degree, is questionable. While results were inconclusive, the study indicated the value of psychological interventions in the cancer process. Further investigation in more controlled studies is needed, as research in this controversial area is only in its infancy.

1335
Lyles JN, Burish TG, Krozely MG, Oldham RK. **Efficacy of relaxation training and guided imagery in reducing the aversiveness of cancer chemotherapy.** J Consult Clin Psychol 50:509-524, 1982.

▶ relaxation, imagery, supportive psychotherapy

50 cancer patients receiving chemotherapy (25 by push injection and 25 by drip infusion) were assigned to 1 of 3 conditions for their chemotherapy treatments: (A) progressive muscle-relaxation training plus guided-relaxation imagery; (B) therapist control, in which a therapist was present to provide support and encouragement but did not provide systematic relaxation training; and (C) no-treatment control. Ss participated in 1 pretraining, 3 training, and 1 follow-up session. Results indicate that during the training sessions, ss who received relaxation training (A) reported feeling significantly less anxious and nauseated during chemotherapy, (B) showed significantly less physiological arousal and reported less anxiety and depression immediately after chemotherapy, and (C) reported significantly less severe and less protracted nausea at home following chemotherapy. Data suggest that relaxation training may be an effective procedure for helping cancer patients cope with the adverse effects of their chemotherapy.

1336
Martin J. **Helping the dying to live—through hypnosis.** JAMA 249:322, 1983. (News)

▶ hypnosis

1337
Meyer J. **Systematic desensitization versus relaxation training and no treatment (controls) for the reduction of nausea, vomiting and anxiety resulting from chemotherapy.** Diss Abstr Int 44:1247-1248, 1983.

▶ systematic desensitization, relaxation

Previously neutral stimuli that are associated with chemotherapy treatments for cancer acquire aversive properties which may serve to produce or compound nausea, vomiting, and anxiety side effects. These symptoms can occur prior to chemotherapy, during administration, and following treatments. Although antiemetic drugs are available, side effects are often refractory to these agents which can produce their own array of distressing side effects. In the present investigation, nausea, vomiting and anxiety occurring during chemotherapy treatments and during the 24-hour recovery period following chemotherapy were examined. Thirteen subjects receiving systematic desensitization, a counterconditioning technique with no known side effects, were compared with 12 subjects receiving relaxation training and with another 12 subjects in a no-treatment control group. It was expected that both systematic desensitization and relaxation training would prove beneficial to patients in controlling side effects. However, it was predicted that desensitization would prove to be a superior symptom control technique. One pretraining, two treatment, and one follow-up session were conducted. Overall, results indicated that both desensitization and relaxation were effective against nausea and anxiety, and somewhat effective against vomiting. For many of the side effects that were controlled through treatments, desensitization proved to be more beneficial to patients than relaxation. The data suggest that behavioral treatments are effective procedures for helping cancer patients cope with the side effects resulting from chemotherapy. Implications of this study are discussed in relation to similar research in this area. Areas for future investigation are identified.

1338

Milne G. **Hypnotic treatment of a cancer patient.** Aust J Clin Exp Hypn 10:123-125, 1982.

▶ hypnosis, autohypnosis, relaxation

A 48-yr-old female cancer patient was treated through hypnosis for depression and severe nausea caused by chemotherapy. Treatment through ego-strengthening suggestions and relaxation exercises followed by self-hypnosis focused on positive imagery ended her nausea and depression and improved her marriage relationship, which had previously deteriorated because of the negative feelings generated by her illness.

1339

Moore K, Altmaier EM. **Stress inoculation training with cancer patients.** Cancer Nurs 4:389-393, 1981.

▶ relaxation, imagery, cognitive therapy

Stress inoculation techniques were taught to outpatient oncology clinic participants during a pilot project at the University of Florida Shands Teaching Hospital. An intervention model developed for use with this population included instruction in coping skills for a variety of problematic situations, such as fear of needles and prechemotherapy vomiting. The pilot sample consisted of nine cancer patients receiving chemotherapy. An inductive thought-listing measurement procedure was used to assess self-statements relevant to the clinic situation. Prior to treatment, four of these patients were assessed as adjusting

well to their clinic experience. The remaining five patients exhibited problematic behaviors, primarily anticipating vomiting. Posttreatment observations indicated that the stress inoculation techniques were beneficial in altering anxiety-related behaviors. Stress inoculation techniques and rationale are discussed. Case examples and suggestions for modification to the model are presented.

1340

Morphis OL. **Hypnosis and its use in controlling patients with malignancy.** Am J Roentgenol 85:897-900, 1961.

▶ hypnosis, autohypnosis

Hypnosis is useful in the care of the majority of patients, but approximately 20 per cent of the patients will not readily go into hypnosis. When these individuals are encountered, one simply goes back to using all the drugs and sedatives that we have used in the past. Hypnosis does not replace good drug therapy. It is an additional therapeutic agent to be used in the management of patients, when indicated.

1341

Morrow GR. **Appropriations of taped versus live relaxation in the systematic desensitization of anticipatory nausea and vomiting in cancer patients.** J Consult Clin Psychol 52:1098-1099, 1984.

▶ relaxation, systematic desensitization

Systematic desensitization has been shown to be an effective treatment for the nausea and vomiting experienced by approximately 25% of cancer patients in anticipation of chemotherapeutic treatments. This biobehavioral intervention could be made more applicable to an oncology clinical setting if it required less professional treatment time. The suggestion that the relaxation part of systematic desensitization could be learned by cancer patients from a prerecorded audiotape prior to meeting a psychologist for treatment was investigated in the present study. Four of 5 cancer patients randomly assigned to a taped-relaxation group experienced nausea while listening to the prerecorded audiotape, whereas none of 5 patients taught muscle relaxation in person reported nausea when subsequently listening to an audiotape made during the live presentation of relaxation.

1342

Morrow GR, Morrell C. **Behavioral treatment for the anticipatory nausea and vomiting induced by cancer chemotherapy.** N Engl J Med 307:1476-1480, 1982.

▶ systematic desensitization, relaxation

The nausea and vomiting experienced by one in four cancer patients in anticipation of chemotherapy is probably a learned response to treatment. To determine whether behavioral approaches for altering learned responses might be useful treatments for these symptoms, we compared the effects of "systematic desensitization" (a behavioral treatment in which relaxation is learned as a response to situations in which patients have had anticipatory nausea and vomiting) with those of counseling and of no treatment. Sixty ambulatory cancer patients with anticipatory nausea and vomiting before their third and fourth chemotherapy treatments were randomized equally to the three groups. Significantly more patients receiving desensitization reported no anticipatory nausea before their fifth and sixth chemotherapy treatments than patients given counseling (P less than 0.05) or no treatment (P less than 0.01). Desensitized patients also reported significantly less severe anticipatory nausea (P less than 0.01) and vomiting (P less than 0.05) and a shorter duration of anticipatory nausea (P less than 0.01). We conclude that systematic desensitization appears to have an antiemetic effect in cancer patients who receive chemotherapy, and may be useful in the management of these problems.

1343

Nesse RM, Carli T, Curtis GC, Kleinman PD. **Pretreatment nausea in cancer chemotherapy: a conditioned response?** Psychosom Med 42:33-36, 1980.

▶ conditioning

Many patients receiving cancer chemotherapy become nauseated as they anticipate their treatments. We studied this phenomenon in eighteen cancer chemotherapy patients. The eight patients who reported pretreatment nausea had more extensive disease than the other patients and had received twice as much chemotherapy. In most cases pretreatment nausea developed only after a number of months of treatment. Nausea was usually precipitated by the odor of the clinic and similar odors elsewhere also caused nausea. Patients continued to experience nausea during follow-up visits after treatment was completed. This syndrome of pretreatment nausea can be understood as a classically conditioned response. Clinical recommendations can be made on this basis.

1344

Nigl AJ. **Electromyograph training to increase oral cavity functioning in a postoperative cancer patient.** Behav Ther 10:423-427, 1979.

▶ biofeedback

S was a 62-yr-old female who underwent several operations to eradicate bilateral mucosal cancer of the lymph node tissue. By receiving auditory and visual feedback regarding her ability to produce above threshold muscle activity, she apparently was able to learn how to use muscles that she previously could not control. The effects of the EMG treatment were seen not only in increased oral cavity functioning, but also in a significant improvement in S's self-esteem and self-confidence.

1345

Pratt A, Lazar RM, Penman D, Holland JC. **Psychological parameters of chemotherapy-induced conditioned nausea and vomiting: a review.** Cancer Nurs 7:483-490, 1984.

▶ review: relaxation, hypnosis, systematic desensitization

Anticipatory nausea and vomiting is now a well-documented phenomenon in a large proportion of patients who receive chemotherapy for cancer. It is explained by the theory of classical conditioning in which powerful nausea-eliciting drugs become paired with innocuous aspects of the treatment situation or the patient's life. After several such pairings, the innocuous events themselves produce emesis without chemotherapy. Much effort has gone into finding effective treatments for anticipatory nausea and vomiting. While some antiemetic drugs have shown efficacy, they have unacceptable side effects. Behavioral psychologists have developed techniques to alleviate anticipatory nausea and vomiting through relaxation, hypnosis, and systematic desensitization. These techniques work by breaking the stimulus pairings between emesis and previously neutral aspects of treatment. This paper will review the literature on anticipatory nausea and vomiting and offer recommendations for controlling this distressing side effect from chemotherapy.

1346

Questad KA. **An empirical study of a rehabilitation program for fatigue related to cancer.** Diss Abstr Int 44:1974-1975, 1983.

▶ behavior therapy

Several studies have shown that fatigue is the single problem most frequently reported by patients receiving treatment for cancer. Despite these studies, no rehabilitation programs have been described for dealing with the specific problem of fatigue. The purpose of this study was to test the effectiveness of a rehabilitation program for reducing three components of fatigue in cancer patients receiving five consecutive weeks of radiotherapy. Patients who agreed to participate were randomly assigned to either a full, immediate treatment condition or an abbreviated, delayed treatment condition. Then the patients completed questionnaires repeatedly, at regular intervals, for four weeks. The questionnaires assessed how tired the patients felt, how much they felt fatigue was interfering with normal activities, and actual activity level along with distress created by cancer symptoms and general mood. Patients in the full treatment condition attended two physical therapy sessions (exercise) and one psychology (stress management) session per week. Patients in the delayed treatment condition filled out forms only for three weeks and then received one week of the treatment. An analysis of the results showed that patients in the full treatment condition reported they felt less tired, and less impaired in their normal activities than patients in the abbreviated treatment condition (p < .05). There were, however, no differences in the levels of actual activity that the two groups reported and no differences in the trends of fatigue or impairment ratings. While the results suggest that patients in the full treatment groups were bothered less by fatigue, it is difficult to determine to what extent the difference was due to extraneous factors such as the different expectations the two groups may have had about the effectiveness of the treatment they received. Further research is needed to clarify what role various factors may plan in determining the immediate effectiveness of the treatment and to see if such treatment helps patients in their long term adjustment care.

1347

Redd WH. **Behavioural analysis and control of psychosomatic symptoms of patients receiving intensive cancer treatment.** Br J Clin Psychol 21:351-358, 1982.

▶ behavior therapy

Examined behavioral symptoms, such as gagging, coughing, and vomiting, commonly observed in cancer patients and sought to determine factors that foster their development. Time-series analyses of patients' behavioral symptoms and assessments of behavioral interventions involving the modification of nurse-patient and family-patient interactions were incorporated. Intervention work with 2 53- and 63-yr-old females and 2 24- and 64-yr-old males is described. Results show that (1) inadvertent social reinforcement by hospital staff and family members fosters the development of behavioral symptoms; (2) personnel associated with treatment can become discriminative stimuli for social attention and thereby evoke symptom behaviors; and (3) by modifying the social reinforcement contingencies associated with treatment protocols the frequency of psychosomatic symptoms can be reduced without changing the quality of medical/nursing care and social interaction.

1348

Redd WH. **Stimulus control and extinction of psychosomatic symptoms in cancer patients in protective isolation.** J Consult Clin Psychol 48:448-455, 1980.

▶ extinction, reinforcement, covert conditioning

Evaluated the use of multiple therapists in the extinction of psychosomatic symptoms (coughing and retching) in 2

acute leukemia patients—a 24-yr-old male and a 63-yr-old female. Baseline assessments of symptom frequency showed that Ss were under stimulus control of ward nurses (WNS). Intervention involved the application of extinction (ignoring symptoms) and differential reinforcement (social attention) by WNS assigned to patient care. The 1st WN to implement these procedures for each patient achieved symptom suppression after 32 (S 1) and 40 (S 2) applications. In the presence of all other WNS, however, symptom occurrence continued. During the next phase a 2nd WN applied these procedures and, after 25 (S 1) and 23 (S 2) entrances, the symptoms were extinguished. However, the symptoms continued in the presence of hospital staff until 4 separate WNS had successfully applied the extinction/differential-reinforcement procedure. Extinction occurred more rapidly (requiring fewer entrances) with each successive WN. At 2-wk and 6-mo follow-up evaluations, the symptoms had not reappeared, and no new problems had developed.

1349

Redd WH. **Control of nausea and vomiting in chemotherapy patients: four effective behavioral methods.** Postgrad Med 75:105-107, 110-113, 1984.

▶ hypnosis, imagery, relaxation, desensitization

Nearly one third of cancer patients who receive chemotherapy experience severe nausea and/or vomiting in anticipation of treatment. Antiemetic drugs are generally of little value in controlling this type of side effect. In this article, Dr. Redd discusses four behavioral methods that have proven effective in reducing the distress associated with cancer chemotherapy. He also encourages physicians to become better acquainted with behavioral intervention as a form of treatment not only of chemotherapy side effects but also of other problems associated with comprehensive cancer therapy.

1350

Redd WH, Andresen GV, Minagawa RY. **Hypnotic control of anticipatory emesis in patients receiving cancer chemotherapy.** J Consult Clin Psychol 50:14-19, 1982.

▶ hypnosis, conditioning

Nausea and vomiting in anticipation of chemotherapy often develop in patients undergoing cancer treatment. In this study, deep muscle relaxation hypnosis controlled these conditioned reactions in 6 female patients (aged 24-56 yrs). Anticipatory emesis recurred when hypnosis was not used. During subsequent sessions in which hypnosis was reinstated, anticipatory emesis was again controlled.

1351

Redd WH, Andrykowski MA. **Behavioral intervention in cancer treatment: controlling aversion reactions to chemotherapy.** J Consult Clin Psychol 50:1018-1029, 1982.

▶ hypnosis, imagery, relaxation, desensitization

During the protracted course of cancer chemotherapy, approximately 25% of patients develop aversion reactions to treatment by becoming nauseated and/or vomiting before their chemotherapy treatments. This phenomenon has been conceptualized as a result of respondent conditioning. Since commonly used antiemetic drugs do not reliably control anticipatory nausea/emesis, behavioral techniques of control have been studied. They include hypnosis used in conjunction with guided-relaxation imagery, progressive muscle relaxation with guided imagery, and systematic desensitization.

1352

Redd WH, Hendler-Cobie S. **Behavioral medicine in comprehensive cancer treatment.** J Psychosoc Oncol 1:3-17, 1983.

▶ behavior therapy

The application of principles of behavioral psychology to treat aversion reactions to chemotherapy, fear of medical procedures, and psychosomatic symptoms in adult and pediatric cancer patients represents a broadening of psychosocial oncology's domain. The authors discuss these applications, focusing on theoretical premises of behavioral medicine and on specific clinical examples. Attention is also given to the integration of behavioral medicine within comprehensive cancer treatment. It is argued that this new area of psychosocial oncology provides an effective means of treating previously unaddressed problems and is compatible with other approaches.

1353

Redd WH, Hendler-Cobie S. **Learned aversions to chemotherapy treatment.** Health Educ Q 10:57-66, 1984.

▶ hypnosis, imagery, relaxation, biofeedback, desensitization

Recent advances in behavioral psychology and its application in medical settings have yielded effective methods for reducing distress in patients undergoing cancer treatment. The present authors discuss the control of anticipatory nausea and vomiting in patients receiving chemotherapy. The development of these symptoms is hypothesized to be of psychopathological or physiological origin, or due to respondent conditioning. Antiemetic drugs are generally unreliable in their control of chemotherapy nausea, especially with conditioned aversions, and may produce side effects of their own. Four behavioral methods—hypnosis used with guided imagery, progressive muscle relaxation training with imagery, biofeedback with imagery, and systematic desensitization—and their uses and results are described. Clinically significant reductions in patient reactions were achieved despite large variations in the type of cancer, stage of the disease, and chemotherapy protocol. The applications of behavioral interventions to other types of cancer treatments are discussed.

1354

Redd WH, Rosenberger PH, Hendler-Cobie S. **Controlling chemotherapy side effects.** Am J Clin Hypn 25:161-172, 1982.

▶ hypnosis, relaxation, imagery

Severe nausea and vomiting are commonly experienced by cancer patients after receiving chemotherapy treatments. Moreover, approximately 25% of these patients develop conditioned aversions to treatment and become nauseated before they receive their chemotherapy injections. The use of deep muscle relaxation hypnosis in conjunction with guided imagery to control pre- and postchemotherapy nausea and emesis is discussed. Theoretical and clinical issues raised by this application of hypnosis in cancer treatment are also addressed.

1355

Rosenberg SW. **Hypnosis in cancer care: imagery to enhance the control of the physiological and psychological "side-effects" of cancer therapy.** Am J Clin Hypn 25:122-127, 1982.

▶ hypnosis, imagery

The use of surgery, radiation, and chemotherapy has resulted in increased control of malignancy and prolonged survival for cancer patients. These modalities also carry significant morbidity. Normal physiological homeostasis is often altered by both the neoplasm and its treatment. The diagnosis, treatment, and social stigma of cancer exact profound psychological impact. Hypnosis effectively can control the range of both physiological and psychological ramifications of cancer and its therapy. The author delineates those effects of hypnosis of proven value to the cancer patient. Incorporation of images into each phase of a hypnosis session is demonstrated with an actual case history and annotated transcript. Imagery as a therapeutic modality is discussed, and specific suggestions and images are presented.

1356
Rotman M, Rogow L, DeLeon G, Heskel N. **Supportive therapy in radiation oncology.** Cancer 39:744-750, 1977.

▶ psychotherapy

Measures for supportive care of the radiation therapy patient are presented. These include emotional support prior to and during the course of therapy facilitated by a written interview that allows the radiation oncologist to be a supportive communicator of realistic information. A discussion is made of the support of body tissues affected by combination radiation and chemotherapy. These tissues usually include skin, oral, esophageal and intestinal mucosa, and teeth. Means of maintaining nutritional support following weight loss of patients during therapy are described.

1357
Rowden L. **Relaxation and visualisation techniques in patients with breast cancer.** Nurs Times 80:42-44, 1984.

▶ review: relaxation, imagery

Extracted summary: On a personal note, I have found that relaxation has helped me deal with daunting situations with some success. This is obviously a subjective opinion, as are those held by the patients I meet who use the techniques and feel helped. I recognize the difficulty of assessing such techniques because of the different methods which can be used and the sceptical views of many of our colleagues. The growing demand for a holistic approach to care requires a research programme to evaluate scientifically these previously untested modes of therapy for the cancer patient.

1358
Scott DW, Donahue DC, Mastrovito RC, Hakes TB. **The antiemetic effect of clinical relaxation: report of an exploratory pilot study.** J Psychosoc Oncol 1:71-84, 1983.

▶ relaxation, imagery

10 42-67 yr old women receiving highly emetic cancer chemotherapy received an experimental clinical relaxation program designed to diminish nausea and vomiting. The experimental protocol consisted of pretreatment education-counseling and use of slow-stroke back massage, guided imagery, and progressive relaxation in concert with continuous attendance and coaching by the investigator during the chemotherapy experience. Results indicate that duration of emetic response, frequency of vomiting, intensity of episodic effort, and volume of emesis were reduced substantially when compared to the known clinical course for patients receiving these agents. Further, a pattern of emetic response characterized by 3 phases was identified. This may provide criteria allowing for more precise patient assessment and improved anti-emetic regimen evaluation. In addition, data gathered provide a base for development of an emetic response rating scale.

1359
Smith MS, Kamitsuka M. **Self-hypnosis misinterpreted as CNS deterioration in an adolescent with leukemia and vincristine toxicity.** Am J Clin Hypn 26:280-282, 1984.

▶ hypnosis, suggestion

A thirteen-year-old girl with leukemia was taught self-hypnosis techniques for symptom control. She was hospitalized with probable vincristine toxicity and a superimposed hyperventilation syndrome. Her spontaneous use of the self-hypnosis technique was misinterpreted as central nervous system deterioration until her apparently comatose state resolved with suggestions from the therapist.

1360
Stoudemire A, Cotanch P, Lascio J. **Recent advances in the pharmacologic and behavioral management of chemotherapy-induced emesis.** Arch Intern Med 144:1029-1033, 1984.

▶ review: hypnosis, relaxation, desensitization, biofeedback

Chemotherapy protocols that induce severe protracted nausea and vomiting are stressful for cancer patients, and the fear that may be associated with chemotherapy often outweighs other negative aspects of the cancer experience. The clinical management of chemotherapy-induced emesis involves pharmacologic approaches, maintenance of hydration, provision of emotional support, and the possible use of behavioral relaxation techniques. We review the literature on the psychological side effects of chemotherapy and offer recommendations for the pharmacologic, supportive, and behavioral treatment of chemotherapy-induced emesis. More effective management of chemotherapy-induced nausea and vomiting also enhances patient compliance and therefore potentially decreases overall morbidity and mortality.

1361
Wechsler F, Delaney L. **Control of emesis in cancer chemotherapy patients through a self relaxation procedure.** Psychosom Med 46:79, 1984. (abstract)

▶ meditation, relaxation

Four cancer patients were given self relaxation training to inhibit the conditioned emetic responses they had developed to their chemotherapy. Following episodes of emesis before, during, and after a minimum of three consecutive chemotherapy administrations, each patient was interviewed, asked to evaluate their nausea SUDS rating scale as well as their level of depression (Beck Depression Inventory), and then given one training session in self relaxation. The self relaxation procedure was explained as a self control procedure according to instructions given by Benson (1976). They were told to close their eyes, breathe regularly and slowly, and to subvocalize the word one upon each exhalation. Patients were then observed practicing the technique for fifteen minutes and given instructions to practice during chemotherapy sessions and whenever symptoms of nausea occurred. Data was quantified in terms of (1) the occurrence of emesis before, during and after chemotherapy and (2) patients ratings of depression and nausea from pre to post treatment. Results indicated that both anticipatory and reactive emesis was eliminated with self relaxation and that all patients reported feeling less nauseated and depressed. These changes were maintained as long as self relaxation was practiced. No further professional intervention was required for control of emesis. While further studies using control group procedures are needed, these data suggest that self relaxation procedures are effective means of controlling emetic responses in cancer chemotherapy patients particularly when the cost of alternative behavioral treatments (professional time and equipment) are considered.

1362
Weddington WW. **Psychogenic nausea and vomiting associated with termination of cancer chemotherapy.** Psychother Psychosom 37:129-136, 1982.

▶ psychotherapy

Psychogenic (pretreatment) nausea with or without vomiting develops in many patients undergoing chemotherapy for cancer. This phenomenon can be understood as classical aversive conditioning of the gastrointestinal system. Most patients tolerate this side effect of chemotherapy treatment. The author reports 4 patients who were noncompliant or discontinued chemotherapy; each patient alleged that the pretreatment symptoms prompted this behavior. Closer examination revealed that these patients avoided chemotherapy because of multiple issues and used the pretreatment symptoms to explain their behavior. The cases illustrate the phenomenon of pretreatment nausea and methods of working therapeutically with oncologists and their patients.

1363
Weddington WW, Blindt KA, McCracken SG. **Relaxation training for anticipatory nausea associated with chemotherapy.** Psychosomatics 24:281-283, 1983.

▶ relaxation

While evaluating cancer patients with prechemotherapy nausea and vomiting, the authors used relaxation training

as an intervention. The cases of a 46-yr-old male and a 58-yr-old male illustrate the use of the approach.

1364
West BL, Goethe KE, Piccionne C. **Cognitive-behavioral techniques in treating anorexia and depression in a cancer patient.** Behav Therapist 5:115-117, 1982.

▶ imagery, cognitive restructuring

Reports the case of a 54-yr-old man who had undergone a prostectomy and 18 mo of anti-neoplastic chemotherapy. S had also experienced a 47-lb weight loss and reported nausea at the mention of food. S was aggressive, especially at mealtimes. A 13-wk treatment program was instituted that began with progressive hierarchical presentation of imaginary scenes consisting of s's consumption of the foods that caused him the least nausea. A cognitive restructuring process was then implemented. S began to use the procedure of imaginary eating scenes to overcome his aversion for other foods. His temperament improved as did his depression (as registered on the Beck depression inventory).

1365
Zeltzer L, Kellerman J, Ellenberg L, Dash J. **Hypnosis for reduction of vomiting associated with chemotherapy and disease in adolescents with cancer.** J Adolesc Health Care 4:77-84, 1983.

▶ hypnosis

Evaluated the effectiveness of hypnosis in reducing vomiting in 9 cancer patients (mean age 14.2 yrs). Ss were administered a battery of tests including the State-Trait Anxiety Inventory and the Rosenberg Self-Esteem Scale. Eight Ss receiving chemotherapy demonstrated significant reductions in the frequency and intensity of emesis. Six of the 8 also demonstrated a shortened duration of emesis. The 9th S, whose vomiting was secondary to her brain tumor, showed a gradual but steady reduction in vomiting with eventual total elimination following hypnosis intervention. Trait anxiety scores for the group were significantly lower at retest 6 mo following hypnosis intervention. Significant changes in scores of health locus of control, impact of illness, or self-esteem were not found. Data support the efficacy of hypnosis for reducing vomiting when used with a comprehensive clinical approach to the cancer patient.

1366
Zeltzer L, LeBaron S, Zeltzer PM. **The effectiveness of behavioral intervention for reduction of nausea and vomiting in children and adolescents receiving chemotherapy.** J Clin Oncol 2:683-690, 1984.

▶ counseling, hypnosis

Fifty-one children 6-17 years of age rated the severity of nausea, vomiting, and the extent to which chemotherapy bothered them during each course of chemotherapy. Sixteen patients had no symptoms and the doses administered to 16 others were not constant so that matched courses could not be assessed. After baseline measurement of two matched courses, the remaining 19 patients were randomized to receive hypnosis or supportive counseling during two more matched courses. An additional course with no intervention was assessed in half of the patients. No significant reduction of symptoms was demonstrated prior to intervention. However, intervention with both hypnosis and supportive counseling was associated with significant reductions in nausea, vomiting, and the extent to which these symptoms bothered patients (all p less than 0.001). Also, after termination of intervention, symptom ratings remained significantly lower than baseline. The data indicate that chemotherapy-related nausea and emesis in children can be reduced with behavioral intervention and that reductions are maintained after intervention has been discontinued.

Treatment of Pain from Disease or Therapy

1367

Ament P. **Concepts in the use of hypnosis for pain relief in cancer.** J Med 13:233-240, 1982.

▶ hypnosis, relaxation

Hypnosis has no single place, but rather a broad range of application of technique and a long standing basis in the philosophy of patient care. We are not purists in any sense of the word. Our use of hypnosis in relief of pain in cases of cancer involves all formal medical procedures enhancing their potential through proper suggestions. We will endeavor to present some techniques of relaxation and pertinent case histories.

1368

Anderson JL. **Nursing management of the cancer patient in pain: a review of the literature.** Cancer Nurs 5:33-41, 1982.

▶ review, behavior therapy

Nurses who care for cancer patients who may be experiencing pain should be aware of current nursing treatment alternatives that are available to help the patient during these times. Through an international review of the literature, alternatives are identified that will help cancer nurses recognize their unique role in pain assessment and management for cancer patients. The following topics, utilizing the nursing process as the organizational framework, are included in this review: 1) the scope of the cancer pain experience; 2) nursing assessment of the patient experiencing pain related to cancer; and 3) nursing interventions, including pharmaceutical and behavioral approaches, which are utilized by nurses in the clinical setting to help the cancer patient modify his pain experience. Pertinent nursing research studies are also cited.

1369

Barber J. **Hypnosis as a psychological technique in the management of cancer pain.** Cancer Nurs 1:361-363, 1978.

▶ hypnosis

1370

Barber J, Gitelson J. **Cancer pain: psychological management using hypnosis.** CA 30:130-136, 1980.

▶ hypnosis

In the treatment of cancer, particularly when pain is a serious symptom, psychological support of a patient is important and can, in fact, facilitate ongoing oncologic treatment. Hypnosis represents a psychological technique of great potency for reducing pain, increasing patients' life-enhancing attitudes, and helping patients deal with death and separation. Ultimately, the value of hypnosis lies in enabling an individual to potentiate inner capacities for creating psychological quiescence and physical comfort. For a suffering cancer patient, relief that comes from within can provide a much-needed experience of personal efficacy and strength.

1371

Butler B. **Hypnosis in care of the cancer patient.** Cancer 7:1-14, 1954. (also Br J Med Hypn 6: in three parts, 1955)

▶ hypnosis, suggestion

1. Pain, anxiety, and organ dysfunction in the cancer patient can be aided by the intensive use of hypnotherapy. The results are proportional to the depth of trance and the efficiency of the program of therapy employed. 2. Patients who easily enter a deep trance can be helped; those who reach only a medium state can be aided, although the more "organic" the complaints, the more ephemeral the response; while patients who, after repeated trials, can only enter a light stage cannot be helped by this means. 3. The main disadvantages of this form of therapy are the few good subjects, the large amount of time required, and the necessity of an experienced and well-trained hypnologist to govern each case. The possible deleterious effect upon the health of the hypnologist and the long period of time required for one patient between onset of symptoms and death, thus limit the number of patients a single therapist could manage. Then, too, public resistance to hypnosis persists. 4. The advantages of hypnotherapy for pa-

tients who enter a deep trance are numerous. Drug requirements are lessened, pain is relieved, organ dysfunction can be corrected as much as possible, and depression, anxiety, and fear are minimized. Life is prolonged and death is approached as is a night's sleep. 5. Prefrontal lobotomy interferes with the induction of the hypnotic state in proportion to the decreased ability of the patient to concentrate and, therefore, appears to be different from the hypnotic state. 6. Narcohypnosis helps to counteract superficial resistance but does not appear to aid otherwise in obtaining greater true hypnotic depth. It does not eliminate all resistance. 7. Future efforts should be expended to learn what hypnosis is and how it alters physiological function. When these fundamentals are understood, its advantages will have a wider and more satisfactory application. 8. There may be a "cancer personality." From a very intensive study of these cases, either an inhibited individual with repressed anger, hatred, and jealousy or a "good" person consumed with self-pity may be prototypes of this personality.

1372

Cangello VW. **The use of hypnotic suggestion for pain relief in malignant disease.** Int J Clin Exp Hypn 9:17-22, 1961.

▶ hypnosis

1. A discussion of the management of severe pain in malignant disease is presented. 2. Twenty-two cases are presented in which pain relief was attempted using hypnotic suggestion. 3. Fifty-nine per cent of these patients showed a decrease in narcotic requirements following the use of this modality. The need for narcotics was reduced seventy-five to one-hundred per cent in eight or thirty-six per cent of the cases, and fifty to seventy-five per cent in five or twenty-three per cent of the cases. There was no change in nine or forty-one per cent of the cases. 4. An average of sixty-six minutes was expended on each of these patients, and the time varied from fifteen minutes to two hours. 5. The length of time of effectiveness of this approach varied from one week to four and one-half months. 6. None of the patients in the failure group who were capable of being hypnotically induced required the chemical or surgical approach, nor appeared to develop a tolerance to the narcotic they were using up to a period of eight weeks that a follow-up was possible. 7. It is concluded that this form of management should be given a trial for the relief of pain in malignant disease before resorting to either chemical rhizotomy or surgical tractotomy since it is relatively simple to perform, has virtually no rate of complication or morbidity, is successful in a satisfactory proportion of the cases, and is not unduly time consuming.

1373

Cangello VW. **Hypnosis for the patient with cancer.** Am J Clin Hypn 4:215-226, 1961-1962.

▶ hypnosis

Extracted summary: The results of this study show that a place exists for the use of hypnotic suggestion in the care of patients with malignant disease. Its use for the relief of pain and mood elevation proved sufficiently successful, not unduly time consuming, and it was free of complications or morbidity. It is especially indicated for pain relief in the patient whose life expectancy is short or for whom chemical and surgical approaches are not suitable. Actually it should be given a trial before resort to these approaches. This study also proves that the time expended is not impractical for the private physician since the initial induction usually required not more than thirty minutes and reinforcement sessions varied from five to fifteen minutes. This work, therefore, could be carried on during a physician's routine hospital or home visits.

1374

Chong TM. **The use of hypnosis in the management of patients with cancer.** Singapore Med J 9:211-214, 1968.

▶ hypnosis

Hypnosis offers an approach to the problem of the cancer patients and may well prove to be the only really practical approach toward solving many of the difficulties encountered in the total care of the cancer patients. Heroic measures of neuro-surgical intervention such as alcohol block, cordotomy, prefrontal lobotomy, hypophysectomy, etc., are rarely useful or necessary.

1375

Cleeland CS. **The impact of pain on the patient with cancer.** Cancer 54:2635-2641, 1984.

▶ behavior therapy

Pain is one of the most feared consequences of cancer. Until recently, however, little has been known about its prevalence, severity, and impact on the patient with cancer. The presence of pain, despite efforts to treat it, represents a continued source of frustration for patient, their families, and the health care team. Although often one of the early indicators of the presence of disease, pain is not a significant problem for the majority of patients in the early stages of disease, with 5% to 10% of patients with solid tumors reporting pain at a level that interferes with mood and activity. But when metastatic disease is present, about one in three patients reports significant pain, and our data and those of others indicate that the majority of patients with end-stage disease will report pain of a severity that interferes with several aspects of the patient's quality of life. Site of tumor is also significantly related to the progression of pain. The relationship between pain intensity and depression and anxiety is examined in detail, and the treatment implications of this relationship discussed. Whereas a modest relationship between pain intensity and depression has been found across several studies, the possibility that depression is a causative factor in the pain experienced by the cancer patient may have been overemphasized. Data on the relief of pain in cancer are reported from the perspective of patients as well as the physicians and nurses who treat them. The majority of physicians and nurses specializing in cancer treatment whom we have surveyed believe that cancer patients in general are undermedicated for pain. Patient survey data indicate that only 50% of cancer patients with pain report 70% or greater pain relief with analgesic medication. Although a number of nonsystemic treatments may be useful for cancer pain management (such as nerve blocks, neurosurgery, and behavioral treatments), they are not widely available and there are few controlled studies of their effectiveness. Teaching patients to report the level of their pain on simple pain intensity scales has proven useful in monitoring the effectiveness of pain management, as well as in helping establish pain control goals for the individual patient.

1376

Eliasberg WG. **Psychotherapy in cancer patients.** JAMA 147:525-526, 1951. (letter)

▶ psychotherapy

1377

Erickson MH. **Hypnosis in painful terminal illness.** Am J Clin Hypn 1:117-121, 1959.

▶ hypnosis

A presentation has been offered of the utilization of hypnosis in terminal painful disease. Three case reports, not entirely typical, have been presented in order to illustrate more adequately the actual possibilities of therapeutic benefits. An effort has been made to describe the therapeutic methodologies employed, but this effort is not fully possible. Hypnotherapeutic benefits, especially in such cases as reported here, are markedly contingent upon a varied and repetitious presentation of ideas and understandings to insure an adequate acceptance and responsiveness by the patient. Also, the very nature of the situation precludes a determination of what elements in the therapeutic procedure are effective in the individual case.

1378

Heiligman RM, Lee LR, Kramer D. **Pain relief associated with a religious visitation: a case report.** J Fam Pract 16:299-302, 1983.

▶ spiritual healing

A 68-year-old black woman tolerated partial colectomy for resection of a carcinoma with minimal postoperative discomfort and without the need of any analgesia. She attributed her positive experience to the presence of protective angels. Psychologic interviews and testing revealed her to be fully in touch with reality. Her experience, as well as those of similar patients reported in the medical literature, has biological, sociocultural, and psychological components. The role of religious belief in the pain experience has received scant attention, but it constitutes a challenging area for future research.

1379

Hilgard JR, Lebaron S. **Relief of anxiety and pain in children and adolescents with cancer: quantitative measures and clinical observations.** Int J Clin Exp Hypn 30:417-442, 1982.

▶ hypnosis

63 6-19 yr olds with cancer, chiefly forms of leukemia, underwent medical treatments that required repeated bone marrow aspirations, normally a painful and anxiety-provoking experience. Ss were then offered the opportunity to volunteer for hypnotic help in pain control. Of the 24 ss who accepted hypnosis, 19 were highly hypnotizable. 10 of the 19 reduced self-reported pain substantially by the 1st hypnotic treatment, and 5 more reduced self-reported pain by the 2nd treatment; none of the 5 less-hypnotizable ss accomplished this. The latter benefitted by reducing their anxiety. Short case reports illustrate the variety of experiences. Analysis of baseline observations before therapeutic intervention revealed age and sex differences. The difference between self-reported and observed pain was significant for ss 10 yrs old and older. There were minor but significant sex differences both in observed and in self-reported pain, with the females reporting more pain.

1380

Holden C. **Pain control with hypnosis.** Science 198:808, 1977.

▶ hypnosis

Much has been learned in recent years about the power of the mind to affect involuntary bodily processes in very specific ways, including the brain's perception of pain. Manifestation of this power is often dismissed as the placebo effect because it is unpredictable, usually temporary, and no one knows how to harness it in a systematic fashion. Yet hypnosis is a technique that can do just that, according to Paul Sacerdote, a New York psychiatrist associated with the oncology service of Montefiore Hospital. Now in his seventies, Sacerdote is one of the most experienced and resourceful hypnotherapists in the country. Unlike most practitioners, he has worked extensively with pain patients, particularly those suffering from pain of cancer and its treatments. In a conversation with Science, Sacerdote said that "at a very minimum one in four people with cancer will respond very well to hypnotherapy for relief of pain." This means that many can do without narcotics altogether and others can have their medications significantly reduced. Sacerdote says it is possible to teach a person how to become hypnotized in only a few sessions: thereafter the patient can hypnotize himself when necessary. He believes almost anyone can derive some benefit from hypnosis, although light trances are hardly different from a simple relaxation state. But many are able to achieve a state so deep as to resemble a stupor.

1381
Kellerman J, Zeltzer L, Ellenberg L, Dash J. **Adolescents with cancer: hypnosis for the reduction of the acute pain and anxiety associated with medical procedures.** J Adolesc Health Care 4:85-90, 1983.

▶ hypnosis

16 cancer patients (mean age 14 yrs) were trained in hypnosis to ease the discomfort and anxiety associated with bone marrow aspirations, lumbar punctures, and chemotherapeutic injections. Ss were administered a battery of measures including the State-Trait Anxiety Inventory and the Rosenberg self-esteem scale. They achieved significant reductions in multiple measures of pain and anxiety after hypnosis training. Preintervention data showed no pattern of spontaneous remission or habituation, and, in fact, an increasing anticipatory anxiety was observed before hypnotic treatment. Significant reductions were also found in trait anxiety. A nonsignificant trend toward greater self-esteem was present, but predicted changes in locus of control and general illness impact were not found. Comparisons between hypnosis rejectors and successful users showed higher levels of pretreatment anxiety in the former.

1382
Lea PA, Ware PD, Monroe RR. **The hypnotic control of intractable pain.** Am J Clin Hypn 3:3-8, 1960-1961.

▶ hypnosis, suggestion, doctor-patient relationship

Twenty unselected patients with chronic intractable pain were referred for treatment by hypnotherapy. Only one of this group did not obtain at least a light hypnotic trance, and two others could not be evaluated for extraneous rea-

sons. Of the remaining 17, three improved sufficiently to be taken off all medications and nine significantly improved, in that the character of the pain was changed and less medication was needed. Of the five failures, four had severe complicating psychiatric problems. A somnambulistic trance was not necessary with the technique we used; often as much was accomplished with medium or even light hypnosis. Responses to post-hypnotic suggestions were delayed from several hours to as much as a week. It is desirable to work with patients before pain becomes so intense that heavy sedation or narcosis is necessary; but, whether patients are physiologically addicted or not, one should not threaten to take away their medication. The chronic pain of these patients becomes an integral part of their lives, so that one has to understand the total life situation to use hypnosis effectively, as the patient often has considerable secondary gains from his illness. It is difficult to know exactly how much benefit is derived from hypnosis itself or how much from such extraneous factors as extra personal attention. In either case, this represents an intense doctor-patient relationship, which considerably enhances the patient's suggestibility. Nevertheless, it is our impression that hypnosis is a useful adjunct to medical therapy in the control of chronic pain.

1383
Margolis CG. **Hypnotic imagery with cancer patients.** Am J Clin Hypn 25:128-134, 1982.

▶ hypnosis, psychotherapy, suggestion, imagery, relaxation

Presents 6 case examples of 27-54 yr olds to describe the use of hypnotic imagery to reduce pain and discomfort in cancer patients. Deep relaxation, ego strengthening, imagery, and suggestions for changes in perception and awareness are the principal techniques used. Hypnotic intervention in these cases is described, with emphasis on the ease with which positive transference is established and the effectiveness with which it may be used to enhance therapeutic effects.

1384
Mizuguchi T. **Management of pain in lung cancer: (I) Chemotherapy and psychotherapy.** Kokyu To Junkan 31:841-845, 1983. (in Japanese: no English abstract)

▶ review: psychotherapy

1385
Mun CT. **The use of hypnosis in the management of patients with cancer.** Singapore Med 9:211-214, 1968.

▶ hypnosis, autohypnosis

Hypnosis offers an approach to the problem of the cancer patients and may well prove to be the only really practical approach toward solving many of the difficulties encountered in the total care of the cancer patients. Heroic measures of neuro-surgical intervention such as alcohol block, cordotomy, prefrontal lobotomy, hypophysectomy, etc., are rarely useful or necessary.

1386
Munro S, Mount B. **Music therapy in palliative care.** Can Med Assoc J 119:1029-1034, 1978.

▶ music therapy, imagery, relaxation

Initial observations regarding the use of music therapy at one hospital in the palliative care of patients with advanced malignant disease are presented. In the hands of a trained music therapist, music has proven to be a potent tool for improving the quality of life. The diversity of its potential is particularly suited to the diversity of the challenges—physical, psychosocial and spiritual—that these patients present.

1387
Noyes R. **Treatment of cancer pain.** Psychosom Med 43:57-70, 1981.

▶ review: supportive psychotherapy, relaxation, hypnosis, hospice

A review of the literature indicates that research in the area of cancer pain is urgently needed. Undertreatment of cancer pain results not only from the limited expectations of patients but also from the inadequate knowledge of many physicians. Successful management of this pain requires awareness of the importance of emotional factors and detailed knowledge of various treatment options. When indicated, analgesic drugs should be administered according to a regular schedule and in sufficient dose to prevent the emergence of pain. Psychological techniques including supportive psychotherapy, relaxation training, hypnosis, and the hospice milieu may contribute to a comprehensive approach to pain. Likewise, psychotropic drugs including phenothiazines and tricyclic antidepressants may be useful adjuncts when administered along with appropriate analgesic medication.

1388
Olness K. **Imagery (self-hypnosis) as adjunct therapy in childhood cancer: clinical experience with 25 patients.** Am J Pediatr Hematol Oncol 3:313-321, 1981.

▶ imagery, autohypnosis

Clinical experience with 25 pediatric cancer patients referred by oncologists for imagery exercises (self-hypnosis) at Minneapolis Children's Health Center suggests that this modality is valuable adjunct therapy for symptom relief, such as reduction of pain and nausea, especially among those patients who begin these exercises at the time of their initial diagnosis. Twenty-one of these patients agreed to use the exercises and 19 demonstrated substantial symptom relief associated with their practice. This experience suggests the need for more research regarding the optimal use of this modality in children with cancer, and for better understanding of how psychological factors contribute, if at all to the development and course of malignancies. A 5-year prospective study of imagery as adjunct therapy in childhood cancer is now in process.

1389
Pahnke WN, Kurland AA, Goodman LE, Richards WA. **LSD-assisted psychotherapy with terminal cancer patients.** Curr Psychiatr Ther 9:144-152, 1969.

▶ psychotherapy, doctor-patient relationship

Therapist enthusiasm, both verbal and non-verbal, is a powerful factor, as in many forms of psychotherapy. Because of the psychological power of the LSD reaction, few patients are disappointed when they are promised an unusual and compelling psychological experience. The dramatic positive changes in attitude and behavior when the treatment is successful are more than enough to keep the enthusiasm of the therapist at an effective level, even in the face of what is at best a grim reality situation. As a final caution to those who may attempt psychedelic psychotherapy with cancer patients, we definitely would not advise its use without specialized training under supervision from those already familiar with the reactions facilitated by this powerful psychoactive drug. Given adequate training, however, our clinical experience so far suggests that skilled use of the psychedelic procedure can be a relatively safe and promising approach in an area which has been most discouraging up to the present.

1390
Pahnke WN, Kurland AA, Unger S, Savage C, Grof S. **The experimental use of psychedelic (LSD) psychotherapy.** JAMA 212:1856-1863, 1970.

▶ psychotherapy

Extracted summary: Use of LSD is not a substitute for skilled psychotherapy. Experiments where LSD was used primarily as a chemotherapeutic agent or with a minimum of psychotherapy have not shown any greater efficacy regarding therapeutic outcome, especially with alcoholics, than control groups. The evidence from the psycholytic use of LSD by European researchers and psychedelic-peak therapy as practiced at the Maryland Psychiatric Research Center indicates that LSD can be an enhancer of skilled psychotherapy when integrated with an intensive psychotherapeutic program of sufficient duration (30 to 50 hours). (Includes case report of a patient with breast cancer.)

1391
Peter B, Gerl W. **Hypnotherapy in the psychologic treatment of cancer.** Hypn Kognition 1:56-68, 1984. (in German)

▶ hypnosis, psychotherapy

A report of the authors' psychotherapeutic and hypotherapeutic work with cancer patients. Among the topics discussed are hypnotherapy for the control of pain and other side effects of the disease and its treatment, hypnotherapeutic activation of the body's immune system and unconscious coping mechanism, hypnotherapeutic stimulation of the will to live, and hypnotherapy as a means to support the patient in coping with the illness.

1392
Sacerdote P. **The use of hypnosis in cancer patients.** Ann NY Acad Sci 125:1011-1019, 1966.

▶ hypnosis, suggestion, supportive psychotherapy

Extracted summary: A certain patient exposed to hypnotherapy on a certain day and hour needs only to be told firmly and authoritatively that he has no pain and he will have no pain; that same patient at another time, or a different patient will be able to relinquish his pain only if the (experimenter) physician can proffer certain "ideas" with which the patient's mind will be able to work at different levels of awareness. One patient may only need to be taught to "relax" and thereby learn to tolerate or largely ignore severe pain; another will be capable upon direct suggestion of developing anesthesia wherever and whenever needed, and to maintain such anesthesia as a posthypnotic suggestion; a third one will only be able to do so by hallucinating a healthy body-image; a fourth one only by achieving complete dissociation. The physician will provoke favorable changes—emotionally and physically—on the vast majority of cancer patients only if he is continuously aware of their various and variable needs and of the non-verbalized demands, and if he finds ways of meeting such needs at levels acceptable to them.

1393
Sacerdote P. **Additional contributions to the hypnotherapy of the advanced cancer patient.** Am J Clin Hypn 7: 308-319, 1965.

▶ psychotherapy, hypnosis

Extracted summary: If, as it seems probable, the inclusion of psychiatry and hypnosis in the treatment of cancer will prove to have more than pain-relieving or antidepressive effects, then it will be important to investigate how these effects are engineered and relayed through neurological, bio-chemical and hormonal interventions. This vast new area of clinical and experimental investigation will be usefully supplemented by experimental studies in lower animals where various changes in behavior and in bio-chemistry following applications of modalities which increase or decrease "stress" can be applied to the study of the reactions of the hosts to the tumors, and to the study of effect of the tumors on the hosts.

1394
Sacerdote P. **Theory and practice of pain control in malignancy and other protracted or recurring painful illnesses.** Hypnosis 18:160-180, 1970.

▶ hypnosis, behavior therapy

Recent neuroanatomical and neurophysiological experimental data suggest absence or presence of pain and changes in pain intensity as expressions of the balance between sensory (peripheral) and central (centrifugal) inputs at synaptic stations. Psychological activities by contributing to the centrifugal input influence conduction, transduction, and perception of pain stimuli. Hypnotically induced analgesia and anesthesia are therefore acceptable as neurophysiological realities. Methods for hypnotic alterations of pain based upon these premises are described. They utilize neurophysiological mechanisms, psychodynamic changes, establishment of new behavioral patterns, or changes in time-space concepts and percepts. A series of case presentations illustrates some of these multiple psychological and physiological approaches to pain control.

1395
Schafer DW. **The management of pain in the cancer patient.** Compr Psychiatry 10:41-45, 1984.

▶ hypnosis, autohypnosis, doctor-patient relationship, meditation, biofeedback, consultation-liaison, spiritual healing

Extracted summary: The primary physician should probably be the leader of those involved in the treatment of cancer pain victims. Other specialists can be consulted, including the anesthesiologist, the neurosurgeon, and the pharmacologist. However, there are many others who may be used adjunctively to help the patient. Special reference must be given to practitioners trained in areas of mental health. Especially when the primary physician finds the patient to be conflicted about his own past and present, or is having difficulty coping with his family or his death, a mental health practitioner would be invaluable. The choice ranges from psychiatrists through psychologists, psychiatric social workers, and marriage, family, and child counselors. The physician's personal familiarity with these practitioners should help him select the proper person to augment the physical treatment of the patient. This is especially true if the primary physician is not conversant with hypnosis, and a mental health practitioner is.

1396

Schafer DW. **Pain, emotions, and the cancer patient.** Surg Annu 16:57-67, 1984.

▶ hypnosis, autohypnosis, biofeedback, meditation, doctor-patient relationship

Pain and emotions in cancer patients work against each other if the emotions are negative. This chapter has tried to explain the kind of pain that cancer patients feel, and to show that the compassionate physician can help those patients cope with pain as well as with other symptoms, and thereby help the patient if the patient is to die with dignity. All treatment must consider the emotional condition of patients in their overall milieu. The state of knowledge of physicians, as well as their emotions, must be responsible for unintentionally contributing to the death of a patient.

1397

Schon RC. **Addendum to "Hypnosis in painful terminal illness."** Am J Clin Hypn 3:61-62, 1960.

▶ hypnosis

Extracted summary: Conscious awareness of impending death by the patient seems to be a prerequisite for help through hypnosis in terminal illness. Unawareness points to excessive repression, to dread of reality. Many terminal cancer patients do not admit to being moribund. Because they dread death they cling to the illusion that they can get well again. Clandestinely, they grope for a miracle cure, and hypnosis, in popular belief, is just that. Unconsciously, however, they know that they have a fatal disease. During trance, to their horror, they find that this unconscious knowledge is laid bare. This they had not bargained for, and they will not let this knowledge pass into consciousness. Hence they reject hypnosis, either outright or by blocking at the next induction, because during trance they had felt helplessly exposed to the reality they find too threatening and too painful to face.

1398

Spiegel D. **The use of hypnosis in controlling cancer pain.** CA 35:221-231, 1985.

▶ hypnosis

Pain is frequently, although not inevitably, associated with cancer. The degree of pain depends on a variety of factors, of which the site and extensiveness of the primary tumor and metastases are but two. The pain experience of cancer patients—and, therefore, to a great extent their quality of life—is also influenced by such psychological factors as mood disturbance and beliefs about the disease and its relation to pain. This paper examines the role of psychological factors in the experience of cancer pain and dis-

cusses the rationale for incorporating hypnosis into a pain management program.

1399

Spiegel D, Bloom JR. **Group therapy and hypnosis reduce metastatic breast carcinoma pain.** Psychosom Med 45:333-339, 1983.

▶ group therapy, autohypnosis

Studied the pain and mood disturbance of 54 women with metastatic carcinoma of the breast over 1 yr. 30 Ss (mean age 54 yrs) were offered weekly group therapy during the year, with or without self-hypnosis training directed toward enhancing their competence at mastering pain and stress related to cancer. Both treatment groups demonstrated significantly less self-rated pain sensation and suffering than the control sample. Those who were offered the self-hypnosis training as well as group therapy fared best in controlling pain. Pain frequency and duration were not affected. Changes in pain measures were significantly correlated with changes in self-rated total mood disturbance on the profile of mood states and with its anxiety, depression, and fatigue subscales. Possible mechanisms for the effectiveness of these interventions are discussed.

1400

Wagner FF. **Metastatic pain influenced by hypnotic suggestion.** Ugeskr Laeger 129:393-395, 1967. (in Danish)

▶ hypnosis, suggestion, relaxation

In order to test the claimed beneficial effect of hypnotic suggestions upon severe, intractable pain, two of the hospital's most desolate cancer patients were selected. The application of a simple "relaxation technique" as well as more refined methods such as "time distortion," "body-mind dissociation" and "pain-heat conversion" offered the patients considerable relief until two weeks prior to death. Not only anxiety and depression decreased dramatically but the patients' general somatic condition improved remarkably for a fairly long period of time.

1401

Zeltzer L, LeBaron S. **Hypnosis and nonhypnotic techniques for reduction of pain and anxiety during painful procedures in children and adolescents with cancer.** J Pediatr 101:1032-1035, 1982.

▶ hypnosis, behavior therapy

Hypnosis was compared with nonhypnotic behavioral techniques for efficacy in reducing pain and anxiety in 27 children and adolescents during bone marrow aspiration and in 22 children and adolescents during lumbar puncture. The patients and independent observers each rated (scale of 1 to 5) pain and anxiety during one to three procedures prior to intervention and one to three procedures with intervention. Prior to intervention for both groups, pain during bone marrow aspiration was rated as more severe (p less than 0.01) than pain during lumbar puncture. During bone marrow aspiration pain was reduced to a large extent by hypnosis (p less than 0.001) and to a smaller but significant extent by nonhypnotic techniques (p less than 0.01), and anxiety was significantly reduced by hypnosis alone (p less than 0.001). During lumbar puncture only hypnosis significantly reduced pain (p less than 0.001); anxiety was reduced to a large degree by hypnosis (p less than 0.001) and to a smaller degree by nonhypnotic techniques (p less than 0.05). Thus hypnosis was shown to be more effective than nonhypnotic techniques for reducing procedural distress in children and adolescents with cancer.

1402
Zeltzer L, LeBaron S. **Behavioral intervention for children and adolescents with cancer.** Behav Med Update 5:17-22, 1983.

▶ review: hypnosis, behavior therapy

Reviews interventions for pain caused by the medical procedures and chemotherapy used to treat cancer in children and adolescents. Most investigations of interventions for reducing pain and anxiety in these children have focused on hypnotic techniques. Various studies have shown that (1) hypnotic susceptibility is related to pain relief, (2) hypnosis is more effective than supportive counseling in reducing pain, and (3) techniques of hypnosis must be varied according to the age of the child. The severe nausea and vomiting caused by chemotherapy cause many children to terminate chemotherapy prematurely. A few small studies have shown hypnosis to be helpful in reducing the side effects of chemotherapy. Other behavioral techniques used successfully with adults are not applicable to children because of developmental differences between the 2 age groups. For example, children often have difficulty in concentrating on relaxing because their attention span is so short.

Treatment of Sexual Dysfunction from Disease or Therapy

1403
Capone MA, Good RS. **Sex counseling for cancer patients.** Obstet Gynecol 15:131-140, 1980.

▶ counseling

We found that sexual functioning of newly diagnosed patients was improved by counseling. Sex counseling by physicians in a clinical setting need not be complex but should be ongoing throughout treatment and follow-up. Because gynecologists see cancer patients for regularly scheduled visits, they are in an ideal position to anticipate areas of concern, repeatedly provide appropriate information, and encourage and assume responsibility for incorporating this material into total care.

1404
Capone MA, Good RS, Westie KS, Jacobson AF. **Psychosocial rehabilitation of gynecologic oncology patients.** Arch Phys Rehabil 61:128-132, 1980.

▶ counseling

This investigation studied the effectiveness of in-hospital, individual counseling on the psychosocial adjustment of patients with newly diagnosed gynecologic malignancies. Levels of psychologic distress, sexual functioning, and return to employment were assessed at 3, 6, and 12 months after counseling. The counseled patients were compared with a similar control group that was assessed but not counseled. In this study, levels of psychologic distress reported by cancer patients were similar to those reported in normal populations. However, at 3 months post-treatment, counseled cancer patients reported significantly less confusion and contradiction within areas of self-perception than did the noncounseled patients. Return to employment and sexual activities were both shown to be adversely affected by the diagnosis and treatment of genital cancer. Results suggested that counseling had a positive effect in enhancing return to normal vocational and sexual functions during the 1st year after treatment.

1405
Capone MA, Westie KS, Good RS. **Sexual rehabilitation of the gynecologic cancer patient: an effective counseling model.** Front Radiat Ther Oncol 14:123-129, 1980.

▶ counseling

Our study has demonstrated the efficacy of psychosexual counseling as a means of facilitating the sexual rehabilitation of women with genital malignancies. When initiated shortly after diagnosis, the crisis-oriented sexual rehabilitation program utilized in this project proved extremely effective in promoting early return to pre-disease levels of sexual function, as well as dramatically reducing the incidence of cessation of sexual activity in the patient with gynecologic cancer. Our experience on a gynecologic oncology service leads us to conclude that successful incorporation of this model into the regular care of the patient requires some adjustment in staff and service organization. The oncology team should include a mental health professional, or a specially trained team member, to serve as a consistent provider of psychosexual care and to assist other team members in improving their rehabilitative interactions with the patient. It is also important that a sexual rehabilitation focus be included in medical rounds and staff conferences to increase awareness of patients' sexual concerns and problems, and to encourage consistent treatment planning for this area of patient care. In conclusion, it is clear that the adoption of an effective psychosexual counseling model helps to provide the kind of comprehensive and holistic care that improves the quality of life for the woman with gyncecologic cancer.

1406
Cheek D. **Hypnotherapy for secondary frigidity after radical surgery for gynecological cancer: two case reports.** Am J Clin Hypn 19:13-19, 1976.

▶ hypnosis, psychotherapy

Shows how ideomotor questioning methods combined with light hypnosis can be used successfully to permit return of orgasmic sexual responses after radical gynecological surgery for cancer. It is concluded that the dividend of improved self respect and hope for the future justify the effort. Steps of therapy are outlined as used with 2 young women.

1407
Derogatis LR, Kourlesis SM. **An approach to evaluation of sexual problems in the cancer patient.** CA 31:46-50, 1981.

▶ counseling

A treatment plan does not have to be a formal set of strategies based on the latest knowledge of human sexual functioning, it should use common sense and be based on a thorough knowledge of the patient and his or her sexual functioning. Many problems will be solved by just the chance to discuss them; patients need to hear that their sexual concerns are completely normal. Patients with other problems may require information about the limitations of performance inherent in the condition. They should be given the opportunity to become desensitized to a surgical mutilation or alteration. Some problems will resist simple strategies based upon acceptance, information giving, and new learning; the oncology team should refer these patients to competent specialists in the treatment of sexual dysfunction. Regardless of how the sexual problems of the cancer patient are addressed, the most fundamental step we must take is to accept sexuality as an inherent and important aspect of being human. We should work to treat the problems that arise in this area with the same excellence and commitment we devote to other aspects of cancer care.

1408
Donahue CV, Knapp RC. **Sexual rehabilitation of gynecologic cancer patients.** Obstet Gynecol 49:118-121, 1977.

▶ counseling

The gynecologic oncologist's obligation encompasses more than cure or successful palliation of pelvic malignancy. The sexual rehabilitation of such patients is vital and must be done sensitively lest one's own concepts of "adequate sexuality" be imposed. Instruction in coital technics and alternative modes of sexual expression can be provided simply and effectively.

1409
Gorzynski JG, Holland JC. **Psychological aspects of testicular cancer.** Semin Oncol 6:125-129, 1979.

▶ supportive psychotherapy, group therapy, doctor-patient relationship

After a diagnosis of cancer is confirmed by orchiectomy, patient and spouse may have adequate opportunity to dis-

cuss again the diagnosis and future treatment. Emotional response at this point is crucial: the diagnosis is cancer. Suddenly, the cultural meaning of the term cancer must be confronted: disfigurement, pain, and possibly death. In addition, the association of cancer of the genital organs and sex, a topic that has been cloaked in folklore and myth and has long been taboo in our society can lead to various misconceptions and apprehensions in both men and women. Emotionally, some patients or their partners view genital cancers as punishment for some real or imagined sexual thoughts or acts or retributions for "excessive" or "aberrant" sexual activities. During this period, shame, guilt and fear, particularly of transmitting the disease, may produce transient psychologically-induced sexual dysfunction, diminished libido, and erectile difficulties. The physician can dispel unnatural concerns and reassure the patient that his symptoms are of not uncommon and emotional origin, and will disappear. Although anxiety is the normal response to a diagnosis of cancer, extreme anxiety may result in patients denying the diagnosis of cancer and thereby in their refusing treatment. Some patients become depressed or pessimistic and refuse therapy because "if it's cancer, there is no use in treatment." Disruption of sleep, work interest, and continued disinterest in sex may occur and only when a therapeutic alliance is forged with the doctor who optimistically outlines a treatment plan does the acute emotional turmoil abate.

1410
Lamb MA, Woods NF. **Sexuality and the cancer patient.** Cancer Nurs 3:137-144, 1981.

▶ counseling

Relatively little attention has been given to the effects that cancer and its treatment may have on the meaning of sexuality for the cancer patient and his/her partner. This article discusses how living with cancer can influence sexuality and sexual expression. In addition, guidelines for sexual assessment, interventions to promote sexual health, and alternate ways of expressing physical love are included.

1411
Lamont JA, DePetrillo AD, Sargeant EJ. **Psychosexual rehabilitation and exenterative surgery.** Gynecol Oncol 6:236-242, 1979.

▶ counseling

Exenterative surgery for pelvic malignancy involves loss of tissue which is sexually responsive. Loss of sexual function however, is more likely to be related to the patient feeling unattractive, to lack of information, or to lack of support in dealing with postoperative psychological reactions. A team approach has been established at our institution to ensure complete care and rehabilitation of these patients. The sexual counselor is involved in a preoperative assessment, during hospital stay and during the postoperative period. This paper described our results with 12 exenterative patients and our particular approach to their psychosexual rehabilitation.

1412
Schain WS. **Role of the sex therapist in the care of the cancer patient.** Front Radiat Ther Oncol 15:168-183, 1980.

▶ counseling, psychotherapy

The need for health professions to assist cancer patients in working through difficulties pertaining to sexuality and in adjusting to changes in self image is discussed. Some of the sexual problems caused by breast cancer, gynecological cancer, colostomy, prostatectomy, and orchiectomy are explored. Comprehensive cancer management should include members of the medical discipline which provide holistic and humanistic treatment. One team member should be both a qualifed sex therapist and psychotherapist. This individual should be introduced to patients at the onset of treatment. Early intervention might avert or minimize some of the sexual morbidity associated with this disease. In general, the sex therapist should provide supportive therapy, explore the problem with the patient, suggest answers, educate the patient, and refer patients when necessary for psychiatric consultation and more extensive psychotherapy.

1413
Schain WS. **Sexual functioning, self-esteem and cancer care.** Front Radiat Ther Oncol 14:12-19, 1980.

▶ counseling, psychotherapy, desensitization

The issue of training health professionals who want to work in this field of sexual counseling is a matter of burgeoning concern predicated on the needs of the patient population which one sees and the resources and responsibilities the professional wishes to actualize. There are good resources today for the health care provider who is interested in acquiring training in sex therapy. There are also a number of consciousness raising experiences (workshops, courses) which can elevate one's sense of awareness to these concerns as well as enhance his/her skills of inquiry and counseling. Helpful procedures extend from just listening and giving the patient permission to ask questions or ventilate sexual fears to the more uncovering dynamic psychotherapies as well as the systematically designed desensitization techniques. It is not essential for any one health professional to do all these therapies; it is only critical to be apprised of their existence and their usefulness in order to provide appropriate referrals to a patient. Cancer is a terrible disease which wrecks havoc with one's body, diminishes one's personal and financial

resources, interferes with family life and often disrupts sexual functioning. While we are making strides in reducing mortality, extending survival, and enhancing the quality of longevity, we are ignoring both the patient's potential for sexual gratification as well as evidence of problems in obtaining sexual pleasure. Holistic health care requires that caregivers understand: (1) what the degree of sexual dysfunction is in patients with cancer in different organ sites and at different life stages; (2) what the resulting disability associated with specific treatments is, and (3) what degree of emotional morbidity reported by the patient regarding quality of life is related to his/her sexual dysfunction. Professional attention must be focused on patient's sexual health as a major component of cancer management in order to optimize quality of life.

1414
Schover LR, Von Eschenbach AC. **Sexual and marital counseling with men treated for testicular cancer.** J Sex Marital Ther 10:29-40, 1984.

▶ counseling

Testicular cancer patients are at risk for sexual and marital problems because their cancer and its treatment reduce their fertility and disrupt intimate relationships at a crucial life stage (ages 15-34 yrs). Chemotherapy, radiotherapy, and surgery have successfully increased survival rates, but at the price of infertility and sexual dysfunction. A survey of 121 men (mean age 32 yrs) treated for nonseminomatous tumors revealed that 20% had low levels of sexual activity, 10% had erectile dysfunction, 6% had difficulty reaching orgasm, and 38% reported decreased orgasmic pleasure. Sexual anxiety related to cancer treatment accounted for much of this dysfunction, but organic factors such as hormonal, vascular, or neurologic damage may have also contributed. Reactions of couples to infertility and marital conflicts common in this group are discussed, and suggestions for sexual and marital counseling are offered.

1415
Schover LR, Von Eschenbach AC, Smith DB, Gonzalez J. **Sexual rehabilitation of urologic cancer patients: a practical approach.** CA 34:66-74, 1984.

▶ psychotherapy

Sexual rehabilitation is an important aspect of preserving a patient's quality of life after treatment for urogenital cancer. Sexual rehabilitation does not usually require a specialized program, but can be an integral part of cancer treatment. Members of the health care team can provide sexual information for the patient and partner, as well as assess the need for more intensive marital or sex therapy. This paper presents specific sexual issues related to prostate, bladder, testicular, and penile cancers.

1416

Shipes E, Lehr S. **Sexuality and the male cancer patient.** Cancer Nurs 4:375-381, 1982.

▶ counseling

Sexuality and its importance in our lives are topics of ongoing concern and interest. Societal role expectations, i.e., our concepts of what is "male" and what is "female" have a profound impact on every area of living. In a health care setting, these role expectations impact both patients and caregivers and greatly affect the care which is given and received. This article addresses the issue of male gender and sexual roles in health and illness, the effects of cancer and cancer therapies on male sexuality, and implications for therapeutic care.

1417

Stoudemire A, Techman T, Graham SD. **Sexual assessment of the urologic oncology patient.** Psychosomatics 26:405-410, 1985.

▶ counseling

Profound psychological ramifications may occur in the patient faced with the diagnosis of urologic malignancy. Disturbances may occur in body image, self-esteem, sexual identity, and sexual functioning. This article reviews the impact of treatment for urologic cancer on sexual functioning as well as psychodynamic factors that should be considered. Guidelines for psychological and sexual assessment of the urologic cancer patient are presented.

1418

Wise TN. **Sexual functioning in neoplastic disease.** Med Aspects Hum Sex 12:16-31, 1978.

▶ counseling

While the patient with cancer must be viewed as an individual with sexual feelings and needs, this must be in the context of the total human experience. All individuals who have neoplastic disease do not need sexual treatment or therapy. Some individuals or sexual partners, however, will develop sexual dysfunctions. Attention to their sexual behavior is needed if their quality of life is harmed or treatment compliance is limited. Recognition of the three parameters—the psychological effects of an illness, the organic performance factors due to the illness itself, and the effects of treatment on sexual enjoyment—provide a useful and easy approach to evaluating the sexual activity of the patient with cancer.

1419

Wise TN. **Effects of cancer on sexual activity.** Psychosomatics 19:769-775, 1978.

▶ counseling

Cancer of any type can affect sexual behavior through the physical and emotional impact of the disease itself and through the effects or chemotherapy of surgery. Major factors to be considered in assessing and treating these problems include the site and characteristics of the particular type of cancer, the patient's life stage and previous psychosocial functioning, and the prognosis. Malignancies of the genital organs may be particularly devastating.

Books and Book Chapters on Cancer

1420
Abse DW. **Investigative psychotherapy and cancer.** In: DM Kissen, LL LeShan (eds.), Psychosomatic Aspects of Neoplastic Disease. London: Pitman, 1963.

1421
Achterberg J, Lawlis GF. **Cancer: the ultimate mystery.** In: J Achterberg, GF Lawlis, Bridges of the Body Mind: Behavioral Approaches to Health Care. Champaign, Illinois: Institute for Personality and Ability Testing, Inc., 1980.

1422
Achterberg J, Lawlis GF. **Imagery of Cancer.** Champaign, Illinois: Institute for Personality and Ability Testing, 1978.

1423
Bahnson CB. **Characteristics of a psychotherapeutic treatment program for cancer patients.** In: HE Nieburgs (ed.), Prevention and Detection of Cancer. Vol. 2. New York: Marcel Dekker, 1978.

1424
Baltrusch HJF. **Psychotherapy with cancer patients: developments, results and limitations.** In: F Antonelli (ed.), Therapy in Psychosomatic Medicine. Rome: Pozzi, 1977.

1425
Baltrusch HJF. **Psychosomatic cancer research: present status and future vistas with special reference to gynecological cancer.** In: L Carenza, P Pancheri, L Zichella (eds.), Psychoneuroendocrinology in Reproduction. London: Academic Press, 1979.

1426
Bond MR. **Psychologic and psychiatric techniques.** In: JJ Bonica, V Ventafridda (eds.), Advances in Pain Research and Therapy. Vol. 2. New York: Raven, 1979.

1427
Booth GC. **Cancer and humanism (psychosomatic aspects of evolution).** In: DM Kissen, LL LeShan (eds.), Psychosomatic Aspects of Neoplastic Disease. London: Pitman, 1963.

1428
Brautigam W, Meerwein F (eds.). **The Therapeutic Talk with Cancer Patients: Progress in Psychooncology.** Bern: Huber, 1985.

1429
Burish TG, Carey MP. **Conditioned responses to cancer chemotherapy: etiology and treatment.** In: BH Fox, BH Newberry, Impact of Psychoendocrine Systems in Cancer and Immunity. Lewiston, New York: Hogrefe, 1984.

1430
Burish TG, Levy SM, Meyerowitz BE (eds.). **Cancer, Nutrition, and Eating Behavior: A Biobehavioral Perspective.** Hillsdale, New Jersey: Lawrence Erlbaum, 1985.

1431
Burke LD. **A national planning program for cancer rehabilitation.** In: JH Burchenal, HF Oettgen (eds.), Cancer Achievements, Challenges, and Prospects for the 1980s. Vol. 2. Orlando, Florida: Grune & Stratton, 1981.

1432
Chapman CR. **Psychologic and behavioral aspects of cancer pain.** In: JJ Bonica, V Ventafridda (eds.), Advances in Pain Research and Therapy. Vol. 2. New York: Raven, 1979.

1433
Cotanch PH. **Relaxation techniques as antiemetic therapy.** In: J Laszlo (ed.), Antiemetics and Cancer Chemotherapy. Baltimore: Williams & Wilkins, 1983.

1434
Crasilneck HB, Hall JA. **Hypnosis: its use with cancer patients.** In: HB Crasilneck, JH Hall (eds.), Clinical Hypnosis: Principles and Applications. Orlando, Florida: Grune & Stratton, 1973.

1435
Crue BL. **Some philosophical considerations of pain—suggestions, euthanasia, and free will.** In: BL Crue (ed.), Pain Research and Treatment. New York: Academic, 1975.

1436
Cunningham AJ. **Should we investigate psychotherapy for physical disease, especially cancer?** In: SM Levy (ed.), Biological Mediators of Behavior and Disease: Neoplasia. New York: Elsevier, 1982.

1437
Dash J. **Hypnosis for symptom alleviation.** In: J Kellerman (ed.), Psychological Aspects of Childhood Cancer. Springfield, Illinois: Thomas, 1980.

1438
Doolittle MJ. **Stress and cancer: new directions in treatment.** In: EH Rosenbaum, IR Rosenbaum (eds.), A Comprehensive Guide for Cancer Patients and their Families. Palo Alto, California: Bull Publishing, 1980.

1439
Elliotson J. **Cure of a True Cancer of the Female Breast with Mesmerism.** London: Walton and Mitchell, 1848.

1440
Finer B. **Hypnotherapy in pain of advanced cancer.** In: JJ Bonica, V Ventafridda (eds.), Advances in Pain Research and Therapy. Vol. 2. New York: Raven, 1979.

1441
Fotopoulos SS. **Psychophysiologic control of cancer pain.** In: JJ Bonica, V Ventafridda (eds.), Advances in Pain Research and Therapy. Vol. 2. New York: Raven, 1979.

1442
Fotopoulos SS, Cook MR, Graham C, Cohen H, Gerkovich M. **Cancer pain: evaluation of electromyographic and electrodermal feedback.** In: Progress in Clinical and Biological Research: 13th International Cancer Congress. Part D. New York: Alan R. Liss, 1983.

1443
Gendler ET, Grindler D, McGuire M. **Imagery, body, and space in focusing.** In: AA Sheikh (ed.), Imagination and Healing. Farmingdale, New York: Baywood, 1984.

1444
Goldberg JG (ed.). **Psychotherapeutic Treatment of Cancer Patients.** New York: Free Press, 1981.

1445
Grossarth-Maticek R, Schmidt P, Vetter H, Arndt S. **Psychotherapy research in oncology.** In: A Steptoe, A Mathews (eds.), Health Care and Human Behaviour. London: Academic, 1984.

1446
Hall H. **Imagery and cancer.** In: AA Sheikh (ed.), Imagination and Healing. Farmingdale, New York: Baywood, 1984.

1447
Helmkamp M, Paul H. **Psychosomatic Cancer Research.** Bern: Huber, 1984.

1448
Hilgard ER, Hilgard JR. **Cancer.** In: ER Hilgard, JR Hilgard, Hypnosis in the Relief of Pain. Los Altos, California: Kaufman, 1975.

1449
Hilgard JR, LeBaron S. **Hypnotherapy of pain in children with cancer.** Los Altos, California: Kaufmann, 1984.

1450
Hilgard JR, Morgan AH. **Treatment of anxiety and pain in childhood.** In: FH Frankel, HS Zamansky (eds.), Hypnosis at its Bicentennial. New York: Plenum, 1978.

1451
Holland JC. **Advances in psychologic support.** In: JH Burchenal, HF Oettgen (eds.), Cancer Achievements, Challenges, and Prospects for the 1980s. Vol. 2. Orlando, Florida: Grune & Stratton, 1981.

1452
Holland JCB. **Coping with cancer: a challenge to the behavioral sciences.** In: JW Cullen, BH Fox, RN Isom (eds.), Cancer: The Behavioral Dimensions. New York: Raven, 1976.

1453
Kellerman J. **Night terrors in a leukemic child.** In: J Kellerman (ed.), Psychological Aspects of Childhood Cancer. Springfield, Illinois: Thomas, 1980.

1454
Kroger WS. **Hypnosis in oncology.** In: WS Kroger, Clinical and Experimental Hypnosis in Medicine, Dentistry, and Psychology. 2nd ed. Philadelphia: Lippincott, 1977.

1455
Lansky B, Lowman JT, Gyulay J, Briscoe K. **A team approach to coping with cancer.** In: JW Cullen, BH Fox, RN Isom (eds.), Cancer: The Behavioral Dimensions. New York: Raven, 1976.

1456
LeShan LL. **You Can Fight for Your Life.** New York: Evans, 1977.

1457
Levenson BS. **A multidimensional approach to the treatment of pain in the oncology patient.** In: JM Vaeth (ed.), Frontiers of Radiation Therapy and Oncology. New York: Karger, 1981.

1458
Levy SM. **The expression of affect and its biological correlates: mediating mechanisms of behavior and disease.** In: L Temoshok, L Zegans, C Van Dyke (eds.), Emotions in Health and Illness: Applications to Clinical Practice. Orlando, Florida: Grune & Stratton, 1984.

1459
Lucas R, Brown C. **Assessment of cancer patients.** In: FJ Keefe, JA Blumenthal (eds.), Assessment Strategies in Behavioral Medicine. Orlando, Florida : Grune & Stratton, 1982.

1460
Maguire P. **The will to live in the cancer patient.** In: B Stoll (ed.), Mind and Cancer Prognosis. New York: Wiley, 1979.

1461
Meerwein F (ed.). **Introduction to Psychooncology.** Bern: Huber, 1981. (in German)

1462
Panagis DM. **Supportive therapy: goals and methods.** In: B Stoll (ed.), Mind and Cancer Prognosis. New York: Wiley, 1979.

1463
Sacerdote P. **Terminal cancer: pain relief through hypnotherapy (a detailed clinical report).** In: DM Kissen, LL LeShan (eds.), Psychosomatic Aspects of Neoplastic Disease. London: Pitman, 1963.

1464
Sacerdote P. **Hypnosis and terminal illness.** In: GD Burrows, L Dennerstein (eds.), Handbook of Hypnosis and Psychosomatic Medicine. New York: Elsevier, 1980.

1465
Sacerdote P. **The uses of hypnosis in cancer patients.** In: EM Weyer, H Hutchins (eds.), Psychophysiological Aspects in Cancer. New York: New York Academy of Sciences, 1966.

1466
Sacerdote P. **Erickson's contribution to pain control in cancer.** In: JK Zeig (ed.), Ericksonian Approaches to Hypnosis and Psychotherapy. New York: Brunner/Mazel, 1980.

1467
Sachs BC. **Hypnotherapy with cancer patients.** In: HJ Wain (ed.), Clinical Hypnosis in Medicine. Miami, Florida: Symposia Specialists, 1980.

1468
Saunders C. **The nature and management of terminal pain and the hospice concept.** In: JJ Bonica, V Ventafridda (eds.), Advances in Pain Research and Therapy. Vol. 2. New York: Raven, 1979.

1469
Schain WS. **Sexual problems of patients with cancer.** In: VT DeVita (ed.), Cancer: Principles and Practice of Oncology. Philadelphia: Lippincott, 1982.

1470
Simonton OC, Matthews-Simonton S. **Stress, self-regulation, and cancer.** In: EM Goldwag, Inner Balance: The Power of Holistic Healing. Englewood Cliffs, New Jersey: Prentice-Hall, 1979.

1471
Simonton OC, Matthews-Simonton S. **Therapeutic applications.** In: J Achterberg, OC Simonton, S Matthews-Simonton (eds.), Stress, Psychological Factors, and Cancer. Fort Worth: New Medicine Press, 1976.

1472
Simonton OC, Matthews-Simonton S, Creighton J. **Getting Well Again.** Los Angeles: Tarcher, 1978.

1473
Sontag S. **Illness as Metaphor.** New York: Farrar, Straus & Giroux, 1978.

1474
Stoll BA. **Mind and cancer prognosis.** In: BA Stoll (ed.), Mind and Cancer Prognosis. Chichester, England: Wiley, 1979.

1475
Stoll BA. **Restraint of growth and spontaneous regression of cancer.** In: BA Stoll (ed.), Mind and Cancer Prognosis. Chichester, England: Wiley, 1979.

1476
Stoll BA. **Is hope a factor in survival?** In: BA Stoll (ed.), Mind and Cancer Prognosis. Chichester, England: Wiley, 1979.

1477
Udupa KN. **Stress and cancer.** In: KN Udupa, Disorders of Stress and Their Management by Yoga. Varanasi, India: Banaras Hindu University Press, 1978.

1478
Von Eschenbach AC, Rodriquez DB (eds.), **Sexual Rehabilitation of the Urologic Cancer Patient.** Boston: Hall, 1981.

1479
Von Eschenbach AC, Schover LR. **Sexual rehabilitation of cancer patients.** In: AE Gunn (ed.), Cancer Rehabilitation. New York: Raven, 1984.

Journal Assessment Index

We have prepared this index to help the reader form a general assessment of the journals cited in this collection. The reader's own critical appraisal is, of course, the best measure for judging the importance of a particular article.

We have characterized each journal by up to five descriptive items. The first item, the parenthetical number after the title, indicates the number of times that we cite the journal, and is a rough measure of the frequency with which a journal publishes articles in this field.

The next possible item, "B," indicates whether the journal is listed on the Brandon List, 1985-86, a guide for small or medium-sized libraries to journals of general scientific interest.

The third possible item, the acronym "AIM," indicates that a journal is in the *Abridged Index Medicus*, March 1985, a list of 117 biomedical journals indexed for the practicing physician. AIM, in other words, denotes clinically oriented material.

The next possible item, "P," indicates that the journal is in the 1984 PsycINFO list of 1,300 journals covered by *Psychological Abstracts*. P, then, denotes journals relevant to fields of psychology and behavior.

The last possible item, which always contains a decimal, is a journal's "impact factor" as devised by the Institute for Scientific Information (see the *Journal Citation Report*, 1983). This factor, which represents the frequency with which an article in a journal is cited in a given year, is a rough measure of the impact that a journal has on the scientific community. (The factor is calculated from the ratio of the number of cited articles in a calendar year to the number of articles published by the journal in that year, a procedure that corrects for the advantage that larger journals have over smaller ones.) The range of the impact factors varies from .000 to 30.214, although most factors fall between .000 and 1.000.

Some older journals are not on any of the last four indexing lists because the journals ended publication before the lists were developed. Readers should also note that some journal articles are significant primarily for their historic or innovative contribution.

Act Nerv Super (Praha) (1)
Acta Allerg (Kbh) (2)
Acta Allergol (3)
Acta Allergol Suppl (1)
Acta Derm Venereol (Stockh) (1) .971
Acta Hipnol Lat Am (3)
Acta Hipnol Latino Tomo (1)
Acta Med Orient (1)
Acta Paediatr Acad Sci Hung (1)
Acta Paediatr Scand (Suppl) (1) 1.068
Acta Psychother (3)
Acta Tuberc Pneumol Belg (4)
Actas Luso Esp Neurol Psiquiatr (1) P
Adolescence (2) P
Adv Asthma Allergy (1)
Adv Psychosom Med (1)
Advances (6)
Akad Beloruss (Minsk) (1)
Allerg Asthma (Leipz) (8)
Allerg Immunol (Leipz) (1)
Allergol Immunopathol (Madr) (1) .088
Allergol Immunopathol (Madr) Suppl (2)
Allergy (1) 1.472
Am J Clin Hypn (51) P
Am J Dis Child (2) B 1.220
Am J Med (2) B, AIM 4.896
Am J Med Sci (2) B, AIM .763
Am J Obstet Gynecol (1) B, AIM 1.892
Am J Orthopsychiatry (7) P .962
Am J Pediatr Hematol Oncol (1)
Am J Psychiatry (8) B, P, AIM 3.209
Am J Psychother (3) P .414
Am J Roentgenol (1) AIM 2.343
Am Pract (2)
Am Rev Resp Dis (4) B, AIM 4.063
Am Rev Tub (3)
Ann Allergy (35) B .756
Ann Clin Res (1) P .586
Ann Dermatol Syphiligr (Paris) (1)
Ann Intern Med (2) B, AIM 7.002
Ann Med Psychol (2) P .037
Ann NY Acad Sci (5) P 1.222
Arch Allergy (1)
Arch Allergy Appl Immunol (1)
Arch Belg Dermatol (1)
Arch Dermatol (9) B, AIM 1.688
Arch Dermatol Syph (22)
Arch Dis Child (2) AIM 1.622
Arch Gen Psychiatry (3) B, AIM 6.113
Arch Intern Med (3) B, AIM 1.819
Arch Klin Exp Dermatol (1)

Arch Neurol Psychiatry (1)
Arch Phys Med Rehabil (3) AIM, .665
Arch Phys Rehabil (1)
Arch Phys Ther (Leipz) (1)
Arch Psychiatr Nervenkr (1) .597
Arerugi (1)
Ariz Med (1)
Army Med Corps (1)
Arthritis Rheum (1) B, AIM 3.673
Arztl Forsch (1)
Arztl Fortbild (1)
Aust Fam Physician (3)
Aust J Clin Exp Hypn (1) P
Aust J Clin Hypnother Hypn (1) P
Aust NZ J Psychiatry (1) P .538
Australas J Dermatol (2)

BTTA Rev (1)
Behav Anal Mod (1)
Behav Med Update (2) P
Behav Neuropsychiatry (1)
Behav Res Ther (7) P
Behav Ther (3) P
Behav Ther Exp Psychiatry (1)
Behav Therapist (1) P
Bibl Haemotol (1)
Bibl Psychiatr Neurol (1)
Biofeedback Self Regul (9)
Biol Psychiatry (1) P 2.857
Blood (1) B, AIM 6.159
Bol Assoc Med Puerto Rico (1)
Bol Brasil Soc Int Hipn Clin Exp (1)
Bol Med Hosp Infant Mex (1)
Br J Clin Psychol (1) P
Br J Dermatol (11) 1.845
Br J Dermatol Syph (3)
Br J Dis Chest (1) 1.097
Br J Hosp Med (1) .399
Br J Med Hypn (8)
Br J Med Psychol (9) P .602
Br J Psychiatry (3) P 2.388
Br Med J (26) B, AIM 2.769
Bronches (2)
Bull Menninger Clin (4) P
Bull NY Acad Med (3)
Bull Rheum Dis (1)
Bull Soc Fr Dermatol Syphiligr (2)
Bull Tufts N Engl Med Center (1)
Bull Tulane Univ Med Fac (1)
Burns (1) .217

CA (7) AIM 2.632
CARIH Res Bull (1)
Calif Med (4)
Can Med Assoc J (11) B, AIM 1.086
Can Nurse (2)
Can Psychiatr Assoc J (1)
Can Psychol Rev (1)
Cancer (4) B, AIM 2.649
Cancer Nurs (8)
Cancer Res (1) 3.788
Cesk Dermatol (1)
Cesk Psychiatr (1) P
Child Welfare (1)
Ciba Found Symp (1) 1.533

Clin Gerontol (1)
Clin Pediatr (1)
Clin Pediatr (Phila) (4) B, P, AIM .393
Clin Proc Child Hosp (2)
Clin Psychol Rev (1) P
Clin Res (1) .144
Clin Rev Allergy (1)
Clinics (1)
Clinique (Par) (1)
Compr Psychiatry (1) P
Conn Med (1) .051
Conn Med J (1)
Contemp Psychoanal (1) P
Curr Psychiatr Ther (2)
Cutis (3) .495

Del Med J (1)
Dermatol Wochenschr (11)
Dermatol Z (1)
Dermatologica (3) .452
Deutsch Gesundheitswes (1)
Dis Chest (1)
Dis Nerv Syst (3)
Diss Abstr Int (13) P
Dtsch Gesundheitswes (2)
Dtsch Med Wochenschr (6)
Dtsch Militararzt (1)

Egypt Yearbook Psychol (1)
Eur J Cancer (2) 2.888
Eur J Respir Dis (Suppl) (1).808
Evol Psychiatr (1) P

Fam Process (1) P
Familiendynamik (2)
Folia Psychiatr Neurol Jpn (1) .261
Folia Psychiatr Neurol Neurochir Med (1)
Fortschr Med (1) .182
Front Radiat Ther Oncol (3)
Fukuoka Igaku Zasshi (1)

G Ital Dermatol (1)
Gac Med Mexico (1)
Gen Hosp Psychiatry (1) P .701
Geriatrics (1) B, AIM .271
Gerontol Clin (Basel) (1)
Gruzlica (1)
Guy's Hosp Rep (3)
Gynecol Oncol (1) 1.186

HNO (1) .127
Haematologia (Budap) (2) .463
Harefuah (2)
Hautarzt (4) .557
Health Educ Q (1)
Health Psychol (1)
Heart Lung (1) B, AIM .361
Hemophilia Lett (1)
Hippokrates (3)
Hosp Pract (1) B, AIM, .562

Hypn Kognition (2)
Hypnosis (1)

Int (1)
Int Arch Allergy (2)
Int Arch Allergy Appl Immunol (7) 1.262
Int Clin (1)
Int J Child Psychother (1)
Int J Clin Exp Hypn (13) P .845
Int J Dermatol (1) .721
Int J Eclectic Psychother (1) P
Int J Fam Ther (1) P
Int J Group Psychother (3) P
Int J Psychoanal (6) P
Int J Psychoanal Psychother (2) P
Int Ment Health Res Newsletter (1)
Int Pharmacopsychiatry (1) P
Int Z Psychoanal (1)

J Abnorm Psychol (1) P
J Abnorm Soc Psychol (1)
J Adolesc Health Care (5) P
J Allergy (2)
J Allergy Clin Immunol (3) B, AIM, 3.378
J Am Acad Child Psychiatry (7) 1.336
J Am Acad Dermatol (5) B, 1.981
J Am Acad Psychoanal (1)
J Am Dent Assoc (1) B, .617
J Am Diet Assoc (1) B, .772
J Am Inst Hypn (3)
J Am Med Wom Assoc (1)
J Am Soc Psychosom Dent Med (8)
J Appl Behav Anal (1) P
J Appl Rehabil Counseling (1)
J Asthma (5) P .178
J Asthma Res (38)
J Behav Med (4) P
J Behav Ther Exp Psychiatry (10)
J Behav Ther Exp Psychol (1)
J Child Asthma Res Inst Hosp (4)
J Child Psychol (1)
J Child Psychol Psychiatry (1) P
J Chronic Dis (1) 1.368
J Clin Exp Hypn (1)
J Consult Clin Psychol (9) P
J Consult Psychol (1)
J Dis Child (1)
J Fam Pract (1) B, P .652
J Fla Med Assoc (1)
J Indiana State Med Assoc (1)
J Invest Dermatol (3) 3.544
J Irish Med Assoc (1)
J Med (1) .522
J Med Assoc Ga (1)
J Med Sci (1)
J Med Soc NJ (4)
J Ment Sci (2)
J Mt Sinai Hosp (2)
J Nerv Ment Dis (12) B, P, AIM 1.577
J Oral Surg Anesth Hosp Dent Serv (1)
J Pediatr (2) B 2.668
J Pediatr Psychol (1) P
J Proj Tech (1)
J Psychiatr Treat Eval (1) P .154

J Psychol (1) P
J Psychosoc Nur Ment Health Serv (2) P
J Psychosoc Oncol (2) P
J Psychosom Res (29) P .789
J R Soc Med (1)
J Rheumatol (2) 1.672
J Sex Marital Ther (1) P
J Soc Casework (1)
J Transpersonal Psychol (1) P
J Urol Nephrol (Paris) (1)
JAMA (19) B, AIM 3.382
Jahrb Psychoanal Psychopathol (1)
Jpn J Hypn (1)
Jpn J Med Progr (1)

Kinderarztl Prax (2)
Klin Med (Mosk) (2) 2.5
Klin Wochenschr (1)
Kokyu To Junkan (1)
Krankenpflege (Frankfurt) (2)
Ky Med J (1)

Lakartidningen (2)
Lancet (19) B, AIM 12.250
Lond Clin Med J (1)

MMW (1)
Med Ann DC (1)
Med Aspects Hum Sex (1)
Med Cir Farm (Rio de Janeiro) (1)
Med Clin N Am (3) B, AIM 2.147
Med Cutan Iber Lat Am (1)
Med J Aust (18) .856
Med J Malaya (1)
Med J Rec (2)
Med Klin (4) .222
Med Ped Oncol (1) .623
Med Press (1)
Med Psicosom (1)
Med Rec (2)
Med Times (1)
Med Welt (2) .173
Medicamenta (Madr) (1)
Medicine (1) B, AIM
Ment Hygiene (1)
Minerva Dermatol (1)
Minerva Med (7)
Mitt Ges Bek Krebskr Nordrhein-
  Westfalen (1)
Mod Med (1)
Mod Treat (2)
Monatsh Prakt Dermatol (1)
Monatsschr Kinderheilkd (3) .235
Mt Sinai J Med (1) .198
Munch Med Wochenschr (2) 1.69

N Engl J Med (8) B, P, AIM 16.465
NY Med J (1)
NY Med J Med Rec l (1)
NY St J Med (7) P .265
Nagoya Med J (1)
Nebr Med J (1)
Ned Tijdschr Geneeskd (11) P

Ned Tijdschr Psychol (1)
Nerv Child (3)
Neurobiologia (1) P
Neurol Neurocir Psiquiatr (1) P
Nord Medicin (1)
North Am (1)
Northwest Med (3)
Nurs Mirror (2)
Nurs Res (2) P, AIM .401
Nurs Times (4)

Obstet Gynecol (2) B, AIM 1.663
Oncol Nurs Forum (3)
Orv Hetil (3)

Paediatrician (1) .154
Pain (1) P 3.318
Pediatr Ann (2) .263
Pediatr Clin North Am (6) B, AIM .679
Pediatr Med Chir (1)
Pediatrics (3) B, AIM 2.563
Penn Med J (3)
Perspect Biol Med (2) .390
Phys Ther (1) B, .265
Plast Reconstr Surg (3) B, AIM 1.268
Postgrad Med (2) B, AIM .393
Postgrad Med J (2) .435
Practitioner (8) .213
Prax Kinderpsychol Kinderpsychiatr (6) P
Prax Pneumol (1)
Prensa Med Argent (1)
Proc R Soc Med (3)
Proc Staff Meet Mayo Clin (1)
Prof Psychol (1) P
Psyche (Stuttg) (2) P
Psychiatr Clin North Am (1) P
Psychiatr Fenn (Helsinki) Suppl: (1)
Psychiatr J Univ Ottawa (1) P
Psychiatr Neurol Med Psychol (Leipz) (1)
  P
Psychiatr Pol (2) P
Psychiatr Q (5) P
Psychic (1)
Psychoanal Prax (1)
Psychoanal Q (2) P
Psychoanal Rev (7) P
Psychoanal Study Child (2) P
Psychol Bull (1) P 3.605
Psychol Rep (4) P
Psychol Today Sept (1)
Psychophysiology (1) P 1.665
Psychosom Med (55) P 2.238
Psychosomatics (26) P .892
Psychother Private Pract (1) P
Psychother Psychosom (15) P .495
Psychother Psychosom Med Psychol (1)
Psychother Theory Res Pract (1) P
Public Health Rep (1) B, AIM
Public Health Rev (1)

Q J Med (1) 2.043
Q J Studies Alcohol (1)
Q Rev Allergy (1)
Q Rev Pediatr (1)

Radiography (1)
Rehabl Lit (1) P
Rehabilitation (Stuttg) (1)
Rep Chron Rheumat Dis (1)
Respir Ther (3)
Respiration (1) .493
Rev Allergy (1)
Rev Brasil Tuberc (1)
Rev Fr Odontostomatol (1)
Rev Fr Psychanal (1)
Rev Gastroenterol (1)
Rev Med Chile (1) .310
Rev Med Chir Soc Med Nat Iasi (1)
Rev Med Psychosom (4)
Rev Med Suisse Romande (1)
Rev Neuropsychiatr Infant (2)
Rev Psicol Norm Patol (1)
Rheumatism (1)
Rheumatol Int (1) .866
Rheumatol Rehabil (1) .551
Rinsho Hoshasen (1)
Riv Sper Freniatr (1) P
Rocky Mt Med J (2)

S Afr Med J (2) .536
Scand J Behav Ther (1) P
Schweiz Med Wochenschr (3) .558
Schweiz Z Psychol Anwendung (1)
Science (1) B, P 7.407
Sem Hop Paris (2) .154
Sem Hop Paris Ther (1)
Semana Med (1)
Semin Oncol (1) 1.696
Semin Psychiatry (1)
Shinryo Shitsu (1)
Singapore Med (1)
Singapore Med J (2)
Skin (1)
Soc Casework (2) P
Soc Sci Med (2) P
Somatics (1)
South Med J (2) AIM .283
Sov Med (1) .108
Surg Annu (1)

Ter Arkh (1)
Tex Med (2) .083
Tex State J Med (1)
Ther Ggw (4)
Ther Umsch (1)
Therapeutique (1)
Therapie (1) .393
Thromb Diath Haem (1)
Tijdschr Geneeskd (1)
Top Clin Nurs (1)
Trans All-India Inst Mental Health (1)
Trans St Johns Hosp Dermatol Soc (1)

US Armed Forces Med J l (1)
Ugeskr Laeger (2)
Ulster Med J (1)
Union Med Can (1) .053
Urol Cutan Rev (3)

Va Med Monthly (2)
Verh Dtsch Ges Inn Med (1)
Verh Dtsch Ges Rheumatol (1)
Vestn Dermatol Venerol (7) .195
Vojnosanit Pregl (1)
Vopr Kurortol Fizioter Lech Fiz Kult (1)
Vopr Okhr Materin Det (1)
Vrach Delo (2)

W Va J Med (1)
Western Med (1)
Wiad Lek (2)

Wien Klin Wochenschr (1) .186
Wien Med Wochenschr (1) .075
Wis Med J (1)

Yoga Mimamsa (1)

Z Allgemeinmed (1)
Z Erkr Atmungsorgane (1)
Z Gesamte Inn Med (1)
Z Gesamte Neurol Psychiatr (1)
Z Haut Geschlechtskr (1)

Z Hautkr (2) .379
Z Klin Med (2)
Z Klin Psychol Psychother (1) P
Z Neurol Psychiatr (1)
Z Physiother (1)
Z Psychosom Med (4)
Z Psychosom Med Psychoanal (9) P .441
Z Psychosom Psychoanal (1)
Zentrabl Inn Med (2)
Zentralbl Haut Geschlechtskr (1)
Zentralbl Psychoanal (1)
Zentralbl Psychother (1)
Zh Nevropatol Psikhiatr (1) P .191

Acknowledgments to Publishers

The following abstracts are reprinted with permission of Academic Press:

Lamont JA, DePetrillo AD, Sargeant EJ. Psychosexual rehabilitation and exenterative surgery. Gynecol Oncol 6:236-242, 1979.

Ludwig AO. Emotional factors in tuberculosis. Public Health 63:883-888, 1948.

Schafer DW. The management of pain in the cancer patient. Compr Psychiatry 10:41-45, 1984.

The following abstracts are reprinted with permission of Almindelige Danske Laegejorening—Danish Medical Association:

Moller P. Psychosomatic dermatology. Ugeskr Laeg 112:892-895, 1950. (in Danish)

Wagner FF. Metastatic pain influenced by hypnotic suggestion. Ugeskr Laeger 129:393-395, 1967. (in Danish)

The following abstract is reprinted with permission of Almqvist & Wiksell Int'l.:

Moller P. Psychotherapy for pruritus. Acta Derm Venereol (Stockh) 31:267–271, 1951.

The following abstracts are reprinted with permission of Amer. Academy of Pediatrics and reproduced by permission of pediatrics:

Bernstein IL, Allen JE, Kreindler L, Ghory JE, Wohl TH. A community approach to juvenile intractable asthma. Pediatrics 26:586-595, 1960.

Rosenthal MJ. A psychosomatic study of infantile eczema (I): The mother-child relationship. Pediatrics 10:581-591, 1952.

Zeltzer L, Dash J, Holland JP. Hypnotically induced pain control in sickle cell anemia. Pediatrics 64:533-536, 1979.

The following abstracts are reprinted with permission of Amer. Cancer Society:

Barber J, Gitelson J. Cancer pain: psychological management using hypnosis. CA 30:130-136, 1980.

Derogatis LR, Kourlesis SM. An approach to evaluation of sexual problems in the cancer patient. CA 31:46-50, 1981.

Levy SM. Biobehavioral interventions in behavioral medicine: an overview. CA 50:1939-1943, 1982.

Schover LR, Von Eschenbach AC, Smith DB, Gonzalez J. Sexual rehabilitation of urologic cancer patients: a practical approach. CA 34:66-74, 1984.

Spiegel D. The use of hypnosis in controlling cancer pain. CA 35:221-231, 1985.

The following abstract is reprinted with permission of American College of Chest Physicians:

Anderson AS. Psychogenic factors in chest diseases. Dis Chest 19:570-576, 1951.

The following abstracts are reprinted with permission of American College of Physicians:

Cassileth BR, Lusk EJ, Strouse TB, Bodenheimer BJ. Contemporary unorthodox treatments in cancer medicine: a study of patients, treatments, and practitioners. Ann Intern Med 10:105-112, 1984.

Mufson I. An etiology of scleroderma. Ann Intern Med 39:1219-1227, 1953.

Scherr MS. Camp Bronco Junction—second year of experience. Ann Allergy 28:423-432, 1970.

The following abstracts are reprinted with permission of American Congress of Rehabilitation Medicine:

Capone MA, Good RS, Westie KS, Jacobson AF. Psychosocial rehabilitation of gynecologic oncology patients. Arch Phys Rehabil 61:128-132, 1980.

Varni JW. Behavioral medicine in hemophilia arthritic pain management: two case studies. Arch Phys Med Rehabil 62:183-187, 1981.

The following abstracts are reprinted with permission of American Journal of Nursing Co.:

Dixon J. Effect of nursing interventions on nutritional and performance status in cancer patients. Nurs Res 33:330-335, 1984.

Hoffman AL. Psychological factors associated with rheumatoid arthritis: review of the literature. Nurs Res 23:218-234, 1974.

The following abstracts are reprinted with permission of American Lung Association:

Ben-Zvi Z, Spohn WA, Young SH, Kattan M. Hypnosis for exercise-induced asthma. Am Rev Respir Dis 125:392-395, 1982.

Lewis RA, Lewis MN, Tattersfield AE. Asthma induced by suggestion: is it due to airway cooling? Am Rev Respir Dis 129:691-695, 1984.

Smith MM, Colebatch HJ, Clarke PS. Increase and decrease in pulmonary resistance with hypnotic suggestion in asthma. Am Rev Respir Dis 102:236-242, 1970.

Spector S, Luparello TJ, Kopetzky MT, Souhrada J, Kinsman RA. Response of asthmatics to methacholine and suggestion. Am Rev Resp Dis 113:43-50, 1976.

The following abstract is reprinted with permission of American Medical Women's Association:

Christensen BE. The psyche and the skin. J Am Med Wom Assoc 10:117-122, 1955.

The following abstracts are reprinted with permission of American Orthopsychiatric Association, Inc.:

Benjamin JD, Coleman JV, Hornbein R. A study of personality in pulmonary tuberculosis. Am J Orthopsychiatry 18:704-707, 1948.

Blom GE, Nicholls G. Emotional factors in children with rheumatoid arthritis. Am J Orthopsychiatry 24:588-601, 1954.

Coolidge JC. Asthma in mother and child as a special type of intercommunication. Am J Orthopsychiatry 26:165-178, 1956.

Dubo S. Psychiatric study of children with pulmonary tuberculosis. Am J Orthopsychiatry 20:520-528, 1950.

Friend MR, Pollak O. Psychosocial aspects in the preparation for treatment of an allergic child. AM J Orthopsychiatry 24:63-72, 1954.

Gaudet EL. Dynamic interpretation and treatment of asthma in a child. Am J Orthopsychiatry 20:328-345, 1950.

The following abstract is reprinted with permission of American Physcial Therapy Association:

Merenstein A, Schenkman M. Pernicious anemia: the disease and physical therapy management: a case report. Phys Ther 64:1076-1077, 1984.

The following abstracts are reprinted with permission of American Psychiatric Association:

Forester B, Kornfeld DS, Fleiss JL. Psychotherapy during radiotherapy: effects on emotional and physical distress. Am J Psychiatry, Vol. 142, pp. 22-27, 1985. Copyright 1985, the American Psychiatric Association. Reprinted by permission.

French TM. Psychogenic factors in asthma. Am J Psychiatry, Vol. 96, pp. 87-101, 1939. Copyright 1939, the American Psychiatric Association. Reprinted by permission.

Handford AH, Charney D, Ackerman L, Eyster ME, Bixler EO. Effect of psychiatric intervention on the use of antihemophilic factor concentrate. Am J Psychiatry, Vol. 137, pp. 1254-1256, 1980. Copyright 1980, the American Psychiatric Association. Reprinted by permission.

Jessner L, Long RT, Lamont JH, Whipple B, Bandler L, Blom GE, Burgin L. A psychosomatic study of allergic and emotional factors in children with asthma. Am J Psychiatry, Vol. 114, pp. 890-899, 1958. Copyright 1958, the American Psychiatric Association. Reprinted by permission.

Lerro FA, Hurnyak MM, Patterson C. Successful use of thermal biofeedback in severe adult asthma. Am J Psychiatry, Vol. 137, pp.735-736, 1980. Copyright 1980, the American Psychiatric Association. Reprinted by permission.

Liebman R, Minuchin S, Baker L. The use of structural family therapy in the treatment of intractable asthma. Am J Psychiatry, Vol. 131, pp. 535-540, 1974. Copyright 1974, the American Psychiatric Association. Reprinted by permission.

Shoemaker RJ, Levine MI, Shipman WG, Mally MA. A search for the affective determinants of chronic urticaria. Am J Psychiatry, Vol. 119, pp. 358-359, 1962. Copyright 1962, the American Psychiatric Association. Reprinted by permission.

The following abstracts are reprinted with permission of American Psychological Association:

Bowers KS, Kelly P. Stress, disease, psychotherapy, and hypnosis. J Abnorm Psychol 88:490-505, 1979. Copyright 1979 by the American Psychological Association. Reprinted (or Adapted) by permission of the publisher.

Creer TL. Asthma. J Consult Clin Psychol 50:912-921, 1982. Copyright 1982 by the American Psychological Association. Reprinted (or Adapted) by permission of the publisher.

Miklich DR. Health psychology practice with asthmatics. Prof Psychol 10:580-588, 1979. Copyright 1979 by the American Psychological Association. Reprinted (or Adapted) by permission of the publisher.

Morrow GR. Appropriations of taped versus live relaxation in the systematic desensitization of anticipatory nausea and vomiting in cancer patients. J Consult Clin Psychol 52:1098-1099, 1984. Copyright 1984 by the American Psychological Association. Reprinted (or Adapted) by permission of the publisher.

Surwit RS. Behavioral treatment of Raynaud's syndrome in peripheral vascular disease. J Consult Clin Psychol 50:922-932, 1982. Copyright 1982 by the American Psychological Association. Reprinted (or Adapted) by permission of the publisher.

The following abstract is reprinted with permission of American Rheumatism Association:

Emery H, Schaller JG, Fowler RS. Biofeedback in the management of primary and secondary Raynaud's phenomenon. Arthritis Rheum 19:795, 1976.

The following abstracts are reprinted with permission of American Society of Clinical Hypnosis:

Aston EE. Treatment of allergy by suggestion: an experiment. Am J Clin Hypn 1:163-164, 1959.

August RV. Hypnotic induction of hypothermia: an additional approach to postoperative control of cancer recurrence. Am J Clin Hypn 18:52-55, 1975.

Cangello VW. Hypnosis for the patient with cancer. Am J Clin Hypn 4:215-226, 1961-1962.

Cohen SB. Warts. Am J Clin Hypn 20:157-159, 1978. (editorial)

Collison DR. Hypnotherapy in the management of asthma. Am J Clin Hypn 11:6-11, 1968.

Diamond HH. Hypnosis in children: the complete cure of forty cases of asthma. Am J Clin Hypn 1:124-129, 1958.

Dubin LL, Shapiro SS. Use of hypnosis to facilitate dental extraction and hemostasis in a classic hemophiliac with a high antibody titer to factor VIII. Am J Clin Hypn 17:79-83, 1974.

Erickson MH. Hypnosis in painful terminal illness. Am J Clin Hypn 1:117-121, 1959.

Fredericks LE. The use of hypnosis in hemophilia. Am J Clin Hypn 10:52-55, 1967.

Goodman HP. Hypnosis in prolonged resistant eczema: a case report. Am J Clin Hypn 5:144-145, 1962-1963.

Gould SS, Tissler DM. The use of hypnosis in the treatment of herpes simplex II. Am J Clin Hypn 26:171-174, 1984.

Hammond DC, Keye WR, Grant CW Jr. Hypnotic analgesia with burns: an initial study. Am J Clin Hypn 26:56-59, 1983.

Hollander MB. Excoriated acne controlled by post-hypnotic suggestion. Am J Clin Hypn 1:122-123, 1959.

Kaye JM. Hypnotherapy and family therapy for the cancer patient: a case study. Am J Clin Hypn 27:38-41, 1984.

Lea PA, Ware PD, Monroe RR. The hypnotic control of intractable pain. Am J Clin Hypn 3:3-8, 1960-1961.

Lucas ON. Dental extractions in the hemophiliac: control of the emotional factors by hypnosis. Am J Clin Hypn 7:301-307, 1965.

Margolis CG, Domangue BB, Ehleben C, Shrier L. Hypnosis in the early treatment of burns: a pilot study. Am J Clin Hypn 26:9-15, 1983.

Moore LE, Kaplan JZ. Hypnotically accelerated burn wound healing. Am J Clin Hypn 26:16-19, 1983.

Moorefield CW. The use of hypnosis and behavior therapy in asthma. Am J Clin Hypn 13:162-168, 1971.

Perloff MA, Spiegelman J. Hypnosis in the treatment of a child's allergy to dogs. Am J Clin Hypn 15:269-272, 1973.

Sacerdote P. Additional contributions to the hypnotherapy of the advanced cancer patient. Am J Clin Hypn 7:308-319, 1965.

Sacerdote P. Hypnotherapy in neurodermatitis: a case report. Am J Clin Hypn 7:249-253, 1965.

Schon RC. Addendum to "Hypnosis in painful terminal illness." Am J Clin Hypn 3:61-62, 1960.

Secter II, Barthelemy CG. Angular cheilosis and psoriasis as psychosomatic manifestations. Am J Clin Hypn 7:79-81, 1964.

Smith MS, Kamitsuka M. Self-hypnosis misinterpreted as CNS deterioration in an adolescent with leukemia and vincristine toxicity. Am J Clin Hypn 26:280-282, 1984.

Surman OS, Gottlieb SK, Hackett TP. Hypnotic treatment of a child with warts. Am J Clin Hypn 15:12-14, 1972.

Twerski AJ, Naar R. Hypnotherapy in a case of refractory dermatitis. Am J Clin Hypn 16:202-205, 1974.

Wakeman RJ, Kaplan JZ. An experimental study of hypnosis in painful burns. Am J Clin Hypn 21:3-12, 1978.

Wink CAS. A case of Darier's disease treated by hypnotic age regression. Am J Clin Hypn 9:146-150, 1966.

The following abstracts are reprinted with permission of American Society of Psychosomatic Dentistry and Medicine:

Hossri CM. The treatment of asthma in children through acupuncture massage. J Am Soc Psychosom Dent Med 23:3-16, 1976.

Meares A. The quality of meditation effective in the regression of cancer. J Am Soc Psychosom Dent Med 25:129-132, 1978.

Meares A. Remission of massive metastasis from undifferentiated carcinoma of the lung associated with intensive meditation. J Am Soc Psychosom Dent Med 27:40-41, 1980.

Sanders S. Hypnotic self control strategies in hemophilic children. J Am Soc Psychosom Dent Med 28:11-21, 1981.

The following abstract is reprinted with permission of Arizona Medical Association:

Schulte HJ, Abhyanker VV. Yogic breathing and psychologic states. Ariz Med 36:681-683, 1979.

The following abstract is reprinted with permission of L'Association des Medecins de Langue Francaise du Canada:

Smith H. The psychosomatic factor in dermatology. Union Med Can 80:1399-1402, 1951. (in French: no English abstract)

The following abstract is reprinted with permission of Association for the Advancement of Psychotherapy:

LeShan LL, Gassmann ML. Some observations on psychotherapy with patients suffering from neoplastic disease. Am J Psychother 12:723-734, 1958.

The following abstracts are reprinted with permission of Australasian College of Dermatologists:

Ironside W. Eczema, darkly mirror of the mind. Australas J Dermatol 15:5-9, 1974.

Whitlock FA. Skin disorders and the mind. Australas J Dermatol 14:5-10, 1973.

The following abstracts are reprinted with permission of Baillere Tindall:

Smith J.M., Burns C.L.C. The treatment of asthmatic children by hypnotic suggestion. British Journal of Diseases of the Chest 54:78-81, 1960.

Varni J.W., Gilbert A. Self-regulation of chronic arthritic pain and long-term analgesic dependence in a haemophiliac. Rheumatology and Rehabilitation 21:171-174, 1982.

The following abstracts are reprinted with permission of Bohn Scheltema en Holkema:

Arndt JL, Polano MK. The psychotherapeutic treatment of a case of pruritis vulvae. Ned Tijdschr Geneeskd 3:2675-2678, 1950. (in Dutch)

Fleischer D. Psychotherapy of disorder of the skin, probably lupus erythematosus. Ned Tijdschr Geneeskd 85:566-567, 1941. (in Dutch)

Kuijpers BR. Constitutional eczema: clinico-psychological findings. Ned Tijdschr Geneeskd 112:976-981, 1968.

Kuypersen BR, Bar LH. The psychologist in the dermatological clinic: methods and possibilities of treatment. Ned Tijdschr Geneeskd 116:1268-1271, 1972. (in Dutch)

Mook J, Van der Ploeg HM. Behavior therapy in bronchial asthma: systematic desensitization applied to 3 patients. Ned Tijdschr Geneeskd 120:1065-1069, 1976. (in Dutch)

Musaph H. Behavior therapy in psychodermatology. Ned Tijdschr Geneeskd 116:1769-1771, 1972.

Stokvis B., Welman AJ. Group therapy and sociotherapy as adjuvants in treating asthma. Ned Tijdschr Geneeskd 99:693-703, 1955.

Van der Hal I. Treatment of asthma by imitation of asthmatic breathing. Ned Tijdschr Geneeskd 100:767-769, 1966.

Van der Ploeg HM, Mook J. Behavior therapy in bronchial asthma. Ned Tijdschr Geneeskd 120:1083-1087, 1976.

The following abstracts are reprinted with permission of Brentwood Publishing Company:

Creer TL. Psychologic aspects of asthma. Respir Ther 7:15-18, 86, 88, 1977.

Honsberger R, Wilson AF. Transcendental meditation in treating asthma. Respir Ther 3:79-81, 1973.

Kinsman RA, Dirks JF, Schraa JC. Psychomaintenance in asthma: personal styles affecting medical management. Respir Ther 11:39-46, 1981.

The following abstracts are reprinted with permission of California Medical Association:

Mandell AJ, Younger CB. Asthma alternating with psychiatric symptomatology. Calif Med 96:251-253, 1962. Reprinted by permission of the Western Journal of Medicine.

Obermayer ME. Psychotherapy of functional dermatoses: its value and limitations as applied to neurodermatitis. Calif Med 1:28-30, 1949. Reprinted by permission of the Western Journal of Medicine.

Selesnick ST, Friedman DB, Augenbaum B. Psychological management of asthma. Calif Med 100:406-411, 1964. Reprinted by permission of the Western Journal of Medicine.

Sirmay EA. The role of psychotherapy in allergy: credits and debits. Calif Med 78:456-458, 1953. Reprinted by permission of the Western Journal of Medicine.

The following abstracts are reprinted with permission of the Canadian Medical Association:

August RV. Hypnotic induction of hypothermia: an additional approach to postoperative control of cancer recurrence. Am J Clin Hypn 18:52-55, 1975.

Cormia FE, Slight D. Psychogenic factors in dermatoses. Can Med Assoc J 33: 527-530, 1935.

Cormier BM, Wittkower EO, Marcotte Y, Forget F. Psychological aspects of rheumatoid arthritis. Can Med Assoc J 77:539-541, 1957.

Detweiler HK. The psychogenic factor in asthma. Can Med Assoc J 62:128-130, 1950.

Edgell PG. The psychology of asthma. Can Med Assoc J 67:121-125, 1952.

Henderson AT. Psychogenic factors in bronchial asthma. Can Med Assoc J 55:106-111, 1946.

Munro S, Mount B. Music therapy in palliative care. Can Med Assoc J 119:1029-1034, 1978.

Napke E. Hypnosis in infertility and allergy. Can Med Assoc J 107:496, 1972. (letter)

Robinson EG. Emotional factors and rheumatoid arthritis. Can Med Assoc J 77:344-345, 1957.

Wittkower ED, Hunt BR. Psychological aspects of atopic dermatitis in children. Can Med Assoc J 79:810-816, 1958.

The following abstracts are reprinted with permission of Canadian Nurses Association:

Ferguson RG, Webb A. Childhood asthma: an outpatient approach to treatment. Can Nurse 75:36-39, 1979.

McFadyen C. The respiratory nurse in action. Can Nurse 74:30-31, 1978. (case report)

The following abstract is reprinted with permission of Canadian Psychiatric Association:

Gervais L. Bronchial asthma and identification with the aggressor. Can Psychiatr Assoc J 11:497-500, 1966.

The following abstract is reprinted with permission of Cancer Research, Inc.:

Holland JC, Rowland J, Plumb M. Psychological aspects of anorexia in cancer patients. Cancer Res 37:2425-2428, 1977.

The following abstracts are reprinted with permission of Charles B. Slack, Inc.:

Mackenzie JN. The production of the so-called "rose cold" by means of an artificial rose: with remarks and historical notes. Am J Med Sci 91:45-57, 1886.

Sadler JE Jr. Coordinated pediatric care through a liaison team. Pediatr Ann 1:72-78, 1972.

Schmidt LM. Warts: their diagnosis and treatment. Pediatr Ann 5:782-790, 1976.

Silverman AJ. Psychiatric factors in dermatologic disorders. Am J Med Sci 226:104-110, 1953.

Zahourek RP. Hypnosis in nursing practice—emphasis on the "problem patient" who has pain (I). J Psychosoc Nurs Ment Health Serv 20:13-17, 1982.

Zahourek RP. Hypnosis in nursing practice—emphasis on the "problem patient" who has pain (II). J Psychosoc Nurs Ment Health Serv 20:21-24, 1982.

Zeltzer L, Le Baron S, Barbour J, Kniker WT, Littlefield L. Self-hypnosis for poorly controlled adolescent asthmatics. Clin Res 28:862A, 1980. (abstract)

The following abstracts are reprinted with permission of Chiggott Publishing Company:

Abramson HA, Peshkin MM. Psychosomatic group therapy with parents of children with intractable asthma: sibling rivalry and sibling support. Psychosomatics 6:161-165, 1965.

Brodsky CM. 'Allergic to everything': a medical subculture. Psychosomatics 24:731-742, 1983.

Chang JC. Nausea and vomiting in cancer patients: an expression of psychological mechanisms? Psychosomatics 22:707-709, 1981.

Daniels DK. Treatment of urticaria and severe headache by behavior therapy. Psychosomatics 14:347-351, 1973.

Garfinkel R. Treatment of a psychosomatic ailment in an elderly woman. Psychosomatics 21:1015-1016, 1980.

Jorgenson JA, Brophy JJ. Psychiatric treatment of seriously burned adults. Psychosomatics 14:331-335, 1973.

Katz ER. Conditioned aversion to chemotherapy. Psychosomatics 23:650-651, 1982. (letter)

Keegan DL. Chronic urticaria: clinical psychophysiological and therapeutic aspects. Psychosomatics 17:160-163, 1976.

Khan AU. Present status of psychosomatic aspects of asthma. Psychosomatics 14:195-200, 1973.

Leibenluft E. An atypical eating disorder following cancer chemotherapy. Psychosomatics 26:147-148, 1985.

Lerer B, Jacobowitz J. Treatment of essential hyperhidrosis by psychotherapy. Psychosomatics 22:536-538, 1981.

Poussaint A. Emotional factors in psoriasis: report of a case. Psychosomatics 4:199-202, 1963.

Reckless J. A behavioral treatment of bronchial asthma in modified group therapy. Psychosomatics 12:168-173, 1971.

Reed JW. Emotional factors in bronchial asthma. Psychosomatics 3:57-66, 1962.

Sanger MD. Psychosomatic allergy. Psychosomatics 11:473-476, 1970.

Schwartz LH, Marcus R, Condon R. Multidisciplinary group therapy for rheumatoid arthritis. Psychosomatics 19:289-293, 1978.

Shocket BR, Lisansky ET, Shubard AF, Fiocco V, Kurland S, Pope M. A medical psychiatric study of patients with rheumatoid arthritis. Psychosomatics 10:271-279, 1969.

Simonton OC, Matthews-Simonton S, Sparks TF. Psychological intervention in the treatment of cancer. Psychosomatics 221:226-233, 1980.

Stoudemire A, Techman T, Graham SD. Sexual assessment of the urologic oncology patient. Psychosomatics 26:405-410, 1985.

Udelman HD, Udelman DL. Rheumatology reaction pattern survey. Psychosomatics 19:776-780, 1978.

Wise TN. Effects of cancer on sexual activity. Psychosomatics 19:769-775, 1978.

Yorkston NJ, Eckert E, McHugh RB, Philander DA, Blumenthal MN. Bronchial asthma: improved lung function after behavior modification. Psychosomatics 20:325-327, 330-331, 1979.

The following abstract is reprinted with permission of College of Radiography:

Goss EO. Wart charming. Radiography 22:75-77, 1956.

The following abstract is reprinted with permission of Colorado Medical Society:

Friedman MM. Hypnotherapy in advanced cancer. Rocky Mt Med J 57:33-37, 1960.

The following abstracts are reprinted with permission of The Committee on Medical Education & Publications:

Jonas DL. Psychiatric aspects of hemophilia. Mt Sinai J Med 44:457-463, 1977.

Joseph ED, Peck SM, Kaufman MR. A psychological study of neurodermatitis with a case report. J Mt Sinai Hosp 15:360-366, 1949.

Lorand S. The psychogenic factors in a case of angioneurotic edema. J Mt Sinai Hosp 2:231-236, 1936.

The following abstract is reprinted with permission of Connecticut State Medical Society:

Peshkin MM. The treatment of institutionalized children with intractable asthma. Conn Med 24:766-770, 1960.

The following abstracts are reprinted with permission of Editorial Garsi:

De Vicente P, Posada JL. Medical sophrology and yoga respiration in the physiotherapy of bronchial asthma. Allergol Immunopathol (Madr) 6:297-310, 1978. (in Spanish)

Freour P, De Boucaud M. Psychological aspects of asthma in children: phenomenological approach. Allergol Immunopathol (Madr) Suppl 9:103-107, 1981. (in French: no English abstract)

Ghory JE. Physical rehabilitation of the asthmatic child. Allergol Immunopathol (Madr) Suppl 9:95-98, 1981.

The following abstract is reprinted with permission of Family Process:

Ritterman MK. Hemophilia in context: adjunctive hypnosis for families with a hemophiliac member. Fam Process 21:469-476, 1982.

The following abstracts are reprinted with permission of Family Service Association of America:

Bellak L. Psychiatric aspects of tuberculosis. Soc Casework 31:183-189, 1950.

Nitzberg H. The social worker in an institution for asthmatic children. Soc Casework 33:111-116, 1952.

The following abstract is reprinted with permission of Fr. Tijdschrift voor Geneeskunde ASBL:

Van Moffaert M. Psychiatric consultation in the dermatology clinic. Tijdschr Geneeskd 31:587-595, 1975. (in Dutch)

The following abstract is reprinted with permission of Georg Thieme Verlag:

Menger W. Possibilities of rehabilitation in children with bronchial asthma. Rehabilitation (Stuttg) 11:199-208, 1972. (in German)

The following abstracts are reprinted with permission of Grune and Stratton, Incorporated:

Gorzynski JG, Holland JC. Psychological aspects of testicular cancer. Semin Oncol 6:125-129, 1979.

Kremer WB, Mengel CE, Nowlin JB, Nagaya H. Recurrent ecchymoses and cutaneous hyperreactivity to hemoglobin: a form of autoerythrocyte sensitization. Blood 30:62-73, 1967.

Surwit RS. Biofeedback: a possible treatment for Raynaud's disease. Semin Psychiatry 5:483-490, 1973.

The following abstracts are reprinted with permission of Human Sciences Press:

Allendy R. A case of eczema. Psychoanal Rev 19:152-163, 1932.

Bien E. The clinical psychogenic aspects of pruritus vulvae. Psychoanal Rev 20:186-196, 1933.

Burns KL. Behavioral health care in asthma. Public Health Rev 10:339-381, 1982.

Jabush M. A case of chronic recurring multiple boils treated with hypnotherapy. Psychiatr Q 43:448-455, 1969.

Montgomery L. Psychoanalysis of a case of acne vulgaris. Psychoanal Rev 23:274-285, 1936.

Muhl AM. Fundamental personality trends in tuberculous women. Psychoanal Rev 10:380-430, 1923.

Prout CT. Psychiatric aspects of asthma. Psychiatr Q 25:237-250, 1951.

Purchard PR. Neurodermatitis with a case study. Psychiatr Q 38:518-527,1964.

Richardson HB. Raynaud's phenomenon and scleroderma: a case report and psychodynamic formulation. Psychoanal Rev 42:24-38, 1955.

Sampliner RB. Psychic aspects of bronchial asthma: review and synthesis of the literature. Psychiatr Q 13:521-533, 1939.

Schilder P. Remarks on the psychology of the skin. Psychoanal Rev 23:274-285, 1936.

Thoma H. The lack of specificity in psychosomatic disorders exemplified by a case of neurodermatitis with a twenty year follow up. Psyche (Stuttg) 34:589-624, 1980. (in German)

The following abstracts are reprinted with permission of Jason Aronson, Inc.:

Karol C. The role of primal scene and masochism in asthma. Int J Psychoanal Psychother 8:577-592, 1980.

Wilson CP. Parental overstimulation in asthma. Int J Psychoanal Psychother 8:601-621, 1980.

The following abstracts are reprinted with permission of Johann Ambrosius Barth:

Barinbaum M. A preliminary report on the significance of Freudian psychoanalysis in dermatology. Dermatol Wochenschr 95:1066-1067, 1932. (in German)

Bunneman O, Jadassohn J, Jolowicz E, Memmesheimer AM, Sack WT, Werther J. Successes and limits of psychotherapy in skin diseases. Dermatol Wochenschr 94:20-26, 1932. (in German)

Cernelc D, Skuber P, Kos S. The medical and psychological study of children with asthma—controlled study of allergic and psychological background of asthmatic children. Allerg Asthma (Leipz) 14:33-43, 1968.

Findeisen DG. Kind, value and risks of known relaxation techniques in bronchial asthma. Z Erkr Atmungsorgane 157:345-354, 1981. (in German)

Hodek B, Skretova K, Skreta M. On psychic factors in the development of bronchial asthma. Allerg Asthma (Leipz) 11:178-202, 1965. (in German)

Levendel L, Lakatos M. Application of the biofeedback method in asthmatic patients. Allerg Immunol (Leipz) 27:35-39, 1981. (in German)

Samek J. Suggestive healing of warts. Dermatol Wochenschr 93:1853-1857, 1932. (in German)

The following abstract is reprinted with permission of Journal of Rheumatology Publishing Company, Ltd.:

Yocum DE, Hodes R, Sundstrom WR, Cleeland CS. Use of biofeedback training in treatment of Raynaud's disease and phenomenon. J Rheumatol 12:90-93, 1985.

The following abstract is reprinted with permission of Journal of the Florida Medical Association:

Bloom FL, Spangler DL, McMichael JE, Wittig HJ, Upson P. Sunshine station—Florida's first camp for children with asthma. J Fla Med Assoc 63:710-713, 1976.

The following abstract is reprinted with permission of Journal of the Indiana State Medical Association:

Adair JR, Theobald DE. Raynaud's phenomenon: treatment of a severe case with biofeedback. J Indiana State Med Assoc 71:990-993, 1978.

The following abstract is reprinted with permission of Kanehara Shuppan Co. Ltd.:

Ishikawa H. The psychotherapy of advanced cancer. Rinsho Hoshasen 24:1115-1119, 1979. (in Japanese)

The following abstracts are reprinted with permission of S. Karger AG, Basel:

Capone MA, Westie KS, Good RS. l Sexual rehabilitation of the gynecologic cancer patient: an effective counseling model. Front Radiat Ther Oncol 14:123-129, 1980.

French TM. Emotional conflict and allergy. Int Arch Allergy 1:28-40, 1949.

Gunnarson S. Asthma in children as a psychosomatic disease. Int Arch Allergy Appl Immunol 1:103-108, 1950.

Haydu GG. Integrative psychotherapy in rheumatoid arthritis and allied states. Adv Psychosom Med 3:196-202, 1963.

Kuypers BRM. Atopic dermatitis: some observations from a psychological viewpoint. Dermatologica 136:387-394, 1968.

Leigh D. Asthma and the psychiatrist: a critical review. Int Arch Allergy Appl Immunol 4:227-246, 1953.

Lucas ON. Hypnosis and stress in hemophilia. Bibl Haemotol 34:73-82, 1970.

Miller H, Baruch DW. Some paintings by allergic patients in group psychotherapy and their dynamic implications in the practice of allergy. Int Arch Allergy Appl Immunol 1:60-81, 1950.

Miller H, Baruch DW. The psychosomatic aspects of management of asthmatic children. Int Arh Allergy Appl Immunol 13:102-111, 1958.

Miller ML. Allergy and emotions: a review. Int Arch Allergy Appl Immunol 1:40-49, 1950.

Musaph H. Psychogenic pruritus. Dermatologica 135:126-130, 1967.

Peshkin MM. Intractable asthma of childhood: rehabilitation at the institutional level with a follow-up of 150 cases. Int Arch Allergy 15:91-112, 1959.

Schatia V. The role of emotions in allergic disorders. Int Arch Allergy Appl Immunol 1:93-102, 1950.

Schain WS. Role of the sex therapist in the care of the cancer patient. Front Radiat Ther Oncol 15:168-183, 1980.

Schain WS. Sexual functioning, self-esteem and cancer care. Front Radiat Ther Oncol 14:12-19, 1980.

Sontag LW. A psychiatrist's view of allergy. Int Arch Allergy Appl Immunol 1:50-60, 1950.

Van Moffaert M. Psychosomatics for the practising dermatologist. Dermatologica 15:73-87, 1982.

Wilson AF, Honsberger R, Chiu JR, Novey HS. Transcendental meditation and asthma. Respiration 32:74-80, 1975.

The following abstract is reprinted with permission of Karl Alber GmbH:

Sauer J, Schnetzer M. Personality profile of asthmatics and its changes in the course of various treatment methods. Z Klin Psychol Psychother 26:171-180, 1978. (in German)

The following abstract is reprinted with permission of Laegeforeningens Forlag Esplanaden:

Lange-Nielsen AF, Retterstol N. Group therapy in asthmatic patients in a medical department: preliminary experience. Nord Medicin 61:270-273, 1959. (in Norwegian)

The following abstract is reprinted with permission of Lakartidningen:

Gustafsson P. Psychological and family dynamic aspects of bronchial asthma in children. Lakartidningen 78:1878-1880, 1981. (in Swedish)

The following abstracts are reprinted with permission of Lancet Ltd.:

Bethune HC, Kidd CB. Psychophysiological mechanisms in skin disease. Lancet 2:1419-1422, 1961.

Day G. Observations on the psychology of the tuberculous. Lancet 251:703-706, 1946.

Day G. The psychosomatic approach to pulmonary tuberculosis. Lancet 1:1025-1028, 1951.

MacKenna RMB, Macalpine I. Application of psychology to dermatology. Lancet 1:65-68, 1951.

Mason AA, Black S. Allergic skin responses abolished under treatment of asthma and hayfever by hypnosis. Lancet 1:877-879, 1958.

Meares A. Mind and cancer. Lancet 1:978, 1979. (letter)

Munro DGM. The psycho-pathology of pulmonary tuberculosis, with special reference to treatment. Lancet 201:556-557, 1921.

Robertson G. Emotional aspects of skin disease. Lancet 2:124-127, 1947.

Sergeant HGS. Verbal desensitization in the treatment of bronchial asthma. Lancet 2:1321-1323, 1969.

Sinclair-Gieben AHC, Chalmers D. Evaluation of treatment of warts by hypnosis. Lancet 2:480-482, 1959.

Strauss EB. Psychogenic asthma. Lancet 1:962, 1927.

Wittkower E. Psoriasis. Lancet 1:566-569, 1946.

The following abstract is reprinted with permission of Lawrence Erlbaum Associates, Inc.:

Wisely DW, Masur FT, Morgan SB. Psychological aspects of severe burn injuries in children. Health Psychol 2:45-72, 1983.

The following abstracts are reprinted with permission of Libra Publishers, Inc.:

Piazza EU. Comprehensive therapy of chronic asthma on a psychosomatic unit. Adolescence 16:139-144, 1981.

Rathus SA. Motoric, autonomic, and cognitive reciprocal inhibition of a case of hysterical bronchial asthma. Adolescence 8:29-32, 1973.

The following abstracts are reprinted with permission of J.B. Lippincott Co.:

Butler B. Hypnosis in care of the cancer patient. Cancer 7:1-14, 1954. (also Br J Med Hypn 6: in three parts, 1955)

Cleeland CS. The impact of pain on the patient with cancer. Cancer 54:2635-2641, 1984.

Cobb S, Miles HHW. Psychiatric conference. Am Pract 3:407-411, 1949.

Combrinck-Graham L. Structural family therapy in psychosomatic illness: treatment of anorexia nervosa and asthma. Clin Pediatr (Phila) 13:827-833, 1974.

Fialkov MJU, Miller JA. Severe psychosomatic illness in children: effect on a pediatric ward's staff. Clin Pediatr (Phila) 20:792-796, 1981.

Friedman DB, Silesnick ST. Clinical notes on the management of asthma and eczema: when to call the psychiatrist. Clin Pediatr 4:735-738, 1965.

Fritz GK. Psychological aspects of atopic dermatitis: a viewpoint. Clin Pediatr (Phila) 18:360-364, 1979.

Hurst A, Henkin R, Lustig GJ. Some psychosomatic aspects of respiratory diease. Am Pract 1:486-492, 1950.

Levy SM, Morrow GR. Biobehavioral interventions in behavioral medicine. Cancer 50:1936-1938, 1982.

Renshaw DC. Sex and the dermatologist. Int J Dermatol 19:469-471, 1980.

Richards W, Church JA, Roberts MJ, Newman LJ, Garon MR. A self-help program for childhood asthma in a residential treatment center. Clin Pediatr (Phila) 20:453-457, 1981.

Rotman M, Rogow L, DeLeon G, Heskel N. Supportive therapy in radiation oncology. Cancer 39:744-750, 1977.

The following abstracts are reprinted with permission of Macmillan Journal Ltd.:

Edwards H. Alternative medicine: the science of spiritual healing. Nurs Times 71:2008-2010, 1975.

Houghton HE. Hypnotherapy in asthma. Nurs Times 61:482-483, 1965.

Lincoln PJ. Serological investigation of a faith healer's patient. Nurs Times 71:2011-2012, 1975.

Rowden L. Relaxation and visualisation techniques in patients with breast cancer. Nurs Times 80:42-44, 1984.

The following abstracts are reprinted with permission of MacMillan Press Ltd.:

Bar LHJ, Kuypers BRM. Behaviour therapy in dermatological practice. Br J Drmatol 88:591–598, 1973.

Bonjour J. Influence of the mind on the skin. Br J Dermatol Syph 41:324–326, 1929.

Calnan CD, O'Neill D. Itching in tension states. Br J Dermatol 64:274–280, 1952.

Cohen SI. Psychological factors in asthma. Postgrad Med J. 47:533–540, 1971.

Cormia FE. Basic concepts in the production and management of the psychosomatic dermatoses. Br J Dermatol 63:83–92, 129–151, 1951.

Duller P, Gentry WD. Use of biofeedback in treating chronic hyperhidrosis: a preliminary report. Br J Dermatol 103:143–146, 1980.

Hellier FF. The treatment of warts with x-rays: is their action physical or psychological? Br J Dermatol 63:193–194, 1951.

Jelliffe AM, Soutter C, Meara RH. An investigation into the treatment of acne vulgaris with Grenz x-rays. Br J Dermatol 81:617–620, 1969.

Kidd C. Congenital ichthyosiform erythroderma treated by hypnosis. Br J Dermatol 78:101–105, 1966.

Macalpine I. Is alopecia areata psychosomatic? A psychiatric study. Br J Dermatol 70:117–131, 1958.

Macalpine I. Psychiatric observations of facial dermatosis. Br J Dermatol Syph 65:177–182, 1953.

Miller RM, Coger RW. Skin conductance conditioning with dyshidrotic eczema patients. Br J Dermatol 101:435–440, 1979.

Robertson IM, Jordan JM, Whitlock FA. Emotions and skin (II): The conditioning of scratch responses in cases of lichen simplex. Br J Dermatol 92:407–412, 1975.

Rogerson CH. Role of psychotherapy in the treatment of asthma-eczema-prurigo complex in children. Br J Dermatol 4:368–378, 1934.

Sack WT. On the psychic and nervous components of the so-called allergic skin diseases and their treatment. Br J Dermatol Syph 40:441–445, 1928.

Waxman D. Behaviour therapy of psoriasis. Postgrad Med J 49:591–595, 1973.

Wittkower E, MacKenna RMB. The psychological aspects of seborrhoeic dermatitis. Br J Dermatol Syph 59:281–293, 1947.

Woodhead B. The eczema-asthma syndrome: psychiatric considerations. Br J Dermatol 67:50–52, 1955.

The following abstracts are reprinted with permission of Marcel Dekker Inc.:

Abramson HA. Reassociation of dreams (III): LSD analysis of a threatening male-female dog dream and its relation to fear of lesbianism. J Asthma Res 14:131–158, 1977.

Abramson HA. The father-son relationship in eczema and asthma (II). J Asthma Res 1:173–206, 1963.

Abramson HA. The father-son relationship in eczema and asthma (III). J Asthma Res 1:317–349, 1964.

Abramson HA. The father-son relationship in eczema and asthma (IV). J Asthma Res 2:65–94, 1964.

Abramson HA. The father-son relationship in eczema and asthma (V). J Asthma Res 2:147–174, 1964.

Abramson HA. The father-son relationship in eczema and asthma (VI). J Asthma Res 5:29–81, 1967.

Ago Y, Ikemi Y, Sugita M, Takahashi N, Toyama N. Treatment of bronchial asthma. J Asthma Res 14:33–35, 1976.

Bentley J. A psychotherapeutic approach to treating asthmatic children in a residential setting. J Asthma Res 12:21–25, 1974.

Bentley J, Wilmerding JW. Individual psychotherapy with asthmatic children as an adjunct to milieu therapy: two case studies. J Asthma Res 15:163–169, 1978.

Bien RF. Remission of intractable asthma in a child during psychotherapy of the mother. J Asthma Res 7:47–51, 1969.

Brown EA. The treatment of bronchial asthma by means of hypnosis: as viewed by the allergist. J. Asthma Res 3:101–119, 1965.

Chong TM. The management of bronchial asthma. J Asthma Res 14:73–89, 1977.

Ghory JE. The short-term patient in a convalescent hospital asthma program. J Asthma Res 3:243–247, 1966.

Goyeche JR, Ago Y, Ikemi Y. Asthma: the yoga perspective (I): The somatopsychic imbalance in asthma: towards a holistic therapy. J Asthma Res 17:111–121, 1980.

Green M, Green E. A tour of four residential centers for the care of asthmatic children in Europe. J Asthma Res 3:299–304, 1966.

Hindi-Alexander M. The team approach in asthma. J Asthma Res 12:79–85, 1974.

Kapotes C. Emotional factors in chronic asthma. J. Asthma Res 15:5–14, 1977.

Kobayashi M. Psychotherapy for tuberculosis patients. Shinryo Shitsu 6:459–465, 1954.

Lubens HM. A psychotherapeutic technique for allergic patients. J Asthma Res 1:167–171, 1963.

Lubens HM. Self analysis: a practical method of psychotherapy for allergic patients. J. Asthma Res 9:87–97, 1971.

Mascia AV. Progress in the treatment of the asthmatic child in a convalescent setting. J Asthma Res 3:239–241, 1966.

Mascia AV. The goals and philosophy of a residential treatment center for asthmatic children. J Asthma Res 8:43–50, 1970.

Mascia AV, Reitner SR. Group therapy in the rehabilitation of the severe chronic asthmatic child. J Asthma Res 9:81–85, 1971.

Peshkin MM. Analysis of the role of residential centers for children with intractable asthma. J Asthma Res 6:59–92, 1968.

Peshkin MM. The emotional aspects of asthma in children. J Asthma Res 3:265–177, 1966.

Peshkin MM. The role of emotions in children with intractable bronchial asthma. J. Asthma Res 2:143–146, 1964.

Peshkin MM, Friedman I. Residential asthma centers in the United States and problems in relation to them. J Asthma Res 12:129–175, 1975.

Sandler, N. Working with families of chronic asthmatics. J Asthma Res 15:15–21, 1977.

Vaugh VC. Emotional undertones in eczema in children. J Asthma Res 3:193–197, 1966.

Wohl, TH. Behavior modification: its application to the study and treatment of childhood asthma. J Asthma Res 9:41–45, 1971.

Wohl TH. Current concepts of the asthmatic child's adjustment and adaptation to institutional care. J Asthma Res 7:41–45, 1969.

Wohl TH. The group approach to the asthmatic child and family. J Asthma Res 4:237–239, 1967.

Zelesnik C. Some implications of concepts of multi-causality in the etiology and treatment of chronic intractable bronchial asthma. J Asthma Res 5:123–128, 1967.

Zivitz N. Evaluation of intractable asthma of children in a new residential treatment center. J Asthma Res 3:291–297, 1966.

The following abstracts are reprinted with permission of
Massachusetts Medical Society:

Cousins N. Anatomy of an illness (as perceived by the patient). N
Engl J Med 295:1458-1463, 1976.

Kutz I, Borysenko JZ, Come SE, Benson H. Paradoxical emetic
response to antiemetic treatment in cancer patients. N Engl J Med
303:148, 1980. (letter)

Morrow GR, Morrell C. Behavioral treatment for the anticipatory
nausea and vomiting induced by cancer chemotherapy. N Engl J Med
307:1476-1480, 1982.

Nissen HA. Chronic arthritis and its treatment. N Engl J Med
210:1109-1115, 1934.

Nissen HA, Spencer KA. The psychogenic problem in chronic
arthritis. N Engl J Med 214:576-587, 1936.

The following abstract is reprinted with permission of The
Mayo Clinic:

Walsh MN, Kierland RR. Psychotherapy in the treatment of
neurodermatitis. Proc Staff Meet Mayo Clin 22:578-584, 1947.

The following abstracts are reprinted with permission of
McGraw-Hill Publications Co.:

Redd WH. Control of nausea and vomiting in chemotherapy patients:
four effective behavioral methods. Postgrad Med 75(5):105-107, 110-
113, 1984.

Waisman M. Atopic dermatitis: clinical aspects and treatment.
Postgrad Med 52(5):180-184, 1972.

The following abstract is reprinted with permission of
Medical Society of Delaware:

Weinstein AG. Crying-induced bronchospasm in childhood asthma:
combined pharmacologic and behavioral management. Del Med J
56:473-476, 1984.

The following abstracts are reprinted with permission of
Medical Society of the State of New York:

Abramowitz EW. The use of placebos in the local therapy of skin
diseases. NY State J Med 48:1927-1930, 1948.

Lewis GM, Cormia FE. Office management of the neurodermatoses.
NY State J Med 47:1889-1894, 1947.

Luparello TJ, McFadden ER, Lyons HA, Bleecker ER. Psychologic
factors and bronchial asthma. NY State J Med 71:2161-2165, 1971.

Oberndorf CP. The psychogenic factors in asthma. NY State J Med
35:41-48, 1935.

Sharlit H. The impact of psychiatry on therapy in dermatology. NY
State J Med 50:1926-1928, 1950.

Weissberg G. Practical aspects of psychosomatic dermatology. NY
State J Med 61:2420-2427, 1961.

The following abstract is reprinted with permission of MMW
Medizin Verlag GMBH:

Bosse K, Hunecke P. The pruritus of endogenous eczema patients.
MMW 123:1013–1016, 1981.

The following abstracts are reprinted with permission of
Modern Medicine Publications, Inc.:

Reed JW. Group therapy with asthma patients. Geriatrics 17:823-830,
1962.

Walsh MN, Kierland RR. Minor psychotherapy in dermatology. Mod
Med 123:123-125, 1950.

The following abstracts are reprinted with permission of
Morgan Grampian Ltd.:

Dreaper R. Recalcitrant warts on the hand cured by hypnosis.
Practitioner 220:305-310, 1978.

McGregor HG. The psychological factor in rheumatic disease.
Practitioner 143:627-636, 1939.

Meares A. Meditation: a psychological approach to cancer treatment.
Practitioner 222:119-122, 1979.

Meares A. Stress, meditation and the regression of cancer.
Practitioner 226:1607-1609, 1982.

Morwood JMB. Relaxation by gramophone in asthma. Practitioner
170:400-402, 1953.

O'Neill D. Asthma as a stress reaction: its diagnosis and treatment.
Practitioner 169:273-280, 1952.

Rogerson CH. Psychological factors in skin diseases. Practitioner
142:17-35, 1939.

Staukler L. A critical assessment of the cure of warts by suggestion.
Practitioner 198:690-694, 1967.

The following abstracts are reprinted with permission of C. V.
Mosby Co.:

Eyermann C. Emotional component of bronchial asthma. J Allergy
9:565-571, 1938.

French AP. Treatment of warts by hypnosis. Am J Obstet Gynecol
116:887-888, 1973. (letter)

Gould WM, Gragg TM. A dermatology-psychiatry liaison clinic. J Am
Acad Dermatol 9:73-77, 1983.

Graham DT. Psychology, behavior, and the treatment of asthma. J
Allergy Clin Immunol 60:273-275, 1977. (editorial)

Hochstadt NJ, Shepard J, Lulla SH. Reducing hospitalizations of
children with asthma. J Pediatr 97:1012-1015, 1980.

Janson-Bjerklie S, Clarke E. The effects of biofeedback training on
bronchial diameter in asthma. Heart Lung 11:200-207, 1982.

Klapper M. Condylomata acuminata and hypnosis. J Am Acad
Dermatol 10:836-839, 1984. (letter)

Levine MI, Geer JH, Kost PF. Hypnotic suggestion and the histamine
wheal. J Allergy Clin Immunol 37:246-250, 1966.

Miklich DR, Renne CM, Creer TL, Alexander AB, Chai H, Davis MH,
Hoffman A, Danker-Brown P. The clinical utility of behavior therapy
as an adjunctive treatment for asthma. J Allergy Clin Immunol 5:285-
294, 1977.

Rapini RP. Treatment of venereal warts using hypnosis. J Am Acad
Dermatol 10:837, 1984. (letter)

Schulte MB, Cormane RH, Van Dijk E, Wuite J. Group therapy of
psoriasis: duo formula group treatment (DFGT) as an example (I). J
Am Acad Dermatol 12:61-66, 1985.

Straatmeyer AJ, Rhodes NR. Condylomata acuminata: results of treatment using hypnosis. J Am Acad Dermatol 9:434-436, 1983.

Wittkower E. Psyche and allergy. J Allergy 23:76-86, 1952.

Zeltzer L, LeBaron S. Hypnosis and nonhypnotic techniques for reduction of pain and anxiety during painful procedures in children and adolescents with cancer. J Pediatr 101:1032-1035, 1982.

The following abstract is reprinted with permission of National Easter Seal Society:

Creer TL, Renne CM, Christian WP. Behavior contributions to rehabilitation and childhood asthma. Rehab Lit 37:226-232, 1976.

The following abstracts are reprinted with permission of Ned. Tijdschr. Geneesk. (Dutch Medical Journal):

Arndt JL, Polano MK. The psychotherapeutic treatment of a case of pruritus vulvae. Ned Tijdschr Geneeskd 3:2675–2678, 1950.

Fleischer D. Psychotherapy of disorder of the skin, probably lupus erythermatosus. Ned Tijdschr Geneeskd 85:566–567, 1941.

Kuijpers BR. Constitutional eczema: clinico-psychological findings. Ned Tijdschr Geneesk 112:976–981, 1968.

Kuypersen BR, Bar LH. The psychologist in the dermatological clinic: methods and possibilities of treatment. Ned Tijdschr Geneeskd 116:1268–1271, 1972.

Mook J, Van der Ploeg HM. Behavior therapy in bronchial asthma: systematic desensitization applied to 3 patients. Ned Tijdschr Geneeskd 120:1065–1069, 1976.

Musaph H. Behavior therapy in psychodermatology. Ned Tijdschr Geneeskd 116:1769–1771, 1972.

Musaph H. Psychiatric study of chronic urticaria patients. Ned Tijdschr Geneeskd 100:3169–3174, 1956.

Stokvis B, Welman AJ. Group therapy and sociotherapy as adjuvants in treating asthma. Ned Tijdschr Geneeskd 99:693–703, 1955.

Van der Hal I. Treatment of asthma by imitation of asthmatic breathing. Ned Tijdschr Geneeskd 100:767–769, 1966.

Van der Ploeg HM, Mook J. Behavior therapy in bronchial asthma. Ned Tijdschr Geneeskd 120:1083–1087, 1967.

The following abstracts are reprinted with permission of New York Academy of Medicine:

Abramson HA. Therapy of asthma with reference to its psychodynamic pharmacology. Bull NY Acad Med 25:345-363, 1949.

Sperling M. Psychologic desensitization of allergy. Bull NY Acad Med 44:587-591, 1968.

Weiss E. Psychosomatic aspects of allergic disorders. Bull NY Acad Med 23:604-630, 1947.

The following abstracts are reprinted with permission of New York Academy of Sciences:

Bowers KS. Hypnosis: an informational approach. Ann NY Acad Sci 296:222-237, 1977.

Feder SL. Psychological considerations in the care of patients with cancer. Ann NY Acad Sci 125:1020-1027, 1966.

Lucas ON. The use of hypnosis in hemophilia dental care. Ann NY Acad Sci 240:263-266, 1975.

Lucas ON, Tocantins LM. Problems in hemostasis in hemophilic patients undergoing dental extractions. Ann NY Acad Sci 115:470-480, 1964.

Sacerdote P. The use of hypnosis in cancer patients. Ann NY Acad Sci 125:1011-1019, 1966.

The following abstracts are reprinted with permission of Oncology Nursing Society:

Burish TG, Carey MP, Redd WH, Krozely MG. Behavioral relaxation techniques in reducing the distress of cancer chemotherapy patients. Oncol Nurs Forum 10:32-35, 1983.

Howard RJ, Miller NJ. Unproven methods of cancer management (II): Current trends and implications for patient care. Oncol Nurs Forum 11:67-73, 1984.

Kaempfer SH. Relaxation training reconsidered. Oncol Nurs Forum 9:15-18, 1982.

The following abstract is reprinted with permission of Oxford University Press:

Rogerson CH. The psychological factors in asthma-prurigo. Q J Med 6:367-394, 1937.

The following abstracts are reprinted with permission of Panstnowy Zaklad Wydawnictw Lekarskich:

Burns KL. Behavioral health care in asthma. Public Health Rev 10:339-381, 1982.

Czubalski K. Psychotherapy and psychopharmacotherapy in the treatment of chronic urticaria. Psychiatr Pol 5:65-68, 1971. (in Polish)

The following abstracts are reprinted with permission of Pergamon Press:

Alexander AB. Systematic relaxation and flow rates in asthmatic children: relationship to emotional precipitants and anxiety. J Psychosom Res 16:405-410, 1972.

Allen KE, Harris FR. Elimination of a child's excessive scratching by training the mother in reinforcement procedures. Behav Res Ther 4:79-84, 1966.

Barendregt JT. A psychological investigation of the effect of group psychotherapy in patients with bronchial asthma. J Psychosom Res 2:115-119, 1957.

Bradley LA, Young LD, Anderson KO, McDaniel LK, Turner RA, Agudelo CA. Psychological approaches to the management of arthritis pain. Soc Sci Med 19:1353-1360, 1984.

Cooper AJ. A case of bronchial asthma treated by behavior therapy. Behav Res Ther 1:351-356, 1964.

Creer TL. The use of a time-out from positive reinforcement procedure with asthmatic children. J Psychosom Res 14:117-120, 1970.

Danker PS, Miklich DR, Pratt C, Creer TL. An unsuccessful attempt to instrumentally condition peak expiratory flow rates in asthmatic children. J Psychosom Res 19:209-213, 1975.

Dekker E, Pelser HE, Groen J. Conditioning as a cause of asthmatic attacks: a laboratory study. J Psychosom Res 2:97-108, 1957.

Erskine J, Schonell M. Relaxation therapy in bronchial asthma. J Psychosom Res 23:131-139, 1979.

Franks CM, Leigh D. The theoretical and experimental application of a conditioning model to a consideration of bronchial asthma in man. J Psychosom Res 4:88-98, 1959.

Gibbs DN. Reciprocal inhibition therapy of a case of symptomatic erythema. Behav Res Ther 2:261-266, 1965.

Groen JJ, Pelser HE. Experiences with, and results of group psychotherapy in patients with bronchial asthma. J Psychosom Res 4:191-205, 1960.

Godfrey S, Silverman S. Demonstration of placebo response in asthma by means of exercise testing. J Psychosom Res 16:293-297, 1973.

Kelly E, Zeller B. Asthma and the psychiatrist. J Psychosom Res 13:377-395, 1969.

Khan AU. Effectiveness of biofeedback and counterconditioning in the treatment of bronchial asthma. J Psychosom Res 21:97-104, 1977.

Kotses H, Glaus KD, Bricel SK, Edwards JE, Crawford PL. Operant muscular relaxation and peak expiratory flow rate in asthmatic children. J Psychosom Res 22:17-23, 1978.

Kotses H, Glaus KD, Crawford PL, Edwards JE, Scherr MS. Operant reduction of frontalis EMG-activity in the treatment of asthma in children. J Psychosom Res 20:453-459, 1976.

Lukeman D. Conditioning methods of treating childhood asthma. J Child Psychol Psychiatry 16:165-168, 1975.

Morgenstern H, Gellert GA, Walter SD, Ostfeld AM, Siegel BS. The impact of a psychosocial support program on survival with breast cancer: the importance of selection bias in program evaluation. J Chronic Dis 37:273-282, 1984. (Also Advancews 1(4):65-66, 1984)

Moore N. Behaviour therapy in bronchia asthma: a controlled study. J Psychosom Res 9:257-276, 1965.

Phillip RL, Wilde GJS, Day JH. Suggestion and relaxation in asthmatics. J Psychosom Res 16:193-204, 1972.

Pinkerton P. Correlating physiologic with psychodynamic data in the study and management of childhood asthma. J Psychosom Res 11:11-25, 1967.

Rakos RF, Grodek MV, Mack KK. The impact of a self-administered behavioral intervention program on pediatric asthma. J Psychosom Res 29:101-108, 1985.

Ratliff RG, Stein NH. Treatment of neurodermatitis by behavior therapy: a case study. Behav Res Ther 6:397-399, 1968.

Sclare AB, Crocket JA. Group psychotherapy in bronchial asthma. J Psychosom Res 2:157-171, 1957.

Sirota AD, Mahoney M. Relaxing on cue: the self-regulation of asthma. J Behav Ther Exp Psychiatry 5:65-66, 1974.

Straker N, Tamerin J. Aggression and childhood asthma: a study in a natural setting. J Psychosom Res 18:131-135, 1974.

Strupp HH, Levenson RW, Manuch SB. Effects of suggestion on total respiratory resistance in mild asthmatics. J Psychosom Res 18:337-346.

Watson DL, Tharp RG, Krisberg J. Case study in self-modification suppression of inflammatory scratching while awake and asleep. J Behav Ther Exp Psychiatry 3:213-215, 1972.

White HC. Hypnosis in bronchial asthma. J Psychosom Res 5:272-279, 1961.

Yorkston NJ, McHugh RB, Brady R, Serber M, Sergeant HGS. Verbal desensitization in bronchial asthma. J Psychosom Res 18:371-376, 1974.

The following abstracts are reprinted with permission of Physicians Postgraduate Press:

Norris A, Huston P. Raynaud's disease studies by hypnosis. Dis Nerv Syst 17:163-165, 1956.

Scarborough LF. Neurodermatitis from a psychosomatic viewpoint. Dis Nerv Syst 9:90-93, 1948.

Schneck JM. Ichthyosis treated with hypnosis. Dis Nerv Syst 15:211-214, 1954.

The following abstract is reproduced with kind permission from PJD Publications Limited, Westbury, N.Y. 11590, U.S.A.:

Ament P. Concepts in the use of hypnosis for pain relief in cancer. J Med 13:233-240, 1982. Copyright 19 by PJD Publications Ltd.

The following abstracts are reprinted with permission of Plenum Press:

Bird EI, Colbourne GR. Rehabilitation of an electrical burn patient through thermal biofeedback. Biofeedback Self Regul 5:283-287, 1980.

Burish TG, Lyles JN. Effectiveness of relaxation training in reducing adverse reactions to cancer chemotherapy. J Behav Med 4:65-78, 1981.

Burish TG, Shartner CD, Lyles JN. Effectiveness of multiple muscle-site EMG biofeedback and relaxation training in reducing the aversiveness of cancer chemotherapy. Biofeedback Self Regul 6:523-535, 1981.

Freedman RR, Ianni P, Wenig P. Behavioral treatment of Raynaud's phenomenon in scleroderma. J Behav Med 7:343-353, 1984.

Freedman RR, Lynn SJ, Ianni P, Hale PA. Biofeedback of Raynaud's disease and phenomenon. Biofeedback Self Regul 6:355-365, 1981.

Haynes SN, Wilson CC, Jaffe PG, Britton BT. Biofeedback treatment of atopic dermatitis: controlled case studies of eight cases. Biofeedback Self Regul 4:195-209, 1979.

Hock RA, Bramble J, Kennard DW. A comparison between relaxation and assertive training with asthmatic male children. Biol Psychiatry 12:593-596, 1977.

King NJ. The behavioral management of asthma and asthma-related problems in children: a critical review of the literature. J Behav Med 3:169-189, 1980.

Kotses H, Glaus KD. Applications of biofeedback to the treatment of asthma: a critical review. Biofeedback Self Regul 6:573-593, 1981.

Surwit RS, Allen LM III, Gilgor RS, Duvic M. The combined effect of prazosin and autogenic training on cold reactivity in Raynaud's phenomenon. Biofeedback Self Regul 7:537-544, 1978.

Taub E, Stroebel CF. Biofeedback in the treatment of vasoconstrictive syndromes. Biofeedback Self Regul 3:363-373, 1978.

Thomas JE, Koshy M, Patterson L, Dorn L, Thomas K. Management of pain in sickle cell disease using biofeedback therapy: a preliminary study. Biofeedback Self Regul 9:413-420, 1984.

Walker LJS, Healy M. Psychological treatment of a burned child. J Pediatr Psychol 5:395-404, 1980.

Wernick RL, Jaremko ME, Taylor PW. Pain management in severely burned adults: a test of stress innoculation. J Behav Med 4:103-109, 1981.

The following abstract is reprinted with permission of
Psychiatria Fennica:

Baltrusch HJF, Stangel W. Psychosomatic aspects of polycythaemia vera. Psychiatr Fenn (Helsinki) Suppl: 133-142, 1981.

The following abstracts are reprinted with permission of W.B. Saunders:

Bakwin RM. Essentials of psychosomatics in allergic children. Pediatr Clin North Am 1:921-928, 1954.

Bukantz SC, Peshkin MM. Institutional treatment of asthmatic children. Pediatr Clin North Am 6:755-773, 1959.

Creak M, Stephen JM. The psychological aspects of asthma in children. Pediatr Clin North Am 5:731-747, 1958.

Falliers CJ. Psychosomatic study and treatment of asthmatic children. Pediatr Clin North Am 16:271-286, 1969.

Landau LI. Outpatient evaluation and management of asthma. Pediatr Clin North Am 26:581-601, 1979.

Ludwig AO. Psychiatric considerations in rheumatoid arthritis. Med Clin North Am 39:447-458, 1955.

Mattsson A. Psychologic aspects of childhood asthma. Pediatr Clin North Am 22:77-88, 1975.

Obermayer ME. Treatment of pruritis. Med Clin North Am 26:113-122, 1942.

Sadler JE Jr. Childhood asthma from the point of view of the liaison child psychiatrist. Psychiatr Clin North Am 5:333-343, 1982.

Sadler JE Jr. The long-term hospitalization of asthmatic children. Pediatr Clin North Am 22:173-183, 1975.

Walsh MN, Kierland RR. Correlation of the dermatologic and psychiatric approaches to the treatment of neurodermatitis. Med Clin N Am 34:1009-1017, 1950.

The following abstracts are reprinted with permission of Schwabe und Co. AG:

Bonjour J. The cure of warts by suggestion. Schweiz Med Wochenschr 57:980-981, 1927. (in French: no English abstract)

Bonjour J. Warts: their etiology demonstrated by cure through suggestion. Schweiz Med Wochenschr 54:748-751, 1924. (in French: no English abstract)

Courteheuse C. Educating the asthmatic patient. Schweiz Med Wochenschr 114:1336-1339, 1984. (in German)

The following abstract is reprinted with permission of Science:

Holden C. Pain control with hypnosis. Science 198:808, 1977.

The following abstract is reprinted with permission of Societe Francaise d'Investissemente:

Zamotaev IP, Rozhnov VE, Sultanova A. Role of psychotherapy in the treatment of bronchial asthma taking into account the "internal picture of the disease." Ter Arkh 55:34-37, 1983. (in Russian)

The following abstract is reprinted with permission of Society for Psychophysiological Research:

Freedman R, Ianni P, Hale P, Lynn S. Treatment of Raynaud's phenomenon with biofeedback and cold sensitization. Psychophysiology 16:182, 1979. (abstract)

The following abstracts are reprinted with permission of Southern Medical Association:

Michael JC. Emotional stress and allergic cutaneous manifestations. South Med J 22:282-283, 1929.

Wright CS. Psychosomatic factors in dermatology. South Med J 42:951-958, 1949.

The following abstract is reprinted with permission of State Medical Society of Wisconsin:

Squier TL. Emotional factors in allergic states. Wis Med J 40:793-796, 1941.

The following abstracts are reprinted with permission of Texas Medical Association:

Davis HK. Psychiatry, immunology, and cancer. Tex Med 81(2):49-52, 1985.

LeBaron S, Zeltzer L. The treatment of asthma with behavioral intervention: does it work? Tex Med 79(7):40-42, 1983.

The following abstract is reprinted with permission of Transpersonal Institute:

Simonton OC, Simonton SS. Belief systems and management of the emotional aspects of cancer. J Transpersonal Psychol 7:29-47, 1975.

The following abstract is reprinted with permission of The Ulster Medical Journal:

Knox SJ. Psychiatric aspects of bronchial asthma: a critical review and case reports. Ulster Med J 29:144-157, 1960.

The following abstracts are reprinted with permission of University Microfilms International, publishers of "Dissertation Abstracts International" (copyright 1985 by University Microfilms International), and may not be reproduced without their prior permission:

Brown BW. Treatment of acne vulgaris by biofeedback-assisted cue-controlled relaxation and guided cognitive imagery. Diss Abstr Int 42:1163, 1981.

Devine JE. Relaxation and parent training in the treatment of bronchial asthma: a clinical study. Diss Abstr Int 40:1887, 1979.

McElroy SR. Psychoanalgesic remediation of sickle cell anemia painful crisis. Diss Abstr Int 41:1118, 1980.

McGraw PC. Rheumatoid arthritis: a psychological intervention. Diss Abstr Int 40:1377, 1979.

Meyer J. Systematic desensitization versus relaxation training and no treatment (controls) for the reduction of nausea, vomiting and anxiety resulting from chemotherapy. Diss Abstr Int 44:1247-1248, 1983.

Orme GC. Hypnosis, pain control and personality change in rheumatoid arthritic patients. Diss Abstr Int 41:3192, 1981.

Randich SR. Evaluation of stress inoculation training as a pain management program for rheumatoid arthritis. Diss Abstr Int 43:1625, 1982.

Shertzer CL. Hypnosis in the treatment of urticaria. Diss Abstr Int 42:3003, 1982.

The following abstract is reprinted with permission of University of Chicago Press:

Ellerbroek WC. Hypotheses toward a unified field theory of human behavior with clinical application to acne vulgaris. Perspect Biol Med 16:240-262, 1973.

Immune System

The following abstract is reprinted with permission of Verlag Klett-Cotta:

Thomae H. The lack of specificity in psychosomatic disorders exemplified by a case of neurodermatitis with a twenty year follow up. Psyche (Stuttg) 34:589-624, 1980. (in German)

The following abstract is reprinted with permission of W. Virginia State Medical Assoc.:

Mitchell JH, Curran CA. A method of approach to psychosomatic problems in allergy. W Va J Med 42:271-279, 1946.

The following abstracts are reprinted with permission of Williams & Wilkins Co.:

Bernstein ET. The emotional factor in skin diseases. J Nerv Ment Dis 89:1-13, 1938.

Booth GC. Personality and chronic arthritis. J Nerv Ment Dis 85:637-662, 1937.

Clarke GHV. The charming of warts. J Invest Dermatol 45:15-21, 1965.

Dudek SZ. Suggestion and play therapy in the cure of warts in children: a pilot study. J Nerv Ment Dis 145:37-42, 1967.

Finer BL, Nylen BO. Cardiac arrest in the treatment of burns, and report on hypnosis as a substitute for anesthesia. Plast Reconstr Surg 27:49-55, 1961.

Gauthier Y, Fortin C, Drapeau P, Breton JJ, Gosselin J, Quintal L, Weisnagel J, Lamarre A. Follow-up study of 35 asthmatic preschool children. J Am Acad Child Psychiatry 17:679-694, 1978.

Gauthier Y, Fortin C, Drapeau P, Breton JJ, Gosselin J, Quintal L, Weisnagel J, Tetreault L, Pinard G. The mother-child relationship and the development of autonomy and self-assertion in young (14-30 months) asthmatic children: correlating allergic and psychological factors. J Am Acad Child Psychiatry 16:109-131, 1977.

Kelman H, Field H. Psychosomatic relationships in pruriginous lesions. J Nerv Ment Dis 88:627-643, 1938.

Klauder JV. Psychogenic aspects of skin diseases. J Nerv Ment Dis 85:249-273, 1936.

McLean JA, Ching AYT. Follow-up study of relationships between family situation and bronchial asthma in children. J Am Acad Child Psychiatry 12:142-161, 1973.

Metzger FC. Allergy and psychoneurosis. J Nerv Ment Dis 109:240-245, 1949.

Minuchin S, Fishman HC. The psychosomatic family in child psychiatry. J Am Acad Child Psychiatry 18:76-90, 1979.

Mohr GJ, Tausend H, Selesnick S, Augenbraun B. Studies of eczema and asthma in the preschool child. J Am Acad Child Psychiatry 2:271-291, 1963.

Pennisi VR. On behavior modification therapy in the recalcitrant burned child. Plast Reconstr Surg 58:216, 1976. (letter)

Schneider E. Psychodynamics of chronic allergic eczema and chronic urticaria. J Nerv Ment Dis 120:17-21, 1954.

Schneider E, Kesten B. Polymorphic prurigo: a psychosomatic study of three cases. J Invest Dermatol 10:205-214, 1948.

Seitz PFD. An experimental approach to psychocutaneous problems. J Invest Dermatol 13:199-205, 1949.

Sperling M. Asthma in children: an evaluation of concepts and therapies. J Am Acad Child Psychiatry 4:44-58, 1968.

Stamm J, Drapkin A. The successful treatment of a severe case of bronchial asthma: a manifestation of an abnormal mourning reaction and traumatic neurosis. J Nerv Ment Dis 142:180-189, 1966.

Straker N, Bieber J. Asthma and the vicissitudes of aggression: two case reports of childhood asthma. J Am Acad Child Psychiatry 16:132-139, 1977.

Treuting TF, Ripley HS. Life situations, emotions and bronchial asthma. J Nerv Ment Dis 108:380-398, 1948.

Yalom ID. Plantar warts: a case study. J Nerv Ment Dis 138:163-171, 1964.

The following abstract is reprinted with permission of Yale University Press:

Jessner L, Lamont J, Long R, Rollins N, Whipple B, Prentice N. Emotional impact of nearness and separation for the asthmatic child and his mother. Psychoanal Study Child 10:353-375, 1955.

The following abstract is reprinted with permission of Yen Folia Publishing Society:

Kaneko Z, Takaishi N. Psychosomatic studies on chronic urticaria. Folia Psychiatr Neurol Jpn 17:16-24, 1963.

The following abstracts are reprinted with permission of Zeitschrift Hautkrankheiten HG:

Breitbart EW. Modern treatment of warts. Z Hautkr 57:27-37, 1982. (in German)

Leuteritz G, Shimshoni R. Psychotherapy in psoriasis—results at the Dead Sea. Z Hautkr 57:1612-1615, 1982. (in German)

Author Index

Crawford PL 44,371, 372,384
Creak M 222
Crede R 827
Creer TL 3-6,17,34, 35,43,167,352,591- 594
Creighton J 1472
Crocket JA 81
Crodel HW 676
Cropp GJ 141
Crouzatier A 725
Crue BL 1435
Cunningham AJ 1230,1436
Curran CA 463
Curtis GC 1343
Cushing RT 345
Cutler M 1274
Cutler R 1274
Czirr R 506
Czubalski K 414,424, 896

D'Auteuil 678
Dahinterova J 7890
Dahlem NW 370
Dahmbe B 382
Daman HR (eds 673
Damme S 193
Daniels DK 415
Danker P 43
Danker PS 6
Danker-Brown P 17
Darlas F 145
Darquey J 353
Dash J 124,713, 1213,1307,1365, 1381,1437
Davidson S 322
Davies JHT 1144
Davis HK 1231
Davis MH 17,35,594
Davis R 1120
Day G 726,727
Day JH 380
De Boucaud M 235, 353
De Clement F 795
De Freitas O Jr 728
De Piano FA 1185
De River JP 488
De Vicente P 354
De la Parra R 98
DeLeon G 1356
DePetrillo AD 1411
Deenstra H 355
Dekker E 7
Delaney L 1361
Dempster CR 1304
Dengrove E 897,915
Denicola MA 1299
Dennis M 125,595
Derner GF 596
Derogatis LR 1407
Deter HC 59
Detweiler HK 223

Deutsch F 224,438, 1146
Devine JE 356
Diakonov MF 1000
Diamond HH 99
Diespecker D 708
Dietrich M 1327
Dietrich SL 700
Dilley JW 597
Dinard E 225
Dionne P 678
Dirks JF 226,257, 263,370,1183,1184
Dixon J 1305
Dixon JK 1299
Dobes RW 824
Dogs W 227,507
Dolan J 1306
Domangue BB 796
Donahue CV 1408
Donahue DC 1358
Doolittle MJ 1438
Dorn L 712
Douady D 729
Doust JWL 274
Dowling SJ 1232
Drapeau P 61,62
Drapkin A 321
Dreaper R 946
Dubin LL 677
Dubinkow EI 825, 826
Dubo S 730
Duchaine J 168
Dudek S 972
Dudek SZ 947
Dudley DL 598,599
Dufour J 678
Dugois P 898
Duguid K 310
Duller P 1001
Dunbar A 827
Dunbar F 600
Dunkel ML 866
Dunn ME 1120
Durner A 1327
Duvic M 568
Dymond AM 851

Eccles D 1330
Eckert E 31
Edgell PG 228,229, 862
Edwards G 100,601
Edwards H 1186
Edwards H 1186
Edwards JE 371,372
Ehleben C 796
Eisenberg BC 117
Eisenlohr E 957
Eissing KW 1085
El-Kholy MK 230
Eletsky VY 1002
Eliasberg WG 1376
Elitzur B 550
Elizur A 322
Ellena V 1133

Ellenberg L 1307, 1365,1381
Eller JJ 1003
Ellerbroek WC 772
Elliotson J 1439
Ellman P 508
Emery H 551
Engels D 1215
Engels WD 1004
England R 918
English OS 671, 1005,1173,1214
Epstein KN 916
Erickson MH 1377
Erskine J 146
Erskine-Milliss J 357
Escande JP 1006
Espin Montanez J 899
Estes SA 1103
Estrin J 900
Ettinger MP 570
Evans E 736,919
Ewin DM 790,812, 1147
Eyermann C 358
Eyre MB 731
Eyster ME 681

Falliers CJ 166,169, 231
Fashingbauer TJ 345
Feder SL 1233
Feinstein A 1308
Feldman GM 36
Ferguson J 1165
Ferguson RG 359
Fernandez GR 1007, 1008
Fezler WD 624,1155
Fialkov MJU 170
Field H 841
Findeisen DG 147, 232
Finer B 1440
Finer BL 732
Finesinger JE 831
Finkelmann A 690
Fiocco V 536
Fiore N 1234
Fireman BH 535
Fisch RI 1183
Fischer E 215
Fischer L 439
Fischer-Williams M 1148
Fishman HC 74
Flarsheim A 733
Fleischer D 1105
Fleiss JL 1311
Foerster K 1309, 1310
Fogelman MJ 788
Ford RM 171
Forester B 1311
Forget F 505
Forth MW 60
Fortin C 61,62

Fotopoulos SS 1441, 1442
Fowler RS 551
Frankel FH 917
Franks CM 8
Frazier CA 1204
Fredericks LE 679
Freed SC 1156
Freedman R 552,602
Freedman RR 553, 554
Freeman EH 440
Freeman J 603,1106
French AP 813
French TM 233,234, 441,604-607
Freour P 235
Freud E 172
Freytag-Klinger H 155
Friedman DB 319, 410
Friedman I 190
Friedman MM 1312
Friend MR 442
Fritz GK 386,828
Fross KH 226
Frost L 462
Frumess GM 1009
Fry L 113,1187
Fukatsu K 738
Fulton JE 774
Fung EH 680

Gachie JP 353
Gajwani AK 1107
Gallagher D 506
Gardey F 236
Gardner GG 1235
Gardner JE 9
Garfinkel R 360
Garnett RW Jr 237
Garon MR 194
Gassmann ML 1245
Gaudet EL 238
Gauthier Y 61,62
Gay Prieto J 1010
Geer JH 450
Geiger AK 63
Gellert GA 1270
Gendler ET 1443
Gentry WD 1001
Geocris K 760
Gerard MW 239,608
Gerber L 555
Gerkovich M 1442
Gerl W 1272,1391
Geronazzo G 930
Gervais L 240
Gettner HH 406
Ghory JE 64,162,173
Gibbs DN 1108
Gilbert A 699,700
Gilgor RS 568
Gillespie RD 241
Gitelson J 1370
Glaus KD 39,371

Glaust KD 372
Godfrey S 101,609
Goethe KE 1364
Goldberg JG 1444
Goldenberg E 783
Goldman L 948
Goldsmith D 918 Golod ER 1068
Gonen JY 702
Gonzalez J 1415
Good RS 1403-1405
Goodman HP 829
Goodman LE 1315, 1389
Gordon AM 1313, 1314
Gordon H 1011
Gordon N 192
Gorzynski JG 1409
Gosman JS 1060
Goss EO 949
Gosselin J 61,62
Gottesman AH 1012
Gottlieb SK 967,968
Gould SS 761
Gould WM 1013
Goyeche JR 148,149
Graf-Best AM 416
Gragg TM 1013
Graham C 1442
Graham DT 361
Graham SD 1417
Grant CW Jr 791
Grant IW 242
Gray S 1151
Gray SC 830
Green E 174
Green M 174
Greenhill MH 831
Greenson RR 959
Greer S 1236
Grindler D 1443
Grodek MV 22
Groen J 7,587
Groen JJ 65,172,443, 610-612
Grof S 1315,1390
Grossarth-Maticek R 1237,1445
Grossbalt TA 1149
Gruber L 417
Gruen GE 1194
Grumach L 950
Gunnarson S 243
Gustafsson P 66
Guy WB 832,833
Gybels J 1316
Gyulay J 1455

Haas A 613
Haas B 1284,1290
Hachez E 1014
Hackett TP 558,967- 969
Hailey BJ 1317

Haiman JA244,444
Hajos MK 245
Hakes TB 1358
Hale P 552
Hale PA 554
Hall H 1446
Hall HR 1188
Hall JA 1145,1434
Hall MD 1238
Hall-Smith P 1163
Halliday JL 246
Hallowitz D 175
Hamberger LK 1318
Hamm J 247
Hammond DC 791
Handford AH 681
Hansen K 248
Hardcastle DH 310
Harding AV 37
Harling J 45
Harms E 614
Harrell EH 914
Harris FR 891
Hartmann von Monakow K 556
Hartz J 734,764
Hau TF 209,249
Haydu GG 509
Haynal A 250,251
Haynes SN 834
Healy M 804
Hecht M 1150
Hedge AR 1239
Heigl-Evers A 835
Heiligman RM 1378
Hellier FF 951,1015
Helmkamp M 1447
Henderson AT 252
Hendler-Cobie S 1352-1354
Hendricks CM 765
Henkin R 735
Hepburn S 176
Hershkoff H 142
Heskel N 1356
Higgins G 1307
Higuchi K 1017
Hilgard ER 1448
Hilgard JR 1379, 1448-1450
Hilliard J 386
Hinid-Alexander M 362
Hirai M 200
Hirt M 595
Hobler WR 867
Hochstadt NJ 10
Hock RA 363,364
Hodek B 253
Hodes R 548
Hoffman A 17
Hoffman AL 510
Hoffman ML 1319
Hoffmann F 1284
Holden C 1380
Holland JC 1240, 1320,1345,1409,1451
Holland JCB 1452
Holland JP 713

Hollander MB 773
Holmes R 323
Holton C 1330
Homburger A 836
Honsberger R 250, 160
Hora J 1274
Horan JS 868
Hornbein R 719,723
Hornig-Rohan M 1206
Horenstein OP 1016, 1110,1134
Hossri CM 102
Houghton HE 103
Howard RJ 1241
Howard WA 131
Howell JD 448
Huebschmann H 557, 776
Hughes H 774,1151
Hughes HH 918
Hunecke P 821
Hunt BR 863
Hurley HJ 1152
Hurnyak MM 40
Hurst A 723,724,735
Hurwich SB 172
Huston P 561

Ianni P 552-554
Ikemi Y 148,149, 342,430,445,615, 616,1017,1111
Iles JD 1189
Imado Y 430
Iranzo Prieto V 899
Ironside W 837
Isbister C 72,176
Ishikawa H 1242
Israel L 838
Izak M 784

Jabush M 1112
Jackson M 60,254
Jacobi E 104
Jacobowitz J 118
Jacobson AF 1404
Jacobson AM 558
Jadassohn J 991
Jaffe PG 834
Janicki MP 762
Janson-Bjerklie S 38
Jaremko ME 807
Jeanguyot MT 729
Jelliffe Am 775
Jelliffe SE 736,919
Jensen RA 225
Jessner L 177,256, 277
Johnson A 511
Johnson AM 607
Johnson RF 952
Johnson SB 640
Johnstone D 166
Jokipaltio L 780

Jolowicz E 991
Jonas DL 682
Jones NF 257,370
Jordan JM 1126
Jores A 617
Joregensen JA 792
Jorgenson JA 793
Joseph ED 869
Julich H 258

Kaempfer SH 1321
Kagan H 172
Kalachnikoff P 737
Kaminski Z 365
Kamitsuka M 1359
Kaneko Z 418
Kaplan JZ 798,803
Kapotes C 178
Karol C 259
Kartamischew AJ 839,920,1018,1113, 1114,1153
Kaszuk C 840
Kattan M 92
Katz ER 1213,1322
Katz RM 133
Katzenelbogen S 512
Kaufman MR 869
Kaufman W 446,489
Kaye JM 1323
Kaywin L 419
Kearney J 1274
Keefe FJ 559
Keegan DL 420
Kellerman J 1205, 1307,1324,1325, 1365,1381,1453
Kelley WE 1019
Kellner K 366
Kelly E 260
Kelly P 1181
Kelman H 841
Kemper KA 261
Kennard DW 363, 364
Kenner C 1139
Kepecs JG 842
Kerekjarto V 617
Kerschnar H 133
Kersten W 262
Kesten B 909
Keye WR 791
Khan AU 11,12,367, 368
Kidd C 1115
Kidd CB 987
Kierland RR 887, 888,1086
Kihara H 430
King NJ 369
Kinnell HG 105
Kinsman RA 130, 257,263,370,1184
Kirkpatrick RA 544, 545
Kishimoto K 738
Klapper M 814

Klauder JV 1020-1022
Kleeman ST 264
Klein RF 702
Kleinman PD 1343
Kleinsorge H 265, 266
Kline HS 1023
Kline MV 870,921
Klinge JE 843,1024
Klopfer B 1243
Klosinski G 1326
Klumbies G 267
Knapp PH 153,268-271,618-622
Knapp RC 1408
Knapp TJ 13
Knight JA 639
Kniker WT 139
Knox SJ 272
Kobayashi M 739
Koblenzer CS 1025
Kohle K 1327
Kohli DR 922
Koldys KW 844
Konig KJ 953
Kopetzky MT 130
Kordova E 1064
Kornfeld DS 1311
Kos S 348
Koshy M 712
Kost PF 450
Kotses H 39,371,372
Kourlesis SM 1407
Kraepelien S 623
Krafchik H 1026
Kraft B 447,448
Kraft BK 421
Kramer D 1378
Krantz W 1116
Kreindler L 162
Krejci E 67
Kremer WB 703
Krisberg J 889
Kroger WS 449,624, 1154-1156,1454
Krozely MG 1293, 1335
Kubo C 430
Kuijpers BR 845
Kulchar GV 429
Kurland AA 1315, 1389,1390
Kurland S 536
Kusano T 616
Kutz I 1328
Kuypers BRM 846, 981
Kuypersen BR 1027

LaBaw WL 638-85, 794,1329,1330
Lacalmontie J 729
Lachman SJ 625,626, 1157
Lachmann W 258
Lakots M 41,42,152
Lamarre A 62

Lamb MA 1410
Lamont J 256
Lamont JA 1411
Lamont JH 177,277
Lamontagne Y 901
Landau LI 373
Lange-Neilsen AF 68
Lansky B 1455
Lansky P 1244
Lantz JE 902
Lascio M 1360
Lask A 627
Lask B 69,587
Latimer PR 1117
Laudenheimer R 106
Laugie H 737
Laugier P 923,1133
Lawlis GF 494,576, 774,830,1421,1422
Lazar BS 680
Lazar RM 1345
LeBaron S 14,139, 686,1331,1366,1401, 1402,1449
LeShan LL 1245, 1456
Lea PA 1382
Lebaron S 1370
Leclerc C 347
Leclerc P 737
Lee LR 1378
Lefer J 513
Leffert F 628
Lehman RE 871
Lehr S 1416
Leibenluft E 1332
Leidman IuM 954, 955
Leigh D 8,273,274, 374,629,630
Lengrand J 737
Leonenko PM 1028
Lerer B 1118
Lerner M 1246
Leroy PE 275
Lerro FA 40
Leuteritz G 924
Levendel L 41,42, 151,152
Levenson BS 1457
Levenson RW 132
Levine GF 653,1168
Levine MI 428,450
Levy SM 1247,1248, 1333,1430,1458
Lewis GM 1029
Lewis MN 107
Lewis RA 107
Lewiston NJ 386
Liagushkina MP 1127
Lichstein PR 1249
Lichtenberg JD 779
Liebman R 70
Lincoln PJ 514
Lindahl MW 704
Lindquist I 515
Lisansky ET 536
Liss A 1334

Littlefield L 139
Lo Presti G 1030
Locke SE 1206
Lofgren LB 276
Long R 256
Long RT 177,277
Lorand S 1119
Loras O 278
Loune RS 131
Lowenstein J 279
Lowman JT 1455
Lubens HM 451,452
Lubman A 1235
Lucan ON 687-692, 709
Lucas R 1459
Ludwig AO 516,517, 631,632,740
Lukeman D 15
Lulla SH 10
Luparello T 115
Luparello TJ 108, 130,518
Lusk EJ 1228
Lustig F 613
Listig GJ 735
Lustig-Juon E 1250
Luthe W 714,1158, 1207
Luz A 131
Lyles JN 1294,1295, 1297,1335
Lynn S 552
Lynn SJ 554
Lyons H 115
Lyons HA 108,518
Lyons JW 652

MacDonald N 113
MacKenna RMB 1031,1032,1137
Macalpine I 781, 1032,1033
Macaulay B 453
Macedo de Queiroz A 280
Mack KK 22
Mackenzie JN 490
Maeda K 200
Magarey C 1251
Magonet AP 109,633
Maguire P 1460
Maher KR 37
Maher-Loughnan G 110
Maher-Loughnan GP 111-113,634,635
Mahoney M 158
Malament IB 1120
Malcolm R 1300
Mally MA 428
Mandell AJ 281
Manferto G 1034
Mann T 767
Mannon JM 1159
Mansmann JA 282
Manuck SB 132
Manuso JS 847

Marchal J 1190
Marchesi C 114
Marcotte Y 505
Marcus R 533
Margolis CG 795, 796,1252,1383
Margolis H 636
Mariz J 848
Marks JB 741
Marley E 630
Martin C 136
Martin J 693,1336
Maruki K 200
Marx E 283
Marx JR 462
Mascia AV 71,179-181,637
Mason AA 113,454, 455,638,1335,1121, 1122,1187,1191
Mastrovito RC 1358
Masur FT 808
Mathe AA 621
Matthew D 69
Matthews-Simonton S 1281,1470-1472
Mattsson A 284,285
Mayer L 721,176
Mayer S 286
McCracken SG 1363
McCrane EJ 788
McCue K 1325
McDaniel LK 500
McDowell JJ 1102
McDowell M 956
McElroy SR 710
McFadden ER 518
McFadden ER Jr 108,115
McFadyen C 116
McGovern JP 639
McGraw PC 519
McGregor HG 520
McGuire M 1443
McHugh RB 31,32
McLaren WR 117
McLaughlin J 849
McLaughlin JT 833
McLean AF 1192
McLean JA 73
McMichael JE 164
Mcgraw P 494
Meara RH 775
Meares A 1253-1269
Meerwein F 1428, 1461
Meijer A 172,287
Melamed BG 640
Memmesheimer AM 957,991
Mengel CE 703
Menger W 375
Menninger K 1012, 1036
Merenstein A 711
Merz B 797
Mesirca P 46
Metzger FC 456
Meurs J 192

284   Immune System

Meyer J 1337
Meyer RP 844
Meyerowitz BE 1430
Michael JC 1037
Mijatovic M 288
Miklich DR 6,16,17,
43,142,159,289
Milberg IL 872,1038
Miles HHW 220,504
Milgrom H 1292
Miller BD 218
Miller H 290-292,
437,457-460,583,
641-643
Miller JA 170
Miller ML 461,873,
1193
Miller NJ 1241
Miller RM 850,851
Millikin LA 546
Millman HL
653,1168
Milne G 1338
Minagawa RY 1350
Minor CL 742
Minuchin S 70,74
Mirakhmedov UM
1039
Miroir R 182
Mirvish I 852
Misch RC 917
Mitchell AJ 462
Mitchell JH 463
Mitchell SD 508
Mitsubayashi T 200
Mittelman B 1040,
1208
Mizuguchi T 1384
Moan ER 422
Mohr GJ 411
Molhuysen-van der
Walle SMC 1124
Molk L 192
Moller P 903,1041
Monroe RR 1382
Monsour KJ 293
Montgomery L 776
Mook J 18,28
Joore F 20
Moore K 1339
Moore LE 798
Moore N 19
Moorefield CW 376
Moorman LJ 743
Moraes Passos AC
118,119
Morgan AH 1450
Morgan SB 808
Morgenstern H 1270
Morphis OL 1340
Morrell C 1342
Morrow GR 1248,
1341,1342
Morwood JMB 120
Motoda K 853
Mount B 1386
Mufson I 560
Muhl AM 744,745
Mullins A 464

Mullins JF 1123
Mun CT 121,122,
1385
Munjal GC 925
Munro DGM 746
Munro S 1386
Murphy WF 1146
Murray N 1123
Musaph H 423,904,
905,1042,1043,1124,
1160-1162
Muser J 192
Mushatt C 269-271,
622
Myers WK 1044

Naar R 1132
Naber J 294,295
Nachin C 935
Nadell R 438
Nagakawa S 1017
Nagata S 430
Nagaya H 703
Nagyova H 1064
Nakagawa S 445,
616,1111
Nakayama Y 200
Napke E 123
Neinstein LS 124
Neisworth JT 20
Nemetz SJ 269-271,
622
Neraal A 75
Nesse RM 1343
Neumann J 1045
Newbold G 1141
Newman LJ 194
Newman M 694
Newton-Bernauer W
1271
Nicholls G 497
Nickel WR 874
Nigl AJ 1148,1344
Nissen HA 521,522
Nitzberg H 183
Noda HH 523
Nolan M 524
Nolte D 21,296,644
Noonberg AR 645
Norris A 561
Norton A 1163
Novey HS 160
Novotny F 926
Nowlin JB 703
Joyes R 1387
Nylen BO 732

O'Neill D 297,894
Obermayer ME 875,
906,958,959,1046,
1164
Oberndorf CP 298
Ogston D 705
Ogston WD 705
Oldham RK 1335
Olen E 1151

Ollendick TH 1194
Olness K 1388
Olson DL 11
Olton DS 645
Orme GC 525
Ostfeld AM 1270
Otop J 526
Overbeck A 76
Overbeck G 76

Pahnke WN 1389,
1390
Paley A 226
Paragis DM 1462
Panush RS 570
Panzani R 377
Papentin F 1209
Pardoe R 811
Pariente R 251
Parrow J 299
Pasqua MC 782
Patterson C 40
Patterson L 712
Paul H 1447
Pearson GHJ 1125
Pearson RSB 1187
Peck LW 91
Peck SM 869
Peek LA 1300
Pelletier KR 1210
Pelser HE 7,65
Perman D 1345
Pennisi VR 799
Peper E 378
Perloff MA 465
Peshkin MM 48-50,
77,165,184-191,379,
646
Peter B 1272,1391
Peterson LL 562
Petow H 303,338
Philander DA 31
Philippus M 125
Phillip RL 380
Phillips J 45
Philpott OS 1138
Piazza EU 381
Piccionne C 1364
Pillsbury DM 429,
1077
Pilon RN 559
Pinard G 61
Pines D 854
Pinkerton P 300-302,
647
Pinney EL 300-302,
647
Pinney EL 747,748
Pipineli-Potamianou A
527
Piscicelli U 126
Planson C 55
Plumb M 1320
Podoswa-Martinez G
855
Polano MK 892
Pollak O 442

Pollnow H 303
Polonsky WH 153
Pope M 536
Portnoy ME 412
Posada JL 354
Posipisil J 1325
Poussaint A 927
Pozner H 304
Pratt A 1345
Pratt C 6,43
Prentice N 256
Preston K 1047
Prick JJG 528
Prior HJ 466
Prout CT 305
Purcell K 192
Purchard PR 876

Quarles van Ufford
WJ 193
Questad KA 1346
Quintal L 61,62

Rabin A 842
Rachelevsky GS 133
Rackemann FM 306
Rafael Toledo J 1151
Raines GN 307
Rainwater N 648
Rakos RF 22
Randich SR 529
Rapaport HG 467
Rapini RP 815
Rathus SA 23
Ratliff RG 877
Ratnoff OD 701,706
Reckless J 78,79
Redd WH 1293,
1296,1347-1354
Reddi C 364
Redondo D 127
Reed JMW 649
Reed JW 80,308
Reitner SR 71
Renne CM 5,17,593
Renneker RE 1273,
1274
Renshaw DC 1048
Retterstol N 68
Rhodes NR 816
Rich E 393
Richards W 194
Richards WA 1315,
1389
Richardson HB 563
Richter R 382
Rieger R 131
Rigler D 1325
Riley J 136
Rimon R 530
Ripley HS 391
Risch C 1165
Ritterman MK 695
Roberts MJ 194
Robertson G 878
Robertson IM 1126

Robin M 842
Robinson EG 531
Roden RG 707
Rodgers CH 364
Rodriquez DB 1478
Rogerson CH 309,
310,468,1049,1195
Rogow L 1356
Rohrer T 143
Rolando D 930
Rollins N 256
Ronconi GF 46
Rook A 1166
Rook AJ 1062
Rosembaum SB 729
Rosenbaum M 827,
907
Rosenbaum MS 879
Rosenberg SW 1355
Rosenberger PH
1354
Rosenthal MJ 856
Rosman B 650
Ross IM 651
Rostenberg A Jr 857
Rotman M 1356
Rowden L 1357
Rowe WS 960
Rowland J 1320
Rozhnov VE 394
Rubin JM 673
Rudzki E 424
Ruiz KN 532
Russell B 1176
Russell BF 1050
Russell JD 1051
Russo DC 715,802,
1103
Ryzhkova EI 1127

Sacerdote P 880,
1275,1392-1394,
1463-1466
Sachs BC 1467
Sack WT 991,1052,
1053,1167,1196
Sadger J 1054
Sadler JE 84
Sadler JE Jr 195,
311,312
Salazar Mallen M
469
Salerno EV 908
Salkin D 756
Salzberg HC 1185
Samek J 961
Sampliner RB 313
Sanderford LD 1299
Sanders S 696
Sandler N 383
Sanger MD 470
Sannomiya A 200
Sargeant EJ 1141
Sauer J 154
Saul LJ 425,471,652,
763,1197
Saunders C 1468
Saunders DR 35,594

Savage C 1390
Scalettar HE 314
Scarborough LF 881
Scarf M 1276
Schaefer CE 653,
1168
Schaeffer G 155
Schafer DW 800,
1395,1396
Schain WS 1412,
1413,1469
Schaller JG 551
Schatia V 472
Schechter MD 882
Schenkman M 711
Scherbel AB 315
Scherding JP 749
Scherr MS 44,196,
197,362,384,654
Schild R 564
Schilder P 1055
Schmidt G 1284
Schmidt LM 962
Schmidt P 1445
Schneck JM 1128
Schneer HI 655
Schneider E 909,
1056
Schnetzer M 154
Schoenberg B 883
Schon RC 1397
Schonell M 146,357
Schonfelder T 770
Schover LR 1414,
1415,1479
Schowalter JM 426
Schraa JC 263
Schuller CF 198
Schulte HJ 156
Schulte MB 928
Schultis K 296
Schultz JH 316,317,
714,1158,1207
Schur M 1129
Schwartz GE 153
Schwartz LH 533
Schwobel G 318
Sclare AB 56,81
Scott A 656
Scott DG 538
Scott DL 538
Scott DW 1358
Scott MJ 1057,1169,
1170,1211
Searle C 1277
Secheny S 1278
Secter II 1058
Sehgal VN 1107
Seidel JV 1183,1184
Seidenfeld MA 750
Seitz PFD 910,1059,
1060,1171
Selesnick S 411,657
Selesnick ST 319
Selinsky H 473
Selvey HA 1279
Serber M 32
Sergeant HGS 24,32
Sergent CB 44

Shafii M 929
Shafii SL 929
Shands HC 220
Shapiro A 1280
Shapiro EM 1123
Shapiro LB 511
Shapiro SS 677
Sharlit H 1061
Sharonov BG 1065
Sharp OB 534
Shartner CD 1297
Sheehan DV 963
Shepard J 10
Sherman C 1149
Shern MA 535
Shertzer CL 427
Shevarova VN 1065
Shimshoni R 924
Shipes E 1416
Shipman WG 428
Shocket BR 536
Shoemaker R 849
Shoemaker RJ 428, 832,833,858
Shorkey CT 801
Shorvon HJ 1062
Shrier L 796
Shubard AF 536
Shultz IT 751
Sichel JP 157
Siegel BS 1270
Siegel SC 133
Siegel SE 1325
Silesnick ST 410
Silver S 1003
Silverberg EL 558, 968
Silverman AJ 1063
Silverman S 101
Simons C 1327
Simonton OC 1281, 1282,1470-1472
Simonton SS 1282
Sinclair-Gieben AHC 964
Sirmay EA 474
Sirota AD 158,658
Sivak VP 884
Skalicanova M 1064
Shorkey CT 801
Shorvon HJ 1062
Shrier L 796
Shubard AF 536
Shultz IT 751
Sichel JP 157
Siegel BS 1270
Siegel SC 133
Siegel SE 1325
Silesnick ST 410
Silver S 1003
Silverberg EL 558, 968
Silverman AJ 1063
Silverman S 101
Simons C 1327
Simonton OC 1281, 1282,1470-1472
Simonton SS 1282

Sinclair-Gieben AHC 964
Sirmay EA 474
Sirota AD 158,658
Sivak VP 884
Skalicanova M 1064
Sklarofsky AB 406
Skreta M 253
Skretova K 253
Skripkin IuK 885
Skryleva TN 1065
Skuber P 348
Slany E 1066
Slight D 1104
Slorach J 1067
Smirnov LD 1068
Smith CM 702
Smith DB 1415
Smith H 1069
Smith JM 128
Smith MM 129
Smith MS 1359
Smith SJ 565
Sneddon IB 1070
Sobrado EA 930
Sokolianskii MN 1071
Solanch LS 581
Sonneck HJ 911
Sontag LW 475,777
Sontag S 1473
Souhrada J 130
Soutter C 775
Sovine DL 1148
Spangler DL 164
Sparer PJ 768
Sparks TF 1281
Spector S 130
Speer F 659
Spencer KA 522
Sperber Z 657
Sperling M 320,476
Spevack M 25
Spiegel D 1398,1399
Spiegelman J 465
Spohn WA 92
Sporkel H 385
Squier TL 477
Sribner VA 26
Staerk M 12
Stamm J 321
Stang RE 131
Stangel W 1222
Staukler L 965
Stein NH 877
Steiner H 386
Steiner M 322
Steinhardt MJ 1072
Steinhausen HC 387
Stenlin JS Jr 1283
Stephen JM 222
Steptoe A 45,323
Stern A 660
Stern E 912
Stewart H 1198
Stierlin H 1284,1290
Stirman JA 788

Stoesser AV 255
Stokes JH 429,1073-1077,1130
Stokvis B 82,83,388, 478,479,661,662
Stoll BA 1474-1476
Stoudemire A 1360, 1417
Stowe JE 783
Straatmeyer AJ 816
Straker N 199,324
Straube W 537
Strauss A 280
Strauss EB 325,326, 389
Stroebel CF 547
Strosberg IM 1285
Strouse TB 1228
Strupp HH 132
Struthers GR 538
Studt HH 209,327, 752,1199
Sugita M 342,616
Sultanova A 138,394
Sulzberger MB 966
Sundstrom WA 548
Surman OS 558,967, 968
Surwit RS 559,566-568
Suvorova KN 1065
Suzuki I 200
Swade R 1182
Swanton C 390
Szyrynski V 480

Takahashi N 342
Takaishi N 418
Tal A 159
Tamerin J 199
Taneli S 85
Tashkin DP 133
Tasini MF 969
Tattersfield AE 107
Taub E 547
Tausend H 411
Taylor JE 801
Taylor PW 807
Taylor RL 970
Techman T 1417
Teichmann AT 1078
Tenzel JH 970
Teshima H 430
Tetreult L 61
Tewell K 1330
Thal AB 501,502
Tharp RG 889
Theobald DE 543
Theopold A 328
Thibier R 729
Thibier R 729
Thoma H 886,1079
Thomas JE 712
Thomas K 712
Thompson BA 753
Thulesius O 569
Thurn A 1131

Tinkelman DG 84
Tissler DM 761
Tobia L 1080
Tocantins LM 690-692
Toyama N 342
Tredgold AF 663
Treuting TF 391
Trojanek S 754
Tsuboi H 738
Tuft HS 191,664, 1200
Tunsater A 392
Turner RA 500
Twerski AJ 1132

Udelman DL 539-541
Udelman HD 539-541
Udupa KN 665,666, 1477
Uglov FG 134
Ullman M 971,972
Ulrich I 85
Unger S 1390
Uno R 1325
Upson P 164

Vachon L 393,621
Van Dijk E 928
VanMoffaert M 1081-1083
Van Pelt SJ 135
Van Stegmann A 329
Van de Klashorst GO 193
Van der Hal I 27
Van der Ploeg HM 18,26
Varni JW 697-700, 715,802,1103,1205, 1212,1213
Vaugh VC 859
Vaughan B 176
Vetter H 1445
Vittouris N 1133
Vogel PG 931,1084
Volkmann H 1085
Vollmer H 973,974
Volmat R 1133
Von Eschenbach AC 1414,1415,1478,1479
Von Leupold W 330
Vorhies C 562
Vorobeva ZV 138

Wagner FF 1400
Wahl CW 481,667
Waisman M 860
Wakeman RJ 803
Walker LJS 804
Walsh MN 887,888, 1086

Walter SD 1270
Walton D 668,1172
Waltz M 1223
Ware PD 1382
Warga C 1286
Warter P 542
Watson DL 889
Waxman D 932
Weaver CM 647
Webb A 359
Weber A 331
Weber G 1284,1290
Wechsler F 1361
Weddington WW 1362,1363
Weidlich S 1327
Weigel BJ 755
Weiker A 1045
Weiner H 669
Weinstein AG 29
Weinstein DJ 805
Weinstock C 1227, 1287,1288
Weintraub A 670
Weisnagel J 61,62
Weiss E 332,333, 482,671,1173,1214
Weiss JH 136
Weissberg G 1087
Weisz AE 806
Weitz RD 1289
Wellisch E 334
Wells LA 13
Welman AJ 388,662
Wendt H 86
Wenig P 553,602
Wernick RL 807
Werther J 991
West BL 1364
Westie KS 1404, 1405
Whalen BT 1304
Whedbee JS 724
Whipple B 177,256, 277
White HC 137
White JG 1317
Whitlock FA 1088, 1126,1174,1175
Wilbur BM 756
Wilde GJS 380
Wilkening K 975
Wilkes WO 757
Wilkinson DS 1062, 1166
Williams DH 861
Wilmerding JW 213
Wilsch L 1134
Wilson AF 150,160
Wilson BJ 788
Wilson CC 834
Wilson CP 335,336, 651
Wilson E 570
Wilson GW 491
Wink CAS 1135, 1136
Winkler F 913

Winkler WT 492
Wirsching B 1284, 1290
Wirsching M 1284, 1290
Wisch JM 933
Wise TN 1418,1419
Wisely DW 808
Wittich GH 337
Wittig HJ 164
Wittkower E 303, 338,483,505,862, 934,1089,1137
Wittkower ED 769, 863,1090,1091,1176, 1215
Wohl TH 30,87,88, 162,201
Wolf J 966
Wolff HH 339
Wolpe J 1177
Woodburne AR 1138
Woodhead B 413, 1201
Woods NF 1410
Woolhandler HW 890
Wooley-Hart A 1291
Worth G 262
Wright CS 1092-1094
Wright GL 340
Wuite J 928

Yalom ID 976
Yaron M 550
Yocum DE 548
Yorkston NJ 31,32, 672
Yoshida GN 84
Young LD 500
Young SH 92,673
Younger CB 281

Zahourek RP 809, 810
Zaidens SH 1095
Zamotaev IP 138,394
Zander W 571
Zanus L 46
Zealley AK 208,577
Zelesnik C 395
Zeller B 260
Zeltzer L 14,139, 713,1307,1331,1365, 1366,1381,1401,1402
Zeltzer LK 686
Zeltzer PM 1366
Zheltakov MM 1178
Zhukov IA 1179
Zide B 811
Ziskind E 341
Zivitz N 202
Ziwar M 484
Zoller JE 203
Zuili N 935
Zwick KG 977

Subject Index

Entries are derived from the text rather than the abstracts of the articles. Numbers refer to abstracts not pages.

asthma and, 310, 340, 396–413, 575, 657
behavior therapy for, 820, 824, 853
biofeedback for, 844, 850, 851
   with relaxation, 830, 834, 847
family therapy for, 817
group therapy for, 832, 833, 858
hypnosis for, 823, 825, 826, 829, 839
   with behavior therapy, 853
   with psychotherapy, 842, 843, 852
   with relaxation, 843
psychotherapy for, 818, 819, 821, 822, 827, 828, 831, 835–838, 840, 841, 845, 846, 848, 849, 854–857, 859–863, 1193
   with family therapy, 817
   with group therapy, 832, 883, 858
   wwith hypnosis, 842, 843, 852
   with relaxation, 843
relaxation for
   with behavior therapy, 820
   with biofeedback, 830, 834, 844, 847
   with hypnosis, 843
   with psychotherapy, 843
suggestion for, 445
Education. *See* Patient education
Ego
in asthma, 63, 178, 183
in psoriasis, 930
in tuberculosis, 730, 733
Eidetic imagery, for cancer pain, 1388
Electroencephalography, in neurodermatitis, 885
Electromyography
for asthma, 141, 384
for cancer or cancer therapy side effects, 1293, 1297, 1344
for eczema, 830, 834
for rheumatoid arthritis, 523
Electronarcosis
for combined skin disorders, 1000
for neurodermatitis, 865, 885
Electrotherapy, for cancer pain, 1316
Emesis. *See* Vomiting, from chemotherapy
Emotions
in acne, 777
in allergy, 639
   with family therapy, 462, 466, 480
   with group therapy, 437, 458, 459, 480
   with milieu therapy, 444
   with psychotherapy, 433, 434, 437, 439, 441, 444, 446, 447, 456, 458, 461, 462, 466, 470, 472–477, 480, 483, 489, 1197
in aphthous ulcerations, 762
in asthma, 577, 628, 660
   with behavior therapy, 159, 346, 349, 358
   with biofeedback, 346
   with group and family therapy, 64, 73, 81, 88, 175, 176, 178, 189, 379
   with hypnosis, 94, 113, 129, 349, 358, 391, 392
   with imagery, 153
   with milieu therapy, 88, 171, 175–178, 185, 188, 213, 347, 379, 444
   with psychotherapy, 73, 178, 185, 188, 206, 209, 211, 213, 223, 229, 231, 233, 234, 237, 239, 244, 246, 250, 252, 255, 256, 264, 268, 269, 271, 277, 280, 282, 284, 285, 290, 292, 297, 301, 304–308, 315, 319, 320, 326, 332, 339, 340, 342,

347, 349, 351, 358, 379, 391, 392, 434, 444
   with relaxation, 129, 131, 140, 149, 159, 346
   with suggestion, 115, 131, 349, 358
   with yoga, 148, 149
in burns, 788, 794, 807
in cancer, 1233, 1234, 1282, 1458
   with behavior therapy, 1221, 1333
   with hypnosis, 1289, 1312
   with imagery, 1289
   with meditation, 1291
   with psychotherapy, 1221, 1274, 1287, 1308
   with relaxation, 1225, 1247, 1291
   with suggestion, 1312
in cancer or cancer therapy side effects
   with behavior therapy, 1324
   with family therapy, 1334
   with hypnosis, 1334
   with psychotherapy, 1311, 1315, 1334
   with relaxation, 1293–1295
   with suggestion, 1334
in cancer pain, 1387, 1392, 1396
in cheilitis glandularis, 1138
in colds, 763
in combined immunologic disorders, 1192, 1198, 1200
in combined skin disorders, 979, 1003, 1140, 1176,
   with group therapy, 1038
   with hypnosis, 987, 1024
   with psychotherapy, 986, 993, 995, 1004, 1005, 1009, 1012, 1016, 1024, 1026, 1033, 1036, 1037, 1040, 1046, 1050, 1055, 1067, 1072, 1075–1077, 1086, 1092, 1104
   with relaxation, 1026
   with suggestion, 986–988, 1024, 1086
in diffuse obstructive pulmonary syndrome, 599
in eczema, 857
   with behavior therapy, 820
   with biofeedback, 850
   with group therapy, 832, 833
   with hypnosis, 842
   with psychotherapy, 822, 827, 828, 831–833, 837, 842, 846, 859–863, 1193
   with relaxation, 820
in hay fever, 603
in hemophilia
   with family therapy, 681
   with group therapy, 688
   with hypnosis, 679, 681, 687, 688, 691
   with psychotherapy, 674, 681, 688
in herpes simplex, 762
in inflammatory skin lesions, 1125
in lichen simplex, 1126
in neurodermatitis, 867, 874–876, 878, 1193
in pruritus, 894–896, 905, 906, 909, 910
in psoriasis, 915, 921, 927, 934
in purpura, 701, 703, 706
in Raynaud's disease, 561, 563
in rheumatoid arthritis
   with group therapy, 539
   with hypnosis, 525, 542, 546
   with psychotherapy, 495, 497, 498, 504, 512, 517, 520, 522, 531, 539, 542
   with social casework, 531

in rosacea, 1130
in scleroderma, 563
in sexual dysfunction in cancer, 1409, 1413, 1419
in sickle cell anemia, 710
in Sjogren's syndrome, 550
in tuberculosis
   with counseling, 731, 751
   with milieu therapy, 720, 726, 751
   with psychotherapy, 716, 720, 725, 726, 733, 736, 740, 744, 751
   with social casework, 740
in urticaria, 418, 419, 425, 428–430
in warts, 937, 971
Enmeshment, in asthma, 170
Environment. *See* Climate; Social environment
Epidermolysis bullosa, 1124
Erythema, 1108
Erythroderma, ichthyosiform, 1115, 1121, 1135
Ewing's tumour, 1232
Exercise therapy, for psoriasis, 922
Exhibitionism
in combined skin disorders, 1023, 1056, 1072
in neurodermatitis, 876
in psoriasis, 919
Existentialism, in asthma, 235
Expectations, in cancer treatment, 1308
Extinction
in asthma, 11, 78, 79, 167
for cancer or cancer therapy side effects, 1348
in lichen simplex, 1126
Extroversion
in asthma, 8
in rheumatoid arthritis, 510
in tuberculosis, 745

Facial muscle relaxation, for asthma, 39
Factor VIII, in hemophilia, 675, 677, 681, 697, 700
Faith healing
for allergy, 444, 1191
for ankylosing spondylitis, 549
for cancer, 1232, 1240, 1246, 1250, 1251
   with hypnosis, 1189
   with imagery, 1228
   with meditation, 1264, 1266
   with suggestion, 1189
for cancer pain, 1378, 1395
for combined immunologic disorders, 1186, 1189, 1191
for rheumatoid arthritis, 514, 538
Family
in asthma
   with assertiveness training, 363
   with family therapy, 63, 75, 76
   with group therapy, 353
   with milieu therapy, 170
   with psychotherapy, 63, 231, 320, 353
   with relaxation, 363
in cancer, 1221, 1290
in eczema, 835, 842, 862
in hemophilia, 695
in pruritus, 902

Immune System

with biofeedback, 33
with imagery, 146
with relaxation, 33, 146
for cancer, 1240, 1246, 1251–1269, 1278, 1279
with imagery, 1217, 1224, 1253
with psychotherapy, 1224
with relaxation, 1224, 1291
with spiritual healing, 1266
for cancer or cancer therapy side effects, 1361
for cancer pain, 1269, 1395, 1396
for combined immunologic disorders, 1209
for hemophilia, 697–700
for warts, 949
Melancholy, in asthma, 269, 270
Menopause, pruritis in, 896
Mental healing, *See* Faith healing
Milieu. *See* Social environment
Milieu therapy
for allergy, 435, 44, 464, 467
for asthma, 161–203, 464, 623, 627, 654, 664
with behavior therapy, 4, 5, 16, 30, 166, 167
with biofeedback, 44, 384
with group and family therapy 49, 50, 72, 77, 84, 88, 162, 173, 175, 176, 178, 181, 186, 189, 345, 348, 379, 381, 383, 386, 390, 395
with hypnosis and suggestion, 91, 395
with psychotherapy, 162, 163, 166, 173, 178, 185, 187, 188, 191, 195, 203, 206, 213, 257, 277, 285, 301, 302, 313, 321, 343, 344, 347, 348, 351, 362, 367, 373–375, 379, 381, 386, 395, 444
with relaxation, 384
for asthma and eczema, 408
for cancer pain, 1387, 1468
for combined immunologic disorders, 1200
for combined skin disorders, 994, 1065, 1068, 1179
for neurodermatitis, 884
for pruritus, 909
for psoriasis, 926
for tuberculosis, 742
with group therapy, 754, 756
with psychotherapy, 720, 726, 727, 729, 751, 755
Minnesota Multiphasic Personality Inventory (MMPI)
in asthma, 154, 226, 253
in cancer, 1315, 1378
in combined immunologic disorders, 1183
in rheumatoid arthritis, 510, 525
in sickle cell anemia, 710
Modeling
in asthma, 9
in burns, 792, 793
Molluscum contagiosum, 1097, 1098, 1116
Mood
in asthma, 323
in burns, 785
in cancer, 1373, 1375, 1399
in hay fever, 603
in herpes simplex 761
in rheumatoid arthritis, 506
Morale, in burns, 785, 786, 800
Mother-child relationship. *See also* Parent-child relationships

in allergy, 433, 441, 460, 462, 471
in alopecia areata, 778
in asthma
with autogenic training, 157
with group and family therapy, 54, 57, 61–63, 67, 72, 348, 353, 386
with milieu therapy, 72, 177, 347, 348, 386
with psychotherapy, 54, 58, 61–63, 72, 157, 234, 235, 237, 238, 243, 252, 256, 259, 277, 292, 293, 298, 309, 319, 322, 335, 344, 347, 348, 353, 386, 642
with relaxation, 54
in combined skin disorders, 1054, 1078
in dermatitis, 1132
in eczema
with hypnosis, 842, 843
with psychotherapy, 827, 840, 842, 843, 849, 854, 861
with relaxation, 843
in neurodermatitis, 876
in purpura, 704
in rheumatoid arthritis 497, 527
in tuberculosis, 725
Motivation, in cancer treatment, 1218, 1281
Mouth cancer, 1344
Mud packs, for skin disorders, 1068
Multiple sclerosis, 1190
Muscle contraction, in asthma, 39, 102
Muscle relaxation. *See also* Deep muscle relaxation; Progressive muscle relaxation; Relaxation
in asthma, 39, 40, 149, 354
in cancer or cancer therapy side effects, 1297, 1354
in hemophilia, 700
Muscle tension. *See* Tension
Muscle tonus, in arthritis, 571
Music therapy, for cancer pain, 1386

Narcissism
in eczema, 854
in perioral dermatitis, 1131
in tuberculosis, 718, 725, 733
Narcohypnosis, for cancer pain, 1371
Narcotherapy, for asthma, 253, 353
Natural killer cells, in cancer, 1221, 1225
Nausea, from chemotherapy
behavior therapy for, 1317, 1331, 1343, 1352
with biofeedback, 1353, 1360
with hypnosis, 1296, 1319, 1345, 1349–1351, 1353, 1360
with imagery, 1349, 1351, 1353, 1364
with relaxation, 1296, 1306, 1337, 1341, 1342, 1345, 1349, 1351, 1353, 1360
with suggestion, 1306
biofeedback for, 1297, 1353, 1360
hypnosis for, 1307, 1402
with behavior therapy, 1296, 1319, 1345, 1349, 1360
with biofeedback, 1360
with counseling, 1366
with imagery, 1349, 1388
with relaxation, 1296, 1338, 1345, 1349, 1360
imagery for

with behavior therapy, 1349, 1351, 1353, 1364
with biofeedback, 1353
with hypnosis, 1349, 1351, 1353, 1354, 1388
with psychotherapy, 1335
with relaxation, 1335, 1349, 1351, 1353, 1354
meditation for, 1361
placebo for, 1301
psychotherapy for, 1301, 1335, 1362, 1366
relaxation for, 1303, 1363
with behavior therapy, 1293, 1296, 1306, 1337, 1341, 1342, 1345, 1349–1351, 1353, 1360
with biofeedback, 1293, 1297, 1353, 1360
with hypnosis, 1293, 1296, 1338, 1345, 1349–1351, 1353, 1354, 1360
with imagery, 1295, 1335, 1349, 1351, 1353, 1354
with meditation, 1361
with psychotherapy, 1335
with suggestion, 1306
suggestion for, 1306
Neoplasms. *See* Cancer
Neurodermatitis, 864–890, 1152
behavior therapy for, 877, 879, 889, 1172, 1177
biofeedback for, 834
group therapy for, 872
hypnosis for, 865, 868–871, 880, 885, 1034
milieu therapy for, 884
psychotherapy for, 864, 867, 873–876, 878, 881–883, 886–888, 890, 1002, 1193
with hypnosis, 868–871
with imagery, 870
with milieu therapy, 884
with suggestion, 869
relaxation for, 834, 877
social casework for, 866
Neurotic disorders
asthma as, 208, 249, 327, 394
combined skin disorders as, 1066
eczema as, 845
hemophilia as, 676
pruritus as, 899
Nightmares, in cancer, 1324, 1453. *See also* Sleep disorders, in cancer
Nondirective therapy, for rheumatoid arthritis, 526
Nursing management
of asthma, 385
of cancer, 1241, 1250, 1277, 1291
of cancer or cancer therapy side effects
with behavior therapy, 1293, 1339, 1345
with biofeedback, 1293, 1321
with hypnosis, 1293, 1321, 1345
with imagery, 1321, 1339, 1357
with relaxation, 1293, 1302, 1303, 1305, 1321, 1339, 1345, 1357
of cancer pain, 1368, 1369
of sexual dysfunction in cancer, 1410, 1416
Nutrition. *See* Anorexia; Cachexia; Eating disorders, in cancer

---

Object relationships
in alopecia areata, 778
in asthma, 256, 321

Immune System

Immune System

Respiratory disease, 588, 626, 671
Respiratory function tests
  with behavior therapy, 208
  with biofeedback, 141
  with family therapy, 69, 173, 176
  with group therapy, 173
  with hypnosis, 124
  with milieu therapy, 173, 176
  with psychotherapy, 124, 173, 208, 245
  with relaxation, 141
Respiratory resistance. *See* Airway
  resistance
Rest, in asthma, 129, 354
Retching. *See* Vomiting, from chemotherapy
Reversal learning, for neurodermatitis,
  879
Reward. *See* Reinforcement
Rheumatic disorders, 493–571
Rheumatoid arthritis, 493–542, 600, 631,
  636, 656, 670
  autogenic training for, 507, 537
  behavior therapy for, 493, 500, 506, 529,
    576
  biofeedback for, 494, 500, 503, 519, 523
  faith healing for, 514, 538
  group therapy for, 500, 533, 535, 539, 540
    with autogenic training, 537
    with behavior therapy, 493
    with psychotherapy, 493, 541
  hypnosis for, 501, 525, 546
    with autogenic training, 507
    with imagery, 524
    with psychotherapy, 502, 542
    with relaxation, 524
  imagery for, 500, 532
    with behavior therapy, 529
    with biofeedback, 503
    with hypnosis, 524
    with psychotherapy, 1190
    with relaxation, 503, 524, 529
    with yoga, 503
  placebo for, 518
  play therapy for, 515
  psychotherapy for, 495–499, 504, 505, 508–
    513, 516, 517, 520–522, 526–528, 530,
    534, 536, 564, 571, 632
    with behavior therapy, 493
    with couples therapy, 539
    with group therapy, 493, 539, 541
    with hypnosis, 502, 542
    with imagery, 1190
    with social casework, 531
  relaxation for, 500
    with behavior therapy, 529
    with biofeedback, 494, 503, 519
    with hypnosis, 524
    with imagery, 503, 524, 529
    with yoga, 503
  social casework for, 531
  yoga for, 503, 665
Rhinitis, 228, 440, 445, 490–492
Rigidity
  in asthma, 170
  in eczema, 842
  in rheumatoid arthritis, 509
Role rehearsal, in cancer treatment, 1247.
  See also Sick role
Rorschach test
  in alopecia areata, 778

  in asthma, 282, 334
  in eczema, 842
  in neurodermatitis, 883
  in rheumatoid arthritis, 505, 510
  in urticaria, 418
Rosacea, 1127, 1130

Schizoid personality disorder
  in asthma, 327
  in psoriasis, 931
Schizophrenia
  with asthma, 274
  with skin disorders, 1095
Scirrhous carcinoma, 1260
Scleroderma
  autogenic training for, 547, 553, 568
  behavior therapy for, 602
  biofeedback for, 547, 548, 553, 570
  hypnosis for, 561
  psychotherapy for, 560, 561, 563
Scratching, 1160
  behavior therapy for, 820, 824, 1102, 1103,
    1117, 1126
  hypnosis and suggestion for, 1132
  psychotherapy for, 1132
  relaxation for, 820
Seasons, and asthma, 375, 384
Seborrhea, 322, 1137
Security
  in asthma, 238, 391
  in rheumatoid arthritis, 516, 517
  in scleroderma, 560
  in urticaria, 423
Self-assertiveness, in asthma, 61, 71, 237
Self-concept
  in asthma, 28, 71, 74
  in burns, 794
  in cancer, 1404, 1406, 1411, 1412
  in combined skin disorders, 1078
  in eczema, 854
  In tuberculosis, 725, 752
Self-consciousness, in asthma, 148, 149
Self-esteem
  in asthma, 139
  in burns, 810
  in cancer, 1223, 1365, 1381, 1413, 1417
  in combined immunologic disorders, 1184
  in combined skin disorders, 1040
  in eczema, 841, 862
  in hemophilia, 680
  in herpes simplex, 761
  in tuberculosis, 733
Self-help groups, for asthma, 194
Self-hypnosis. *See* Autohypnosis
Self-management
  of asthma
    with behavior therapy, 2, 4, 22, 346
    with biofeedback, 346
    with family therapy, 22
    with milieu therapy, 4, 213
    with psychotherapy, 213
    with relaxation, 22, 158, 346
  of hemophilia, 696, 699, 700
  of neurodermatitis, 889
  of pruritus, 903
  of psoriasis, 928
  of rheumatoid arthritis, 500, 525

  of sickle cell anemia, 712, 713
Self-mutilation, 770, 1102
Self-pity, in cancer 1371
Self-punishment, in pruritus, 912
Senoi-Dreamwork, for rheumatoid
  arthritis, 532
Separation
  in alopecia areata, 779
  in asthma
    with group and family therapy, 226, 383,
      386
    with milieu therapy, 383, 386
    with psychotherapy, 226, 239, 250, 256,
      319, 386
  in cancer, 1238
  in dermatitis, 1132
  in herpes simplex, 760
  in pruritus, 897
  in rheumatoid arthritis, 531, 536
Sex factors
  in acne, 775
  in asthma, 208, 1199
  in cancer, 1313, 1379
  in tuberculosis, 1199
Sex therapy, in cancer, 1403, 1412–1414
Sexual problems. *See also* Psychosexual
  development
  in asthma and eczema, 402–404
  in cancer, 1469, 1478, 1479
    counseling for, 1403–1405, 1407, 1408,
      1410–1414, 1416–1419
    desensitization for, 1413
    group therapy for, 1409
    hypnosis for, 1406
    psychotherapy for, 1406, 1409, 1412,
      1413, 1415
  in combined immunologic disorders, 1199
  in combined skin disorders
    with group therapy, 1023
    with hypnosis, 1024
    with psychotherapy, 1023, 1024, 1048,
      1056, 1075, 1104, 1105
    with suggestion, 1024
  in eczema, 827, 842, 849
  in herpes simplex, 759
  in neurodermatitis, 881
  in pruritus, 912, 913
  in rheumatoid arthritis, 504
Sibling rivalry, in asthma, 48
Sickle cell anemia, 710, 712, 713
Sick role
  in asthma
    with autogenic training, 59
    with group and family therapy, 59, 60, 63,
      76
    with hypnosis and suggestion, 326
    with milieu therapy, 170
    with psychotherapy, 60, 63, 252, 326, 335
    with relaxation, 59
  in cancer, 1309, 1362
Sjogren's syndrome, 550
Skin conductance. *See* Galvanic skin
  response
Skin disorders, 770-n1179
  acne, 770–777
  alopecia areata, 778–783
  atopic dermatitis, 817–863
  burns, 784–811

combined disorders, 978–1095, 1149, 1161,
1162, 1164, 1166, 1168, 1171, 1173,
1175
  autogenic training for, 1041, 1158
  behavior therapy for, 981, 1027, 1042,
1082, 1155, 1157, 1165
  biofeedback for, 983, 1001, 1148
  group therapy for, 996, 1023, 1038, 1064
  hypnosis for, 980, 982, 983, 985, 987,
990, 992, 1000, 1007, 1008, 1011,
1018, 1024, 1028, 1034, 1035, 1041,
1052, 1057–1059, 1063, 1071, 1080,
1141, 1142, 1145, 1153–1155, 1169,
1170, 1174, 1179, 1185
  imagery for, 983
  milieu therapy for, 994, 1065, 1068, 1179
  patient education for, 1021
  placebo for, 978, 983
  psychotherapy for, 978, 984, 989, 991,
993, 995, 997–999, 1002, 1004–1006,
1009–1017, 1019–1027, 1029–1033,
1036, 1037, 1039–1041, 1043–1056,
1059–1064, 1066, 1067, 1069, 1070,
1072–1079, 1081–1095, 1099, 1104,
1150, 1151, 1163, 1167
  relaxation for, 1001, 1021, 1026, 1073,
1074, 1094
  suggestion for, 982, 983, 987, 988, 992,
1000, 1007, 1010, 1011, 1018, 1021,
1022, 1024, 1028, 1052, 1058, 1059,
1063, 1064, 1071, 1086, 1153
condyloma acuminata, 812–816
eczema, 817–863
neurodermatitis, 864–890
pruritus, 891–913
psoriasis, 914–935
warts, 936–977
Skin resistance. *See* Galvanic skin response
Skin temperature
in asthma, 40, 141
in burns, 787
in cancer treatment, 1218
in eczema, 844, 847
in hemophilia, 698
in psoriasis, 914, 916, 918
In Raynaud's disease
  with autogenic training, 553, 559, 568
  with biofeedback, 551–554, 558, 559, 562,
570
  with hypnosis, 558
in rheumatoid arthritis, 519, 523
in scleroderma, 570
in vasoconstrictive syndromes, 547, 548
Sleep disorders, in cancer, 1453. *See also*
Insomnia; Nightmares
behavior therapy for, 1306
group therapy for, 1330
hypnosis for, 1330
relaxation for, 1306
suggestion for, 1306
Sleep therapy. *See* Electronarcosis;
Narcohypnosis; Narcotherapy
Social casework
for allergy, 442, 462
for asthma
  with group and family therapy, 175, 181,
228, 315, 345, 359
  with hypnosis and suggestion, 131
  with milieu therapy, 175, 181, 183, 345
  with psychotherapy, 73, 228, 272, 315

  with relaxation, 131
for asthma and eczema, 411
for neurodermatitis, 866
for rheumatoid arthritis, 531
for scleroderma, 560
for tuberculosis, 718, 724, 740
Social environment
in asthma, 610
  with behavior therapy, 208
  with group and family therapy, 63, 85
  with hypnosis and suggestion, 109, 326
  with psychotherapy, 63, 85, 208, 231, 326
in cancer, 1237, 1240, 1333
in combined skin disorders, 1015, 1025,
1027, 1078
in rheumatoid arthritis, 636
in seborrhoeic dermatitis, 1137
Social skills training, in eczema, 820
Sociotherapy
for asthma, 82, 167, 388
for cancer, 1237
for scratching, 1102
Spiritual healing. *See* Faith healing
Spirometry
with hypnosis and suggestion, 94, 129
with psychotherapy, 242
with relaxation, 129
Spondylitis, ankylosing, 549, 564
Spontaneous remission
in cancer, 1475
  with faith healing, 1189
  with hypnosis, 1189, 1226
  with meditation, 1255, 1258–1260, 1262,
1264–1266, 1278
  with psychotherapy, 1279, 1287
  with suggestion, 1189
in rheumatoid arthritis, 501, 517
in warts, 936, 971, 972, 974, 977
Sports therapy, for asthma, 147. *See also*
Exercise therapy; Gymnastics
Stimulus control
for cancer or cancer therapy side effects,
1348
for hemophilia, 697
**Stimulus generalization, of cancer or
cancer therapy side effects,** 1318
Stress
in acne, 777
in allergy, 475
in aphthous ulcerations, 762
in asthma
  with behavior therapy, 14
  with biofeedback, 14, 370
  with group and family therapy, 189
  with hypnosis and suggestion, 14, 326, 392
  with milieu therapy, 189, 301, 347
  with psychotherapy, 253, 264, 271, 297,
301, 304, 308, 310, 326, 340, 341, 347,
360, 392, 610
  with relaxation, 14, 360, 370
  with yoga, 665, 666
in asthma and eczema, 400
in cancer, 1438, 1470, 1471, 1477
  with behavior therapy, 1221, 1223, 1229,
1333
  with family therapy, 1284
  with hypnosis, 1226, 1289, 1393
  with imagery, 1238, 1247, 1289
  with meditation, 1251, 1261, 1262, 1291

  with psychotherapy, 1220–1222, 1231,
1393
  with relaxation, 1225, 1238, 1247, 1291
  with spiritual healing, 1251
  with yoga, 1477
from cancer or cancer therapy side effects
  behavior therapy for, 1346, 1360
  biofeedback for, 1360
  group therapy for, 1399
  hypnosis for, 1320, 1360, 1399
  psychotherapy for, 1313, 1356
  relaxation for, 1302, 1308, 1360
in combined immunologic disorders, 1181,
1188
in combined skin disorders
  with hypnosis, 987, 1007
  with psychotherapy, 1015, 1016, 1036,
1037, 1072, 1083, 1086
  with suggestion, 987, 1007, 1086
in eczema, 844, 849
in hemophilia, 674, 679, 688, 689
in herpes simplex, 761, 762
in neurodermatitis, 874, 876
in pruritus, 894
in psoriasis, 916, 924
in purpura, 701, 703, 706
in rheumatoid arthritis
  with attention control 529
  with behavior therapy, 493, 529
  with biofeedback, 494
  with group therapy, 493, 535
  with imagery, 529
  with psychotherapy, 493, 517, 531
  with relaxation, 494, 529
  with social casework, 531
in tuberculosis, 720, 731, 752, 768
in urticaria, 430
in warts, 937
Stress inoculation training
for burns, 807
for cancer or cancer therapy side effects,
1339
for rheumatoid arthritis, 529
Stress management
for cancer, 1234, 1241
for cancer or cancer therapy side effects,
1302, 1321, 1346
for psoriasis, 918
for rheumatoid arthritis, 535
Suggestion
for acne, 772, 773, 775
for allergy, 436, 445, 449, 450, 490, 1191
for arsphenamine dermatitis, 1113
for asthma, 92–94, 97, 100, 102, 103, 107–
109, 115, 116, 119, 122, 125, 127–132,
135, 136, 138, 445, 518, 638, 1192
  with behavior therapy, 19, 27, 349, 358,
377, 380
  with biofeedback, 350
  with group and family therapy, 83, 350,
395
  with milieu therapy, 395
  with psychotherapy, 241, 253, 282, 286,
326, 339, 349, 350, 358, 374, 377, 391,
394, 395
  with relaxation, 102, 119, 129, 131, 350,
380
for burns, 785, 788, 791, 796, 810
for cancer, 1189, 1231, 1234, 1237, 1243

in Raynaud's disease
  autogenic training for, 547, 559
  behavior therapy for, 567
  biofeedback for, 543, 547, 544, 559, 567
  hypnosis for, 561
  psychotherapy for, 561
  relaxation for, 567
in scleroderma, 560, 561
Venereal warts, 812–816
Verbal behavior
  in asthma 268
  in purpura, 704
Viral disorders
  combined skin disorders, 980
  condyloma acuminata, 812–816
  warts, 936–877
Visualization. *See* Imagery
Vital capacity
  with behavior therapy, 380
  with hypnosis, 90, 124
  with relaxation, 380
  with suggestion, 380
Vitamin therapy
  for ankylosing spondylitis, 549
  for rheumatoid arthritis, 524
Vitiligo, 1100, 1107
Vocational rehabilitation
  for asthma, 375
  for tuberculosis, 751
Vomiting, from chemotherapy
  behavior therapy for, 1317, 1331, 1347, 1348, 1352
    with hypnosis, 1296, 1319, 1345, 1349–1351, 1353
    with imagery, 1339, 1349, 1351, 1353
    with relaxation, 1296, 1337, 1339, 1341, 1342, 1345, 1349, 1351, 1353
  biofeedback for, 1353

classical conditioning in, 1328
group therapy for, 1330
hypnosis for, 1307, 1365, 1402
  with behavior therapy, 1296, 1319, 1345, 1349–1351, 1353, 1360
  with biofeedback, 1353, 1360
  with counseling, 1366
  with group therapy, 1330
  with imagery, 1349, 1351, 1353, 1354
  with relaxation, 1296, 1345, 1351, 1353, 1354, 1360
imagery for
  with behavior therapy, 1339, 1349, 1351, 1353
  with biofeedback, 1353
  with hypnosis, 1349, 1351, 1353, 1354
  with relaxation, 1339, 1349, 1351, 1353, 1354, 1358
meditation for, 1361
placebo for, 1301
psychotherapy for, 1301, 1362, 1366
relaxation for, 1294, 1303, 1318, 1363, 1433
  with behavior therapy, 1293, 1296, 1337, 1339, 1341, 1342, 1345, 1349, 1351, 1353, 1360
  with biofeedback, 1293, 1353, 1360
  with hypnosis, 1293, 1296, 1345, 1349, 1351, 1353, 1354, 1360
  with imagery, 1295, 1339, 1349, 1351 1353, 1354, 1358
  with meditation, 1361
Von Willebrand's disease, 680
Vulnerability
  in allergy, 473
  in asthma, 308, 360

Warts, 936–977. *See also* Condyloma acuminata; Molluscum contagiosum
conditioning for, 963

folk medicine for, 937, 949
hypnosis for, 946, 960, 961, 967–969, 1182, 1226
  with meditation, 952
  with psychotherapy, 942, 954
  with suggestion, 941, 945, 952, 955, 956, 958, 959, 964, 970–972
meditation for, 952
play therapy for, 947
psychotherapy for, 936, 943, 962, 976, 1143
  with hypnosis, 942, 954
suggestion for, 938–940, 944, 948, 950, 951, 953, 957, 965, 966, 973–975, 977
  with conditioning, 963
  with folk medicine, 937
  with hypnosis, 941, 945, 952, 955, 956, 958, 959, 964, 970–972
  with meditation, 952
  with placebo, 947
  with play therapy, 947
Weather, and asthma, 375. *See also* Climate
Will to live, in cancer, 1272, 1308, 1391, 1460
Witchcraft. *See* Folk medicine
Withdrawal
  in cancer, 1221, 1314
  in eczema, 832

Yoga
  for asthma, 144, 585, 666
    with biofeedback, 156
    with breathing exercises, 148, 149, 354
    with imagery, 156
    with relaxation, 149, 156, 354
  for cancer, 1240, 1246, 1477
  for rheumatoid arthritis, 503, 665